OXFORD MEDICAL PUBLICATIONS

Brain's clinical neurology

Brain's Clinical Neurology

Sixth edition

Revised by

SIR ROGER BANNISTER

C.B.E., Hon. LL.D., Hon. D.Sc., M.A., M.Sc., D.M. (Oxon), F.R.C.P.
*Physician, The National Hospital for Nervous Diseases,
Queen Square, London; Physician, The Department of Neurology,
St. Mary's Hospital, London; Neurologist,
Western Ophthalmic Hospital, London*

London   New York   Tokyo

OXFORD UNIVERSITY PRESS

1985

Oxford University Press, Walton Street, Oxford OX2 6DP

London New York Toronto
Delhi Bombay Calcutta Madras Karachi
Kuala Lumpur Singapore Hong Kong Tokyo
Nairobi Dar es Salaam Cape Town
Melbourne Auckland

and associates in
Beirut Berlin Ibadan Mexico City Nicosia

OXFORD *is a trade mark of Oxford University Press*

© *Oxford University Press, 1960, 1964, 1969, 1973, 1978, 1985*

FIRST EDITION 1960
SIXTH EDITION 1985

British Library Cataloguing in Publication Data

Brain, Walter Russell, Baron Brain
Brain's clinical neurology. —6th ed. —(Oxford
medical publications).
1. Nervous systems—Diseases
I. Title   II. Bannister, Sir, Roger
616.8   RC346
ISBN 0–19–261455–X
ISBN 0–19–261454–1   Pbk

Photoset by Cotswold Typesetting Ltd, Cheltenham
Printed in Great Britain by
Butler and Tanner Ltd, Frome, Somerset

Preface

In preparing the sixth edition of *Brain's Clinical Neurology*, it has still been my aim to preserve Lord Brain's original intention of writing a textbook for physicians, general practitioners, and students which explains clearly how to diagnose and treat common neurological disorders. The present edition includes enough detail to take the medical student and young doctor up to the level required for membership or equivalent general medical specialist qualifications. It aims to be readable and moreover capable of being read within the span of a brief neurological course. In the past five years there have been two exciting developments in particular which have changed the practice of neurology more fundamentally than at any time in the past 20 years: first, the new generation of neurotransmitters and secondly, the new imaging techniques.

Who would have imagined 20 years ago that in addition to the classical transmitters (including substance P and GABA) more than 30 neuropeptides and neurohormones which modulate nerve transmission would be discovered? A new introductory section on neurotransmitters and endorphins has therefore been included with a section reviewing pain perception and some newer techniques for the control of intractable pain.

The second new development has been the rapid advance of diagnostic imaging techniques so that to the latest CT scanners with computer 'reconstruction' programs has been added digital subtraction angiography, nuclear magnetic resonance scanning and positron emission tomography. Some earlier invasive and often painful techniques such as air encephalography have been virtually dropped and cerebral angiography is much less often necessary. The prospect of using these new techniques to link pathological and metabolic changes at precisely localized sites, without hazard to the patient, has become a realistic probability, not just a fanciful dream. Comments on these new techniques have been incorporated in this edition.

The basic text still seeks to emphasize what I believe remains the fundamental attraction of neurology. There is an orderliness in the neat balance between the clinical history, often entwined with subtle psychological aspects, and knowledge of the basic anatomy and physiology of brain function. These basic sections have needed some revision. The neurologist has to make first an anatomical diagnosis, then a pathological diagnosis, and finally a functional assessment in terms of the patient's management. Recently I was rather surprised that a consultant neurologist commented that he did not think it necessary for a general practitioner to do a complete neurological examination because it was so difficult. A careful history is very important but the simple neurological examination cannot be neglected and this book aims to remove any anxieties about the examination techniques. A guide to an abbreviated neurological examination to exclude gross neurological disease has been included in this edition.

My aim has also been to provide some insight into the exciting new scientific developments provided in neurology in the hope that these will stimulate the reader but not divert him too much from the core of basic neurological information.

Neurological treatment, becoming in many diseases a much more complex matter of drug manipulation of receptors, has required extensive revision. For example neurologists are being faced with more problems in the late stages of Parkinson's disease when 'on/off' symptoms and dyskinesias result from different types of pre- and postsynaptic disturbances. In addition, we are only just beginning to see attempts, as yet unsuccessful, to apply the same principles of neurotransmitter modulation to other neuronal degenerations such as Huntington's chorea and Alzheimer's disease. As it is impossible to cover all the advances in neurology, some areas, for example paediatric neurology, which have become neurological specialties in their own right have been abbreviated and are therefore necessarily incomplete. Despite resisting the temptation to attempt to cover all topics the length of the text has had to be increased. In this edition particular attention has also been given to the revision of the sections on the common neurological disorders of dementia, cerebro-vascular disease, and the assessment of coma and brain-death, particularly as the medicolegal and ethical aspects of brain-death have become increasingly a matter of public interest and debate. New material in this edition is also included in sections on c.s.f. globulins and serology, language function and handedness, sleep disorders, virus diseases, myasthenia, hereditary degenera-tion, pituitary tumours and prolactinomas, mitochondrial myopathies, autonomic function, multiple sclerosis, and epilepsy.

London   R.B.
August 1984

Acknowledgements

It is a pleasure to acknowledge the debt I owe to my colleagues for many helpful discussions and for material used for illustrations. In addition to the acknowledgements made in previous editions I would like to thank the following: Dr D. Carr, of Harvard Medical School, who kindly advised on the section on neuropeptides, endorphins, and pain and provided Figs. 0.7, 0.8, 0.9 (after Melzack and Wall), and 0.10 (after Fields). Professor J. Z. Young (Fig. 0.4); Dr D. Sutton and Churchill Livingstone for kindly providing most of the radiological illustrations, which appeared in *Textbook of radiology and imaging* 3/e; Miss S. Ford (fundus photographs, Fig. 2.3, Plates 2, 3, and 4), the Department of Audio-Visual Communication at St Mary's Hospital, London, and the Photographic Department at the National Hospital, Queen Square, London; Dr J. A. Morgan Hughes (Plate 8); Dr D. N. Landon (Fig. 20.5); Professor R. F. Schmidt and Springer Verlag (Figs. 3.9, 3.10, 3.2, 4.1, 7.10, 17.2, and 17.2, which appeared in *Human physiology* (ed. Schmidt and Thews 1983); Dr J. A. R. Lenman and Pitman Publishing (Fig. 5.11, which appeared in *Clinical electromyography* 3/e (ed. Lenman and Ritchie));Professor C. D. Marsden and *The Lancet* (Fig. 16.2); Dr J. Gilroy and Macmillans (Figs. 2.4, 2.7, 2.8, and 2.20, which appeared in *Medical neurology* (by Gilroy and Meyer); Professor A. Richens and Churchill Livingstone (Table 7.1, adapted from *A textbook of epilepsy* (ed. Laidlaw and Richens 1982)); Dr A. M. Halliday and Butterworths (Fig. 5.8, which appeared in *Clinical neurophysiology* (ed. Stalberg and Young)); Professor J. W. Lance and Professor J. G. McLeod and Butterworths (Figs. 3.1, 5.10, and 5.11, which appeared in *A physiological approach to clinical neurology*); Dr G. Bydder, Department of Diagnostic Radiology, Royal Postgraduate Medical School, London (all the NMR scans); Dr A. R. Valentine (Fig. 5.9); Dr R. Wise, Physics Isotopes Section, MRC Cyclotron Unit, Royal Postgraduate Medical School, London (Fig. 14.9); Dr B. Pansky and Macmillans (Fig. 2.1, which appeared in *Review of neurosciences* (ed. Pansky and Allen 1980)); Dr T. Nikaido (Fig. 10.4, which appeared in *Archives of Neurology* 25); and Dr M. Rosser and the Update Group (Fig. 16.4, which appeared in *Update*).

Contents

(Plates fall between pp. 246 and 247 of the text.)

x   *Contents*

PART V   PSYCHOLOGICAL FACTORS IN NEUROLOGY

Introduction

THE APPROACH TO THE NEUROLOGICAL DIAGNOSIS

The practical steps which need to be taken to reach a neurological diagnosis may be summarized under four headings:

1. The detailed history

This represents a record of the exact onset and evolution of the symptoms, supported by any observations which may be obtained from witnesses or family. In no branch of medicine is a good history more important than in neurology. It makes all the difference in the diagnosis of a difficult case in which the physical signs may not be in doubt. Time spent on it is well worth while. The poor witness can be helped by leading questions. After taking the detailed history it should be possible to list the probable site or sites of the nervous system affected, from muscle to cerebral cortex. Also, from the course of development of the symptoms (for example, whether episodic or progressive), it should be possible to suggest the likely pathological diagnosis. For example, vascular lesions tend to cause sudden or episodic symptoms, cerebral tumours more often cause slowly progressive symptoms.

2. The general history

This involves the use of leading questions about past life and social and family history which may affect the interpretation of the detailed history.

3. The detailed neurological examination

The patient's symptoms elicited during the detailed history will have pointed to parts of the nervous system which must be examined in great detail, with care and precision. For example, if the patient complains of weakness of the legs, the examination of the tone, the distribution of weakness and any alteration of reflexes will determine with certainty whether the weakness is the result of involvement of the upper motor neurone or lower neurone. In order to answer particular questions about the site of the lesion the examiner may have to invent new tests or modify standard tests. He may be limited by the powers of concentration and attention of the patient, particularly during testing of sensation or when testing higher cerebral functions. The interpretation of signs elicited is more difficult than learning to elicit them.

4. The abbreviated neurological examination

When the parts of the nervous system under suspicion have been examined in detail, the remainder of the examination can be completed more briefly (see p. 33). This also represents the minimum neurological examination in the patient without focal neurological symptoms. With increasing experience the examiner will select for himself the tests he finds most helpful. Of course, this abbreviated examination may at any moment draw the attention of the alert examiner to some unexpected abnormality which will require more detailed investigation. Naturally in practice in any patient the detailed and abbreviated examinations take place concurrently. The suspicions of certain lesions are proved by the detailed examination of a particular part, while the absence of any other disease is confirmed by the more abbreviated general examination.

From repeated examination of this kind, in every patient seen, an invaluable and partly unconscious knowledge of the range of the 'normal' will eventually be acquired. At first clinical signs may be missed by the student and significance may be attached to false signs. But eventually a proper balance will be achieved and the correct reliance placed on each sign. It will be appreciated, for example, that fundi can have suspicious margins without the patient having papilloedema and in the aged the ankle jerks may be absent and the appreciation of vibration sense in the feet lost without the patient having subacute combined degeneration of the cord, or tabes.

In Part I of this book there is a methodical account of symptoms that point to disease of a particular part of the nervous system and the relevant questions that should be asked of the patient, followed by an account of the detailed examination needed to elicit confirmatory physical signs.

With practice the examiner will be able to infer with reasonable confidence the level of the nervous system involved. By deduction, from the history of the evolution of the symptoms, the probable pathological diagnosis can then be made and treatment and management determined.

SOME GENERAL PRINCIPLES OF STRUCTURE AND FUNCTION

Certain disturbances of brain function are determined by the fact that brain is relatively incompressible but easily distorted, and is suspended by arachnoid and dural membranes within the rigid skull (Figs. 0.1 and 0.2). When the brain is enlarged by inflammation, tumour, or haemorrhage, it can to some extent be accommodated by displacement of cerebrospinal fluid or venous blood, but there are limits to this adjustment and obstruction to the venous drainage or cerebrospinal fluid circulation can then result in brain compression. The soft consistency of the brain determines the rotational and shearing stresses and hence the damage caused by head injuries.

Blood supply

The brain receives about one-fifth of the total cardiac output and its blood flow is kept remarkably constant within a wide range of arterial pressures by baro-

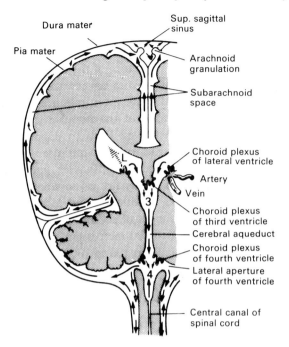

Fig. 0.1. Diagrammatic cross-section of the brain to show support by dura and cerebro-spinal fluid.

receptor reflexes and local autoregulation. The metabolic requirements of neurones are ensured by supporting glia which have some processes attached to capillary walls and other processes which end on neurones (Fig. 0.3). The limitation to transport of metabolites is provided by the blood–brain barrier and depends on active cellular transport mechanisms and not mere transudation.

Nerve transmission

The chemical basis of nerve transmission along a nerve fibre is a sudden increase in conductance of the nerve membrane. The resting potential is caused by a gradient with an extracellular sodium concentration some ten times the intracellular concentration and maintained by active transport of sodium ions. Passage of the impulse leads to an influx of sodium and the electrical field generated leads to depolarization of the adjacent membrane and hence propagation of an impulse. In a myelinated fibre excitation occurs only at the nodes of Ranvier and conduction is saltatory and takes place some 50 times as fast as in unmyelinated fibres. Damage to the myelin sheath blocks conduction and local anaesthetics act by inhibiting the activation of the changes of sodium conductance.

Conduction velocities vary from 2 to 100 metres per second, according to fibre size, and the impulse rates range from 100 to 1000 impulses per second. The overall complexity of nervous integration may be judged from a few simple

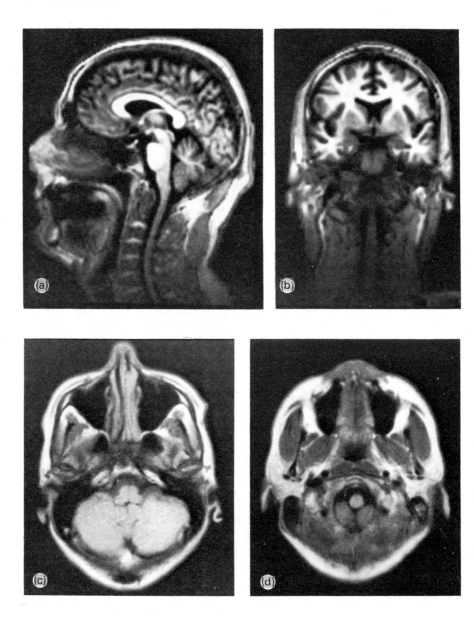

Fig. 0.2. Nuclear magnetic resonance scans of normal brain to show brain anatomy. (a) Sagittal; (b) coronal; (c) high medulla (showing cerebellar tonsils); (d) low medulla.

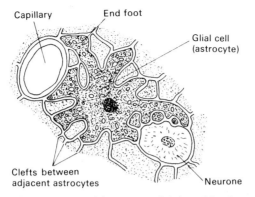

Fig. 0.3. Drawing of an astrocyte with processes joining a blood vessel and a neurone.

facts. The central nervous system has been estimated to contain some 10 billion neurones, and 100 billion glia. On each of 10 million Purkinje cells in the cerebellum there are some 300 000 synaptic endings. In a major descending path, the pyramidal tract, there are about one million fibres, but it has been estimated that there are some 20 times this number of fibres from the cortex to lower brain structures indirectly modulating movement.

Synaptic transmission in the central nervous system

This differs from impulse propagation along a nerve fibre by being mediated chemically, not electrically. The main transmitters are noradrenaline, acetylcholine, dopamine, serotonin, GABA, substance P, and glycine. Transmission is unidirectional and sub-threshold activation of many synaptic terminals leads to summation (Figs. 0.4 and 0.5). Neuronal links are known to give some measure of feedback control by the processes of pre- and postsynaptic inhibition. Chemical mediators transmit excitation by increasing permeability to sodium or inhibition by increasing the permeability of the postsynaptic membrane to chloride, and so stabilize the resting potential. The same neurone may respond to different transmitters released on its surface whose influence may be excitatory or inhibitory. The complexity of these synaptic contacts permits an almost infinite number of influences to play on the neurone and affect its rate of firing. This is the basis of the 'integrative action' of the nervous system and the capacity for feeling, thought, and muscular action.

Though human behaviour cannot imaginably be equated to the sum of the transmission of myriads of nerve cells at any one moment, neurologists think theoretically in terms of these complex patterns, just as they have to use the almost equally abstracted and remote evidence of tendon jerks when examining patients.

Each transmitter is released from synaptic vesicles (see Fig. 0.6) into the

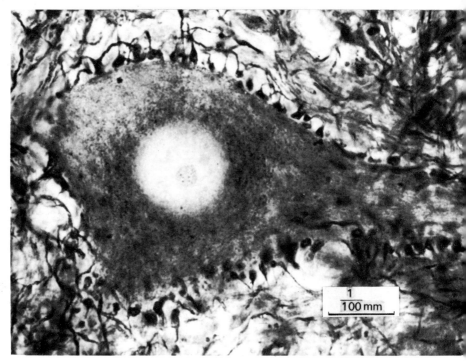

Fig. 0.4. A living neurone with dendrites and covered with synaptic endings dissected from the brain of a rabbit.

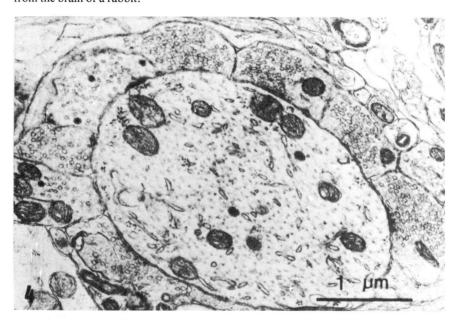

Fig. 0.5. Electron microscopic appearance of a dendrite completely covered by synaptic contacts with axonal boutons.

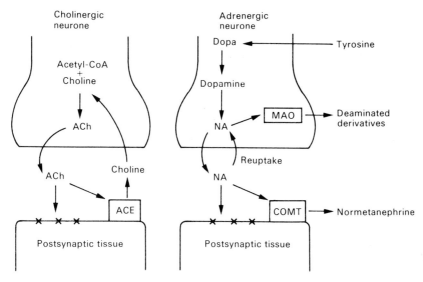

Fig. 0.6. Diagram of biochemical events at cholinergic and adrenergic endings (ACh, acetylcholine; ACD, acetylcholinesterase; NA, noradrenaline; X, receptor; MAO, monoamine oxidase; COMT, catechol-O-methyl transferase).

synaptic cleft where it either depolarizes or stabilizes the postsynaptic membrane. The transmitter is then removed, either by active re-uptake or destruction, specific enzymes being involved for different transmitters. The receptors, which are proteins bound to the synaptic membrane, are specific for each transmitter or its analogues, the number of receptors being much in excess of the normal quantal release of transmitter by an impulse. It seems likely that the amount of impulse traffic can modify the number of available receptors, so causing changes which may underlie processes such as 'learning'. Just as there are internuncials and collateral branches which give a negative feedback control to motor neurones, there is a chemical feedback process by which presynaptic receptors can inhibit the release of transmitters.

The main transmitters may be inhibited or enhanced by certain drugs. The general principles are similar for each transmitter. Its action is enhanced if more of its precursor is provided, if its release is triggered by another chemical, if a receptor agonist is provided or if the inactivating enzyme or re-uptake mechanism is blocked. Alternatively the effectiveness of transmission is reduced if its synthesis is reduced, its release blocked, or if the receptor is blocked.

Classical neurotransmitters

The discovery of the co-existence of more than one peptide alongside a classical transmitter in a single neurone has thrown doubt on the classical Dale concept of 'one neurone–one transmitter'. The precise receptor mechanisms differ for different transmitters but in general the receptor can be thought of as an organized molecular surface which when presented with a chemical messenger triggers off a cascade of biochemical changes which by amplification initiates a maximal response. Cyclic AMP or GMP may be generated not only by classical monoamine transmitters such as acetylcholine, noradrenaline, and dopamine, but also by peptides such as ACTH, TRH, glucagon, and AVP. The same transmitter may influence different types of receptors using adenyl cyclase and the second messenger system. There are certain special mechanisms of action for each transmitter. For *noradrenaline* the target cell membrane is coupled to the enzyme adenyl cyclase which converts ATP to cyclic AMP or GTP to GMP. The cyclic nucleotide then initiates the physiological response. This second messenger system amplifies the response to the transmitter. *Acetylcholine* functions differently at peripheral and central synapses. At the peripheral synapses, there is a simple ionic flow effect whereas centrally a second messenger molecule is involved. For *dopamine* there are two types of receptors, effects upon the D1 receptors requiring cyclic AMP and these upon the D2 receptors not requiring it. In addition to the direct excitation or inhibition of target neurones, transmitters may act presynaptically on adjacent receptors to alter the amount of transmitter released.

Besides the neuroanatomical links between different parts of the brain established by classical fibre staining and electrophysiological techniques there are now important connections which have been identified from the basis of common transmitter systems. The speed and specificity of these systems differs according to the transmitter involved. The monoamines are present in small groups of neurones chiefly in the brainstem and they have diffuse ascending and descending pathways modulating the activity of a large number of target cells. Destruction of the system in experimental animals with the neurotoxin 6-hydroxydopamine has remarkably little effect on the survival or behaviour of the laboratory animal. *Dopamine* is present in neurones of the substantia nigra and ventral tegmentum which project to the forebrain and is involved in emotional responses as well as the important pathways to the corpus striatum whose degeneration causes Parkinson's disease. *Serotonin* is present mainly in midline raphe nuclei of the brainstem. These have ascending projections but also a descending system to the dorsal horns of the spinal cord which modulates the sensitivity of the spinal cord to pain inputs from the periphery. *Acetylcholine* acts as the fast transmitter as in neuromuscular transmission peripherally but cholinergic neurones are also abundant in the basal ganglia. Diffuse ascending projections largely derived from the nucleus basalis of Meynert seem to correspond to what was previously described as the 'ascending activating reticular system' causing cortical arousal. Impairment of the system, which utilizes mainly muscarinic receptors in the brain, may as in Alzheimer's disease disrupt memory function. The amino acid GABA appears to be the main inhibitory transmitter in the brain and may be used by as many as one-third of all synapses in brain, being used in fast point-to-point neuronal circuits. It rapidly inhibits practically all neurones when applied locally and it does so by increasing the cell permeability to choride ions, thus stabilizing the resting membrane potential near the chloride equilibrium level. Receptors for benzodiazepine anxiolytic drugs are closely associated with the GABA receptor and chloride channel.

The classification of a particular compound as either a neurotransmitter, neuromodulator or neurohormone can now no longer be precisely made. Classical transmission involves release of a chemical agent presynaptically which causes postsynaptic depolarization or hyperpolarization. Transmitters act on subsynaptic membranes to open pores or channels of a certain diameter, though which all ions with a smaller diameter can pass. If the wall of the pore is electrically charged, this charge can obstruct similarly charged ions. Neuromodulation is defined as the alteration of receptor coupled membrane conductance without the direct activation of such conductance. A neurohumoral regulator is an active compound released by nerve endings but carried by the blood to its sites of action. A compound that functions as a neurotransmitter at one site may act as a neuromodulator at another and as a neurohormone at a third. Also it seems probable that one neurone can release both a transmitter and neuromodulators. The brain, through the pituitary and pineal glands, controls endocrine mechanisms, responds to hormone synthesized in the periphery, and utilizes many molecules centrally that also act as hormones peripherally.

Neuropeptides

Neuropeptides, comprised of a sequence of amino acids, differ in structure from other previously identified transmitters which are usually amines or individual amino acids. Biologically active peptides originally found in the gut (e.g. substance P, VIP, and cholecystokinin) are also present in the central nervous system. Conversely peptides originally found in the brain (e.g. somatostatin, neurotensin, and enkephalin and corticotrophin-releasing factor) are also found in the gut. It may be due to opportunism in the evolutionary process by which a molecule that serves one function may be adapted to serve another function at a different place and time. Neuropeptides are present widely in the animal kingdom, even in unicellular organisms. They have a modulatory effect on the behaviour of the whole organism. For example in animals an injection of small amounts of angiotensin into the ventricular system causes drinking behaviour, LHRH triggers female sexual behaviour, and, most interesting from the neurological point of view, vasopressin has been reported to improve learning behaviour in animals. The total list of neuropeptides now exceeds 30 and is probably incomplete. In addition there are trophic peptides, for example nerve growth factor, which are essential for the differentiation and survival of peripheral sensory and sympathetic neurones and which may also be involved in maintaining central monoaminergic neurones. Other trophic factors operating for other types of nerve cells are likley to determine which cells survive and function out of the vastly greater number of primitive cells in the earliest development of the nervous system. It is by no means improbable that other endogenous counterparts of other potent groups of drugs which are not themselves transmitters may be discovered.

REFERENCES

Bloom, F.E. (1982). Neurotransmitters and CNS disease: the future. *Lancet* **ii**, 1381–5.

Hoehn-Saric, R. (1982). Neurotransmitters in anxiety. *Archs gen. Psychol.* **39**, 735–42.

Hökfelt, T., Johansson, O., Ljungdahl, A., Lundberg, J.M., and Schultzberg, M. (1980). Peptidergic neurones. *Nature, Lond.* **284**, 515–21.

Hughes, J., Smith, T.W., Kosterlitz, H.W., Fothergill, L.A., Morgan, B.A., and Morris, H.R. (1975). Identification of two related pentapeptides from the brain with potent opiate agonist activity. *Nature, Lond.* **258**, 577–9.

Iversen, L.L. (1982). Neurotransmitters and CNS disease: introduction. *Lancet* **ii**, 914–18.

Krieger, D.T. and Martin, J.B. (1981). Brain peptides. *New Engl. J. Med.* **304**, 944–51.

Praag, H.M. van (1982). Neurotransmitters and CNS disease: depression. *Lancet* **ii**, 1259–64.

Roth, J., Le Roith, D., Schiloach, J., Rosenzweig, J.L., Lesmiak, M.A., and Havrankova, J. (1982). The evolutionary origins of hormones, neurotransmitters and other extracellular messengers: implications for mammalian new biology. *New Engl. J. Med.* **306**, 523–7.

Endorphins and pain

Endorphins are a naturally occurring group of neuropeptides with morphine-like properties which may act as neurotransmitters, neuromodulators, or neurohormones. Knowledge of these substances started with the demonstration first that radiolabelled narcotic agonists act on specific opiate receptors in particular brain regions, particularly the peri-aqueductal grey matter. If such receptors exist in the brain then the brain must presumably produce naturally occurring substances with an affinity for these receptors. A search by Hughes and Kosterlitz yielded in 1975 two pentapeptides, leucine and methionine 'enkephalin', that is literally 'in the head', now abbreviated to leu- and met-enkephalin. They share an amino acid sequence in common with another endorphin, beta-endorphin, derived from a previously isolated larger molecule called beta-lipotrophin which is itself part of a pre-hormone that also gives rise to ACTH and beta-MSH (Fig. 0.7). At present, three families of endogenous opioids are recognized. All share certain portions of their amino acid sequence, but are derived from three separate precursor molecules termed pro-opio-melanocortin ('POMC') or pro-ACTH-endorphin, pro-enkephalin, and pro-dynorphin. Plasma beta-endorphin arises from the pituitary gland whereas plasma enkephalins are secreted from the adrenal medulla with noradrenaline and adrenaline. However, their principal interest in neurology lies in their

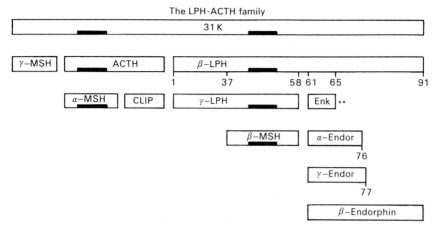

Fig. 0.7. The lipotrophic–ACTH family of precursors of endorphins.

localization in various parts of the brain and their function as modulators in the pain pathways. In addition their action at higher levels of brain function is now being investigated. A disorganization of these neural hormones during injury such as shock may release active peptides causing the complex hallucinations of the near death experience which resembles the disturbances with limbic dysfunction (p. 354). We almost certainly have not yet come to the end of the list of endogenous opiate peptides. It is also probable that other endogenous substances may be discovered which correspond to the sites of other potent groups of drugs which are not themselves transmitters, for example benzo-diazepines and the anticonvulsants (see p. 187).

The pain pathways and endorphins

Pain impulses are carried in small-diameter myelinated fibres (Aδ) and unmyelin-ated (C) axons but not in larger fibres (Fig. 0.8). The small fibres are susceptible to local anaesthetic block whereas larger fibres are more susceptible to pressure block. At the root entry zone these fibres conducting pain impulses end in the substantia gelatinosa of the dorsal horn and are thought to release transmitter substance P. Axons of the spinal neurones with which they synapse cross the midline and ascend to the reticular formation, midbrain, tegementum, and central grey matter eventually passing to the thalamic nuclei and the somato-sensory and association cortex. Enkephalin is found in high concentration in small neurones close to the nociceptive input and opiate receptors are also found in areas where there are substance-P-containing nerve terminals. Studies of the isolated preparation of the trigeminal nucleus in animals have shown that met-enkephalin blocks the effect of substance P and this effect is itself blocked by naloxone, an opiate antagonist. At high concentrations substance P appears to excite the nociceptive pathway and so oppose the analgesic effects of endorphins. It has been speculated that it might be possible

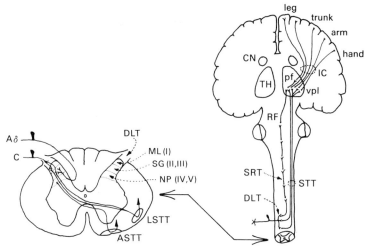

Fig. 0.8. Pain pathways

STT spinothalamic tract (A = anterior; L = lateral)
DLT dorsolateral tract
RF reticular formation
IC internal capsule
CN caudate nucleus
TH thalamus
v.p.l. ventral posterolateral nucleus
SRT spinoreticular tract
SG substantia gelatinosa.

to develop a substance P antagonist which might be a non-opiate analgesic drug. The original Melzack and Wall hypothesis in 1965 postulated that large- and small-diameter afferent fibres converge in the dorsal horn both on a spinal neurone that transmits the painful stimuli onwards and on an interneurone which itself has a gating or inhibitory effect on transmission (Fig. 0.9). The interneurone is also under the control of descending pathways which can therefore exert, from the midbrain or medullary level, inhibitory control of the 'gate' mechanism. The precise location of the postulated spinal inhibitory neurones and the part played by postsynaptic inhibition of these neurones is uncertain but endorphin release is likely to have a critical inhibitory modulatory role.

In the region of the periventricular grey matter there are rich concentrations of met-enkephalin and leu-enkephalin and in the limbic system and hypothalamus there is also a high concentration of enkephalin receptors (Fig. 0.10). At these higher levels pain transmission is now thought to be regulated by both short- and long-term feedback mechanisms. Stimulation of stereotactically implanted electrodes in the peri-aqueductal grey matter in man produced dramatic and often complete abolition of painful impulses. The descending pathways from the peri-aqueductal grey matter pass to the posterior horn indirectly via the

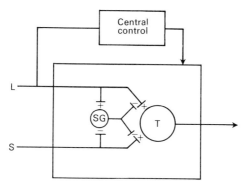

Fig. 0.9. Gate hypothesis of Melzack and Wall. Schematic diagram of dorsal horn.
L large myelinated fibre
S small unmyelinated fibre
SG inhibition substantia gelatinosa interneurone
T transmission cell in dorsal horn.

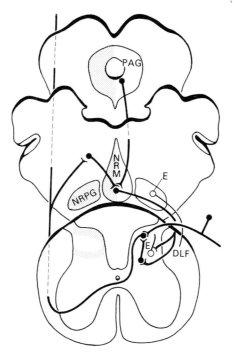

Fig. 0.10. Endorphins and the pain pathways. Endogenous opiates (stippled areas) demonstrated at three levels: (a) the midbrain; (b) the medulla and (c) the spinal cord.

PAG periaqueductal grey matter
NRPG nucleus reticularis paragigantocellularis
NRM nucleus raphe magnus
DLF dorsolateral fasciculus
E endorphin.

brainstem raphe serotonergic neurones which are a crucial link from the peri-aqueductal grey matter to the dorsolateral horn of the spinal cord. The hyperalgesic state which sometimes follows brainstem, spinal or diencephalic lesions could result from the absence of the descending inhibition and such pain, as would be expected, is refractory to narcotic analgesics. One would also expect drugs enhancing serotonin to have an analgesic effect. Certainly some painful states such as migraine are helped by tricyclic antidepressants which also block serotonin uptake.

There are several critical sites along the pain pathway at which the passage of impulses may be modulated. At the peripheral receptor endings bradykinin, histamine, prostaglandins, and possibly other endogenous analgesic substances exert synergistic effects. Sympathetic fibres exert a positive feedback upon nociceptors, probably by ephaptic non-synaptic contacts with adjacent primary afferent fibres. Experimental studies of nerve lesions in animals have thrown light on some beneficial clinical effects of sympathetic block in man, now often achieved by the intravenous guanethidine infusion technique rather than by surgical sympathectomy.

Acupuncture and electrical stimulation in the treatment of chronic pain

It has always been a puzzling fact that on the battlefield or sports field or after a car crash pain perception may be delayed after a severe injury. It is said that acupuncture was discovered several thousand years ago in China when a soldier pierced by an arrow only felt the pain when the arrow was removed. Recently the beneficial effects of acupuncture, with or without low-frequency electrical stimulation, has been recognized in a variety of pain syndromes. Though the precise mechanism of its action still eludes us, a number of clues have been provided by electrical stimulation of the midbrain and a study of narcotic addiction.

Electrical stimulation of the animal brain in the region of the peri-aqueductal grey matter produces analgesia without a generalized behavioural depression of the animal and also causes a rise in c.s.f. endorphin. It appears to act by liberating peptides from this region. It has been shown that analgesia induced in animals by electrical stimulation can be transferred to recipient animals by the transfer of post-electro-acupuncture cerebrospinal fluid. The specific opiate antagonist drug naloxone reverses the electro-acupuncture analgesia of low-frequency electrical stimulation, but not of high frequency. In 1975 Venn reported that symptoms of heroin withdrawal could be alleviated by electro-acupuncture. C.s.f. met-enkephalin levels in heroin addicts are normal rather than reduced as might be expected on theoretical grounds but they are high after successful acupuncture treatment. In narcotic addiction it has been suggested that opiates, as artificial agonists, inhibit the normal synthesis of endorphin by means of a homeostatic negative feedback mechanism. The sudden cessation of the opiate might then precipitate transient insufficiency of endorphins that could be responsible for the withdrawal syndrome. Abrupt withdrawal of the opiate might also cause excessive release of cyclic AMP which has been inhibited by the opiate.

The management of chronic pain

Many chronic pain syndromes have an organic basis in the first instance but through lack of treatment or lack of understanding of the mechanisms involved a secondary psychological disturbance becomes added to the original lesion. In the management of the chronic pain syndrome an attempt at precise diagnosis must always precede treatment. Neurological types of chronic pain include 'central' pain, causalgia, sympathetic dystrophy, phantom pain and post-herpetic pain. The true nature of the pain is often difficult to diagnose. For example, if the precise history of the nature of the pain has not been taken, the migrainous neuralgic headache syndrome, which responds specifically to ergotamine, may be mistaken either for classical migraine or even sometimes for the entirely different type of brief stabbing pain which occurs in trigeminal neuralgia and which responds to carbamazepine. In chronic pain syndromes there is often unwillingness to try some of the more complex new treatment techniques such as acupuncture, electrical stimulation, or dorsal root entry zone thermocoagulation. There have also been recent attempts at dorsal column implantation of stimulators which have been of some benefit. Biofeed-back and relaxation with operant conditioning can also be considered. Such methods may provide continuing relief for some patients, though often it is not possible to predict in advance which patients will benefit. If the pain has a causalgic-like quality then regional intravenous guanethidine sympathetic block is often helpful. In the treatment of pain perhaps the most surprising discovery is that placebos release some endogenous opiates and can be blocked by naloxone. Although only 5 per cent of subjects with experimental pain respond to a placebo a third of patients with clinical pain have relief from a placebo, thereby countering the belief that only 'imaginary' pain responds to a placebo. The placebo effect suggests that the expectation of relief is capable of triggering the release of endorphins when clinically significant pain is present. Anti-depressants, antispasmodics, and antinauseants all play their part in contri-buting to the treatment designed to affect transmission of pain through pain pathways. In the future, the development of endorphin analogues may permit greater selectivity of analgesic effects including lower risk of respiratory depression or addictiveness.

REFERENCES

Basbaum, A.I. and Fields, H.L. (1978). Endogenous pain control mechanisms: review and hypothesis. *Annls Neurol.* **4**, 451–62.
Carr, D.B. (1983). Endorphins in contempory medicine. *Comp. Ther.* **9**, 40–5.
Hannington-Kiff, J.G. (1974). Intravenous regional sympathetic block with guanethidine. *Lancet* **i**, 1019–20.
Jessell, T.M. (1982). Neurotransmitters and CNS disease: pain. *Lancet* **ii**, 1084–7.

Loh, L. and Nathan, P.W. (1978). Painful peripheral states and sympathetic blocks. *J. Neurol. Neurosurg. Psychiat.* **41**, 664–71.

—— —— and Schott, G.D. (1981). Pain due to lesions of central nervous system removed by sympathetic block. *Br. med. J.* **282**, 1026–8.

—— —— —— and Wilson, P.G. (1980). Effects of regional guanethidine infusion in certain painful states. *J. Neurol. Neurosurg. Psychiat.* **43**, 446–51.

Mann, F. (1973). Treatment of intractable pain by acupuncture. *Lancet* **ii**, 57–60.

Melzack, R. and Wall, P.D. (1965). Pain mechanisms: a new theory. *Science, NY* **150**, 971–9.

SOME IMMUNOLOGICAL PRINCIPLES

The unique and 'privileged' position of the brain immunologically appears to result from the *blood–brain barrier*, which is formed by tight junctions of specialized endothelium of brain capillaries, which prevent the leakage of antibodies into the brain. The choroid plexus is lined by cuboidal endothelium with tight junctions and cerebrospinal fluid drains away by bulk drainage, therefore reducing the concentration of protein in the cerebrospinal fluid. Immunoglobulins and lymphocytes do not usually pass into the brain unless infection, infiltration, or neoplasia damage the blood–brain barrier. This prevents the development of the kind of self-tolerance which occurs in other body tissues. The consequences include the easy sensitization to autologous brain tissue, and one disadvantage is that once a foreign agent such as a virus has reached the brain, the immune mechanisms to eliminate it are defective, especially if the patient is for some reason immunosuppressed as for example after renal transplantation or has immunodeficiency or is immunocompromised for some other reason. There is also a *blood–nerve barrier*. This is relevant in the development of acute inflammatory polyneuropathy (the Guillain–Barré syndrome) in which there is a predominant radicular pattern of damage, a site where the blood–nerve barrier has been shown in the experimental animal model to become defective.

In the nervous system, as elsewhere in the body, it is not always easy to distinguish between immunological mechanisms which are aetiologically causal, those which are the effects of cell damage and those which are merely epiphenomena. The responses to antigens can be of several kinds, different mechanisms usually acting concurrently. The humoral responses result in the production of antibodies by plasma cells derived from B lymphocytes. The second type of immune response is the cell-mediated or delayed-hypersensitivity response which is under the influence of thymic T lymphocytes which can result in a greater degree of cell damage. Both the humoral and cell-mediated responses may be directed against external antigens or viruses, or against normal or subtly altered 'self' antigens in the nervous system, so producing auto-immune disturbances. The end result of this kind of response is usually perivenous lymphocytic infiltration, and this is the type of reaction which is thought to cause sub-acute sclerosing panencephalitis (see p. 452). Immune complexes are sometimes formed and may trigger the complement system; this can damage the small blood vessels and cause a vasculitis and even widespread brain lesions as, for example, in lupus erythematosis. The full criteria for identifying a neurological disease as auto-immune in aetiology require the demonstration of antigens which attack preparations of the tissue *in vitro* with a high degree of specificity, as has been shown in myasthenia gravis. At a less certain level there is a strong suspicion that auto-immune factors play a part in the development of Sydenham's chorea, post-viral encephalopathy, acute inflammatory polyneuropathy, polymyositis, systemic lupus erythematosus, orbital pseudo-tumour, polyarteritis nodosa, and Wegener's granulomatosis.

If the antigen is a virus persisting within the brain, as for example in the Creutzfeldt–Jakob disease, a more complex immune disturbance may occur in which the lymphocytic infiltration or inflammatory changes usually associated with immune disease are not seen. Such a response might bring within the realm of immunology some of the hitherto unexplained neuronal degenerative disorders such as motor neurone disease and idiopathic Parkinsonism in which there are no inflammatory changes.

In cases of malignancy (p. 525) even in the absence of overt neurological disorders, lymphocytic sensitization may occur to both central and peripheral nerve proteins. These proteins may share some antigenic determinants present on the surface of the neoplastic cells, so causing the 'immune' neuropathies. At the same time other neurological complications of a carcinoma or lymphoma, such as progressive multi-focal leuco-encephalopathy (p. 454), may be the result not of hypersensitivity but of immunological depression as a result of treatment, but in many neurological diseases in which immune mechanisms are involved we are left with the dilemma of whether immune responses should be suppressed or stimulated.

SOME GENERAL PRINCIPLES OF TREATMENT

Diseases of immunity

The main aims of treatment of neurological disorders of immunity are to limit damage to brain tissue and to reduce brain swelling.

Steroids

Steroids have several probable effects including suppression of local inflammatory cell infiltration, reduction of local oedema, suppression of circulating lymphocytes and to a lesser extent the inhibition of antibody formation. Some of the common neurological conditions which have been treated with steroids are multiple sclerosis, acute polyneuritis, Bell's palsy, polymyositis, and cranial arteritis. There is no convincing evidence that ACTH is in general better than prednisolone or prednisone. Prednisolone has a sodium-retaining effect and if given in large doses for a long time should be given with a low-salt diet and potassium supplements. Alternate-day as opposed to continuous treatment causes less suppression of the hypothalamic–pituitary–adrenal system if long-term high-dose treatment is needed. Single daily or alternate-day doses are insufficient for cranial arteritis and patients with myasthenia may feel significantly weaker on non-steroid days. Side-effects of prednisolone in addition to weight gain and changes in mood include gastrointestinal upsets including even gastric haemorrhage, the risk of which is reduced by giving enteric-coated tablets.

Immunosuppressant treatment

Immunosuppressant drugs block the division of inflammatory cells in various ways. Mercaptopurine (Purinethol) and azathioprine, both interfere with nucleic acid synthesis, while methotrexate (Amethopterin) blocks folate metabolism. All have adverse effects which determine the dose which can be tolerated. Effective trials have rarely been reported of sufficiently high doses given for sufficient time to ensure total immunosuppression. Preliminary studies in multiple sclerosis have highlighted the danger of relapse on ceasing treatment. The possible increased vulnerability to the presumed virus has to be considered as well as the increased susceptibility to infection and neoplasia caused by immunosuppression.

Treatment of brain swelling

Experimental studies in animals indicate that there are various types of brain swelling. Certain toxins cause mainly white-matter oedema, whereas local freezing causes extracellular oedema fluid resembling plasma exudate. Experimental ischaemia causes oedema affecting the grey matter more than white matter but the nature of the damage depends on the relative degree of underperfusion and the subsequent abnormality of endothelial permeability after the initial anoxic damage has occurred.

In a variety of neurological conditions, treatment aims to reduce the local and generalized effects of brain swelling. In addition to encephalitis or cerebral tumour, the other commonest conditions are vascular disease with hypertensive encephalopathy or infarction, sometimes cerebral abscess, metabolic disease such as liver failure or carbon dioxide retention, toxic disease such as lead encephalopathy, and diseases with brain swelling of unknown cause such as benign intracranial hypertension.

Dexamethasone, a potent glucocorticoid with only mild salt-retaining properties, reduces cerebral oedema by several mechanisms. It probably modifies certain cell membranes, inhibits formation of prostaglandin endoperoxidases, and reduces arachidonic acid release and degradation to free radicles which may be produced in excess. Steroids are most effective when there is oedema around a subacute or chronic focal lesion, associated with an increase in the permeability of the blood–brain barrier, rather than with disturbed cellular processes with an excess of intracellular water, such as occurs in early ischaemic damage or after water intoxication. There is no proof of the effect of steroids in reducing the formation of cerebrospinal fluid as for example in benign intracranial hypertension. Dexamethasone is most useful in the treatment of brain tumours in order to 'buy' time while neurosurgery is planned or to reduce the likelihood of post-operative swelling. It may reduce cerebrospinal fluid production, decrease the extracellular space of white matter, inhibit the swelling of astrocytes and interfere with entry of water and salt into the brain. After high initial doses of 8 mg i.v. or i.m. followed by 4 mg six-hourly for a week, the dose may then be reduced to a maintenance level of 1 mg daily by mouth for many months or even years, usually without serious side-effects developing. Hypertonic solutions such as glycerol, frusemide, or mannitol may be as effective over 24 hours but are sometimes followed by a rebound rise of pressure which does not seem to occur with maintained dexamethasone treatment.

Manipulation of neurotransmitters in treatment

Recent advances in knowledge of neuropeptides and neurotransmitters raise new possibilities for modifying brain function in disease. The brain is largely unable to synthesize acetylcholine, serotonin, and catecholamines *de novo* and so the plasma concentration of their respective precursors, choline and amino acids tryptophan and tyrosine, determine the brain concentration and hence the rate of transmitter synthesis from them. In a number of diseases there are specific defects which are known. For example in Huntington's chorea post-mortem studies have shown a loss of inhibitory neurones in the corpus striatum which normally contain GABA. Unfortunately there is no GABA analogue which is capable of crossing the blood–brain barrier. However, in *Huntington's chorea* there are also cholinergic defects and antimuscarinic drugs such as benzotropine exacerbate the chorea while physostigmine tends to improve it. Attempts at treatment have been made with oral choline which has not so far shown any benefit, presumably because multi-neuronal damage and extensive pre- and postsynaptic cholinergic destruction has occurred. Choline chloride has been given in a dose of 10 to 20 mg per day in *dyskinesias* and has been thought to suppress these involuntary choreic movements on some occasions. Lecithin has also been used and is less unpleasant to take and may raise the plasma choline level for longer than oral choline chloride. In *Alzheimer's disease* there is a major defect of cholinergic function. Attempts have therefore been made using choline and lecithin for treatment but these have not yet proved successful. Physostigmine, which augments synaptic ACh by slowing its degradation, may have promise, however. There has also been an interesting attempt, in view of the knowledge that vasopressin improves learning behaviour in animals, to increase memory function in patients with Alzheimer's disease using vasopressin, but this again has not so far been successful. There is evidence from the c.s.f. levels of 5HIAA, the metabolite of serotonin, of a defect of serotonin in *post-hypoxic intention myoclonus*. 5-Hydroxytryptophan (5HT) in a dose of 10–12 mg has helped in the treatment of this disorder. However, the disease in which replacement of the neurotransmitter loss has proved on the whole most effective is still *parkinsonism*, with the use of levo-dopa which crosses the blood–brain barrier. When given with a dopa decarboxylase inhibitor it does not cause such marked systemic effects (see p. 343).

The management of anxiety, depression, and other 'psychiatric' disorders has become more scientific as knowledge of transmitters has increased. Anxiety in man resembles fear in animals and appears to be mediated by parts of the brainstem, hypothalamus, limbic system, and cerebral cortex. Benzo-diazepine receptors are functionally linked to the GABA recognition sites in the brainstem and, together with the noradrenaline and serotonergic transmitters systems have a specific relation to anxiety. Two clinical types of anxiety can be recognized, the panic attacks which respond to tricyclics or monoamine oxidase inhibitors and a more generalized tension which responds to benzodiazepines.

In some *depressives* is has been suggested that defective serotonin metabolism is a factor because its metabolite 5HIAA is deficient in the cerebrospinal fluid. Trials of 5HT in a dose of 3 to 5 mg daily have been inconclusive. The transmitter defects in *schizophrenia* are complex. An excessive release of dopamine by amphetamine may lead to schizophrenic symptoms in man. This has led to the hypothesis that schizophrenia may be due to an overactivity of the dopamine system and antidopaminergic drugs have been used as part of the treatment of schizophrenia.

Various psychoactive drugs mimic the effects of natural transmitters on their receptors. For example LSD mimics the effect of serotonin. Caffeine increases the amount of cyclic AMP and therefore increases the concentration of mono-amines. Monoaminoxidase inhibitors like phenelzine (Nardil) and tranyl-cypromine (Parnate) potentiate the effect of noradrenaline; dopamine and serotonin and enhance excitement and reverse depression. They also permit dangerous hypertension by release of tyramine from foods and by alpha-receptor agonists. Tricyclic antidepressants and cocaine block the uptake of monoamines and so increase the effects of noradrenaline and serotonin.

Care of the chronic neurological patient

The principles of rehabilitation have until recently been relatively neglected but in chronic neurological disease where cure is not possible much can be done to relieve neurological symptoms. As patients develop an increasingly sophisti-cated knowledge of their illness, often through the lay press, it can be helpful to refer patients to societies set up to advance the interests of patients with neuro-logical diseases, including Parkinson's disease, multiple sclerosis, motor neurone disease, Alzheimer's disease, migraine, and Huntington's chorea. Sometimes it may be wise to refer them to an increasing number of books written for the benefit of the patients, often written by patients themselves.

REFERENCES

Bradbury, M. (1979). *The concept of a blood–brain barrier.* Wiley, New York.
Calne, D.B. (1980). *Therapeutics in neurology,* 2nd edn. Blackwell, Oxford.
Fishman, R.A. (1978). The pathophysiology and treatment of brain oedema. In

Recent advances in clinical neurology, No. 2 (ed. W.B. Matthews and G.M. Glaser). Churchill-Livingstone, Edinburgh.

—— (1980). *Cerebrospinal fluid in diseases of the nervous system.* Saunders, Philadelphia.

Graham, J. (1981). *Multiple sclerosis, a self-help guide to its management.* Thorsons, Wellingborough.

Illis, L.S., Segwick, E.M., and Glanville, H.J. (eds.) (1982). *Rehabilitation of the neurological patient.* Blackwell, Oxford.

Meinig, G., Aulich, A., Wende, S., and Reulen, H.J. (1976). The effect of dexa-methasone and diuretics on peritumour brain oedema; comparative study of tissue water content and computerized tomography. In *Dynamics of brain oedema* (ed. H.N. Pappins and W. Feindel) pp. 301–5. Springer, Berlin.

Saunders, C.M. (1978). *Management of terminal disease.* Arnold, London.

Wiles, C.M. (1982). Steroids in neurology. *Br. J. hosp. Med.* **28,** 308–22.

Wilson, B. (1982). Battling with motor neurone disease. *Br. med. J.* **284,** 34–5.

GENERAL REFERENCES AND FURTHER READING

Adams, R.D. and Victor, M. (1981). *Principles of neurology,* 2nd edn. McGraw-Hill, New York.

Blackwood, W. and Corsellis, J.A.N. (eds.) (1976). *Greenfield's neuropathology,* 3rd edn. Arnold, London.

Cooper, J.R., Bloom, F.E., and Roth, R.H. (1983). *The biochemical basis of neuro-pharmacology,* 4th edn. Oxford University Press, New York.

Davison, A.N. and Thompson, R.H.S. (eds.) (1981). *A molecular basis of neuro-pathology.* Arnold, London.

Lance, J.W. and McLeod, J.G. (1981). *A physiological approach to clinical neurology,* 3rd edn. Butterworths, London.

Neuwelt, E.A. and Clark, W.K. (1978). *Clinical aspects of neuro-immunology.* Williams and Wilkins, Baltimore.

Schmidt, R.F. and Thews, G. (eds.) (1982). *Human physiology.* Springer, Berlin.

Spillane, J.A. and Spillane, J.D. (1983). *An atlas of clinical neurology,* 3rd edn. Oxford University Press.

Walton, J.N. (1984). *Brain's diseases of the nervous system,* 9th edn. Oxford University Press.

Weller, R.O., Swash, M., McLellan, D.L., and Scholtz, C.L. (eds.) (1982). *Clinical neuropathology.* Springer, Berlin.

Part I

Disorders of function: symptoms and signs

1 The examination of the patient

THE HISTORY OF THE ILLNESS

In the diagnosis of nervous diseases the history of the patient's illness is often of greater importance than the discovery of his abnormal physical signs. The group of physical signs may be common to several disorders, and only an accurate knowledge of their mode of development may enable the correct diagnosis to be made. The history obtained from the patient should always be supplemented, if possible, by an account of his illness given by a relative or by someone who knows him well. This is essential when the patient suffers from mental impairment and also when his complaint includes attacks in which he loses consciousness, but it is always desirable, since a relative or friend will often remember an important point which the patient himself has forgotten to mention.

First note the patient's name and address, age, and exact details of his occupation. The last-named is often of importance as a source of exposure to injury or to toxic substances. Ascertain if he is right-handed.

It is well to begin by asking the patient of what he complains and when he was last in normal health, in this way fixing, at least provisionally, the date of onset of his symptoms. After this he should be allowed to relate the story of his illness as far as possible without interruption, questions being put to him afterwards to expand his statements and to elicit additional information. In the case of all symptoms it is important to ascertain not only the date but also the mode of onset, whether sudden, rapid, or gradual, whether the symptom since its first appearance has fluctuated in intensity and whether the patient's condition is improving, stationary, or deteriorating at the time of examination.

History of present illness

Inquiry should always be made with regard to the following symptoms, whether or not the patient mentions them spontaneously:

Mental state

The patient's mental history should be ascertained, not only as far as possible from himself, but also from relatives or friends, on the lines laid down below for the examination of his mental condition. If mental abnormality is suspected it is necessary to ascertain the patient's normal level of intelligence and temperament.

25

Sleep

Has he suffered from disturbances of sleep, either from paroxysmal or persistent sleepiness or from insomnia?

Speech

Has he difficulty in speaking? If so, of what nature? Has he been able to understand what is said to him, and to read? Has his writing been affected?

Attacks of loss of consciousness

Has he suffered from attacks of loss of consciousness, with or without convulsions? If so, the following further inquiries should be made.

When did the first attack occur? Was it precipitated by an accident or associated with an acute illness? How soon was it followed by the second? What is the usual interval between the attacks? Are they increasing in frequency? Do the attacks occur in bouts? Has the patient had a series of attacks without recovering consciousness? Do the attacks occur at any special time of the day? Do they occur only by day or only by night? In the case of a woman, are they related to the menstrual periods? Is any factor known to precipitate the attacks? Does the patient have any warning? If so, what, and how long does it precede the attack? How does an attack begin? Is its onset local or general, gradual or sudden? Is consciousness lost? Do convulsive movements occur in the attack? If so, are they symmetrical or asymmetrical? Has the patient injured himself in an attack? Does he bite his tongue and pass urine? How long do the attacks last? What is his condition afterwards? Are the attacks followed by headache, sleepiness, paralysis, or mental disturbance, such as automatism? What treatment has he had and how has he responded to it? Has he at any time suffered from head injury? Was labour difficult? If the attacks did not begin in infancy, did he suffer from infantile convulsions? Is there a family history of epilepsy or of fainting fits or mental disorder?

Headache

Has he suffered from headache? If so, attention must be paid to the following points. How long has the patient suffered from headache? Is it increasing in severity? Is it constant or paroxysmal, and if paroxysmal what is the duration of the paroxysms, and do they occur at any special times of day? Are they precipitated by any circumstance or activity, and how, if at all, can they be relieved? What is the character of the headache, and what is its situation? Is it associated with tenderness of the scalp or skull, with visual disturbances, vomiting, or vertigo? Has there been an injury of the head? Are there symptoms of nasal obstruction or of a discharge, either from the nostrils or into the pharynx? Is there a history of syphilis?

Special senses

Has he had hallucinations of smell or taste or noticed an impairment of these senses? Has he had visual hallucinations? If so, what has been their character and distribution in the visual fields? Has there been any visual impairment: if so, of one or both eyes and of what nature? Has it been transitory or progressive? Has he had double vision? If so, has this been transitory or progressive and has he noticed this symptom when looking in any special direction? Is his hearing impaired? If so, is this unilateral or bilateral and is the deafness associated with tinnitus? Does he suffer from giddiness? If so, he should describe precisely its nature and precipitating factors, and state whether it is associated with a sense of rotation of himself or of his surroundings, and with deafness, tinnitus, or vomiting.

Movement and sensibility

Does he complain of muscular weakness, of loss of control over the limbs or of involuntary movements, and if so, what is the distribution of these symptoms? Has his gait been abnormal, and if so, how? Has he tended to fall, and if so, in what direction? Has he had any spontaneous sensory disturbances, especially pain, numbness, or tingling?

The sphincters and reproductive functions

Has there been any disturbance of sphincter control? Has he experienced difficulty in holding or passing urine or faeces? Has he had polyuria? In the case of a man, are libido and sexual potency normal for his age? In the case of a woman, has there been any abnormality in menstruation, especially amenorrhoea?

Nutrition

Is the weight stationary, diminishing, or increasing?

History of previous illnesses

Inquiry as to previous illnesses should always include, in the case of a male patient, a specific inquiry as to venereal disease. A history of aural discharge or of tuberculosis may be important in relation to intracranial abscess or tuberculous meningitis. A history of convulsions or of meningitis in childhood or of encephalitis lethargica may be significant in relation to a later illness. A history of 'influenza' should be amplified by details of the illness thus described. Inquiry should always be made for a history of accidental injury, especially to the head and spine.

Social history

This should include inquiry as to the patient's educational and occupational career, adjustments to family life, military service career, residence abroad, and personal habits in respect of recreation, tobacco, and alcohol. If alcoholic excess is admitted, its amount and duration should be ascertained.

Family history

The family history is often of great importance, since many diseases of the nervous system are hereditary. The patient should always be asked whether cases of nervous or mental disease have occurred among his relatives and if so the precise nature of the illness should, if possible, be ascertained. Consanguity in the parents should be inquired for. If the patient is married, inquiry should be made as to the state of health of the spouse. Death of husband or wife from general paresis or aneurysm may afford an important clue to a syphilitic disorder in a patient. The number of children and the occurrence of miscarriages and stillbirths should be ascertained.

Genetic mechanisms

Many neurological disorders are inherited. For example Huntington's chorea and tuberose sclerosis are inherited as autosomal 'dominants' and Friedreich's ataxia, Wilson's disease and Refsum's disease as 'recessives', apparently occurring sporadically unless there has been consanguinous marriage. The commonest neurological disease inherited by a sex-linked mechanism, apart from colour-blindness, is the Duchenne type of muscular dystrophy. Leber's optic atrophy is also inherited in this way. It is not always correct to assume that a neurological disorder has only one mechanism of inheritance; different enzymatic defects (and therefore different genetic defects) may result in the same apparent biochemical defect. Chromosomal defects may also cause brain disease, for example an extra chromosome attached to the twenty-first pair (trisomy 21) occurs in mongolism. The value of genetic counselling has become increasingly important in the hope of reducing the incidence of these serious inherited disorders.

In a 'dominant' condition the patient has a one in two chance of transmitting it to his children. For an autosomal recessive condition in which both parents are carriers, demonstrated by the birth of an affected child, there is a one in four risk for further children. For X-linked diseases all the daughters of a male patient are carriers and they have a one in two chance of producing affected sons or carrier daughters. Women carriers of Duchenne dystrophy can often be identified because of raised serum creatine kinase levels, but the spontaneous genetic mutation rate is high, probably occurring in about a third of patients with Duchenne dystrophy. Ataxia telangectasia is an X-linked progressive disorder of infancy with cerebellar signs and skin telangectasia which is associated with immunodeficiency, both humoral and cell mediated. There is evidence that genetic counselling is reducing the number of children in families with Huntington's chorea but as yet there is no way to identify symptomless heterozygotes or to treat the patients successfully who have developed chorea.

There is an association between the histocompatibility phenotypes and susceptibility to neurological disease. Human leucocyte antigens (HLA) are encoded by at least four loci on the sixth chromosome. The antigens most often associated with multiple sclerosis are HLA-A3, HLA-B7, and DR2, depending on the geographical area of residence. The greatest difference in frequency between multiple sclerosis patients and controls has been for HLA-DR2 which is present in 60 per cent of patients with multiple sclerosis and 18 per cent of controls. The comparison of patients with multiple sclerosis in different areas suggests that separate aetiological agents, possibly viruses, are important in the development of multiple sclerosis in different geographic areas. Some multiple sclerosis patients with the HLA-DRw2 antigen have higher mean antibody titres to several viruses, including measles. Diseases in which auto-antibodies are commonly found, are associated with HLA-DR3 antigens; the most important neurological disease with this association is myasthenia gravis in young women (see p. 439).

CLINICAL EXAMINATION

State of consciousness

Is the patient conscious or unconscious? If unconscious, how far does he respond to stimuli, such as pinching the skin? Can he be roused, and if so, when he is roused is his mental condition normal or abnormal? How far can he think with normal clarity and speed, and perceive, respond to, and remember current stimuli? Can he swallow? The following psychological investigations are of course applicable only to conscious patients.

Intellectual functions

Is the patient orientated in space and time? Does he recognize his surroundings and does he know the date? Is his memory normal, and, if impaired, is it better for more remote than for recent events? Does he fill gaps in his memory by confabulating, that is, by relating imaginary events? Retentiveness may be tested by asking the patient to retain and repeat a series of digits – normally seven can be repeated – or retain a person's name, address, and the name of a flower for five minutes.

What is his level of intelligence? Is he in touch with current events? Can he grasp the meaning of a passage which he reads from a newspaper, or of a picture depicting an incident?

Does he suffer from delusions or hallucinations? A delusion is an erroneous belief which cannot be corrected by an appeal to reason and is not shared by others of the patient's education and station. A hallucination is a perceptual impression occurring in the absence of a corresponding external stimulus. A patient may conceal both delusions and hallucinations. The latter may sometimes be suspected on account of his behaviour. For example, a patient who is subject to visual hallucinations may behave as though manipulating invisible objects, while one who is experiencing auditory hallucinations, for example voices, may adopt a listening attitude.

Emotional state

Is the patient's emotional state normal? Is he excited or depressed? If excited, is his condition one of elation, that is excitement associated with a sense of well-being, or of fear and anxiety. Apart from excitement, does he experience an abnormal sense of well-being – euphoria? Is he anxious and, if so, to what does he attribute his anxiety? Is he irritable? Is he emotionally indifferent and apathetic? Does he take normal care of his dress and appearance, or is he indifferent and dirty?

Speech and articulation

Are speech and articulation normal? If there is reason to suspect that the patient is suffering from aphasia, the appropriate tests must be carried out (p. 136).

The cranial nerves

I. Test the sense of smell for each nostril separately (p. 35).

II. Test the visual acuity and visual fields (p. 37). Examine the ocular fundi (p. 39).

III, IV, and VI. Are the pupils equal, central, and regular? Are they abnormally dilated or contracted? Test the reactions to light, both direct and consensual, of each eye separately, and the reaction on accommodation.

Test the ocular movements, upwards and downwards and to either side, and ocular convergence. Is squint, diplopia, or nystagmus present? Note the size of the palpebral fissures. Does the patient exhibit ptosis or retraction of the upper lids? Is exophthalmos present?

V. Is there wasting of the temporal muscles and masseters? Test the jaw movements and the jaw-jerk.

Examine sensibility to light touch, pin-prick, heat and cold, over the trigeminal area, and test the corneal reflexes.

VII. Is the facial expression normal? Is there wasting of the facial muscles? Is the face the site of involuntary movements? Test the following voluntary movements – closure of the eyes, elevation of the eyebrows, frowning, retraction of the lips, pursing the lips, whistling. Test emotional facial movements – e.g. smiling. In some cases of facial paralysis it is necessary to test the sense of taste (p. 80).

VIII. Test the hearing, both air-conduction and bone-conduction. If hearing is defective, apply both Weber's and Rinne's tests (p. 71). In certain cases it may be necessary to test the vestibular reactions (p. 73).

IX and X. Is the soft palate elevated normally on phonation? Test the palatal and pharyngeal reflexes. Examine the movements of the vocal cords, if necessary.

XI. Test the movements of the sternocleidomastoids and trapezii.

XII. Examine the tongue. Is it wasted? Is fasciculation present? Is it tremulous? Is it protruded centrally, or does it deviate to one side?

Note the presence or absence of head retraction and test for cervical rigidity.

The limbs and trunk

The following is a convenient routine for the examination of the limbs and trunk. Examine the upper limbs while the patient is lying down; then ask him to sit up, or, if he is unable to do so, to turn on to one side, and examine the scapular muscles and the back; then ask him to lie down again and examine the front of the thorax and the abdomen, and finally the lower limbs. Sensibility as well as motor functions should first be examined in this order, but in many cases, especially when there is reason to suspect a lesion of the spinal cord, it may be convenient to review the sensibility of the body as a whole.

Muscular power and co-ordination

In examining the limbs note first their *posture* and the presence or absence of *muscular wasting* and *fasciculation*. Next note the presence or absence of *involuntary movements*, of which the following are those most commonly encountered. A tic is a co-ordinated repetitive movement involving as a rule a number of muscles in their normal synergic relationships. Choreic movements are quasi-purposive, jerky, irregular, and non-repetitive, and are characterized by dissociation of normal muscular synergy. Athetosis consists of slow, writhing movements, which are most marked in the peripheral segments of the limbs. Tremor is a rhythmical movement at a joint, brought about by alternating contractions of antagonistic groups of muscles. Myoclonus is a shock-like muscular contraction affecting part or the whole of the muscle independently of its antagonists. If involuntary movements are present, note their relationship to rest, posture, and voluntary movement.

Next examine *muscle tone* by passive movement at the various joints and note the presence or absence of *muscular contractures*. Next test voluntary power by asking the patient to carry out against resistance the movements possible at the various joints, comparing successively the same movement on the two sides of the body. If it is desired to record the degree of power present in a muscle the following scale may be used:

> No contraction, 0
> Flicker or trace of contraction, 1
> Active movement, with gravity eliminated, 2
> Active movement against gravity, 3
> Active movement against gravity and resistance, 4
> Normal power, 5.

Muscular co-ordination is tested in the upper limbs by asking the patient to touch the tip of his nose with the tip of his forefinger, first with the eyes open and then with the eyes closed. He should also be asked to carry out alternating movements of flexion and extension of the fingers, or pronation and supination of the forearms simultaneously on both sides. When the patient is in bed, co-ordination of the lower limbs may be tested by asking him to place one heel on the opposite knee, or to raise the leg from the bed and touch the observer's finger with his toe.

Movements of the abdominal wall are tested by asking the patient to raise his head from the bed against resistance and noting by palpation the degree of contraction of the abdominal muscles and also whether displacement of the umbilicus occurs.

Sensibility

As a routine, the patient's appreciation of light touch, pin-prick, heat and cold, posture, passive movement, and vibration should be tested, attention being paid not only to defective sensibility but also to the presence of tenderness of the superficial and deep structures. In some cases additional tests may be needed (p. 120). Since the spinal segmental areas run longitudinally along the long axis of the upper limbs, sensibility on the ulnar border should be compared with that on the radial border, either by applying successive stimuli transversely to the limb, or by dragging the stimulus, for example a pin, along the skin. On the trunk the segmental areas are distributed almost horizontally. Changes of sensibility are therefore best detected by moving the stimulus from below upwards or vice versa. In the lower limbs the sacral segmental areas, which are represented on the sole and the posterior aspect of the limb, should always be tested.

The reflexes

The following reflexes should be examined as a routine: *in the upper limbs*, the biceps-, supinator- and triceps-jerks; *on the trunk*, the abdominal reflexes; *in the lower limbs*, the knee- and ankle-jerks and the planar reflexes; at the same time tests for patellar and ankle clonus should be carried out.

The sphincters

Note the state of the sphincters and examine the abdomen for evidence of distension of the bladder.

Trophic disturbances

Note the state of the patient's nutrition, especially the presence of wasting or excessive obesity and the condition of the external genitalia. Note the distribution of hair on the body, anomalies of sweating, and the presence or absence of cutaneous pigmentation, naevi, and trophic lesions of the skin, nails, and joints.

The head and spine

Examine the *scalp* and *skull* and also the *spine*, noting the presence of deformity, rigidity, and tenderness in the latter.

A complete general physical examination should be made. Examination of the peripheral blood vessels, especially the carotids, is important. Inequality of carotid pulsation should be noted, and ausculation for a bruit should be carried out over each carotid, mastoid process, and eye. If a bruit is present, can it be abolished by carotid compression? A bruit originating in the vertebral artery may be audible above the clavicle posterolaterally to the carotid artery.

Gait

If the patient is well enough to leave his bed, observe whether he is able to stand without support with the feet together, and whether the steadiness of his stance is affected when he closes his eyes (Romberg's test). Ask him to walk, if necessary with support, and note the presence of spasticity of the lower limbs in walking. Slight disturbances of stance and gait may be detected by asking the patient to stand first on one foot and then on the other, first with the eyes open and then with the eyes closed; and to walk along a line, placing one heel in front of the other toe.

Abbreviated neurological examination

If the neurological examination is sometimes omitted by general practitioners this may be because the formal neurological examination is so lengthy and they are uncertain how to shorten it. A reasonably swift abbreviated examination is possible in the patient in whom no neurological lesion is expected. If competently and carefully performed this may be regarded as a satisfactory screening process, to be amplified into the full formal examination if any abnormalities are revealed.

The mental state will have become apparent during the history taking. The cranial nerve examination is conducted, omitting the test for the sense of smell. Pupils are tested with a torch and fundi examined with an ophthalmoscope. Fields are tested to confrontation with the hands. External ocular movements are checked by getting the patient to follow the torch, thereby excluding nystagmus. Light touch with cotton wool is checked over all the three divisions of the trigeminal nerve territory. Facial grimacing and eye closure are observed. Hearing is tested by repeating numbers softly in each ear while moving a finger over the opposite ear to occlude the sound from this ear. The palate is examined during phonation and the tongue is examined at rest and protruded. The arms are outstretched and any falling away when the eyes are closed is noted. Finger–nose–finger co-ordination is noted and the capacity to perform rapid movements with each hand is tested. In the legs, hip flexion, knee flexion, and dorsiflexion of the feet are tested. The jaw-jerk, deep tendon reflexes, abdominal and plantar responses are then checked. Sensory testing can be restricted to the appreciation of fine touch and pin prick in the hands and feet and the perception of vibration sense at the ankles and wrists. Finally the patient stands and performs Romberg's test and then with his eyes open and gazing straight ahead walks a few steps with the heel–toe gait. If this examination is reliably performed most clues to the grosser types of neurological defects will be noted.

REFERENCES

Baraitser, M. (1982). *The genetics of neurological disorders.* Oxford University Press.

Bickerstaff, E.R. (1980). *Neurological examination in clinical practice,* 4th edn. Blackwell, Oxford.

Bing, R. (1969). *Local diagnosis in neurological diseases,* 5th edn. (ed. W. Haymaker). Mosby, St. Louis.

DeJong, R.H. (1979). *The neurological examination,* 4th edn. Harper and Row, Hagerstown, Md.

Harper, P.S. (1981). *Practical genetic counselling.* Wright, Bristol.

Holmes, G.M. (1968). *Introduction to clinical neurology,* 3rd edn. Livingstone, Edinburgh.

Kety, S.S., Rowland, L.P., Sidman, R.L., and Matthysse, S.W. (1983). Genetics of neurological and psychiatric disorders. *Res. Publ. Ass. Res. nerv. Ment. Dis.* **60,** 1983.

Pryse-Phillips, W. and Murray, T.J. (1982). *Essential neurology,* 2nd edn. Exerpta Medica, New York.

2 The cranial nerves

THE FIRST OR OLFACTORY NERVE

Anatomy and physiology

The filaments of the olfactory nerve carry impulses from the smell receptors in the nasal mucosa to the olfactory bulb, from which the olfactory tract conveys them along the floor of the anterior fossa of the skull to the olfactory area of the cerebral cortex in the neighbourhood of the uncus (uncinate gyrus).

Examination

By the sense of smell we perceive not only scents but also flavours, the sense of taste being concerned only with the recognition of the four primary tastes – sweet, bitter, salt, and acid. To test the sense of smell small bottles containing such substances as oil of peppermint, oil of almond, or a little powdered coffee are applied in turn to each nostril and the patient is asked if he recognizes them. Many normal individuals with an acute sense of smell nevertheless find it difficult to name scents. It may therefore be necessary to ask the patient 'Is it coffee? Is it peppermint? . . .' and so on.

Causes of anosmia

Before concluding that anosmia, or loss of the sense of smell, is due to a nervous lesion, it is necessary to exclude disorders of the nose itself. There are patients who say that they lost their sense of smell many years previously and cannot account for it. In neurological practice there are only two important causes of anosmia. Bilateral loss of smell is sometimes seen after a *head injury*. This is usually not associated with a fracture of the skull, and if improvement does not occur within a few weeks of the injury it is likely to be permanent. Unilateral loss of the sense of smell may be an early sign of a *tumour*, especially a meningioma of the olfactory groove, pressing upon the tract. Such a tumour may eventually lead to bilateral anosmia.

THE OPTIC NERVE AND VISION

Anatomy and physiology

The fibres of the optic nerve are the axons of the ganglion cells of the retina, of which the macula is the region of most acute vision. Within the optic nerve the fibres from the upper quadrants of the retina lie above those from the lower

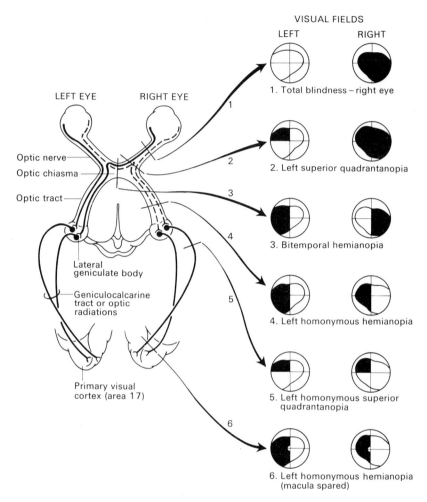

Fig. 2.1. Diagram of central connections of the optic nerve and optic tract and effect of lesions.

ones. There is a partial decussation of the fibres from each optic nerve at the optic chiasma, those from the nasal half of each retina crossing the middle line to join those from the temporal half of the opposite retina (Fig. 2.1). The result of this is that whereas each optic nerve carries impulses from the whole vision field of the same eye, each optic tract carries impulses from the temporal half of the retina on the same side and the nasal half of the retina on the opposite side, and so is concerned with vision in the opposite half of the visual field of each eye. This remains true of the visual pathways between the chiasma and the visual cortex on each side. The optic tract delivers the impulses concerned with vision to the lateral geniculate body on the same side from which the next relay, the optic radiation, originates. Here again, the fibres derived from the upper quadrants of the retinae lie above those from the lower. The optic radiation passes through the posterior limb of the internal capsule, the upper fibres running fairly directly through the subcortical white matter of the occipital lobe to the upper lip of the calcarine sulcus on its medial aspect. The lower fibres take a more circuitous course, dipping down to pass round the tip of the descending horn of the lateral ventricle before turning back again through the subcortical white matter to reach the lower lip of the calcarine sulcus. The cortical areas lying above and below the calcarine sulcus thus comprise the visual cortex, which spreads a little way on to the lateral aspect of the cerebral hemisphere at the occipital pole.

The visual acuity and the visual field

For neurological purposes the visual acuity should be assessed after correction of any refractive error. Distant vision may be estimated by testing the patient's power of reading Snellen's type at a distance of six metres. The visual acuity is expressed as a fraction, the distance of the eye from the type, that is six metres, being divided by the distance at which the patient should be capable of reading the smallest type he can read. Normal visual acuity is thus 6/6ths. If at six metres the patient can only read type which he should be capable of reading at 60 metres, the visual acuity is said to be 6/60ths. Near vision is tested by Jaeger's types.

Perimetry is the term used for mapping the visual field. At the bedside much valuable information can be obtained by confrontation perimetry. The examiner stands or sits opposite to the patient and about a metre away from him. The patient is told to cover one eye with his hand and fix the gaze of his other eye upon the opposite eye of the examiner. The examiner then brings a test object, either his finger or a white or coloured disc on a holder, inwards from beyond the periphery of his own visual field, midway between himself and the patient, who is asked to say when he first sees it. This procedure is carried out above, below, and to either side, and if necessarily intermediately, and so the examiner is enabled to determine the extent of the patient's visual field relative to his own. In special cases it may be necessary to carry the test object across the visual field in various directions, the patient being asked to say if it disappears from view and when it reappears. In this way an area of defective vision within the field, a *scotoma*, may be detected.

In young children and unco-operative, e.g. semiconscious, patients a field defect may sometimes be detected by noticing whether the patient reacts to an object brought in from the periphery in various directions, or whether he blinks in response to a feint with the hand towards the eye – the *menace reflex*.

In order to record the visual field it is necessary to use either a mechanical perimeter or Bjerrum's screen, which is a more delicate method of testing, and may reveal defects not discoverable by other methods.

Visual field defects

When a lesion involves one *optic nerve* it will produce a visual field defect which is limited to the eye concerned. Various types of encroachment on the field from without may be produced by pressure upon the nerve, and a concentric constriction may occur in syphilitic primary optic atrophy. One of the commonest and most important visual field defects is a *central scotoma* (Fig. 2.2) which occurs in optic neuritis. Figure 2.2 shows the area of loss of vision on testing with a circular white disc 3 mm in diameter, two metres from the patient. The visual field defect characteristic of advanced papilloedema and secondary optic atrophy is a concentric constriction.

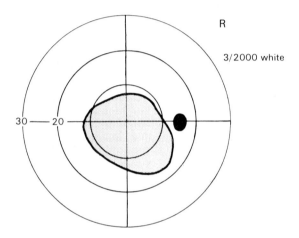

Fig. 2.2. A central scotoma due to retrobulbar neuritis.

The most characteristic visual field defect associated with a lesion of the optic chiasma is a *bitemporal hemianopia* (see Fig. 2.1). This is a characteristic symptom of a pituitary tumour, and it occurs because the upward pressure of the tumour interferes with the blood supply of the decussating fibres in the chiasma, and since, as we have seen, these come from the nasal half of the retinae the resulting field defect is bitemporal. This, however, is only a phase in the course of a progressive lesion which if unrelieved will go on to involve the nasal fields and so produce complete blindness.

Lesions of one *optic tract* produce a crossed homonymous hemianopia, that is to say, if the left optic tract is involved there will be loss of vision in the right half of each visual field. The area of field defect is not always identical on the two sides, and an *incongruous hemianopia* is characteristic of an optic tract lesion.

Lesions involving the *optic radiation* also cause a crossed homonymous hemianopia. Characteristically a temporal lobe lesion, because it damages the lower fibres, is likely to lead to a defect in the crossed upper quadrants only, a crossed upper quadrantic hemianopia, and a lesion of the upper part of the parietal lobe is likely to produce the reverse effect, a crossed inferior quadrantic hemianopia. A lesion of the optic radiation in the occipital lobe usually produces a *complete crossed homonymous hemianopia*, the line dividing the blind from the seeing area passing through the macular region. A lesion of the visual cortex, when complete, as after thrombosis of the posterior cerebral artery, similarly produces a crossed homonymous hemianopia, but in such cases the blind area often spares the macular region (see Fig. 2.1). Bilateral infarction of the occipital lobe causes *cortical blindness* in which pupillary reactions are normal but optokinetic nystagmus (p. 74) is absent. Though completely blind the patient may deny that he is blind, presumably because of destruction of related visual association areas (Anton's syndrome).

Ophthalmoscopy

Examination of the fundus of the eye is of great importance in many medical conditions, but especially in neurology. Except when the pupil is greatly contracted, it is usually possible to examine the optic disc; but to make a complete examination of the retina, the pupil should previously be dilated with homatropine. In examining the optic disc one should note its colour, the state of the physiological cup, the disc edge, the blood vessels, and the presence or absence of haemorrhages or exudate. The normal optic disc is circular and rosy pink in colour, though slightly paler than the surrounding retina (Plate 2(a)). When there is a large physiological cup which reaches to the edge of the disc, such a disc normally looks paler than discs with a smaller cup. The normal appearance of the optic disc can be learned only from experience. The common abnormalities of the disc are:

Papilloedema

Papilloedema means merely swelling of the optic disc. In its early stages the disc is pinker than normal, and the veins appear somewhat full. Next the nasal edge of the disc becomes blurred. Then this blurring extends to the temporal edge, and the physiological cup begins to fill with exudate (Plate 2(b)). Later the swelling lifts the surface of the disc above the level of the surrounding retina. In such cases the veins appear much more congested and tortuous, and flame-shaped haemorrhages and white exudate are likely to appear along the course of the vessels leaving the congested disc (Plate 2(c)). Papilloedema must be distinguished from certain other conditions which may superficially resemble it. Occasionally a leash of pale fibres is seen spreading for a short distance across the retina from one part of the disc, due to medullated nerve fibres (Plate 2(d)). This is a congenital abnormality and has no pathological significance. The discs may appear swollen in hypermetropia, in certain vascular anomalies of the nerve head and when hyaline bodies are partly buried in the nerve head. Fundus photography after intravenous injection of fluorescein shows exudate of the dye around the disc in papilloedema and in doubtful cases is helpful in distinguishing true from false papilloedema (Fig. 2.3).

The papilloedema is due to obstruction to the venous return from the prelaminar region of the optic nerve which is supplied from the posterior ciliary arteries, not the retinal artery (Plate 1). One of the commonest causes of papilloedema is increased intracranial pressure. It is usually bilateral. Such papilloedema is usually due to intracranial tumour, brain abscess, benign intracranial hypertension, or meningitis. If unrelieved it produces concentric constriction of the visual fields and ultimately blindness. Papilloedema also occurs in inflammatory lesions of the optic nerve, i.e. optic neuritis, sometimes called papillitis. This may be unilateral or less frequently bilateral. The swelling of the optic disc is not usually great, but whereas in papilloedema due to increased intracranial pressure visual acuity remains normal for some time, in optic neuritis it is severely depressed from the outset and the characteristic visual field defect is a central scotoma. Papilloedema may also occur in malignant hypertension. In this condition the edge of the optic disc is blurred and there may be some exudate in the physiological cup, but much swelling of the disc is rare. The arteries are thickened and tortuous and patches of white exudate are frequently to be found in the retina.

Optic neuritis

This is the commonest neurological visual disorder. The term implies an inflammatory lesion of the optic nerve or optic nerve head, though the inflammation in most cases is of the indirect kind which occurs in demyelinating disease. The patient, most often a young woman in otherwise good health, notices over a day or so the rapid deterioration in central vision, which may progress towards total loss of vision. The eye is often painful on movement and tender on pressure over the closed eyes. Testing of the visual fields will confirm a central scotoma if the deterioration is not too severe. If the neuritis affects the optic nerve head this will be swollen on ophthalmoscopy, the appearances being virtually indistinguishable from mild papilloedema due to raised intracranial pressure, though the lack of serious impairment of vision in papilloedema is of great practical importance and usually enables a confident distinction to be made between these two critically different conditions. If the neuritis involves the optic nerve behind the eye and the disc appears normal, the special term *retrobulbar neuritis* is often used.

Local or generalized infection is rarely the cause of optic neuritis but needs to be excluded in all cases. An ischaemic lesion of the optic nerve head may mimic optic neuritis due to demyelination but the patient is usually older, may have hypertension and recovery is less complete. Fluorescein studies also help to distinguish the nature of the ischaemic disc swelling (Fig. 2.3; Plate 3(a) and (b)). Syphilitic optic neuritis occurring in secondary syphilis can also usually be distinguished by fluorescein angiography and recovers more slowly and less completely.

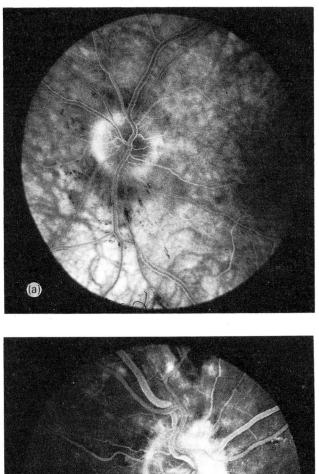

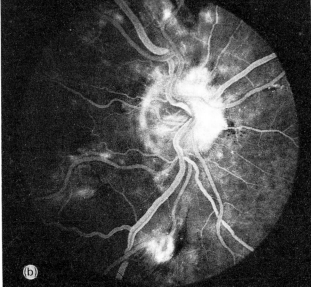

Fig. 2.3. (a) Fluorescein study showing ischaemic optic neuritis with leakage around disc and some small haemorrhages. (b) Fluorescein study of hypertensive retinopathy showing leakage from disc and extensive areas of leakage and some areas of haemorrhage.

Prognosis and treatment

Optic neuritis due to demyelination recovers to nearly normal vision spontaneously in almost all patients. In such patients evoked potentials will reveal a defect even though the visual acuity is normal and the disc fails to show optic pallor. The visual evoked responses (p. 160) will therefore not only confirm the presence of optic neuritis in a doubtful case but may provide further evidence, which may be used with caution, that the other eye has been affected as a result of a previous and possibly asymptomatic episode. This of course increases the chances of the patient developing a further demyelination. Further episodes of optic neuritis may occur in the same or opposite eye and in almost one-half of patients over fifteen years follow-up demyelination develops elsewhere, becoming typical of multiple sclerosis although not necessarily incapacitating. The HLA-DRw2-negative patients are more likely to develop further demyelination. Treatment with prednisolone for optic neuritis is usually given over some three weeks, if vision is seriously impaired. The evidence suggests that it reduces inflammatory swelling but the most recent attempts at controlled trials have not proved its benefit.

Secondary optic atrophy

If increased intracranial pressure is relieved by treatment, or if the inflammatory lesion causing optic neuritis subsides spontaneously, the optic disc may return to normal. If, however, increased intracranial pressure is not relieved in time, the end result of papilloedema is *secondary optic atrophy* (Plate 3(c)). The swelling of the disc diminishes, and it becomes paler. The arteries become constricted and the perivascular lymph spaces thickened. Finally the disc is pale and flat, the physiological cup remaining filled, and the edges of the disc being less distinct than formerly. The arteries are constricted, but the veins often remain congested for a considerable time.

Primary optic atrophy

The term primary optic atrophy is applied to an optic disc which becomes atrophic without having undergone any preliminary visible change. In such cases the optic disc is pale. The pallor may be limited to the temporal half, as in some cases of disseminated sclerosis, or it may involve the whole disc, which is sometimes bluish-white in colour, as in syphilitic optic atrophy (Plate 4(a)). The physiological cup is preserved, and indeed may be deeper than normal, showing the lamina cribrosa at the bottom. The edge of the optic disc is normal. The vessels may also be normal, but there is a tendency for both arteries and veins to be reduced in size. When the optic atrophy is due to obstruction of the central artery of the retina, the vessels are thread-like in calibre.

The visual fields in primary optic atrophy depend upon the causal lesion. After retrobulbar neuritis there may be a residual central scotoma. In syphilitic optic atrophy either the peripheral or the central parts of the visual fields may suffer most.

The most important cause of primary optic atrophy is pressure on the optic nerve by tumour, particularly one in the neighbourhood of the pituitary. It may sometimes follow a head injury involving the frontal region or orbit. Optic atrophy may also follow retrobulbar neuritis or a vascular occlusive lesion of the optic nerve particularly in patients with arteriosclerosis, diabetes or cranial arteritis. Rare causes of optic atrophy include neurosyphilis, especially tabes and general paralysis, and vitamin B_{12} deficiency. It may also follow exposure to a number of toxic substances, including tobacco (tobacco amblyopia), methyl alcohol, lead, arsenic, carbon bisulphide, certain insecticides, and quinine. The most recent addition to the list is clioquinol (contained in Entero-Vioform) which in Japan appears to have caused optic atrophy with more widespread neurological symptoms (subacute myeloptic neuropathy), distinct from multiple sclerosis.

Patients with tobacco amblyopia probably have a defect in the ability to metabolize cyanide. The normal active form of vitamin B_{12} in the blood is methylcobalamin and the proportion of cyanobalamin is raised in many cases. Apart from stopping such patients smoking completely, hydroxocobalamin should be given by intramuscular injection, never cyanocobalamin. A similar defect of cyanide detoxication may occur in Leber's hereditary optic atrophy which should be treated similarly.

Consecutive optic atrophy (Plate 4(b)) is a term used when the disc presents the appearance of primary optic atrophy, but this is consecutive upon lesions of the retina, such as retinitis pigmentosa (Plate 4(c)) or the various forms of choroidoretinitis, which manifest themselves by deposits of scattered black pigmentation in the retina.

Certain abnormalities of the fundus may point to underlying neurological disease, for example subhyaloid haemorrhage in subarachnoid haemorrhage (Plate 4(d)), retinal angiomas in cerebellar haemangioblastoma (Lindau–von Hippel disease), and miliary tubercules in tuberculous meningitis.

THE PUPILS

Anatomy and physiology

The size of the pupil is regulated by two opposing nervous influences, those of the sympathetic and the parasympathetic (Fig. 2.4). The sympathetic fibres are dilator: they run downwards in the tegmentum of the brainstem and in the cervical spinal cord from which they emerge by the anterior roots of the eighth cervical and first and second thoracic segments. They then pass into the cervical sympathetic nerve trunk, up which they travel to enter the skull with the internal carotid artery, and thence to the eye. Damage to these iridodilator fibres at any point in their course leads to a contracted pupil, which, however, still reacts to light, and since the sympathetic fibres also supply the smooth muscle in the upper lid, the small pupil of ocular sympathetic palsy is associated with a slight degree of ptosis of the upper lid (Horner's syndrome) (Fig. 2.5). The iridocon-

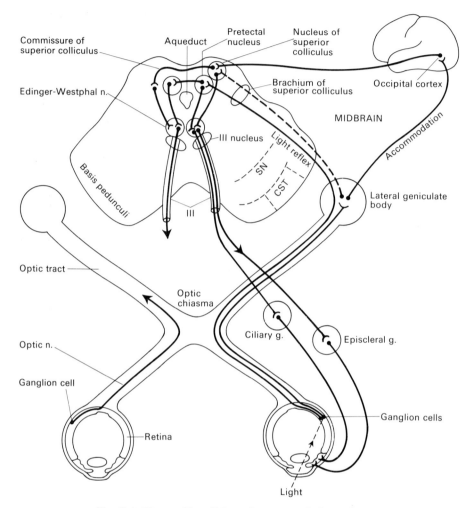

Fig. 2.4. The pupillary light and accommodation reflexes.

strictor fibres originate in the third nerve nucleus in the midbrain. Entering the third nerve they run to the ciliary ganglion and thence to the circular muscle of the iris. Paralysis of the iridoconstrictor fibres either in the nucleus of the third nerve or in the course of the nerve itself causes dilation of the pupil, and the dilated pupil fails to react to light and accommodation. When a lesion damages both the iridoconstrictor and the iridodilator fibres, as may happen when it is situated in the neighbourhood of the cavernous sinus, the pupil is intermediate or cadaveric in size, and fails to react to light and accommodation.

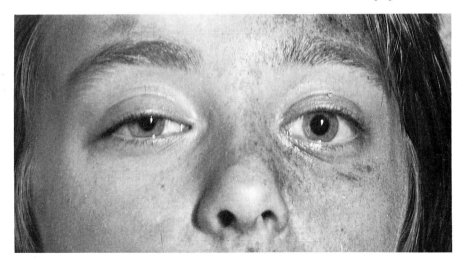

Fig. 2.5. Horner's syndrome with loss of sweating (sweating on normal side marked with quinizarin powder).

Examination of the pupils

The following points require to be noted in the examination of the pupils. Are they equal, central, and regular? Is their size normal, or are they dilated or constricted? Do they react normally to light, accommodation, and convergence?

The pupils are normally smaller in adult life than in childhood, and in old age than middle age.

Dilation of the pupil is produced by a lesion of the iridoconstrictor fibres in the third nerve at any point between the third nerve nucleus and the eye. It is also produced by paralysis of the iridoconstrictor terminals by a mydriatic, such as homatropine. Constriction of the pupil is produced by paralysis of the sympathetic iridodilator fibres at any point in their course.

Inequality of the pupils results from a unilateral lesion of either the iridoconstrictor or the iridodilator fibres. It also occurs when one pupil is intermediate in size and fails to constrict to light and dilate to shade. The affected pupil is then the larger when the normal one is constricted and the smaller when it is dilated.

The reaction to light

If one eye is exposed to light, a constriction of both pupils normally occurs. The response of the pupil of the eye upon which the light fails is called the direct reaction, that of the opposite pupil the consensual reaction. To elicit the light reflex, the patient should be asked to look at a distant object, in order to eliminate the contraction of the pupil on accommodation, and the eye not being tested should be covered in order to eliminate the consensual reaction. A light is then shone on the eye to be tested and the reaction of the pupil observed. When the consensual reaction is to be tested, it is the reaction of the shaded opposite eye which is observed.

The normal range of the contraction of the pupil as a reflex response to light can be learned only by experience. Moreover it is not an all-or-none reaction. An impairment of the reaction will be shown by a reduction in its normal amplitude, and often by a failure to sustain the degree of contraction initially obtained. Loss of the pupillary reaction to light is sometimes called *reflex iridoplegia*.

Loss of the reaction of the pupil to light is the result of a lesion involving the reflex pathway at some point. On the afferent side the reflex runs by the visual pathways described above, to the superior colliculus. Thence internuncial pathways run to the iridoconstrictor part of the third nerve nucleus on both sides, thereby enabling the light stimulus falling upon one eye to evoke a contraction of both pupils. It follows that a lesion which impairs conduction in one optic nerve will diminish or abolish the reaction of both pupils to light. A lesion in the neighbourhood of the cerebral aqueduct (of Sylvius) may have the same effect, usually bilaterally, while, as stated above, a lesion involving the third nerve at any point in its course may interrupt the efferent pathway for the reflex to the ipsilateral eye.

The reaction on accommodation

When the gaze is directed from a distant to a near object, contraction of the medial recti brings about a convergence of the axes of the eyes, and, in association with this, accommodation occurs by contraction of the ciliary muscle, and the pupil contracts. When each eye is tested in this way separately the pupillary reaction is known as the reaction on accommodation; when the two eyes are tested together, it may be called the reaction on convergence. Sometimes it is described jointly as the reaction on accommodation–convergence. In general these two reactions behave in the same way. In these circumstances contraction of the pupil is in the nature of an associated movement, which is probably the outcome of impulses originating in the visual cortex, and descending either directly or by way of the middle frontal gyrus to the midbrain, there to terminate in the iridoconstrictor part of the third nerve nucleus. To elicit this reaction the patient should be asked to look at a distant object and then at the examiner's finger, which is gradually brought to within 5 cm of the eye.

The following are the principal varieties of abnormal pupillary reaction:

The Argyll Robertson pupil

The pupillary abnormality known as the Argyll Robertson pupil was described by that Scottish ophthalmologist as follows. 'The pupil is small . . . constant in size, and unaltered by light or shade; it contracts promptly and fully on convergence and dilates again promptly when the effort to converge is relaxed; it dilates slowly and imperfectly to mydriatics.' To this one might add one further and almost constant abnormality, namely a patchy atrophy and depigmentation of the fibres of the iris which, especially towards its margins, acquire a somewhat opaque and 'ground-glass' appearance. The pupillary abnormality thus described by Argyll Robertson is almost always due to neurosyphilis, being commonly found in tabes and general paresis, and not uncommonly in meningovascular syphilis.

Since the Argyll Robertson pupil reacts to convergence but not to light, it has been argued that the lesion cannot involve the iridoconstrictor fibres in the course of the third nerve, since this pathway is common to both reactions. Some, therefore, would place the lesion due to gliosis near the cerebral aqueduct where it is supposed to interrupt the reflex path of the light reaction between the superior colliculus and the third nerve nucleus, but spares the more ventrally placed accommodation–convergence input. An alternative view is that the lesion lies in the ciliary ganglion which, it is believed, the fibres concerned in the reaction on accommodation bypass, and so escape damage. This view on the whole seems the more satisfactory, and it would also explain the smallness of the pupil as the result of damage to the sympathetic iridodilator fibres, and the commonly associated ptosis of the upper lid as the result of injury to the sympathetic fibres going to the smooth muscle of the upper lid. The associated atrophy of the iris also seems more likely to be the result of a lesion in the ciliary ganglion than of one in the midbrain.

If we extend the term Argyll Robertson pupil to other examples of reflex iridoplegia in which the pupil is not necessarily smaller than normal, we shall have to admit other lesions of the upper part of the midbrain as causes, such as tumour, vascular lesions, and encephalitis.

Tonic pupils and absent tendon reflexes

This disorder, sometimes known as the Holmes–Adie syndrome, is not uncommon, and is important because, though itself benign, it may be confused with the Argyll Robertson pupil or other pupillary abnormalities which may be of serious import.

The tonic pupil, which is found almost exclusively in females and usually in early adult life, may be associated with no symptoms and discovered on routine examination, or it may be brought to attention because the patient complains either of sudden blurring of vision in one eye, or that one pupil has become larger than the other. The abnormality is unilateral in about 80 per cent of cases. The affected pupil is moderately dilated, and is therefore usually larger than its fellow. When tested by ordinary methods the reaction of the affected pupil to light, both direct and consensual, is either completely or almost completely absent. The characteristic feature, however, from which the syndrome derives its name, is the response of the pupil to accommodation. Whereas a hasty examination may suggest that the pupil does not react at all on accommodation, nevertheless, if the patient is made to gaze fixedly at a near object, the pupil, sometimes after slight delay, contracts very slowly through a range which is often greater than normal, so that the affected pupil actually becomes smaller than the normal one. When accommodation is relaxed, dilatation of the pupil begins, either at once or after a slight delay, and proceeds even more slowly than its contraction. This is the tonic pupillary reaction. Sometimes the reaction on accommodation is lost as well as that to light.

Some abnormality in the tendon reflexes is usually present, the ankle-jerks, knee-jerks, and arm-jerks being diminished or lost in this order of frequency. Occasionally the tonic pupil occurs with normal reflexes. If attention is paid to the points described, there should be no difficulty in distinguishing the tonic pupil from the Argyll Robertson pupil. The fact that in both tabes and the Holmes–Adie syndrome some of the tendon reflexes may be absent may also be a source of confusion, but the character of the pupillary abnormalities usually enables the two conditions to be distinguished without difficulty, and in the Holmes–Adie syndrome the patient does not suffer from lightning pains, sensory loss, or ataxia, which are all symptoms commonly found in tabes.

There may be progression with the passage of years so that eventually both pupils become abnormal and reflex loss becomes more widespread. The tonic pupil constricts on conjunctival instillation of Mecholyl (2.5 per cent), while the normal pupil remains unaffected. Such supersensitivity points to impairment of the postganglionic nerve supply according to the principle of denervation hypersensitivity. The ciliary ganglion has been shown to be almost without ganglion cells in the few cases of Adie's syndrome studied at post mortem. In some cases there is evidence of widespread defects of autonomic function in addition to the loss of reflexes and pupillary changes. The cause has not been established. The physical signs are permanent, but have no ill-effect beyond some occasional difficulty in accommodation (see p. 46).

The Hutchinsonian pupil

Jonathan Hutchinson drew attention to the pupillary abnormalities commonly seen in the presence of rapidly rising intracranial pressure in one half of the cranial cavity, for example, in a case of traumatic haemorrhage from the middle meningeal artery. The pupil on the side of the lesion is first contracted and then widely dilated, and the same sequence of events is then to be observed in the pupil on the opposite side.

The innervation of the upper lid

The striated muscle of the upper lid, the levator palpebrae superioris, is inner-vated by the third nerve, but the smooth muscle of the lid receives its nerve supply from the cervical sympathetic. Damage to either of these nerves causes ptosis of the lid. When the ptosis is due to a third nerve palsy, the eye is completely or almost completely closed, and if the patient is asked to look upwards no associated elevation of the paralysed lid occurs. On the other hand, when the ocular sympathetic is paralysed, the drooping of the upper lid is only slight, and its lower level is usually only about 2 mm below that of the lid on the opposite side. When the patient is asked to look upwards, an associated elevation of the affected upper lid occurs as the result of contraction of the levator. The amplitude of this movement is normal, but since the lid starts at a lower level than its opposite fellow it remains at a lower level, relatively, after both have moved upwards. The ptosis of the upper lid resulting from paralysis of the ocular sympathetic is associated with a contraction of the pupil due to the same cause. Ptosis of the upper lid resulting from paralysis of the third nerve is usually associated, on the other hand, with a dilated and fixed pupil, and with paralysis of the external ocular muscles which receive their innervation from the same source.

Ptosis of the upper lid is sometimes encountered as the result of a muscular disorder, especially the disturbance of function at the myoneural junction which occurs in myasthenia gravis. In myasthenia the ptosis is usually bilateral, and becomes worse as the patient grows tired. This point may be demonstrated by asking the patient to look upwards, when the resulting fatigue of the levator leads to drooping of the upper lid which is evident when the patient is asked to gaze horizontally forwards.

Retraction of the upper lid is attributable to a relative or absolute shortening of the elevating muscles, perhaps especially of the smooth muscle. When present it is exaggerated when the patient voluntarily elevates his eyes, and it is responsible for the lag of the upper lid in following the downward movement of the eye, which is known as von Graefe's sign. The common cause of lid retraction is thyrotoxicosis, but it is occasionally a symptom of organic nervous disease, for example tabes or Parkinsonism. Retraction of the upper lid may be unilateral or bilateral, and may occur with or without exophthalmos.

Exophthalmos

The presence or absence of exophthalmos should be noted. In doubtful cases it is best detected by looking down at the patient from above. The commonest causes of exophthalmos are exophthalmic goitre, and exophthalmic ophthalmoplegia, in both of which it is usually but not invariably bilateral. It may also be due to forward displacement of the eye by a space-occupying lesion such as a tumour within or behind the orbit and then is usually unilateral. Proptosis is the term used for protrusion of the eye in unilateral or asymmetrical exophthalmos.

THE EYE MOVEMENTS

Anatomy and physiology

The eyes normally move together, hence their movements are called conjugate. They move in this parallel fashion in any direction except in convergence, when the visual axes no longer remain parallel since the two eyes are medially rotated or adducted. The eye movements commonly tested are conjugate movement laterally to right and left, vertically upwards and downwards, and convergence.

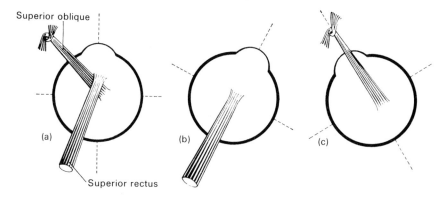

Superior oblique

Superior rectus

(a)   (b)   (c)

Fig. 2.6. Diagram of the line of action of the superior rectus and superior oblique muscles of the right eye when the eye is looking: (a) straight ahead; (b) outwards; (c) inwards.

Usually the patient is asked to follow a moving object with his eyes, such as the observer's finger. He may, however, be asked to look in the required direction on command.

Six muscles move each eye, the four recti, superior and inferior, lateral and medial, and the two obliques, superior and inferior. The lateral rectus moves the eye outwards and the medial rectus inwards in the horizontal plane. The action of the other two recti and the obliques is more complex, as is shown in Fig. 2.6. The actions of the vertical recti and the obliques vary according to the position of the eye, because of the site of insertion of these muscles. Fig. 2.6 shows a simplified diagram of the planes of action of the superior rectus and the superior oblique of the right eye. From this it is clear that if the eye is turned outwards the axis of the eye is in line with the action of the recti and they will act as pure elevators or depressors. If the eye is turned inwards the obliques will act as almost pure elevators or depressors. When their plane of action is at right angles to the axis of the eye, the recti and obliques will have a secondary action as rotators or torters. Intorsion is the term given to a rolling of the top of the eye towards the bridge of the nose and extorsion is its opposite. Thus when the eye is turned inwards torsion is caused by the recti, but when the eye is turned outwards torsion is caused by the obliques. The superior rectus and inferior oblique act together as elevators of the eye, while the inferior rectus and the superior oblique act as depressors. In the conjugate movement there is a harmonious contraction of the appropriate muscles of the two eyes (Fig. 2.7). In lateral conjugate deviation the lateral rectus of one eye and the medial rectus of the other contract together.

The association of the two eyes in conjugate movement depends upon nervous pathways which run from the cerebral cortex to the nuclei of the muscles concerned. Let us consider conjugate deviation of the eyes to the right

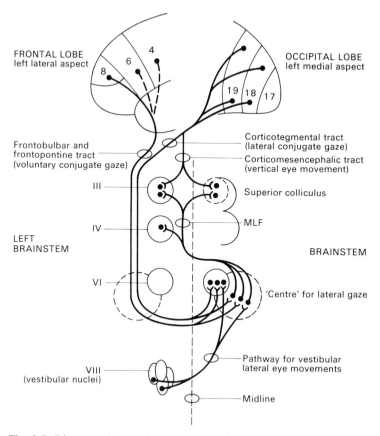

FRONTAL LOBE
left lateral aspect

OCCIPITAL LOBE
left medial aspect

Frontobulbar and
frontopontine tract
(voluntary conjugate gaze)

Corticotegmental tract
(lateral conjugate gaze)

Corticomesencephalic tract
(vertical eye movement)

Superior colliculus

MLF

LEFT
BRAINSTEM

BRAINSTEM

'Centre' for lateral gaze

Pathway for vestibular
lateral eye movements

VIII
(vestibular nuclei)

Midline

Fig. 2.7. Diagram of the pathways concerned in conjugate eye movements.

(Fig. 2.7). The upper motor neurones concerned in this movement start in the posterior part of the middle frontal gyrus on the left side. They then pass downwards through the internal capsule to the upper part of the midbrain, where, like other upper motor neurones, they decussate. To produce the required movement the pathway has to bring into action together the right lateral rectus and the left medial rectus. It does this by descending in the brainstem to the neighbourhood of the right lateral rectus nucleus. In order to link this with the nucleus of the opposite medial rectus, a further pathway now turns upwards in the medial longitudinal fasciculus and crosses the middle line to reach that part of the left third nerve nucleus which innervates the left medial rectus. The upper motor neurones concerned with conjugate lateral movement to the left are the mirror image of those just described. Those concerned with conjugate vertical movements do not need to descend into the pons, but terminate in relation with those parts of both third nerve nuclei which supply the superior and inferior recti and the inferior obliques and with both fourth nerve nuclei which supply the superior obliques.

We now come to the lower motor neurones which innervate the external ocular muscles. They originate in the nuclei of the third, fourth, and sixth cranial nerves. The first two of these lie in the midbrain just anterior to the cerebral aqueduct, and the nucleus of the sixth nerve lies in the pons beneath the floor of the upper part of the fourth ventricle, and partly encircled by the fibres of the seventh nerve. The third nerve emerges from the brainstem on the medial aspect of the crus cerebri and passes forwards to the lateral wall of the cavernous sinus where it lies close to the fourth and sixth nerves and the first division of the fifth nerve, and then it enters the orbit where it supplies the levator palpebrae, the superior, medial and inferior recti, and the inferior oblique, as well as the ciliary muscle and the constrictor of the pupil.

The nucleus of the fourth nerve supplies the opposite superior oblique muscle. Its fibres therefore decussate with those of its fellow before emerging just behind the quadrigeminal bodies. It then winds round the cerebral peduncle (Plate 6), and passes forward to the wall of the cavernous sinus, after which it enters the orbit to supply the superior oblique.

The sixth nerve emerges at the inferior border of the pons (Plate 5) and has a long extracerebral course along the base of the brain before it, too, reaches the lateral wall of the cavernous sinus, thence entering the orbit to supply the lateral rectus muscle.

OPHTHALMOPLEGIA

Ophthalmoplegia means paralysis of the ocular muscles, and from what has already been said it will be clear that this may arise as a result of lesions at many different points. The principal varieties, in terms of disordered anatomy and physiology, are four:

1. Conjugate ophthalmoplegia, in which there is an impairment of conjugate ocular movement.

2. Nuclear ophthalmoplegia, in which the lesion involves the nuclei supplying the ocular muscles.

3. Ophthalmoplegia due to a lesion involving one or more of the third, fourth, and sixth cranial nerves.

4. Ophthalmoplegia of muscular origin, in which the disorder of function lies not in the nervous system but in the ocular muscles themselves.

Conjugate ophthalmoplegia

Paralysis of conjugate movement to one side may occur as a result of a lesion in one of two situations. An extensive subcortical lesion of one cerebral hemisphere may cause loss of conjugate deviation of the eyes to the opposite side. The commonest example of this is a vascular lesion, and when, as often happens, the patient is unconscious, the eyes, and the head, are turned to the side of the lesion by the unopposed action of the healthy cerebral hemisphere. The other common lesion lies in the pons in the neighbourhood of the sixth nerve nucleus. Such a lesion, usually a tumour, causes paralysis of conjugate deviation of the eyes to the same side, and is often associated with facial paralysis on that side. Conjugate vertical movements, upwards and downwards, may be lost as the result of a lesion, usually neoplastic or vascular, involving the upper midpart of the brain just above the third nerve nuclei. In such cases, although the patient cannot voluntarily elevate his eyes or raise them when attempting to follow a moving object, it is often possible to induce elevation of the eyes reflexly by asking him to fix an object and then passively flexing his neck.

Conjugate convergence of the eyes may also be impaired or lost as the result of a lesion of the upper part of the midbrain, and is not uncommonly defective in Parkinsonism and in progressive supranuclear palsy (see p. 343).

Internuclear ophthalmoplegia

A brainstem lesion in the region of the medical longitudinal bundle may interrupt the connections between the third and sixth nerve nuclei (Fig. 2.7). Impulses from the 'centre' for conjugate lateral gaze, which is thought to be near the sixth nerve nucleus, pass to the ipsilateral sixth nerve nucleus but not to the contralateral third nerve nucleus. On attempted conjugate lateral gaze to the same side, the contralateral medial rectus then fails to contract, though the muscles will contact normally on convergence. The abducting eye may show nystagmus. A lesion in this site is characteristic of disseminated sclerosis.

Nuclear ophthalmoplegia

This is not a very common cause of ophthalmoplegia. It is a term usually restricted to lesions involving the nuclei of the third and fourth nerves, of which a neoplasm is probably the commonest. In nuclear ophthalmoplegia the visual axes do not remain parallel as they do in the paralyses of conjugate ocular gaze, but there is a varied degree of paralysis of the various external ocular muscles innervated by the third and fourth nerves, including often the levator palpebrae, which leads to ptosis, and also the iridoconstrictor.

Paralysis of the third, fourth, and sixth nerves

Paralysis of the third nerve

Complete paralysis of the third nerve causes complete ptosis of the upper lid, and complete internal ophthalmoplegia, the pupil being widely dilated and failing to react to light and accommodation, which is also paralysed. There is paralysis of the superior, medial, and inferior recti, and the inferior oblique. The unantagonized lateral rectus causes outward deviation of the eye, and the only remaining ocular movements are abduction, carried out by the lateral rectus, and a movement of depression and intorsion. The ptosis masks the diplopia, which becomes evident to the patient when the eyelid is raised for him. A partial lesion of the third nerve may paralyse the external ocular muscles which it supplies, but spare the fibres which innervate the pupil. When both the third nerve and the ocular sympathetic are injured, as may happen with a lesion just behind the orbit, the pupil is not dilated, because the iridodilator fibres are paralysed as well as the iridoconstrictor. It therefore remains of medium size.

The third nerve may be damaged by the pressure of a tumour or an aneurysm or by trauma to the head. It may be involved in meningitis, in meningovascular syphilis, or by a vascular lesion in elderly atheromatous or diabetic subjects.

Fourth nerve paralysis

Paralysis of the fourth nerve causes weakness of the superior oblique muscle which leads to weakness of downward gaze, more marked when the eye is turned inwards, and to extorsion, especially when the eye is turned downwards. As a result of the defect of downward gaze the patient with a superior oblique paralysis often complains of double vision when walking downstairs. The patient may develop a head tilt to the opposite side in order to compensate for the extorsion and obtain binocular vision.

Sixth nerve paralysis

A lesion of the sixth, or abducens, nerve causes paralysis of the lateral rectus muscle with loss of abduction of the eye, which is deviated inwards by the unantagonized medial rectus. This causes diplopia (p. 56).

When paralysis of the lateral rectus is the result of a lesion of the nucleus of the sixth nerve within the pons there are almost invariably associated signs of lesions of other neighbouring pontine structures, especially the seventh nerve. Isolated paralysis of one lateral rectus, therefore, usually means that the lesion involves the nerve at some point between the pons and the orbit. Owing to its long and rather devious course the sixth nerve is peculiarly susceptible to damage. Apart from the direct pressure of a tumour, it may suffer as the result of a general increase in intracranial pressure, in which case sixth nerve paralysis has been described as a 'false localizing sign'. It may also be compressed by an aneurysm and, like the third nerve, involved in meningovascular syphilis, or by a vascular lesion in an atheromatous subject. It is fairly frequently damaged as the result of head injury and is more liable than the third nerve to be affected in meningitis, pyogenic or tuberculous.

Ophthalmoplegia due to muscular disorders

The principal causes are myasthenia gravis and exophthalmic ophthalmoplegia. Ocular myopathy is rare. The characteristic feature of ophthalmoplegia of muscular origin is a distribution of muscular weakness which cannot be explained in terms of a neurological lesion. Both eyes are often affected. In myasthenia there is usually ptosis, and the ophthalmoplegia ranges from weakness of one ocular muscle of one eye to virtual paralysis of all muscles of both eyes. The weakness rapidly increases with fatigue, and muscular power is improved by neostigmine and similar drugs. In exophthalmic ophthalmoplegia, the muscular weakness, which first affects the elevators and abductors, is usually bilateral, and associated with exophthalmos and retraction of the upper lid. The conjunctivae are oedematous and later congested.

Exophthalmic ophthalmoplegia

In Graves' disease, the commonest cause of exophthalmic ophthalmoplegia, the changes range from mild lid-lag (von Graefe's sign) and lid retraction to chronic inflammation of the muscles, fibro-fatty connective tissue and even lacrimal glands, with venous engorgement and oedema which may threaten the sight. There now appears to be an autoimmune process directed against orbital tissues and antibodies to an eye muscle antigen have been reported in a high proportion of exophthalmic cases and in no thyrotoxic patients without eye disease. Ocular computerized tomographic scans will detect muscle swelling before the onset of clinical signs. There are no thyroid abnormalities in about 10 per cent of patients with endocrine exophthalmos but the full range of thyroid function tests is needed in all cases. In thyrotoxicosis there is an elevation of the circulating biologically active tri-iodothyronine (T_3) in association with a suppressed pituitary thyrotrophin (TSH). An autoimmune disturbance may possibly occur without evidence of thyroid involvement in idiopathic orbital inflammation, the pseudo-tumour or Tolosa–Hunt syndrome which responds to steroids. The management of thyrotoxic exophthalmos remains difficult, mild cases subsiding within a few months, but some patients developing rapidly progressive exophthalmos may require high-dose steroids, immunosuppression with azothiaprine, plasmapheresis, or even orbital decompression.

SQUINT

Squint, or strabismus, is the term applied to a lack of parallelism of the ocular axes. When the movements of one eye are limited by weakness of one or more ocular muscles and the other eye moves normally, squint is bound to occur and is described as convergent or divergent according to the angle made by the ocular axes. This is known as paralytic squint, which is important to distinguish from concomitant or spasmodic squint, which does not indicate nervous disease. Concomitant squint differs from paralytic squint in that it is equal for all positions of the eyes, and, if the fixing eye is covered, the movements of the squinting eye are found to be full. Concomitant squint is not associated with diplopia; paralytic squint, at least in the early stages, usually is.

DIPLOPIA

Diplopia, or double vision, is a very common symptom of ophthalmoplegia. Why does it occur? The retina is an extended sensory surface, each point on which has 'local sign'. When I look at a table and chair I see them as two objects and not one because their two images fall upon different points in my retina. When I look at a single object, I see only one, even though I see it with two eyes, because in my two eyes the two images of the single object fall upon corresponding points, and my nervous system presents them to me as a single image. When a movement of one eye is paralysed, diplopia results because the images of a single object formed by the two eyes no longer fall upon corresponding points of the retinae. For example, in paralysis of the right lateral rectus the right eye is not moved outwards. If the patient attempts to deviate his eyes horizontally to the right, the image of a small object falls in the left eye upon the macula. In the right eye, however, which is not displaced, it falls upon the nasal half of the retina, which is normally the receiving point for images lying to the right of the fixation point. Consequently the patient now sees two images of the single object, and the one produced by the affected eye, which is called the false image, lies to the right of and parallel with the true image. The further the test object is moved to the right, the further into the nasal half of the right retina the image moves, and the further the false image appears to move to the right. From these facts we can deduce two simple rules governing the appearance of diplopia:

1. The separation of the images increases the further the eyes are moved in the normal direction of pull of the paralysed muscle.

2. The false image is displaced in the direction of the plane or planes of action of the paralysed muscle.

It follows from these two rules that when the gaze is so directed that the separation of the images is the greatest, the more peripherally situated image is the false one, derived from the affected eye, which can thus be ascertained. The simplest method is to cover up one eye with a red and the other with a green glass, or a pair of coloured plastic goggles. The patient is then made to look at a light, such as an ophthalmoscope lamp, or a small but well-illuminated piece of white paper. This is moved until the maximal separation of the images is obtained, and they are then distinguishable by their colour. If coloured glasses are not available, an intelligent and co-operative patient is usually able to distinguish the images by noticing which disappears when each eye is covered separately. When the affected eye has been discovered, the paralysed muscle can be determined. It is the muscle which normally displaces the eye in the direction of displacement of the false image.

The causes of diplopia

There are a few practical points which need to be borne in mind in connection with diplopia. No difficulty arises when the ophthalmoplegia is obvious: the cause of the diplopia is then the cause of the ophthalmoplegia. There are, however, numerous cases in which either the patient complains of transitory diplopia which is not present at the time of examination, or of slight double vision, which is present at the time, but the cause of which is not apparent on clinical examination. In such cases the help of the ophthalmologist must be sought. Special tests will usually show which muscle or muscles are at fault, and also whether the diplopia is likely to be due to organic disease or merely to defective balance of the eye muscles, which, unless recognized, may lead to an erroneous diagnosis of a serious nervous disorder. If the appropriate tests establish that the diplopia is nervous in origin, possible causes which should be considered are disseminated sclerosis and myasthenia gravis, and in the elderly cerebral atheroma. Since the fusion of the images of near objects depends upon convergence of the eyes, double vision results if an object is brought so near the patient that he can no longer converge both eyes upon it. This of course is normal, but defective ocular convergence is sometimes the cause of double vision at greater distances. Spasm of convergence sometimes occurs in hysterical patients, and this may cause apparent limitation of ocular movements, and diplopia.

NYSTAGMUS

Nystagmus is a disturbance of ocular posture characterized by a more or less rhythmical oscillation of the eyes. This movement may be of the same rate in both directions, or quicker in one direction than in the other. In the latter case the movements are distinguished as the quick and the slow phases. The quick phase is taken to indicate the direction of the nystagmus, so that if the slow phase is to the left and the quick to the right, the patient is said to exhibit nystagmus to the right. Nystagmus may occur when the eyes are in the position of rest, or only on deviation in certain directions, or on convergence, or only when the head is in a certain position – positional nystagmus. The movement may be confined to one plane, horizontal or vertical, or occur in more than one plane – rotary nystagmus.

The posture of the eyes depends primarily upon two sets of afferent impulses. The first are visual, and are concerned with the regulation of the position of the eyes in relation to the object of visual interest. The second group are labyrinthine, and it is by means of these that the position of the eyes is regulated in relation to the position and movements of the rest of the body and in particular of the head. The posture of the eyes is co-ordinated by a central mechanism which receives these afferent impulses and controls the efferent impulses to the ocular muscles (Fig. 2.8). This may be called the central vestibulocerebellar system. Nystagmus, therefore, regarded as a disorder of ocular posture, may be the result of a disturbance of function of these afferent pathways or their central organization or, less frequently, the efferent pathways, and there remain one or two forms of nystagmus the cause of which has not yet been located.

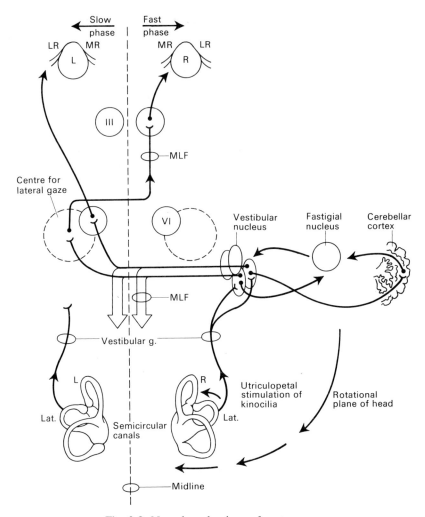

Fig. 2.8. Neural mechanisms of nystagmus.

The principal causes of nystagmus are:

1. NYSTAGMUS OF RETINAL ORIGIN. Amblyopia coming on in early life may cause nystagmus if some vision is retained and especially if macular vision is impaired. Nystagmus of this type is usually horizontal and pendular, with oscillations of approximately equal rate in each direction. The oscillations may be fine or coarse and may fluctuate from moment to moment. Miner's nystagmus has been attributed to the relative inefficiency of macular vision in a dim light resulting in defective fixation. It is also believed, however, that neurosis may play a part in maintaining the disorder.

2. LABYRINTHINE NYSTAGMUS. Nystagmus in relation to tests of labyrinthine function is considered below (p. 74). Nystagmus due to disease of the

labyrinth is usually rotary. Acute lesions of the internal ear cause nystagmus, usually rotary, and with the quick phase as a rule towards the opposite side. The amplitude of the oscillation is increased when the eyes are deviated in the direction of the quick phase, and diminished on fixation in the direction of the slow phase. Chronic labyrinthine lesions often lead to fine rotary nystagmus on lateral fixation to one or both sides, especially to the side of the lesion. A variety of labyrinthine nystagmus is known as positional nystagmus (see p. 74).

3. NYSTAGMUS DUE TO CENTRAL LESIONS. Nystagmus is a common symptom of lesions of the brainstem and cerebellum. With cerebellar lesions it may occur on fixation in any direction, the slow phase being towards the position of rest, and the quick phase towards the periphery with the fast phase to the same side. With a unilateral cerebellar lesion it is present in both eyes, and is most marked on conjugate deviation to the side of the lesion. It may occur as a result of lesions involving the vestibulocerebellar connections in the brainstem. Vertical nystagmus is always due to a central brainstem lesion.

4. CONGENITAL AND FAMILIAL NYSTAGMUS. Congenital nystagmus is usually a fine pendular oscillation of the eyes present at rest and increased on deviation in all directions. It is often familial.

The causes of nystagmus

When nystagmus is due to a visual defect arising early in life the cause is usually obvious. The same is true of congenital nystagmus, which is usually recognized early in life, and is the commonest cause of nystagmus on central fixation. When nystagmus is due to disease of the labyrinth, it is usually associated with paroxysmal vertigo and deafness. The cause of nystagmus of central origin can be ascertained only by considering it in relation to the patient's history and other symptoms and physical signs. Disseminated sclerosis is a common cause, and this type of nystagmus also occurs in cases of hereditary ataxia, syringo-myelia, and tumours and vascular lesions of the brainstem and cerebellum.

THE FIFTH OR TRIGEMINAL NERVE

Anatomy and physiology

The fifth nerve contains both motor and sensory fibres. It arises from the inferior surface of the pons on its lateral aspect by two roots, a large sensory and a small motor root (Plate 5). The two roots pass forwards in the posterior fossa to enter a cavity in the dura mater overlying the apex of the petrous bone. Here the sensory root expands to form the trigeminal (Gasserian) ganglion. This gives rise to three large nerve trunks, which constitute the three divisions of the trigeminal nerve, namely, the ophthalmic or first division, the maxillary or second, and the mandibular or third. The motor root becomes fused with the third division. The cutaneous distribution of the three divisions is shown in Fig. 2.9. The trigeminal nerve also supplies sensation to the nasal mucosa, hard and soft palate, teeth, the anterior two-thirds of the tongue and the buccal

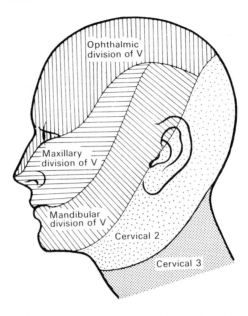

Fig. 2.9. Cutaneous distribution of the three divisions of the trigeminal nerve and the second cervical spinal segment.

mucosa. The most important of the muscles innervated by the motor root are the temporalis, the masseter, the medial and lateral pterygoids, and the tensor veli palatini. When it enters the pons the sensory root of the trigeminal nerve divides. The fibres concerned with the appreciation of light touch and postural sensibility enter the principal sensory nucleus in the pons, while the fibres concerned with the appreciation of pain and temperature pass downwards in the spinal tract, which enters the medulla and reaches as low as the second cervical segment of the spinal cord. These fibres enter the spinal nucleus of the trigeminal nerve, those from the ophthalmic division ending in its lowest part, those from the maxillary division next above, and those from the mandibular division highest. Fibres from this nucleus cross the middle line and eventually join the spinothalamic tract in the pons (see Fig. 3.6, p. 113).

Examination

Examination of the trigeminal nerve involves its sensory, reflex, and motor functions. Light touch is tested by cotton wool, pain by pin-prick, and thermal sensibility by hot and cold tubes, each of the three divisions of the nerve being tested separately.

The two principal reflexes mediated by the trigeminal nerve are the corneal reflex and the jaw-jerk. The *corneal reflex* is tested by applying a wisp of cotton wool to the cornea. This stimulus applied to one eye normally causes blinking of both eyes. If corneal sensibility, supplied by the ophthalmic division of the nerve, is diminished, this response will be reduced, or may be absent. Weakness of the orbicularis oculi, a muscle innervated by the facial nerve, will cause diminution or loss of the corneal reflex on the side stimulated even though corneal sensibility is normal, but in such a case normal blinking will occur on the opposite side.

The *jaw-jerk* is elicited by placing a finger horizontally across the chin, asking the patient to open the mouth slightly and relax, and then tapping the finger with a patellar hammer. The response is a movement of elevation of the jaw. In normal people the jaw-jerk may be somewhat difficult to elicit, and the resulting movement is not very brisk. A pathologically exaggerated jaw-jerk indicates the presence of an upper motor neurone lesion above the level of the pons. The chief diagnostic value of the jaw-jerk arises from comparing it with the tendon reflexes in the upper limbs. If both jaw-jerk and arm-jerks are uniformly exaggerated, the lesion responsible is likely to be above the pons. If, on the other hand, the jaw-jerk is normal but the arm-jerks are exaggerated, it is probably below the foramen magnum.

Lesions of the motor root cause weakness and wasting of the muscles of mastication on the affected side. Wasting of the temporalis muscle and of the masseter leads to hollowing above and below the zygoma, and, when the patient is made to clench his teeth, palpation reveals that contraction of these muscles is less vigorous than on the normal side. When the mouth is opened the jaw deviates to the paralysed side as a result of the unantagonized action of the lateral pterygoid muscle on the opposite side. When the masticatory muscles are paralysed on both sides, the jaw hangs open, as may occur in the late stages of motor neurone disease, and in some cases of myasthenia gravis when these muscles become fatigued.

LESIONS OF THE TRIGEMINAL NERVE

The trigeminal nerve may be damaged either within the brainstem or in its course from the pons to its areas of distribution. The commonest lesions within the brainstem are those which involve the spinal tract and nucleus. Owing to the fact that these structures are concerned with appreciation of pain, heat, and cold over the trigeminal area, damage to them produces dissociated sensory loss over the area concerned, i.e. impairment of the appreciation of pain, heat, and cold with preservation of that of light touch. Since the three divisions of the nerve are represented in inverse order from below upwards in the spinal tract and nucleus, a lesion involving the lowest parts of those structures will cause dissociated sensory loss over the ophthalmic division; one somewhat higher in the medulla will involve the ophthalmic and maxillary divisions, while a lesion just below the point of entry of the nerve will cause dissociated sensory loss over the distribution of all three divisions. The commonest example of such a lesion is thrombosis of the posterior inferior cerebellar artery which supplies the spinal tract and nucleus of the trigeminal, but varies in different individuals in the level at which it does so.

The other common lesion involving the spinal tract and nucleus is syringo-bulbia (syringomyelia involving the medulla). Here we are dealing not with a lesion with a well-defined level like a vascular lesion, but with an elongated pencil of tubular glial tissue extending upwards into the tegmentum of the medulla. When this compresses the spinal tract and nucleus of the trigeminal nerve it involves first those fibres which represent the most caudal parts of the distribution of all three divisions, and, as the pressure slowly increases, the area of dissociated sensory loss creeps cephalad in all three divisions converging upon the tip of the nose and the upper lip (Fig. 2.9).

The sensory root of the nerve which extends from the pons to the trigeminal ganglion may be compressed by a tumour, especially an acoustic neuroma. This may cause a sensation of numbness in the face, and some diminution in appreciation of light touch, pin-prick and temperature in the areas affected, and of the corneal reflex on that side. The motor root may be compressed with the sensory root. Numbness and sensory loss over the trigeminal area may also be due to disseminated sclerosis, when the lesion is probably within the pons at the point of entry of the trigeminal sensory root. The trigeminal ganglion is occasionally the site of a neurofibroma, and the first division especially is liable to be attacked by the virus of herpes zoster.

TRIGEMINAL NEURALGIA

Trigeminal neuralgia is a paroxysmal disorder of unknown aetiology character-ized by brief attacks of severe pain within the distribution of one or more divisions of the trigeminal nerve. It is also known as *tic douloureux*. Exception-ally it may be due to organic nervous disease, especially disseminated sclerosis. Females are affected more often than males, and it is rare before middle life, but may make its appearance in old age.

Symptoms

The characteristic features of trigeminal neuralgia are the paroxysmal character of the pain, its precipitation by some stimulus, its severity, its brevity, and its limitation usually to within the distribution of one sensory division of the nerve, almost always the second or third division. The patient often describes the pain as agonizing, stabbing, shooting, or like an electric shock. It occurs in brief attacks, each of which lasts from a few seconds up to half a minute or so. It is apt to be brought on by certain stimuli such as eating or talking when the third division is involved, blowing the nose when the second division is the site of the pain, or washing the face with either division. This is often a 'trigger spot', a small area within the division affected, touching which is particularly liable to bring on an attack. The pain may evoke a spasm of the face, whence the term *tic douloureux*. The eye may be closed and tears may run from it. In severe cases the attacks may occur many times a day. There is no accompanying objective sensory disturbance within the trigeminal area except that a patient will occasionally indicate that a spot on the skin is more sensitive than the rest. During the early part of the illness the pain may remit for weeks or even months, but it always returns. Later, there are no remissions. A history or the presence of physical signs of other lesions in the nervous system will enable the correct diagnosis to be made in the small proportion of cases in which the cause is disseminated sclerosis. Other causes of facial pain are discussed in Chapter 8.

Treatment

The analgesic and anticonvulsant drugs used in the past have been largely supplanted by carbamazepine (Tegretol). This drug was originally developed because of its anticonvulsant properties but it is remarkably effective in controlling the pain of trigeminal neuralgia and often makes it possible to postpone the necessity for surgical treatment, sometimes indefinitely. Carbamazepine sometimes causes side-effects of nausea, giddiness, and drowsiness and a half tablet (100 mg) should be given initially and the dose increased slowly to three 200 mg tablets a day, over a few days. In common with other anticonvulsants it has been reported to cause aplastic anaemia and so should be discontinued when the attack of neuralgia has abated or if a skin rash occurs.

A variety of surgical procedures are available if medical treatment fails. Lasting relief can be obtained only by blocking the pain fibres from the division of the nerve which is the seat of the painful discharge. This can be done by alcoholic injection of the trigeminal ganglion or by surgical division of the sensory root. Alcoholic injection of the ganglion can usually be relied upon to give relief for eighteen months to two years, or even longer, but in many cases it needs to be repeated. Surgical division of the sensory root gives permanent relief. The preferred surgical procedures are now either selective thermocoagulation through the foramen ovale or open surgery with selective section under direct vision. Particularly in the United States there is increasing use of microvascular decompression operation removing presumed compressing vascular loops in the posterior fossa. The fact that surgical section will cause numbness of the face must be explained to the patient beforehand. Analgesia of the cornea may lead to *neuropathic keratitis,* and the eye needs protection by suitable goggles after the nerve interruption. Paralysis of the muscles innervated by the motor root occurs after ganglion injection, but is of no practical importance.

THE SEVENTH OR FACIAL NERVE

Anatomy and physiology

The facial nerve contains motor fibres only: these supply the muscles of expression. It is accompanied in part of its course, however, by a small number of

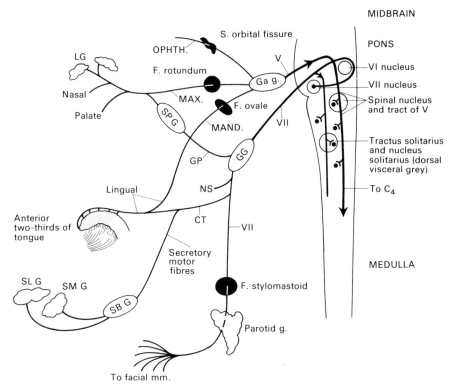

Fig. 2.10. Central and peripheral connections of the seventh nerve.

CT Chorda tympani	MAND. Mandibular division of fifth
GG Geniculate ganglion	SP G Sphenopalatine ganglion
Ga g Gasserian ganglion (semilunar ganglion)	NS Nerve to stapedius
G P Greater superficial petrosal	SB G Submandibular ganglion
LG Lachrymal gland	SM G Submandibular gland
MAX. Maxillary division of fifth	SL G Sublingual gland

sensory fibres going to the external acoustic meatus, by fibres which stimulate salivary secretion, and others which convey taste impulses from the anterior two-thirds of the tongue (Fig. 2.10). The nucleus of the facial nerve is situated in the ventral part of the tegmentum of the pons. Its fibres pass backwards to loop round the nucleus of the sixth nerve before turning forwards to emerge from the lateral aspect of the lower border of the pons, on the medial side of the eighth nerve, from which the seventh is separated by the pars intermedia. The facial nerve crosses the posterior fossa to enter the petrous portion of the temporal bone where it occupies the aqueductus Fallopii or facial canal. Within the bone it turns first outwards then backwards and then downwards to emerge from the skull at the stylomastoid foramen. Where it turns backwards it gives off the parasympathetic lachrymal fibres (greater superficial nerve). It then expands to form the geniculate ganglion, which receives the pars intermedia and contains the ganglion cells of the taste fibres of the chorda tympani, which supply the anterior two-thirds of the tongue with taste. Within the facial canal the facial nerve gives off a branch to the stapedius muscle, and after emerging from the stylomastoid foramen it gives branches to the stylohyoid muscle, to the posterior belly of the digastric and the occipital belly of the occipitofrontalis, and then turns forwards to divide within the parotid gland into a number of branches which innervate the muscles of expression, including the buccinator and the platysma.

Examination

The functions of the upper fibres of the facial nerve are tested by asking the patient to close the eyes, to raise the eyebrows, and to frown. The power of the orbicularis oculi to close the eye can be tested against the resistance of the observer's thumb. The lower fibres of the nerve are tested by asking the patient to retract the angles of the mouth voluntarily, to smile, to purse the lips and blow out the cheeks, and to whistle. The platysma can be tested by asking the patient to draw down the angles of the mouth whilst tightening up the neck muscles.

FACIAL PARALYSIS

The following varieties of facial paralysis, depending upon the site of the lesion responsible, are recognized. Facial paralysis may be due to:

1. A supranuclear or upper motor neurone lesion involving the pyramidal fibres concerned in voluntary facial movement.

2. A supranuclear lesion involving the fibres concerned in emotional movement of the face, leading to mimic paralysis.

3. Lesions involving the lower motor neurones in the nucleus, or facial nerve.

4. Disorders of the facial muscles.

Facial paralysis due to a supranuclear pyramidal lesion is distinguished by the fact that movements of the lower part of the face are affected more severely than those of the upper, owing to the fact that upper facial movements are innervated by both cerebral hemispheres and lower facial movements by the opposite hemisphere only. Moreoever, although voluntary retraction of the angle of the mouth is weak, emotional and associated movements of the face are little, if at all, affected. These are the common findings in hemiplegia from any cause.

The fact that emotional movements of the face are usually spared in hemiplegia indicates that the upper motor neurones concerned in these movements have a course which is separate from that of the pyramidal fibres. When this pathway is damaged alone, which is a somewhat rare occurrence, emotional movements are diminished or lost while voluntary movements are retained – mimic paralysis. This is most likely to happen with a lesion of the opposite frontal lobe. In some cases both emotional and voluntary movements are affected equally.

Lesions involving the lower motor neurones supplying the facial muscles, since they destroy the final common path, are likely to affect to an equal extent both voluntary and emotional movement, and as a rule the upper and lower facial muscles are equally weakened. The symptoms of facial paralysis due to lower motor neurone lesions are described in more detail below, in the section dealing with Bell's paralysis. On closing the eyes they usually turn upwards. After a facial palsy, this upward turning may be clearly seen (Bell's phenomenon) (see Fig. 2.11).

Facial paralysis in relation to the site of the lesion

Within the pons the facial nucleus or the fibres of the facial nerve may be involved in massive lesions, usually neoplastic, which, owing to the anatomical relations of the facial nucleus, are likely also to involve the sixth nerve, causing paralysis of the lateral rectus or the neighbouring centre of conjugate lateral deviation to the same side. Trigeminal sensory and motor loss may also be present and the long sensory and motor pathways may also be affected. Syringobulbia may cause weakness of the facial muscles. Multiple sclerosis sometimes causes transient facial paresis. Selective damage to the motor neurones in the nucleus may occur acutely in poliomyelitis or as part of the slow degenerative process in motor neurone disease.

Within the posterior fossa the proximity of the facial nerve to the pars intermedia and the eighth nerve is responsible for the fact that these nerves usually suffer together. Lesions in the cerebellopontine angle, therefore, of which acoustic neuroma is the commonest, are likely to cause deafness, and loss of taste in the anterior two-thirds of the tongue, in association with the facial paralysis. If the lesion is between the brainstem and the geniculate ganglion there is likely to be loss of lachrymation and loss of taste. Loss of taste with normal lachrymation indicates a lesion between the geniculate ganglion and the origin of the chorda tympani.

Within the temporal bone the facial nerve may be damaged in fractures of the base of the skull. Infections of the middle ear and mastoid and their surgical treatment were a commoner cause of facial palsy in the past than today. Herpes zoster of the geniculate ganglion may cause facial paralysis, the syndrome of Ramsay Hunt (p. 403). Facial paralysis due to a lesion within the petrous bone is associated with loss of taste on the anterior two-thirds of the tongue if the lesion is proximal to the point at which the chorda tympani leaves the facial nerve. The lesion responsible for Bell's paralysis is believed to lie within the facial canal. After leaving the stylomastoid foramen the fibres of the facial nerve are exposed to trauma, and may undergo degeneration in polyneuritis throughout their length. They may also be involved in sarcoidosis.

Muscular disorders responsible for facial paralysis include myasthenia gravis, the facioscapulohumeral type of muscular dystrophy, and dystrophia myotonica. The lesion is bilateral and involves both upper and lower facial muscles.

Bell's facial paralysis

Bell's facial paralysis, named after Sir Charles Bell (1774–1842), is a facial paralysis of acute onset attributed to a non-suppurative inflammation of the facial nerve within the stylomastoid foramen. It may occur at any age from infancy to old age, but appears to be most common in young adults; males are affected more often than females. The cause is unknown. It is sometimes attributed to exposure to a draught, and may follow an infection of the nasopharynx. In a small proportion of cases it has been proved to be due to the virus of herpes zoster, but in most cases no cause is discoverable.

Symptoms

Bell's palsy is almost always unilateral. The onset is sudden and frequently the patient awakens in the morning to find the face paralysed. He or his friends observe that his mouth is drawn to one side. There is frequently pain at the onset, within the ear, in the mastoid region, or around the angle of the jaw.

There is paralysis of the muscles of expression. The upper and lower facial muscles are usually equally affected, and the muscles are paralysed to an equal extent for voluntary, emotional, and associated movements. The eyebrow droops, and the wrinkles of the brow are smoothed out. Frowning and raising the eyebrows are impossible. Owing to paralysis of the orbicularis oculi the palpebral fissure is wider on the affected than on the normal side, and closure of the eye is impossible. Eversion of the lower lid and lack of approximation of the punctum to the conjunctiva impair the absorption of tears, which tend to overflow the lower lid. The nasolabial furrow is smoothed out, and the mouth is drawn over to the sound side (Fig. 2.11). The patient is unable to retract the angle of the mouth or to purse the lips, as in whistling. Owing to paralysis of the buccinator the cheek is puffed out in respiration, and food tends to accumulate between the teeth and the cheek. The displacement of the mouth causes deviation of the tongue to the sound side when it is protruded, and may thus cause paralysis of the tongue to be suspected in error.

When the chorda tympani nerve is involved there is loss of taste on the anterior two-thirds of the tongue, and when the lesion of the facial nerve extends to above the point at which the branch to the stapedius muscle is given off, the patient is likely to complain of hyperacusis, leading to an unpleasant intensification of loud sounds.

Diagnosis

In most cases this is easy, depending upon the sudden occurrence of facial paralysis with or without loss of taste on the anterior two-thirds of the tongue

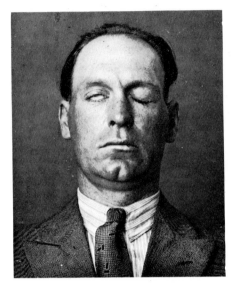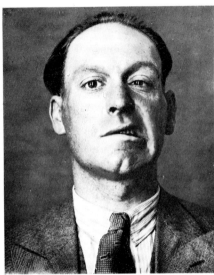

Fig. 2.11. Bell's facial paralysis on the right side. Note weakness of the orbicularis oculi and of the retractors of the angle of the mouth.

as an isolated symptom in an otherwise healthy person. Suppurative otitis can be excluded by investigating the ear. The only two other conditions which may closely simulate Bell's palsy are poliomyelitis and disseminated sclerosis. Poliomyelitis should be suspected as a cause when unilateral facial paralysis occurs during an epidemic of that disease, especially in a child or adolescent, and if it occurs a few days after a febrile illness. In a doubtful case a pleocytosis in the cerebrospinal fluid might provide confirmatory evidence. Multiple sclerosis should be considered as a possible cause when unilateral facial paralysis occurs in a young adult, especially if it is painless, not very severe, and clears up in two or three weeks. This diagnosis is more often made retrospectively than at the time, when it can be made only if other physical signs of the disease are present.

Prognosis

In most patients with Bell's palsy nearly complete recovery eventually occurs, though in a few it may take several months. Permanent severe paralysis is rare. Incomplete recovery ranges from the persistence of some slight degree of facial weakness to the initial paralysis remaining unchanged. In the latter case contracture usually develops in the paralysed muscles, and this does much to improve the appearance of the face at rest, although the paralysis is evident when the patient smiles. In the presence of contracture the nasolabial furrow may become actually deeper on the paralysed side than on the normal side, and the affected eyebrow may be drawn downwards. In cases of incomplete recovery one often finds that when the patient is asked to close the eyes the associated retraction of the angle of the mouth is stronger on the affected than on the normal side, and when he is asked to show his teeth some contraction of the orbicularis oculi muscle occurs on the affected side. Presumably this is because some of the regenerating nerve fibres have become directed to the wrong muscles. Occasionally, regenerating autonomic fibres reach the lachrymal glands instead of the salivary glands which they originally innervated, causing the 'crocodile tears' phenomenon.

Electrophysiological studies are helpful in determining the severity of the lesion and hence the prognosis. If some voluntary facial movement is present within five days of the onset, then functional recovery will be nearly perfect and electrical studies are not necessary. However, if the paralysis is complete after five days, electrical stimulation of the facial nerve may provide useful information. If a muscular response occurs and the latency falls within the normal range then recovery is likely to be complete. An increased latency suggests partial denervation but the prognosis for complete recovery is still good. If the nerve is electrically inexcitable, as it is in some 10 per cent of cases, the denervation is probably complete and recovery is likely to be slow and partial, with a poor final result. Fibrillation does not occur until two to three weeks after the acute denervation in these cases and so its absence at an early stage is of limited help in deciding the prognosis.

Treatment

Symptomatic treatment with analgesics may be necessary during the early stage if the ear is painful. If facial movement is already recovering five days after the onset then no further treatment is necessary. However if there is complete paralysis after five days, especially if the electrical tests confirm denervation, treatment with steroids is advisable. Steroids are presumed to reduce the swelling of the facial nerve in the canal and therefore the likelihood of severe denervation. Prednisolone may be given in an initial dose of 80 mg daily reducing to zero over ten days. While regeneration is occurring, passive movement of the face by massage should be carried out and active exercises started as soon as there is some return of voluntary power. Galvanic stimulation of the facial muscles is frequently recommended though it is doubtful how much this influences the ultimate recovery and it should be discontinued if contracture of the facial muscles occurs. It is important to use protective eye drops if the paralysis prevents blinking. If after two or three weeks have elapsed, there is evidence of complete denervation, it is too late to expect much, if anything, from surgical decompression of the facial nerve in the canal and earlier operation is difficult to justify when most of the cases submitted to operation would recover spontaneously. Plastic surgery may improve the facial appearance when severe paralysis persists after some six months.

CLONIC FACIAL SPASM (FACIAL MYOCLONIA)

This is a disorder of unknown aetiology which chiefly affects middle-aged or elderly women. There are frequent shock-like contractions of the facial muscles, usually limited to one side. It is probably the result of an irritative lesion at some point in the course of the nerve, and has been ascribed to a lesion of the geniculate ganglion. The fact that in some cases taste is lost over the anterior two-thirds of the tongue on the same side lends some support to this view. The twitching usually begins in the orbicularis oculi, which may cause the patient embarrassment as it gives the appearance of winking. The spread of the disorder is extremely slow, but gradually the muscles of the lower part of the face are involved, especially the retractors of the angle of the mouth. Finally, strong facial spasms may involve all the muscles on one side almost continuously. At this stage there is always slight weakness and wasting of the muscles, which occasionally becomes severe.

Facial myoclonia is not likely to be confused with the muscular twitches which are sometimes seen after partial recovery from Bell's paralysis. It has to be distinguished from blepharospasm, prolonged spasm of both orbicularis oculi muscles, which also occurs chiefly in elderly women. In this condition the movements are bilateral and there is no clonic twitching of the lower facial muscles. Facial myokymia is a widespread fasciculation of the facial muscles due to involvement of the facial nucleus or facial nerve by a tumour or demyelination. It should be distinguished from localized peri-ocular myokymia which may occur in normal persons and from facial dyskinesias occurring after treatment with drugs.

In the absence of treatment clonic facial spasm is a slowly progressive disorder, and spontaneous recovery does not occur. In some cases the twitching ceases when there is a severe degree of facial paralysis.

Drugs are of no value. Cure by means of surgery has been reported after relieving compression of the facial nerve in the posterior fossa by the vertebral artery or its branches. Permanent relief can be obtained by nerve block, which can be carried out by alcohol injection, but of course leads to facial paralysis.

THE EIGHTH OR VESTIBULOCOCHLEAR NERVE

THE COCHLEAR FIBRES AND HEARING

Anatomy and physiology

Both the internal ear and the eighth nerve which supplies it have two functions, hearing and equilibrium. The cochlea, concerned with hearing, is supplied by the part of the eighth nerve known as the cochlear part, while the semicircular canals, the utricle and the saccule, which are concerned with the recognition of the position of the head in relation to gravity and its movements in space, are supplied by that portion of the eighth nerve known as the vestibular part. These two parts run together from the internal acoustic meatus to the lateral aspect of the lower border of the pons. In its passage across the posterior fossa the eighth nerve lies on the lateral side of the seventh nerve, from which it is separated by the pars intermedia.

Within the brainstem the cochlear fibres end in the cochlear nucleus, from which relay fibres cross the middle line just beneath the floor of the fourth ventricle. On the opposite side auditory fibres pass upwards in the lateral lemniscus to the inferior colliculus and the medial geniculate body, from which further fibres are distributed to the cortical auditory centre in the transverse temporal gyrus and adjacent portion of the superior temporal gyrus.

Tests of auditory function

Impairment or loss of hearing may be due to a disturbance of the auditory conducting mechanism in the middle ear, or damage to the sensory cells of the spiral organ (of Corti) in the cochlea, or a lesion of the auditory fibres in the eighth nerve, or to the central auditory pathways or their cortical end-stations in the brain. The most important practical distinction is that between 'middle-ear deafness' and 'nerve deafness', though, as we shall see, it has recently been possible to analyse the latter further.

The first step in testing the hearing is to form a rough estimate of its efficiency in either ear. This can most simply be done by recording the distance at which the patient is able to hear a whispered voice with one ear when the opposite external acoustic meatus is blocked. If the whispered voice cannot be heard, the same test can be applied with the spoken voice. The result can be recorded as 'whispered voice at six feet', or 'spoken voice at one foot'.

The following tests are employed to distinguish middle-ear deafness from nerve deafness. In *Weber's test* a vibrating tuning fork (C = 256) is applied to the patient's forehead or vertex in the middle line, and he is asked whether the sound is heard in the middle line or is localized in one ear. In normal individuals the sound appears to be in the middle line. In middle-ear deafness it is usually localized in the affected ear, in nerve deafness in the normal ear. This is due to the fact that in nerve deafness bone conduction of sound is reduced as well as air conduction, whereas in middle-ear deafness air conduction is reduced but bone conduction is relatively enhanced.

Rinne's test is based upon the same fact. A vibrating tuning fork is applied to the patient's mastoid process, the ear being closed by the observer's finger. The patient is asked to say when he ceases to hear the sound, and the fork is then placed at the external acoustic meatus. In middle-ear deafness the sound cannot be heard by air conduction after bone conduction has ceased to transmit it. In nerve deafness, as in normal individuals, the reverse is the case.

A further distinction between nerve deafness and middle-ear deafness is that in the former loss of hearing is most marked for high-pitched tones; in the latter for low-pitched tones.

Loudness recruitment is a phenomenon which is useful in distinguishing between conductive and nerve deafness, and between nerve deafness due to a lesion of the sensory end-organs in the cochlea and that due to damage to the fibres of the cochlear part of the eighth nerve. A patient who is deaf in one ear is tested by presenting to either ear alternately a sound of the same frequency but of different intensities. The patient is then asked to say when the sound heard by the deaf ear appears to be as loud as that heard by the normal ear. In conductive deafness the ratio between intensities of two sounds which appear equally loud to the two ears remains the same, however the intensity is varied. In nerve deafness, however, as the intensity increases the ratio diminishes, so that a point is reached at which sounds of equal intensity appear equally loud in the two ears. This is known as loudness recruitment. It has been shown that loudness recruitment is a characteristic of a lesion involving the cochlear end-organ and it is usually absent when the disorder involves the cochlear nerve fibres.

Lesions responsible for nerve deafness

Nerve deafness may be due to the lesions of the following structures in descending order of frequency:
1. The sensory terminals in the internal ear.
2. The eighth nerve.
3. The nuclei or ascending auditory pathways within the brainstem.
4. The auditory cortical areas.

Lesions of the internal ear include *Ménière's syndrome* and *acute labyrinthitis,* which may be either primary or secondary to *purulent otitis media, meningococcal meningitis,* or *mumps. Trauma* following head injury is also a cause. It is uncertain whether *streptomycin* causes deafness by damaging the eighth nerve or the auditory centres in the pons.

The commonest lesions of the eighth nerve itself are compression by a tumour in the cerebellopontine angle, especially an *acoustic neuroma,* and *trauma*.

Deafness is a rare symptom of lesions within the central nervous system, but may occur in disseminated sclerosis and tumours involving the midbrain. Temporal lobe lesions do not cause deafness unless they are bilateral.

TINNITUS

Tinnitus is a sensation of noise caused by abnormal excitation of the auditory apparatus or its afferent pathways or cortical areas. The noise heard may be high- or low-pitched and is variously described as hissing, whistling or, in severe cases, resembling the noise made by a steam engine or by machinery. It may possess a rhythm corresponding to that of the pulse. The commonest cause of tinnitus is a lesion of the internal ear, in which case it is likely to be associated with deafness and sometimes with vertigo. Drugs may cause tinnitus, especially quinine, salicylates, and streptomycin. Sometimes the origin of the tinnitus appears to be circulatory. Abnormal sounds arising within the cranium, which may also cause a bruit audible to the observer, may be conducted to the ear and so cause tinnitus. Irritation of the eighth nerve may cause tinnitus, but this is a rare symptom of lesions of the auditory nuclei and ascending pathways. Tinnitus may also occur as the result of lesions in the neighbourhood of the auditory cortex in the temporal lobe.

Persistent tinnitus sometimes leads to much distress and depression in elderly people. Its treatment is disappointing. In severe cases in which tinnitus is intolerable it may be justifiable to destroy the cochlea or to divide the eighth nerve, but the patient should be told that complete deafness in the ear thus treated will result, and that tinnitus may persist in spite of the operation. The psychiatric importance of tinnitus in the elderly and aged should always be borne in mind. It may be a symptom of underlying depression.

THE VESTIBULAR FIBRES AND THE FUNCTIONS OF THE LABYRINTH

The part of the labyrinth concerned with equilibrium consists of the semi-circular canals, the utricle, and the saccule. The semicircular canals, three in number, are hollows in the petrous part of the temporal bone, the osseous canals being occupied by membranous tubes filled with endolymph, and separated from the bony walls by perilymph. They are arranged approximately in three planes of space at right angles to one another and are so placed that when the head is inclined 30 degrees forwards from the erect position the lateral canal is horizontal. The anterior canal lies in a plane midway between the frontal and the sagittal planes, with its outermost portion anteriorly, and runs inwards and backwards. The posterior canal lies in a vertical plane at right angles to the anterior canal, with its outermost portion posteriorly, and runs inwards and forwards. Each canal exhibits a dilatation, the ampulla, which contains specialized epithelium, the crista, bearing hair cells which are the vestibular receptors. Somewhat similar receptors exist in the utricle and saccule, but in these the hair cells are in contact with small crystals, the otoliths. The semicircular canals are excited by movement and especially angular movement: the utricle and saccule convey information concerning the position of the head in space, the position of the otoliths with reference to the hair cells varying under the influence of gravity. In addition to responding to movement or change of position, the labyrinths are in a state of continuous tonic activity manifested in a steady discharge of action potentials.

As already stated, the vestibular portion of the labyrinth is innervated by the vestibular division of the eighth nerve. After entering the pons the vestibular fibres end in a series of terminal nuclei, or run directly to the cerebellar cortex by the inferior cerebellar peduncle. Fibres from the vestibular nuclei run upwards to terminate in cortical centres in the posterior parts of the temporal lobes, and downwards in the vestibulospinal tracts to influence motor activity.

Stimulation of the labyrinth

The labyrinth can be stimulated either by rotating the patient, which produces nystagmus in the opposite direction, or by irrigating one ear with hot or cold water. In rotation both labyrinths are stimulated: the caloric tests has the advantage of making it possible to investigate the function of each labyrinth separately. The following is the standard caloric test.

The patient lies on a couch with his head raised 30 degrees so that the horizontal canal becomes vertical. Irrigating the right ear with cold water cools the canal, and so causes a current in the endolymph from above downwards in the patient's existing position, or from before backwards with reference to the normal position of the head. Such a current is the same as that normally evoked by turning the patient to the left, in which case the inertia of the endolymph causes it to move backwards in the right lateral canal. The temperatures used are 30°C and 44°C. Each of these is allowed to flow into the external acoustic meatus from a reservoir for 40 seconds, during which period not less than 250 ml of water should flow. The effects are measured in terms of the time interval between the application of the stimulus and the end of the resulting nystagmus. The observations are carried out in the straight-ahead position of gaze.

Much still remains to be learned about the interpretation of the caloric vestibular tests. Abnormal responses are encountered in almost all cases of Ménière's syndrome and tumours of the eighth nerve. Canal paresis indicates a lesion of the ipsilateral labyrinth or eighth nerve and is often associated with a directional preponderance to the opposite side. Directional preponderance is also a valuable diagnostic sign of lesions of the vestibular areas within the cerebral hemispheres or brainstem.

Positional nystagmus

Sometimes paroxysmal vertigo and nystagmus are related to a particular position of the head and semicircular canals and are then called positional vertigo and nystagmus. To demonstrate this the patient is seated on a couch. The examiner then grasps the patient's head, brings him rapidly into a supine position with the head lowered some 30 degrees below the horizontal at the end of the couch, and turned some 30 to 45 degrees to one side (Fig. 2.12). In this position the vertical canals approach the horizontal plane. A latent period of a few seconds usually precedes the onset of the nystagmus, which is accompanied by vertigo and feelings of general distress.

Optokinetic nystagmus

Optokinetic nystagmus is a term applied to the nystagmus evoked by a succession of moving objects passing before the eyes. Optokinetic nystagmus has been shown to be independent of the vestibular nuclei and to depend upon the angular and supramarginal gyri. It is reduced when the striped drum, at

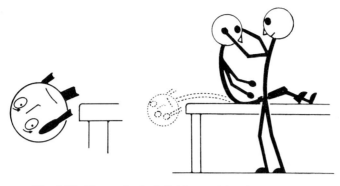

Fig. 2.12. The method of eliciting positional nystagmus.

which the patient is asked to look, is rotated to the same side as the cerebral lesion.

VERTIGO

Vertigo may be defined as the consciousness of disordered orientation of the body in space. The derivation of the term implies a sense of rotation of the patient or of his surroundings, but this, though frequently present, is not the only form of vertigo as just defined. There are three ways in which the spatial orientation of the body may be felt to be disordered. The external world may appear to move, often in a rotatory fashion, but other forms of movement, such as oscillation, may be experienced. The body itself may be felt to be moving, either in rotation or as a sensation of falling, or the movement may be referred to within the body, e.g. within the head. Finally, the postures and movements of the limbs, especially the lower limbs, may be felt to be ill-adjusted and unsteady. The motor accompaniments of vertigo consist of forced movements of the body, such as falling, and disordered orientation of parts of the body, manifested in the eyes as nystagmus. Visceral disturbances, such as pallor, sweating, alterations in the pulse rate and blood pressure, nausea, vomiting, and diarrhoea may be present.

The maintenance of an appropriate position of the body in space depends upon afferent impulses from many sources, of which the labyrinths are the most important, and these afferent impulses are received by central mechanisms, of which the cerebellum, the vestibular nuclei, and the red nuclei are probably the principal ones, and which constitute reflex paths by which the position of the body is normally appropriately orientated. Vertigo may result from the disordered function either of the sensory end-organs, the afferent paths, or the central mechanisms concerned.

The causes of vertigo

Aural vertigo

By far the commonest cause of vertigo is a disturbance of function of the labyrinth. This may be the effect of unaccustomed stimuli acting upon normal labyrinths, as in rotation, and motion-sickness. The commonest, and therefore the most important, form of vertigo arising in the labyrinth is Ménière's syndrome, causing recurrent aural vertigo.

Vestibular neuronitis

Vertigo occurs from time to time in small epidemics, the cause of which is obscure, but presumably infective. The onset is usually abrupt, and may be associated with vomiting and nystagmus. The acute phase usually lasts a few days, but milder feelings of giddiness and unsteadiness may persist for a few weeks. The absence of auditory symptoms and the occasional presence of diplopia suggest that the causative lesion may sometimes be in the nervous system rather than in the labyrinth itself. The caloric tests show an abnormality of vestibular function, though hearing is normal. Treatment is by means of sedation with a drug such as prochlorperazine (Stemetil) and the prognosis for complete recovery within a few weeks is good.

Positional vertigo

Positional vertigo is a benign condition in which giddiness is provoked by head movement, and is usually associated with positional nystagmus (see p. 57). The caloric responses are usually normal. The mechanism is thought to be detachment of calcium carbonate crystals from the otoconia of the otolith organ of the affected utricle. These fall against the cupula of the posterior semicircular canal. Causes include viral infection, trauma and degenerative changes with age. Attacks are provoked by changes of posture but usually subside within a few weeks.

Vertigo due to lesions of the vestibulocerebellar pathways

Lesions of the eighth nerve may cause vertigo, but this is not usually a prominent symptom of acoustic neuromas. Central lesions involving the vestibular nuclei, their connections with the cerebellum, or the cerebellum itself, are responsible for the vertigo which may occur in disseminated sclerosis, syringobulbia, and neoplastic and vascular lesions of the brainstem and cerebellum.

Vertigo of cortical origin

Since the vestibular system has cortical representation in the posterior part of each temporal lobe, disturbance of the function of this part of the brain may cause vertigo. The aura of an epileptic attack may be a feeling of giddiness. Vertigo may also occur in migraine, and in association with localized cerebral lesions, either vascular or neoplastic.

Psychogenic vertigo

'Giddiness' is a common symptom among sufferers from anxiety neurosis. There is usually no sensation of rotation, but the patient complains of a feeling of instability associated with a sense of anxiety, and this is often accompanied by symptoms of overactivity of the sympathetic nervous system. Vertigo may also occur as a conversion symptom in hysteria.

Ménière's syndrome

Recurrent aural vertigo may be due to a variety of causes. Ménière's syndrome now stands out as a definite pathological entity. It is characterized clinically by the recurrence of attacks of severe giddiness leading usually to vomiting and prostration, and associated with tinnitus and increasing deafness. The disorder runs a protracted course with a tendency to disappearance of the vertigo as the deafness increases.

Aetiology and pathology

Men suffer from Ménière's syndrome more often than women, in a proportion of about 3 to 2. It is chiefly a disorder of middle age, especially late middle age, the average age of onset being 49, and more than one-third of all patients are first affected after the age of 60. It has been shown to be the result of a gross dilatation of the endolymph system of the internal ear, without evidence of infection or trauma, and causing degenerative changes in the cochlear and vestibular sense organs. The mechanism of the endolymphatic dilatation remains unexplained.

Symptoms

The usual history is that the patient has suffered from slowly progressive deafness and tinnitus in one or both ears for months, or even years, and then suddenly has an attack of giddiness. This may develop so rapidly that the patient falls; more often it takes a few minutes to become severe. In a severe attack the patient is literally prostrated, and there is an intense sensation of rotation of the surroundings, less often of the patient himself. Vomiting soon develops with severe nausea, and lasts as long as the patient remains very giddy. Sometimes there is also diarrhoea. The pulse may be rapid or slow, and the blood pressure raised or lowered, and there may be profuse sweating. Transitory double vision may occur, and in very severe cases consciousness may be lost. Deafness and tinnitus are sometimes intensified during the attack. The vertigo may last for from half an hour to many hours, and then gradually subsides. On attempting to stand and walk the patient is unsteady and staggers.

During the attack the patient usually lies on the sound side and exhibits a rotary nystagmus which is most evident on looking towards the affected ear. In the intervals between the attacks giddiness is liable to be brought on by sudden movements of the head, and there is often a fine rotary nystagmus on extreme lateral fixation to either side, especially on looking to the affected side. There may be some persistent unsteadiness indicated by an inability to stand steadily with the eyes closed or to walk heal-and-toe. Deafness may be unilateral or bilateral. Both ear- and bone-conduction are usually impaired and there is a selective loss of the higher tones. Recruitment is present.

Caloric tests show in about 50 per cent of cases canal paresis on the affected side, in about 20 per cent directional preponderance, and in another 20 per cent directional preponderance plus canal paresis. In only 10 per cent is the caloric test normal. The electrocochleogram and its response to glycerol dehydration provides a more precise diagnosis.

Diagnosis

Ménière's syndrome may sometimes by confused with *petit mal*, but when giddiness is a symptom of minor epilepsy the attacks last only a few seconds, consciousness is always impaired or lost, and the giddiness disappeares as rapidly as it develops. The severe vomiting in Ménière's syndrome may suggest *migraine*, but in migraine giddiness is rare and when present only slight, and headache is a prominent symptom. In Ménière's syndrome tinnitus and some impairment of hearing are always present, and a lesion which involves both the cochlear and the vestibular functions must be situated either in the internal ear or in the eighth nerve. A *tumour* of the eighth nerve usually interferes with the functions of the trigeminal and the facial nerves on the same side, as well as the cerebellum. When vertigo is due to lesions of the *brainstem* or *cerebellum*, hearing is usually unimpaired, and other symptoms of lesions in these situations are usually present. When vertigo is due to *vestibular neuronitis* hearing is normal and the caloric test indicates selective damage to the vestibular system.

Prognosis

The attacks tend to recur at irregular intervals, and with varying severity. Usually the intervals of freedom last only a few weeks; in rare cases the patient is free from attacks for years. There is a tendency for the attacks to diminish in severity spontaneously and finally cease as the deafness becomes severe. Exceptionally, in the absence of radical treatment, the attacks continue for many years. Eventually half the patients are affected in both ears.

Treatment

The acute attack, if severe, must be treated by rest in bed and sedatives. Dimenhydrinate (Dramamine) promethazine theoclate (Avomine), prochlor-perazine (Stemetil), and cinnarizine (Stugeron) are useful, as they are for motion-sickness. If the vomiting is severe chlorpromazine, 25–50 mg, should be given by intramuscular injection or a sedative dose of diazepam (Valium). Betahistidine hydrochloride (Serc) has been reported to have a specific vasodilator effect on labyrinthine circulation. After the attack has subsided a maintenance dose of phenobarbitone may help to prevent a recurrence. The fact that the dilated endolymph system in the internal ear is sensitive to changes in the osmotic tension of the blood is the basis for treatment by restriction of salt and fluid intake or use of diuretics, but this is not often conspicuously successful. A careful search for focal sepsis in the teeth, tonsils, and nasal sinuses should be carried out, and any infection found appropriately treated. Blockage of the auditory (Eustachian) tube, if present, should be relieved. If the patient shows no response to medical measures, and especially if the vertigo incapacitates him from following his occupation, surgical treatment should be considered. A unilateral labyrinthectomy is the operation of choice, and can now be carried out without impairment of hearing by means of ultrasonic waves. The alternative is an endolymphatic shunt operation. All sufferers from vertigo should be warned of the risks which a sudden attack may involve.

THE NINTH OR GLOSSOPHARYNGEAL NERVE

The glossopharyngeal nerve arises by a series of radicles from the posterior lateral sulcus of the medulla between the fibres of origin of the vagus and accessory nerves (Plate 6). After crossing the posterior fossa it emerges through the anterior compartment of the jugular foramen. Its motor supply to the stylopharyngeus muscle is unimportant. It supplies common sensibility to the posterior third of the tongue, the tonsils, and the pharynx, and taste fibres to the same region, and is concerned in the secretion of saliva, especially by the parotid gland.

Clinically it is tested by investigating sensation over the area of its supply, which is also the receptive field for the pharyngeal or gag reflex (a contraction of the pharynx elicited by touching its walls), and by testing the appreciation of taste on the posterior one-third of the tongue. Isolated lesions of the glossopharyngeal nerve are almost unknown. It is most frequently damaged in association with the vagus and accessory nerves at the jugular foramen.

Glossopharyngeal neuralgia

The glossopharyngeal is occasionally subject to paroxysmal neuralgia, which in its general characteristics resembles the much commoner paroxysmal trigeminal neuralgia. The pain occurs in brief attacks, which may be very severe, usually in the side of the throat radiating down the side of the neck in front of the ear and to the back of the lower jaw. It may begin deep in the ear. Attacks tend to be precipitated by swallowing or by protruding the tongue, and the ear may be extremely sensitive to touch. Treatment consists of surgical avulsion of the nerve, which may be performed in the neck in debilitated subjects, but should usually be carried out intracranially in the posterior fossa.

THE SENSE OF TASTE

Anatomy and physiology

There are only four tastes: sweet, salt, bitter, and acid. All other flavours are olfactory sensations. The peripheral path of the taste fibres is probably as follows. Those carrying impulses from the anterior two-thirds of the tongue pass at first through the lingual nerve to the chorda tympani, through which they reach the facial nerve and the geniculate ganglion, which contains their ganglion cells (see Fig. 2.10). From this they pass to the pons by the pars intermedia. Taste fibres from the posterior one-third of the tongue, from the pharynx, and from the lower border of the soft palate are carried by the glossopharyngeal nerve. After entering the pons the taste fibres psss into the tractus solitarius to terminate in the nucleus of this tract, from which relay neurones cross the middle line and turn upwards in the tegmentum of the pons and medulla to form the gustatory fillet which ascends to the thalamus, from which the taste fibres are further relayed to the cortical centre for taste at the foot of the postcentral gyrus.

Testing the sense of taste

The sense of taste is tested by means of weak solutions of sugar, common salt, quinine, and acetic acid or vinegar. The patient must keep his tongue protruded, and must reply to questions by nodding or shaking his head. It is convenient to have the names of the four tastes written on cards to which he can point. The protruded tongue is dried, and a drop of the testing solution applied to the lateral border on one side. The patient is then asked to indicate what he tastes. The anterior two-thirds and the posterior one-third of the tongue must be tested separately. The tongue is dried between successive tests.

Disturbances of taste sensation

Loss of taste – ageusia – on the anterior two-thirds of the tongue may occur as the result of lesions of the chorda tympani or of the geniculate ganglion. These structures are sometimes impaired in cases of facial paralysis. Lesions of the glossopharyngeal nerve cause loss of taste on the posterior one-third of the tongue. Lesions of the tractus solitarius and its nucleus cause unilateral ageusia, and lesions near the middle line of the pons may cause bilateral loss of taste from destruction of both gustatory fillets. Little is known about loss of taste resulting from cerebral lesions, though it is occasionally lost together with the sense of smell as the result of a head injury. Hallucinations of taste may occur, like those of smell, as the result of an irritative lesion involving the neighbourhood of the uncus (uncinate gyrus). Lesions in this region may also cause parageusia, a perversion of taste in which many substances excite the same unpleasant flavour.

THE TENTH OR VAGUS NERVE

Anatomy and physiology

The vagus nerve contains both sensory and motor fibres. The sensory fibres convey common sensibility to part of the external ear, and carry afferent impulses from the pharynx and larynx and thoracic and abdominal viscera. The motor fibres are of two kinds. Some innervate the thoracic and abdominal viscera through the parasympathetic ganglia. The others are derived from the nucleus ambiguus, an elongated column of grey matter stituated deep in the medulla. Its fibres are distributed through the glossopharyngeal, vagus, and accessory nerves to the striated muscles of the palate, pharynx, and larynx.

The vagus nerve leaves the medulla by a series of radicles at the anterior margin of the inferior cerebellar peduncle and in series with the roots of the glossopharyngeal nerve above and the accessory below (Plate 6). The roots form a single trunk which leaves the skull through the jugular foramen in which it occupies the same compartment as the accessory nerve. Passing down the neck in the carotid sheath it enters the thorax where the courses of the right and left nerves differ somewhat, but both come to lie on the posterior surface of the root of the lung and, passing through the oesophageal opening of the diaphragm, enter the abdomen.

Within the neck the vagus gives off the recurrent laryngeal nerves which pursue a different course on the two sides. The right recurrent laryngeal nerve arises at the root of the neck where the vagus crosses the subclavian artery, around which it passes upwards and immediately behind the subclavian, the common carotid artery, and the thyroid gland. The left recurrent laryngeal nerve leaves the vagus as it crosses the aortic arch, and after passing beneath the arch turns upwards in the superior mediastinum between the trachea and the oesophagus to the neck, where its course is the same as that of the right nerve. The terminal branches of the recurrent laryngeal nerves innervate all the muscles of the larynx except the cricothyroid, which is supplied by the external laryngeal branch of the vagus. The internal laryngeal branch is the principal sensory nerve of the larynx.

Examination

To investigate the motor functions of the vagus nerve note the appearance of the soft palate and pharynx. Ask the patient to phonate and observe whether the soft palate is elevated, and if so whether it moves in the middle line or is drawn to one side. Test the palatal reflex by touching the soft palate on either side and observing the response, which should be the elevation of the palate in the midline. Test the pharyngeal, or gag, reflex similarly. In each case the vagus is responsible for the motor fibres of the reflex arc only, the sensory fibres being supplied by the trigeminal and glossopharyngeal nerves. When necessary, examine the vocal cords and observe their position at rest and their behaviour on inspiration and attempted phonation.

LESIONS OF THE VAGUS NERVE

Nuclear lesions

Lesions of the nucleus ambiguus may occur in posterior inferior cerebellar thrombosis, syringobulbia, medullary tumour, motor neurone disease, and poliomyelitus. They usually cause an associated paralysis of the soft palate, pharynx, and larynx. The lesion is unilateral in the first, and may be either unilateral or bilateral in the remainder.

Lesions in the posterior fossa

Lesions which involve the vagus between its emergence from the medulla and its exit from the skull in the jugular foramen almost invariably affect neighbouring cranial nerves, expecially the ninth, eleventh, and twelfth. Such lesions are not common, and the commonest of them is a tumour, especially a glomus tumour.

Lesions of the recurrent laryngeal nerve

The left recurrent laryngeal nerve, owing to its longer course, is more exposed to damage than the right. Within the thorax it may be compressed by aneurysm of the aorta, and rarely by the large left atrium in mitral stenosis, or by neoplasm of the mediastinum or enlargement of mediastinal glands due to neoplastic metastases or one of the reticuloses. Within the neck both recurrent laryngeal nerves are exposed to trauma, to the pressure of enlarged deep cervical glands, whether malignant or inflammatory, and of an enlarged thyroid, and may be involved in carcinoma of the oesophagus.

A lesion of the recurrent laryngeal nerve may cause total paralysis of the larynx, or paralysis of abduction of the vocal cord on the affected side.

Symptoms of lesions of the vagus nerve

Paralysis of the palate

Unilateral palatal paralysis usually causes no symptoms. It is detected on examination of the throat by the fact that when the patient phonates, for example in saying 'Ah', elevation of the palate fails to occur on the affected side, and the uvula is drawn over to the normal side. Bilateral palatal paralysis causes regurgitation of food into the nose on swallowing, because the palate fails to shut off the nasopharynx. For the same reason the voice acquires a nasal resonance, and there is an alteration in the pronunciation of consonants, for the correct utterance of which the nasopharynx should be occluded. This is most evident in the pronunciation of *b* and *g*, 'rub' becoming 'rum', and 'egg' 'eng'. There is no elevation of the paralysed palate on phonation and the palatal reflex is lost.

Paralysis of the pharynx

Unilateral paralysis of the pharynx as a rule causes no symptoms. On examination the pharyngeal wall droops on the affected side, and the pharyngeal reflex is present only on the normal side. Bilateral pharyngeal paralysis causes marked dysphagia and bilateral loss of the pharyngeal reflex, and saliva accumulates in the pharynx.

Paralysis of the larynx

Little is known regarding the occurrence of paralysis of the larynx as the result of supranuclear lesions. Hemiplegia does not impair the movement of the vocal cords. The following varieties of laryngeal paralysis may occur.

Unilateral paralysis

In this condition there is a paralysis both of abduction and of adduction of one vocal cord, which lies in the intermediate or cadaveric position. This may occur as a result of a unilateral lesion at any point between the nucleus ambiguus and the recurrent laryngeal nerve inclusive. Phonation is not abolished, since the normal cord crosses the middle line to meet the paralysed one, but there is usually some hoarseness and difficulty in coughing.

Bilateral total paralysis

This may be produced by bilateral lesions at any point between the nucleus ambiguus and the inferior ganglion so that both the superior and recurrent laryngeal nerves are involved. Both vocal cords are paralysed in the cadaveric position. Phonation and coughing are lost. There is no dyspnoea, but inspiratory stridor may occur on deep inspiration.

Bilateral abductor paralysis

This may occur as the result of nuclear lesions or of bilateral lesions of the recurrent laryngeal nerves. As the superior laryngeal nerves are spared the tensors are active and some adduction of the vocal cords is possible. In bilateral abductor paralysis both vocal cords lie close together at or near the middle line and fail to abduct on inspiration. The voice is little affected and coughing is normal, but owing to the failure of abduction there is severe dyspnoea, with marked inspiratory stridor.

Bilateral adductor paralysis

This is usually hysterical. The vocal cords are not adducted in phonation, which is therefore lost, and the patient can only whisper. Adduction occurs, however, in coughing, which is unaffected.

THE ELEVENTH OR ACCESSORY NERVE

Anatomy and physiology

The accessory is a purely motor nerve, which arises partly from the medulla and partly from the spinal cord (Plate 6). The accessory portion is derived from cells which are situated in the lower part of the nucleus ambiguus. The spinal portion is derived from cells situated in the lateral part of the anterior horn of grey matter of the spinal cord from the first cervical down to the fifth cervical segment. The spinal rootlets unite to form a trunk which ascends in the spinal canal to the foramen magnum where it joins the accessory portion to form a single trunk which leaves the skull through the jugular foramen in the same compartment as the vagus. There the accessory fibres join the vagus. The spinal portion enters the neck to supply the sternocleidomastoid muscle and the trapezius.

Examination

Wasting of the sternocleidomastoid muscle is detected by absence of the prominence normally due to the stout band crossing the neck obliquely. On flexion of the neck both these muscles normally stand out symmetrically. On lateral rotation to either side the muscle of the side opposite that to which the face is turned becomes prominent. The outer border of the upper part of the trapezius normally forms a gentle curve extending from its origin in the occipital bone downwards and outwards. The trapezius is tested by asking the patient to shrug the shoulders, when the two muscles normally contract symmetrically.

LESIONS OF THE ACCESSORY NERVE

Lesions of the nucleus ambiguus have been described in the preceding section dealing with the vagus nerve. The cells of origin of the spinal fibres of the accessory in the anterior horns of the grey matter of the upper five cervical segments may undergo degeneration in poliomyelitis and motor neurone disease, or may be compressed in syringomyelia or by tumours involving the spinal cord in the cervical region. Within the posterior fossa the nerve trunk may be damaged, especially by the pressure of a tumour, when it usually suffers in association with the neighbouring cranial nerves, especially the ninth, tenth, and twelfth. After emerging from the skull the nerve may be compressed or involved in inflammation by the upper deep cervical nodes, or suffer from trauma. When the lesion is deep to the sternocleidomastoid, both sternocleidomastoid and trapezius are paralysed; when it is in the posterior triangle of the neck, the sternocleidomastoid escapes. Both muscles may be affected in myopathy.

Symptoms of lesions of the accessory nerve

Paralysis of one sternocleidomastoid causes no abnormality in the position of the head at rest. The muscle is wasted and is less salient than its fellow on the opposite side. There is weakness of rotation of the head to the opposite side, and when the patient flexes the neck and chin is slightly turned to the paralysed side by the unopposed action of the normal opposite muscle. A lesion of the accessory nerve causes paralysis of only the upper fibres of the trapezius. This part of the muscle is wasted and the normal curve formed on the back of the neck by its lateral border becomes flattened. The shoulder is lowered on the affected side, and the scapula becomes rotated downwards and outwards, the lower angle being nearer the midline than the upper. There is also slight winging of the scapula, which disappears when the serratus anterior is brought into action. There is weakness of elevation and retraction of the shoulder, and the patient is unable to raise the arm above the head after it has been abducted by the deltoid. It can still be raised above the head in front of the body, however, a movement in which the serratus anterior takes part. Bilateral paralysis of the sternocleidomastoid is usually associated with weakness of the other flexor muscles of the neck. As a result, the head tends to fall backwards when the patient is erect. Weakness and wasting of the sternocleidomastoids of muscular origin is conspicuous in dystrophia myotonica. Paralysis of both trapezii causes weakness of extention of the neck, and the head tends to fall forwards. This is most frequently seen in motor neurone disease, and in myasthenia gravis.

THE TWELFTH OR HYPOGLOSSAL NERVE

Anatomy and physiology

The hypoglossal nerve is the motor nerve of the tongue. Its fibres originate in the hypoglossal nucleus of the medulla, from which they emerge on its ventral aspect between the olive and the pyramid (Plate 6). After a short course across the posterior fossa the nerve passes through the hypoglossal canal to leave the skull. In the neck the nerve passes downwards and forwards and then turns medially to reach the tongue.

Examination

Ask the patient to protrude the tongue, and note whether it is protruded in the middle line or deviated to one side. Ask the patient to move it from side to side when protruded, or to close the mouth and push out the cheek with the tip of the tongue on either side. Observe whether there is any wasting, which is usually seen first along the lateral margin and is manifested in advanced cases by wrinkling of the tongue. See if there is any fasciculation, a fine flickering contraction of muscle bundles. When fasciculation is only slight it may be more evident when the tongue lies on the floor of the mouth than when it is protruded. Note whether the tongue is furred on one side and not on the other. Look for tremor or other involuntary movements.

LESIONS OF THE HYPOGLOSSAL NERVE

Unilateral lower motor neurone lesions of the tongue may occur as the result of lesions involving the nucleus or the fibres of the nerve between the medulla and the hypoglossal canal. Neither is common, but the most frequent cause of unilateral hypoglossal paralysis is compression by a tumour. The commonest cause of a bilateral lower motor neurone lesion is involvement of the medullary nuclei in motor neurone disease – progressive bulbar palsy. In such cases fasciculation is conspicuous as long as active degeneration is occurring. The medullary nuclei may also be attacked in the bulbar form of poliomyelitis.

Symptoms

After a cerebral vascular lesion it is common to find that the patient is unable to protrude his tongue on command, although he can still protrude it in other circumstances. This is an apraxia of protrusion of the tongue. After a unilateral upper motor neurone lesion the tongue deviates to the paralysed side on protrusion, that is the side opposite to the lesion. A unilateral lower motor neurone lesion causes weakness and wasting of the corresponding half of the tongue. The wasting throws the epithelium on the affected side into folds on which fur tends to accumulate more than on the normal side. The median raphe becomes concave towards the paralysed side, to which the tip is deviated, and the tongue deviates to the paralysed side on protrusion. This deviation is greater after a lower motor neurone lesion than after an upper motor neurone lesion. Unilateral paralysis of the tongue does not impair articulation.

Bilateral lower motor neurone lesions cause marked wasting of both sides, associated with fasciculation when the lesion is due to a progressive degeneration of the cells of the nuclei. In severe cases of bilateral paralysis the tongue lies on the floor of the mouth and protrusion is impossible. Dysarthria and some degree of dysphagia are present. In dysarthria due to bilateral palsy of the tongue alone the patient finds it difficult to pronounce *t* and *d*, and the anteriorly produced lingual vowels, *e, a, i*. But bilateral paralysis of the tongue is not usually an isolated phenomenon, and in such cases dysphagia and dysarthria are therefore due in part to paralysis of other muscles.

Bilateral upper motor neurone paralysis of the tongue occurs as the result of lesions involving both corticospinal tracts above the medulla. In such cases the tongue is somewhat smaller than normal, owing to spastic contraction of the muscles, but true wasting does not occur. All movements are weak.

REFERENCES

Ashworth, B. and Isherwood, I. (1981). *Clinical neuro-ophthalmology,* 2nd edn. Blackwell, Oxford.

Bender, M.B. (1980). Brain control of conjugate horizontal and vertical eye movements: a survey of the structural and functional correlates. *Brain.* **103,** 23–69.

Cogan, D.G. (1956). *Neurology of the ocular muscles,* 2nd edn. Thomas, Springfield, Ill.

—— (1966). *Neurology of the visual system.* Thomas, Springfield, Ill.

Glaser, J.S. (1978). *Neuro-ophthalmology.* Harper and Row, Hagerstown, Md.

Hallpike, C.S. (1965). Clinical otoneurology and its contributions to theory and practice. *Proc. R. Soc. Med.* **58,** 185–96.

Hughes, E.B.C. (1954). *The visual fields.* Blackwell, Oxford.

Rudge, P. (1983). *Clinical neurotology.* Churchill Livingstone, Edinburgh.

Sweet, W.H. and Wepsic, (1974). Controlled thermocoagulation of trigeminal ganglion and rootlets for differential destruction of pain fibers. *J. Neurosurg.* **40**, 143–56.

Taylor, W. (ed.) (1973). *Disorders of auditory function.* Academic Press, London.

Walsh, F.B. (1969). *Clinical neuro-ophthalmology,* 3rd edn. Williams and Wilkins, Baltimore.

3 Examination of the limbs and trunk

Examination of the limbs and trunk involves observation of posture, muscle tone, tested by investigating the resistance of muscles to passive movement, the presence or absence of involuntary movements, and of muscular wasting and fasciculation, voluntary power in the various muscle groups, motor co-ordination, the reflexes, and sensation. Neurological disorders also sometimes cause trophic symptoms.

MUSCLE TONE

Muscle tone, as Sherrington showed, is reflex in origin. The muscle spindles are the receptors in the muscles which respond to stretch by sending impulses which travel in the largest afferent fibres from the muscles to the spinal cord. The muscle spindles are themselves innervated by the smallest, gamma, efferent fibres in the anterior spinal roots, and these have been shown to regulate the response of the muscle spindles, acting synergically with external stretch. So by means of the stretch, or myotatic, reflex, and the lengthening and shortening reactions also described by Sherrington, muscle tone is reflexly maintained and adjusted to the needs of posture and movement. Hence interruption of the reflex arc on its afferent or efferent side leads to hypotonia.

The muscle spindles can be regarded as detectors of the difference in length between the intrafusal and extrafusal (or ordinary) fibres, which are in parallel (Fig. 3.1). The spindles are silenced when the extrafusal fibres shorten by themselves and are excited when the extrafusal fibres are lengthened by stretch. If the gamma impulses set the intrafusal fibre to a desired length, then the extrafusal fibres are forced by the subsequent stretch reflex to follow suit. This would automatically adjust the alpha input to the load on the muscle, as, for example, during a change from more isometric to more isotonic contraction. The true situation is known to be much more complicated in that there are 'nuclear bag' and 'nuclear chain' intrafusal fibres. The former are concerned with static and dynamic stretch and the latter only with static stretch. The muscle spindles are innervated by different gamma fibres, which are responsible for the dynamic and static discharges of the spindles. Some spindles, particularly in flexor muscles, are even innervated by alpha fibres. So the spindles are therefore the basis of all movements rather than just the slow tonic reflexes which Sherrington mainly studied.

The spinal reflex mechanisms are profoundly influenced by higher levels of

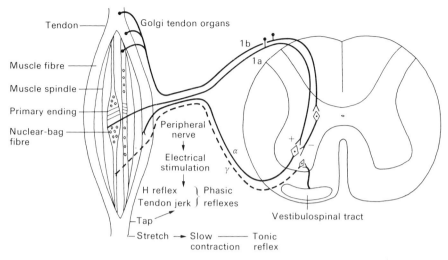

Fig. 3.1. The monosynaptic reflex arc. Group 1a afferent fibres from nuclear-bag and nuclear-chain fibres of the muscle spindle synapse directly upon the large alpha motor neurones in the anterior horn, whose axons cause the muscle fibres surrounding the spindle to contract. The alpha cell is inhibited through an interneurone by group 1b afferent fibres from Golgi tendon organs. The gamma efferent system supplying the contractile ends of muscle spindle fibres is regulated by descending motor pathways, one of which, the vestibulospinal tract, is illustrated.

the nervous system. They may be affected by structural damage and by various drugs. In general the supranuclear control of the alpha and gamma motor neurones is similar, presumably because both act together in the control of movement. The gamma fibres often have a lower threshold than the alpha fibres when natural stimuli are used, as if to 'prepare' the alpha system. There are, however, instances in which the linkage may be broken experimentally, as for example following acute destruction of the anterior cerebellum when rigidity due to alpha motor neurone discharge is produced, as opposed to the decerebrate rigidity caused by release of gamma activity. The spinal reflex mechanisms are depressed by neural shock, hence after an acute lesion of either one cerebral hemisphere or the spinal cord the paralysed limbs remain for a considerable time hypotonic. As the cerebellum is mainly facilitatory to the stretch reflex, cerebellar deficiency causes hypotonia. The reticular formation of the brainstem is also mainly facilitatory, hence removal of higher inhibitory control over the reticular formation leads to decerebrate rigidity. Loss of corticospinal tract influence also causes spasticity. The influence of the corpus striatum is complex, but damage to the substantia nigra causes hypertonia. Chorea, on the other hand, leads to muscular hypotonia.

Lower motor neurone lesions lead to hypotonia by interfering with the efferent pathway of the reflex arc upon which muscle tone depends. The same effect is produced by primary degeneration of the muscles themselves, as in the myopathies, and in benign congenital hypotonia. Interruption of the reflex pathway on the afferent side occurs as the result of lesions of the spinal sensory nerve roots, especially in tabes dorsalis. In polyneuritis both afferent and efferent pathways may be damaged. To sum up, then, the principal causes of muscular hypotonia are:

1. Neural shock, either cerebral or spinal.
2. Lesions of the cerebellum.
3. Chorea.
4. Lower motor neurone lesions.
5. Lesions involving the sensory afferents.
6. Primary degeneration of the muscles themselves.

Muscular hypertonia is to be regarded as a release phenomenon. A cortico-spinal tract lesion at the level of one internal capsule releases from higher control centres in the midbrain and pons, the uncontrolled activity of which produces the distribution of muscular hypertonia characteristic of *hemiplegia.* In the upper limb hypertonia predominates in the adductors of the shoulder, the flexors of the elbow, wrist, and fingers, and the pronators of the forearm. In the lower limb the hypertonia is manifested in the extensor muscles, the plantar flexors of the ankle and toes being physiologically extensors, and the adductors of the hip.

In decorticate rigidity both arms are usually in flexion and adduction but both legs are extended. The lesion, above the superior colliculus, may be at the level of the internal capsule or thalamus. In midbrain lesions there is decere-brate rigidity with a clenched jaw, retracted neck, arms and legs stiffly extended and internally rotated. Fragments of decerebrate posture with extended arms and flexed legs point to mid-pontine lesions. With medullary lesions and low pontine lesions there is usually an abolition of all posture and, because of involvement of the reticular formation, the patient is usually in profound coma.

The same physiological principles apply to the distribution of muscle tone and the resulting posture in paraplegia produced by a lesion of the spinal cord. After a bilateral corticospinal tract lesion, for example in the mid-dorsal region, the posture of the lower limbs produced by the uninhibited action of the remaining descending pathways in the spinal cord, particularly the vestibulo-spinal tracts, is the same as that in hemiplegia or in decerebrate rigidity and, predominating in the extensors, gives rise to *paraplegia-in-extension.* A more extensive lesion of the spinal cord, however, which interrupts the vestibulo-spinal tract as well as the corticospinal tract, thereby cuts off the influences upon which the extensor hypertonia depends, and paraplegia-in-extension gives place to *paraplegia-in-flexion* which is produced by the now uninhibited action of the nociceptive flexor withdrawal reflex (p. 110). The hypertonia which follows a corticospinal tract lesion is commonly called *spasticity.*

Muscular hypertonia due to an extrapyramidal lesion is usually called rigidity. The commonest example of this is *parkinsonian rigidity.* This differs from spasticity in two main respects. As we have just seen, the hypertonia which follows a corticospinal tract lesion is distributed predominantly to one or other of the opposing muscle groups, in hemiplegia, for example, to the flexors of the upper and the extensors of the lower limb. Parkinsonian rigidity is on the whole evenly distributed to opposing muscle groups, with the result that it tends to bring about a posture of the limbs and trunk which is intermediate between flexion and extension. Secondly, if an attempt is made by the observer to overcome by passive movement the hypertonia of a spastic limb, the maximum resistance is experienced at the onset, and when once this has been overcome the hypertonia is much reduced. This has been described as the 'clasp-knife' effect. In parkinsonian rigidity, on the other hand, the resistance encountered by the observer on passively moving a segment of a limb is much the same at all points in the range of movement. Two varieties of parkinsonian rigidity can be recognized, sometimes called 'cog-wheel' and 'lead-pipe'. In cog-wheel rigidity the observer finds that as he passively moves the patient's limb, the resistance he encounters is subject to a series of rapid fluctuations which can be shown to be due to the superimposed effect of tremor causing an alternating contraction and relaxation of the muscle being stretched. In lead-pipe rigidity no such fluctuations occur, and the resistance is uniform. Hypertonia is occasionally of predominantly muscular origin, when it occurs chiefly as the prolongation of a muscular contraction initiated by voluntary effort, as in the myopathic disorders, dystrophia myotonica and myotonia congenita.

Clinical management of spasticity

Spasticity is the velocity sensitive resistance to passive stretch of the muscle. It must be remembered that sometimes spasticity may be useful to a patient, for example a hemiplegic who can use a spastic leg as a prop or to the paraplegic who needs spasticity in order to walk on elbow crutches. In a chair-bound paraplegic, however, flexor spasms can be painful and continue as a major problem in management.

The physiological basis of spasticity is an increased fusimotor innervation of the muscle spindle through the dynamic gamma motor neurones. Other factors are the decreased presynaptic inhibition to control the sensory inflow from the periphery, the loss of reciprocal innervation and a loss of recurrent inhibition mediated by Renshaw cells and an increase in alpha motor neurone excitability from excitatory sources other than the muscle spindles.

Dantrolene sodium (Dantrium) a hydantoin derivative acts directly on the muscle by affecting the excitation-coupling mechanisms of skeletal muscle and the intrafusal fibre, affecting rapidly contracting muscles. It is useful in the treatment of spasticity caused both by cerebral and spinal lesions. The initial dose is 25 mg daily and the maintenance dose is 100–400 mg daily in divided doses. Side-effects include drowsiness or in high doses, muscular weakness. It should be used with caution in patients with pulmonary, myocardial or liver disease.

Baclofen (Lioresal) is a derivative of the inhibitory neurone transmitter GABA and has several actions apart from its ability to release GABA from GABA-ergic synapses and it also blocks the excitatory effect of sensory inputs from limb muscles. It also depresses mono- and polysynaptic reflexes by reducing excitatory postsynaptic potentials and has analgesic properties by blocking the postsynaptic action of substance P. It is most useful in spasticity due to spinal cord lesions such as multiple sclerosis. The initial dose is 5 mg three times a day and the maintenance dose, to be built up slowly, is 60–100 mg daily, with side-effects of nausea, weakness, and confusion. It should not be used in epileptics and sudden withdrawal may cause hallucinations.

Diazepam (Valium), a benzodiazepine, has complex actions partly through brainstem mechanisms and partly by enhancing the actions of GABA at its spinal cord receptors independent of its action on the brain. It is useful in patients with partial or complete spinal lesions in a total dose of 6–40 mg daily. The principal side-effect is drowsiness. The effect of Valium on spasticity lasts longer than its sedative effect and so these unwanted sedative effects can be reduced by giving a daily dose at night.

POSTURE

As has been shown in the preceding paragraphs, there is an intimate relationship between movement, posture, and muscle tone. Movement begins and ends in posture and, as Sherrington said, posture is tonus. Physiologically one of the main functions of muscle tone is the maintenance of posture. As we have seen, in hemiplegia, decerebrate rigidity, paraplegia, and Parkinsonism the posture of the limbs and sometimes of the whole body is determined by the pathological distribution and degree of muscle tone. Conversely, when a limb is hypotonic, as in cerebellar disease and chorea, its maintenance in any posture becomes difficult. All of these, however, are factors operating upon the posture of a limb as a whole. At a lower level of nervous organization, represented by the lower motor neurone, posture is influenced by selective muscular weakness. Posture may then be determined by the effect of gravity when some of the anti-gravity muscles are weak, by the unopposed action of muscles normally antagonistic to those paralysed, and ultimately often by contractures occurring in the healthy muscles. Wrist-drop, finger-drop, and foot-drop are examples of abnormal postures produced by gravity in the presence of paralysis of the extensors of the wrist and fingers and dorsiflexors of the ankle respectively. Ulnar nerve paralysis, median nerve paralysis, and paralysis of both nerves combined lead to characteristic postures of the fingers resulting from the unopposed action of the remaining non-paralysed muscles.

INVOLUNTARY MOVEMENTS

THE DYSKINESIAS

All abnormal movements arising from a disturbance of the extrapyramidal system may be grouped under the term dyskinesia. This term does not imply a particular pathology and includes a range of amplitude from the most violent hemiballismus, through chorea, athetosis, dystonia, and torticollis, to mild tremors. Their mechanism of production in neurophysiological or anatomical terms is less easy to understand than some of the biochemical triggering factors.

Chorea

Choreic movements are best described as quasi-purposive, rather resembling fragments of purposive movement following one another in a disorderly fashion. In the face the movements are always bilateral. Frowning, raising the eyebrows, pursing the lips, smiling, and bizarre movements of the mouth and tongue occur. The protruded tongue may be held between the teeth to prevent its sudden withdrawal. In the upper limb movements occur at all joints, but in the lower limbs they are usually less conspicuous and are most evident at the periphery. The involuntary movements render voluntary movements ataxic. In mild cases speech is not affected, but in severe cases there is considerable dysarthria, and mastication and swallowing may also be disturbed. Respiration is often jerky and irregular. Choreic movements disappear during sleep.

The movements of chorea differ somewhat according to the cause of the disorder. When chorea is congenital it often merges into athetosis. The description given above corresponds to that commonly found in Sydenham's chorea, due to rheumatic fever. In Huntington's chorea the movements often remain for a long time predominantly distal, resembling a coarse static tremor and interfering with co-ordination. Hemiballismus is chorea of unilateral distribution due to a lesion involving the opposite subthalamic nucleus (corpus Luysii). In this condition the movements tend to be violent, often causing wide excursions of segments of the limbs at all joints.

Athetosis

Athetoid movements are slower, coarser, and more writhing than choreic movements. This has been attributed to the release of alternating grasp and avoidance reactions caused by corticostriatial fibre degeneration. One or both halves of the body may be involved. The muscles innervated by the cranial nerves are always much more severely affected when the athetosis is bilateral than when it is unilateral. In bilateral athetosis the patient exhibits frequent grimaces resembling caricatures of normal facial expressions of all kinds. The tongue may be the site of writhing movements of protrusion and withdrawal and in severe cases the involuntary movements of the articulatory and pharyngeal muscles lead to dysarthria and dysphagia. The head may be rotated to one or other side, or extended. In unilateral athetosis the facial movements usually consist of little more than an exaggeration of normal expressions. In the upper limbs the peripheral segments exhibit the involuntary movements to a greater extent than the proximal segments. The limb is usually adducted and internally rotated at the shoulder, and semiflexed at the elbow. The characteristic posture of the hand is one of marked flexion of the wrist, with flexion at the metacarpophalangeal and extension at the interphalangeal joints. This posture is disturbed by slow, writhing movements of flexion and extension at the wrist and fingers with varying degrees of adduction and abduction. Movements may also occur at the shoulder and elbow, leading sometimes to retraction and internal rotation at the shoulder and extension at the elbow. In severe cases of unilateral athetosis the patient characteristically grasps the affected limb with the normal hand to restrain the movement, or even sits on it. Except in the mildest cases the movements completely interfere with the voluntary use of the limb.

The movements of the lower limb are usually less severe than those of the upper and again are most marked in the distal segments. The foot is usually maintained plantar-flexed and inverted with marked dorsiflexion of the great toe. Athetoid movements are always exaggerated by an attempt to use the limbs in voluntary movement, and by nervousness and excitement. They diminish when the patient lies down, and disappear during sleep.

Dystonia

From a functional point of view chorea, athetosis, and dystonia may be regarded as a series of disturbances which merge into one another. Dystonia is a kind of frozen athetosis, characterized by distorted postures of the limbs and trunk resulting from excessive muscular tone in antagonistic muscle groups. It commonly begins in the plantar flexors of the ankle, so that the patient has to walk on his toes. Later the glutei and trunk muscles become involved, causing lordosis of the lumbar spine. The hypertonic muscles offer great resistance to passive stretching, and the muscular contraction itself may cause severe pain. Dystonia musculorum deformans or torsion spasm is a rare striatal disorder, sometimes familial and sometimes manifesting itself sporadically in childhood.

Tremor

Tremor is a more or less rhythmical oscillating movement of a segment of a limb or of the head. It may occur when a limb is at rest, or when it is voluntarily maintained in a certain position – action tremor, or on voluntary movement – intention tremor. In addition to these features points to note about tremor are its distribution, its rate and rhythm, and whether anything increases or lessens its severity. Tremor is a common symptom of nervous disorders. The following are the chief varieties.

Physiological or action tremor

Normal people have a fine tremor of the hands on maintaining a posture. The rate is about 8–12 Hz in young children, increases with maturity to 20 Hz and decreases again with age. It appears to be the result of some central synchronization of motor neurone activity. An action tremor becomes more obvious in old age, fatigue, anxiety, thyrotoxicosis, uraemia, prehepatic coma and intoxication with various poisons including mercury, cocaine, and alcohol. Its reduction in myxoedema may be the result of slowing of the muscle contraction time which is responsible for the 'slow' reflexes.

Parkinsonian tremor

In parkinsonism, in addition to any action tremor there is an alternating tremor which usually begins in one upper limb and later involves the lower limb on the same side, the other side being affected in the same order after a further interval. Rarely it begins in the lower limb. In the upper limb the hand is most affected. Movements of the fingers occur at the metacarpophalangeal joints and may be combined with movements of the thumb – the 'pill-rolling' movement. Movements at the wrist may be flexion and extension, lateral displacement, or pronation and supination. Often the tremor shifts from one to another group of muscles while the patient is under observation. Little movement usually occurs at the joints above the wrist. In the lower limb tremor is most marked at the ankle, at which flexion and extension occur. Parkinsonian tremor often spares the head, but that may become involved in either a nodding or a rotary tremor.

The rate of parkinsonian tremor (Fig. 3.2) lies between 3 and 7 movements a second (Hz), being slower in paralysis agitans than encephalitic parkinsonism. It is present when the patient is at rest, and is usually temporarily suppressed when the limb is voluntarily moved. It can be inhibited for a time by conscious effort. It is increased by emotional excitement and disappears during sleep.

Sporadic or familial intention tremor

Such tremor may be fine and rapid, or slow and coarser, and tends to be increased by emotion and, unlike parkinsonian tremor, by voluntary movement (Fig. 3.2). It is usually, but not invariably, absent at rest. It affects principally the upper limbs but also involves the head more frequently than Parkinsonian tremor. It is not associated with muscular weakness or rigidity. Alcohol, though it often reduces the tremor, carries worse dangers. Treatment with sedative drugs is disappointing, but beta-adrenergic blocking drugs are sometimes helpful. If these fail primidone may be helpful especially if the tremor is in the range of 5–7 Hz.

Cerebellar tremor

Tremor due to cerebellar deficiency is best interpreted as the result of a disturbance of a central 'feedback' mechanism by means of which the smooth

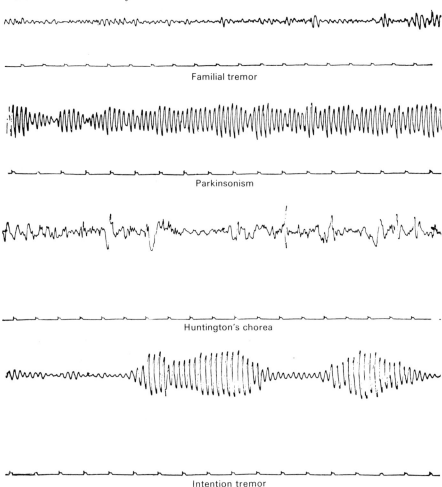

Fig. 3.2. Recordings of four different types of tremor (time marker, seconds).

maintenance of posture and movement is normally regulated. In cerebellar disease static tremor develops if the patient attempts to maintain a limb in a fixed posture, and tremor on voluntary movement is partially the result of faulty fixation of the limb and partly due to a defect of co-ordination which leads to the hand or the foot first deviating in one direction from the ideal course of the intended movement and then by over-correction deviating in another. *Intention tremor* is a variety of tremor in which this disorder of co-ordination becomes evident only as the distal part of the limb approaches its objective, the finger, for example, oscillating more and more violently as it approaches the nose, or the hand in lifting a glass of water to the mouth (Fig. 3.2). This type of tremor, presumably due to a disorder of the cerebellar connections, is most frequently seen in disseminated sclerosis.

Though disease involving the corpus striatum or the cerebellum and its connections is the commonest cause of tremor, tremor may also occur, especially on movement, in patients with lesions of the *frontal lobe,* or diffuse disorders of which *general paresis* is a common example.

Hysterical tremor

A fine tremor may occur on strong emotion, especially fear. Two forms of *hysterical tremor* are encountered; a fine tremor, localized to one limb or generalized, and resembling the shaking of extreme fear; and a coarse, irregular shaking, intensified by voluntary movement. In common with other hysterical symptoms, hysterical tremor is characterized by its irregularity, variability from time to time, and by a tendency to diminish when the patient's attention is distracted and increase when it is directed to the affected part of the body.

Myoclonus

The term myoclonus is applied to a brief, shock-like muscular contraction which may involve the whole muscle or be limited to a small number of muscle fibres. It may affect one or many muscles, either successively or simultaneously, and frequently contractions occur symmetrically in muscles on the opposite sides of the body. The contraction may be too slight to cause movement of a segment of the limb, or may cause such violent movements as to throw the patient to the ground. The commonest form of myoclonus, apart from the occasional jerk in a normal person while falling asleep, is that associated with epilepsy (pp. 187 and 193). Otherwise it is rare, occurring occasionally in encephalomyelitis or encephalopathy; sporadically, involving the soft palate, pharynx, diaphragm and sometimes other muscles; or as the rare paramyoclonus multiplex. There is pathological evidence associating non-epileptic myoclonus with disorders of the olivodentate system.

Neurochemistry of myoclonus

Though it has been suggested that serotonin acts as an inhibitory modulator of sensory input preventing the exaggerated motor responses which constitute myoclonus, it has not yet been possible to localize the abnormal circuits precisely in the brain. Experimental studies also suggest that efferent cerebellar pathways are involved. Patients with post-anonoxic intention myoclonus and progressive myoclonic epilepsy have been shown to have consistently low levels of cerebrospinal 5-hydroxyindolacetic acid (5HIAA), a metabolite of serotonin. This suggests the possibility of a reduced concentration of brain serotonin. Serotonin precursors have proved of benefit in the treatment of certain types of myoclonus. 5-Hydroxytryptophan (5HT) given either with a peripheral decarboxidase inhibitor such as carbidopa or with a monoaminoxidase inhibitor improves several types of myoclonus, including post-hypoxic and palatal myoclonus. Some improvement in myoclonus with epilepsy has been reported with sodium valproate and clonazepam.

MUSCULAR WASTING AND FASCICULATION

Numerous general disorders, especially metabolic abnormalities, may cause generalized muscular wasting, but we are here concerned only with muscular wasting as a symptom of disorders of the nervous system or muscles themselves.

Muscular wasting may be the result of:

1. *Lesions above the level of the lower motor neurone.* Slight muscular wasting may occur as a result of a corticospinal tract lesion, but it is here difficult to distinguish the direct effect of the lesion from the resulting disuse. Conspicuous muscular wasting sometimes occurs, especially in the upper limb, as the result of a lesion of the opposite parietal lobe causing sensory loss of the cortical type: this is sometimes called 'parietal wasting'.

2. *Lesions of the lower motor neurone.* A lesion of the lower motor neurone at any point in its course from the anterior horn cells of the spinal cord or motor nuclei of the brainstem through the peripheral nerves to their ending in the muscles causes wasting of the part of the muscle which it innervates.

3. *Muscular disorders.* Disorders of the muscles independently of their nerve supply may cause muscular wasting. This is seen especially in the myopathies.

4. *Reflex muscular wasting.* This is seen especially in muscles in the neighbourhood of a joint which is the site of a painful lesion, e.g. the shoulder in periarticular fibrositis.

Distribution of muscular wasting

An accurate assessment of the distribution of muscular wasting is of great diagnostic importance.

1. Muscular wasting of cerebral origin is found in those muscles which are the site of the muscular weakness or are affected by the cortical sensory loss.

2. Muscular wasting due to lesions involving the lower motor neurones, comprises those resulting from:

(i) Diffuse damage to motor neurone cells. This develops acutely in poliomyelitis and insidiously in motor neurone disease. Anterior horn cells are affected in a manner which is usually characteristic of the causal disorder and the distribution of the muscular wasting depends upon its distribution, extent, and severity in the neuraxis.

(i) The lesion may involve the motor nerve supply of one or more spinal segments. The muscular wasting then has an anatomical distribution which is determined by the nerve supply of the affected segment or segments (see pp. 116–17). An example of this is the effect of compression of a single spinal anterior nerve root or of two or more consecutive anterior nerve roots.

(iii) In the cervical and lumbosacral regions the spinal anterior nerve roots, having emerged from the intervertebral foramina as the spinal nerves, intermingle to form the cervical, lumbar, and sacral plexuses. The resulting redistribution of lower motor neurones means that injury to some part of a plexus causes muscular wasting with a distribution corresponding to the supply of the part of the plexus affected.

(iv) From plexuses spring the peripheral nerves, each of which has its own characteristic distribution of motor neurones to muscles. There is therefore an anatomical distribution of muscular wasting corresponding to each peripheral nerve (pp. 116–17).

3. Finally, muscular wasting due to disorders of muscles occurring independently of their nerve supply has usually also a characteristic distribution, which is symmetrical and bears no relation to the nerve supply, but is usually characteristic of the particular form of myopathy, and in some is associated with pseudohypertrophy of certain muscles.

FASCICULATION

The term fasciculation is used to describe the isolated fine twitches which are seen in certain disorders of muscular innervation and in severe cases give the whole muscle a flickering appearance, because the twitch involves the contraction of a group, bundle or fascicle of muscle fibres, and a contraction of a single fibre is not visible. Fasciculation is difficult to see in a patient with much subcutaneous fat. Inspection should be made in a good light. The patient should be warm because shivering may be mistaken for fasciculation. In the limbs a good way to bring out fasciculation is to shorten the muscle being inspected by the appropriate passive movement, for example to extend the elbow while looking at the triceps. Percussion of the muscle with the finger tip may also elicit it.

It used to be thought that fasciculation indicates only a degenerative lesion of the motor neurone cells in the nuclei of the brainstem or anterior horns of the spinal cord, but it is now recognized that it may occur as the result of lesions much more widely distributed. It is, however, seen in its most characteristic form as the result of such degeneration in motor neurone disease. It does not occur when the cells of the motor neurones are rapidly injured or destroyed, as in the actue stage of poliomyelitis, but it may be encountered persisting indefinitely in some muscles in patients who have recovered from poliomyelitis, and does not then indicate a progressive lesion. Fasciculation is often to be seen in some muscles in the upper limbs in patients with cervical myelopathy due to spondylosis: it also occurs in syringomyelia, but may be observed only when the disease is in a phase of active progression. Fasciculation sometimes occurs as the result of a lesion of a spinal anterior root, for example in the upper or lower limb when the relevant root is compressed by an intervertebral disc protrusion. It used to be thought that fasciculation did not occur as the result of primary muscular diseases. This is probably true of the hereditary myopathies, but it may certainly be observed in some cases of polymyositis and in thyrotoxic myopathy.

Fascicular twitching of the facial muscles, especially the orbicularis oculi, is common as a transitory occurrence in normal persons – 'live blood', or myokymia – and is also found in clonic facial spasm. Spasmodic facial contractions are also seen after incomplete recovery from facial paralysis. A few isolated muscular twitchings are often observed in bedridden patients, especially in the calves.

Fibrillation is the term applied to the isolated spontaneous contraction of individual muscle fibres. As the contraction of single fibres is not visible to the naked eye, it can only be recognized by electromyography (p. 162). It has the same significance as fasciculation and indicates a lesion of the lower motor neurone. Electromyography is a valuable aid to the interpretation of muscular wasting and fasciculation.

MUSCULAR WEAKNESS

Muscular weakness may be classified in relation to its six important causes, which are:

1. Upper motor neurone lesions.
2. Lower motor neurone lesions.
3. Extrapyramidal lesions, especially parkinsonism and chorea.
4. Cerebellar lesions.
5. Primary muscular disorders.
6. Hysteria.

UPPER MOTOR NEURONE LESIONS

The recognition that muscular weakness is due to an upper motor neurone lesion depends in part upon its distribution and in part upon the presence or absence of certain other signs. The terms upper motor neurone lesion and corticospinal tract lesion are at present used interchangeably, but it should be realized that the corticospinal tract (Fig. 3.3) is certainly derived from larger areas of the cortex than merely the precentral gyrus, and is therefore not identical with the axons of the pyramidal cells.

An upper motor neurone lesion may originate within the brain or within the spinal cord. A *cerebral* lesion may be: (i) cortical; (ii) subcortical; (iii) in the internal capsule, or capsular; (iv) in the brainstem.

1. Owing to the wide surface distribution of the upper neurones in the cerebral cortex (Fig. 3.4) a cortical lesion of a given size will involve fewer such fibres than at any lower level, consequently cortical upper motor neurone lesions usually produce a monoplegia, that is, paralysis of the face or of one limb only, without, or with only slight, implication of adjoining cortical areas. Since the precentral cortex contains the bodies of the pyramidal cells, a cortical lesion in this region may lead to excitation of the corticospinal fibres which expresses itself as a Jacksonian convulsion (p. 190).

2. Subcortical lesions. In the corona radiata the upper motor neurones are

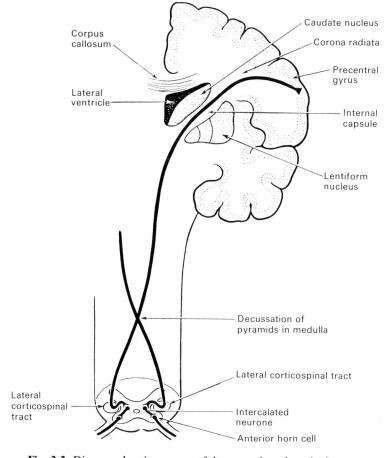

Corpus
callosum

Caudate nucleus

Corona radiata

Precentral
gyrus

Lateral
ventricle

Internal
capsule

Lentiform
nucleus

Decussation of
pyramids in medulla

Lateral corticospinal tract

Lateral
corticospinal
tract

Intercalated
neurone

Anterior horn cell

Fig. 3.3. Diagram showing course of the crossed corticospinal tracts.

converging towards the internal capsule (Fig. 3.3 and Plate 5), and are closer together than in the cortex. Subcortical lesions tend therefore to involve more fibres than cortical lesions of equal size, and it is usual to find that, though the weakness may predominate in one limb, the whole of the opposite side of the body is to some extent involved.

3. Lesions in the internal capsule. Here (Fig. 3.3) the upper motor neurones are more closely crowded together than at higher levels, and a lesion in this situation is therefore likely to produce a crossed hemiplegia.

4. Lesions in the brainstem. Such lesions are also likely to produce a hemiplegia or, since both corticospinal tracts here lie near to each other, a quadriplegia. Hemiplegia due to a lesion of the brainstem can be distinguished from a capsular hemiplegia only be means of the physical signs resulting from damage to other structures in these situations, in the case of the internal capsule the

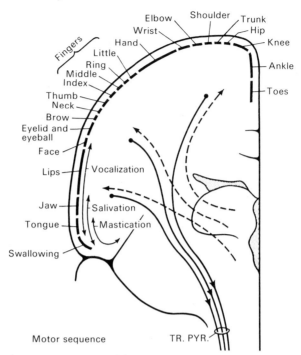

Fig. 3.4. Corticospinal motor pathway (corticospinal tract). Cross-section through right hemisphere along the plan of the precentral gyrus. The sequence of responses to electrical stimulation of the surface of the cortex (from above down, along the motor strip from toes through arm and face to swallowing) is unvaried from one individual to another.

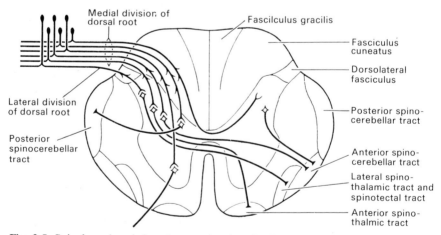

Fig. 3.5. Spinal cord and dorsal root, showing the divisions of the dorsal root, the collaterals of the dorsal root fibres, and some of the connections which are established by them. The lateral and ventral spinothalamic tracts are also called the posterior and anterior spinothalamic tracts respectively.

sensory pathways and the optic radiation which lie behind the corticospinal fibres, and in the case of the brainstem particularly the cranial nerve nuclei and their motor and sensory pathways at the various levels, and also the long ascending sensory tracts.

Cerebral upper motor neurone lesions may of course be at any level, bilateral as well as unilateral.

The upper motor neurones may be injured in the *spinal cord* at any segmental level. If the lesion is above the cervical enlargement both upper and lower limbs will be affected; if below, the weakness will be confined to the lower limbs. The main difference between hemiplegia of cerebral and of spinal origin is that in the latter there is no weakness within the territory of the cranial nerves. (For further details of spinal cord lesions, see pages 358–89.)

What has just been said is concerned with how the distribution of the weakness resulting from an upper motor neurone lesion is related to the anatomical situation of the lesion. Physiologically, as is best seen in the case of a partial or progressive upper motor neurone lesion, it is the more voluntary and the more skilled movements which suffer most, while the less voluntary and less skilled are relatively spared. Thus voluntary movement of the face is more impaired than emotional movement, and the finer movements of the fingers then the grosser movements at the shoulder and elbow. Parallel with this it becomes more difficult for the patient to move a segment of the limb in isolation, so that in any attempted movement the limb tends to move as a whole.

The associated disturbances which are of value in the recognition of upper motor neurone lesions concern muscle tone and wasting. Though disuse may lead to a little loss of volume in the affected muscles, conspicuous wasting does not occur after an upper motor neurone lesion. Muscular tone is characteristically increased (p. 88), the tendon reflexes are exaggerated, clonus is often present, and if the upper motor neurones concerned in movement of the lower limb are involved, the corresponding plantar reflex is extensor. There are, however, exceptional cases in which weakness due to an upper motor neurone lesion is present without hypertonia and even without an extensor plantar response.

LOWER MOTOR NEURONE LESIONS

The characteristics of a lower motor neurone lesion are wasting of the muscles innervated. The distribution of the weakness, or, according to the severity of the lesion, paralysis, of the affected muscles will be identical with that of the wasting, and its characteristics have been described above (p. 98). When the lower motor neurones are involved at a point of their course in which they are anatomically associated with sensory fibres, for example in the spinal nerve, a plexus, or a mixed peripheral nerve, the muscular wasting and weakness will be associated with sensory disturbances having a distribution characteristic of the grouping of the sensory fibres at the point of damage. Fasciculation may be present (p. 99). The tendon reflex mediated by muscles which are the site of a lower motor neurone lesion will be diminished or lost according to the severity of the lesion. If, however, the patient also has an upper motor neurone lesion the enhancing effect of this upon the tendon reflexes may, as long as there are muscle fibres capable of contraction, out-weigh the depressing effect of the lower motor neurone lesion, as is often seen in motor neurone disease.

It should be borne in mind that extrapyramidal and cerebellar lesions may cause muscular weakness as well as lesions of the upper and lower motor neurones. This is of little more than academic importance in the case of cerebellar lesions, but may cause difficulty in diagnosis in two types of extrapyramidal lesion. Slowness and weakness of movement are characteristic of parkinsonism—parkinsonian akinesia—and are sometimes the presenting symptoms of parkinsonism unaccompanied by tremor. Severe muscular weakness may occur in chorea – paralytic chorea – in which case choreic movements will be absent from the paralysed limb.

PRIMARY MUSCULAR DISORDERS

Muscular weakness may occur as the result of disorders which involve the muscles independently of the nervous system. These include myasthenia gravis, the various forms of myopathy, and polymyositis. The characteristic feature of the myopathies is the occurrence of muscular wasting with a distribution which does not correspond to the anatomical supply of any part of the nervous system, but is distinctive for the particular form of myopathy. The wasting is symmetrical, usually begins before the age of 20, is only slowly progressive, and is not uncommonly familial. The characteristic features of myasthenic weakness are its tendency to involve the elevators of the eyelids, the ocular and the facial muscles early, and its striking increase on fatigue. The clinical picture in polymyositis may resemble that of a sporadic case of myopathy, but in the more acute cases the affected muscles are firm and tender, and the skin may be red and swollen.

HYSTERIA

Hysterical muscular weakness ranges from a complete paralysis of the limb to a moderate reduction in muscular power. In cases of moderate weakness commonly encountered the characteristic feature is the innervation of the antagonistic muscles. For example when a patient, lying in bed, is asked to flex the knee against resistance, the quadriceps can be seen and felt to contract simultaneously, instead of, as normally, relaxing. Similarly the attempt to dorsiflex the ankle evokes a simultaneous contraction of the calf muscles. The rather feeble and slightly tremulous grasp characteristic of hysterical weakness of flexion of the fingers is easily recognized. Hysterical muscular weakness is often associated with hysterical sensory loss. Besides these positive features, the hysterical nature of the weakness is confirmed by the presence of normal reflexes in the affected limb and the absence of muscular wasting, except in some very long-standing cases.

MUSCULAR CO-ORDINATION

Anatomy and physiology

By muscular co-ordination is meant the ability to control a movement accurately, considered in isolation from the strength with which the movement is performed. It probably would not occur to us to make this division of function in respect of a normal movement, and it is lesions of the nervous system which have shown that there exist mechanisms of co-ordination which are largely separate from those concerned with voluntary power. Voluntary movement is primarily guided by sensation, especially the sensations which make us aware of the position of the different segments of the limb which is being moved in relation to each other and to the rest of the body. Co-ordination, therefore, depends primarily upon the integrity of the sensory pathways concerned, especially those which terminate in the postcentral convolution. But the discharge of nervous impulses from the motor cortex through the cortico-spinal pathways under the influence of afferent impulses derived from the postcentral gyrus needs to evoke a most complex pattern of nervous activities presided over by the cerebellum.

THE CEREBELLUM

The cerebellum receives afferent fibres from the proprioceptor organs of the body, namely the labyrinths and the muscles. The latter reach the cerebellum by the dorsal and ventral spinocerebellar tracts. Each hemisphere of the cerebellum also receives fibres from the opposite olive, and the corticospinal fibres send collaterals to it.

The cerebellar cortex consists of three principal layers of cells. From the intermediate layer of Purkinje cells fibres are distributed chiefly to the dentate nuclei. From this and the other cerebellar nuclei, efferent pathways are distributed to the opposite red nucleus. The cerebellum exerts its influence upon the spinal cord indirectly through the various pathways descending to the cord from the brainstem.

Animal experiment and observations on man have combined to establish the role of the cerebellum as an unconscious mechanism for graduating and harmonizing muscular contraction both in voluntary movement and in the maintenance of posture in the service of our conscious aims. And it seems that for this purpose it employs an elaborate feedback mechanism whereby the state of contraction or relaxation of the relevant muscles at any moment is influenced by 'information' received from the muscles and other proprioceptors, and the aim of the movement expressed through corticospinal impulses. The lateral lobes of the cerebellum are concerned chiefly with movements of the limbs on the same side of the body, and of the eyes to that side, while the vermis is concerned chiefly with what may be termed axial functions, namely speech, the maintenance of the upright posture of the trunk, standing, and walking.

Symptoms of cerebellar deficiency

The symptoms of cerebellar deficiency are those of a breakdown of the physiological mechanisms just described. *Muscular hypotonia* is due to loss of the facilitatory influence of the cerebellum upon the stretch reflex. It is evident in a diminished resistance to passive movements and in the fact that if the outstretched upper limb receives a sudden tap, it shows a greater displacement than a normal limb. *Static tremor* develops if the patient attempts to maintain a limb in a fixed posture. Disorders of movement are readily understood as the result of a breakdown of the feedback mechanism concerned in their smooth co-ordination. *Ataxia* or *inco-ordination* is one result, fine movements, for example those of the fingers, suffering especially. *Tremor* occurs on voluntary movement. *Dysdiadochokinesis* is the term applied to an inability to carry out alternating movements with rapidity and regularity. For example, the patient cannot smoothly alternately pronate and supinate his forearm or flex and extend his fingers. *Nystagmus* is usually present in cerebellar disease (p. 74). Disturbances of articulation resulting from a lesion of the vermis cause the speech to be jerky and explosive. The syllables tend to be separated from each other, while individual syllables are slurred owing to defective formation of consonants. Disorders of gait are described below.

Tests of co-ordination

Muscular co-ordination is tested in the upper limbs by asking the patient to touch the tip of his nose with the tip of his forefinger, first with the eyes open and then with the eyes closed. He can also be asked, with the eyes open to touch first the tip of his nose and then the observer's finger. He should also be asked to carry out alternating movements of flexion and extension of the fingers, or pronation and supination of the forearms simultaneously on both sides. When the patient is in bed, co-ordination of the lower limbs may be tested by asking him to place one heel on the opposite knee and then move it downwards, keeping it on the shin, or to raise the leg from the bed and touch the observer's finger with his toe. He should then be asked to carry out simultaneously alternating movements of flexion and extension of the toes on both sides.

The causes of inco-ordination

The principal causes of inco-ordination are: (i) sensory loss and (ii) lesions involving the cerebellum or its connections. Loss of postural sensibility leads to inco-ordination which is made worse by closing the eyes. An example of this is the ataxia of the lower limbs occurring in tabes dorsalis. In general, vision compensates better for postural loss in the upper than in the lower limbs. Inco-ordination due to lesions of the cerebellum and its connections is not usually made worse by closing the eyes. It is encountered in patients with a cerebellar tumour, and the hereditary ataxias.

THE REFLEXES OF THE LIMBS AND TRUNK

THE TENDON REFLEXES

A so-called 'tendon reflex' or 'tendon-jerk' is a sharp muscular contraction evoked by suddenly stretching the muscle. The sudden stretch may be brought about by tapping the tendon, or by suddenly displacing the segment of a limb into which the muscle is inserted. The response, a muscular contraction, is most evident in the muscle stretched, but may not be confined to this muscle. The physiological basis of the tendon reflex is the myotatic reflex (p. 88) which is the reflex contraction of a muscle or part of a muscle in response to stretch. It is mediated by a reflex arc consisting of only two neurones with one synapse between them. Table 3.1 gives the principal tendon reflexes, their mode of elicitation, and their innervation. Sluggish reflexes can be reinforced by asking the patient to clench his hand.

Diminution and absence of the tendon reflexes

A tendon reflex is diminished or abolished by a lesion which interrupts the reflex arc either on its afferent or its efferent side. Muscular disease may

Table 3.1. *Principal tendon reflexes*

Reflex	Mode of elicitation	Response	Spinal segment	Peripheral nerve
Biceps-jerk	A blow upon the biceps tendon	Flexion of the elbow	Cervical 5–6	Musculocutaneous
Triceps-jerk	A blow upon the triceps tendon	Extension of the elbow	Cervical 6–7	Radial
Supinator-jerk or radial reflex	A blow upon the styloid process of the radius	Flexion of the elbow	Cervical 5–6	Radial
Flexor finger-jerk	A blow upon the palmar surface of the semiflexed fingers	Flexion of the fingers and thumb	Cervical 7–8	Median and ulnar
Knee-jerk	A blow upon the quadriceps tendon	Extension of the knee	Lumbar 2–4	Femoral
Ankle-jerk	A blow upon the tendon-calcaneus	Plantar flexion of the ankle	Sacral 1–2	Sciatic

diminish or abolish a tendon reflex by rendering the muscle incapable of responding to the nervous impulse, for example in myopathy. The afferent path may be affected alone, for example by a lesion involving the posterior spinal nerve roots, as in tabes dorsalis. The efferent path may similarly be affected alone, for example, by a lesion involving the anterior horn cells of the spinal cord as in poliomyelitis or motor neurone disease. Or both may be affected together, as when the lesion involves the peripheral nerves which carry both the sensory and the motor fibres of the reflex arc. Disorders at higher levels of the nervous system may depress the tendon reflexes; for example, neural shock, coma, and increased intracranial pressure.

The principal causes of diminution or loss of the tendon reflexes are as follows:

1. Polyneuropathy, in which the distal tendon reflexes tend to be affected before the proximal ones.

2. Diabetes mellitus, in which the knee- and ankle-jerks are often lost in the absence of other evidence of polyneuropathy.

3. The Holmes–Adie syndrome, in which some reflexes, particularly the knee- and ankle-jerks, or all of the reflexes may be diminished or lost, the cause being unknown.

4. Tabes dorsalis, in which the ankle-jerks tend to be lost before the knee-jerks and the tendon reflexes in the upper limbs are affected later than those in the lower limbs.

5. Sciatica, in which the ankle-jerk on the affected side is usually diminished or lost.

6. Cervical spondylosis, in which the diminution or loss of tendon reflexes is usually limited to the upper limbs.

7. Syringomyelia, in which the reflex abnormalities are also confined to the upper limbs, though there are in addition other signs of spinal cord involvement.

8. Poliomyelitis, with asymmetrical loss of reflexes.

9. The tendon reflexes, or some of them, are occasionally congenitally absent.

Exaggeration of the tendon reflexes

Some people naturally have tendon reflexes which are brisker than the average, and exaggeration of the tendon reflexes is often seen in states of anxiety which is reflected in increased muscular tension. Apart from this the only important cause of exaggeration of the tendon reflexes is a lesion of the upper motor neurones.

Clonus

Clonus is a rhythmical series of contractions in response to the maintenance of tension in a muscle, and is often elicitable when the tendon reflexes are exaggerated after an upper motor neurone lesion. Clonus of the quadriceps, or patellar clonus, is best elicited by a sudden downward displacement of the patella. Ankle clonus is obtained by sharply dorsiflexing the ankle. Clonus of the flexors of the fingers can sometimes be elicited in response to stretching these muscles by suddenly extending the fingers.

Hoffmann's reflex

To elicit this the patient's hand is pronated and the observer grasps the terminal phalanx of the middle finger between his forefinger and thumb. With a sharp flick the phalanx is passively flexed and suddenly released. A positive response consists of a sharp twitch of adduction and flexion of the thumb and flexion of the fingers. This reflex is physiologically identical with the flexor finger jerk, which is elicited by tapping the palmar surface of the slightly flexed finger. It is an index of muscular hypertonia rather than of an upper motor neurone lesion as such. In states of muscular hypertonia a reflex response may spread beyond the muscles stretched, as when a tap on the styloid process of the radius elicits a contraction not only of the brachioradialis but also of the long flexors of the fingers.

CUTANEOUS REFLEXES

Superficial abdominal reflexes

These are reflexes consisting of a brisk unilateral contraction of a segment of the abdominal wall in response to a cutaneous stimulus, such as a light scratch with a pin. It is convenient to elicit them at three levels on each side – just below the costal margin, at the level of the umbilicus, and at the level of the iliac fossa. The response is mainly segmental, being maximal at the level of the stimulus. Although the superficial abdominal reflexes probably utilize a short spinal reflex arc they are normally dependent upon the integrity of the corticospinal tract. Hence a corticospinal tract lesion is usually associated with diminution or loss of the superficial abdominal reflexes on the same side. If the corticospinal tract defect is slight, the reflexes may be reduced in strength but not completely abolished, those of the lowest segments being most impaired. The loss of the superficial abdominal reflexes is not always proportional to the severity of the corticospinal tract lesion. In disseminated sclerosis, for example, the reflexes may be lost early, at a stage of the disease when other signs of corticospinal tract lesions are slight. In congenital diplegia, on the other hand, they are usually brisk.

The reflex arcs of the superficial abdominal reflexes are situated in the spinal cord from the seventh to the twelfth dorsal segments. Lesions involving the arcs themselves may produce diminution or loss of the reflexes, the commonest being damage to the lower motor neurone by poliomyelitis. Little importance can be attached to diminution of the superficial abdominal reflexes in stout people, after repeated pregnancies or abdominal operations, and after middle life.

The cremasteric reflex

The cremasteric reflex is closely related to the abdominal reflexes. The appropriate stimulus is a light scratch along the inner aspect of the upper part of the thigh and the response is a contraction of the cremaster muscle, with elevation of the testicle. This reflex, the arc of which runs through the first lumbar spinal segment, is diminished or abolished by a lesion of the corticospinal tract. It is usually extremely brisk in children, in whom it may sometimes be elicited by a stimulus applied to any part of the lower limb. It is usually diminished or absent in a patient with varicocele.

The flexor plantar reflex

The flexor plantar reflex is the normal response after the first year of life to a scratch with a pin or a firm blunt object such as a key upon the sole of the foot. It consists of plantar flexion of the toes, usually associated with dorsiflexion of the foot at the ankle, contraction of the tensor fasciae latae muscle, and other variable muscular contractions. It is a spinal segmental reflex mediated by the first sacral segment of the cord, and akin to the abdominal reflexes.

The extensor plantar reflex

Babinski, a Parisian of Polish origin, in 1896 first pointed out that in the presence of a corticospinal tract lesion the normal flexor plantar reflex is replaced by an upward, extensor movement of the great toe. It has been shown that the extensor plantar reflex is not an isolated phenomenon, but is part of a more widespread nociceptive reflex flexion of the whole lower limb. The afferent focus, i.e. the region from which the reflex is most easily elicited, is the outer border of the sole. The motor focus, or minimal response, is a contraction of the inner hamstring muscles. In its fully developed form the reflex consists of flexion at all joints of the lower limb with dorsiflexion of the great toe and abduction or fanning of the other toes. 'Positive Babinski reflex' and 'upgoing toe' are alternative terms which are sometimes employed. Ther terms flexor and extensor are misleading in that an abnormal (extensor) response results from a released nociceptive reflex due to withdrawal or physiological flexion and shortening of the limb, including the great toe.

When testing the plantar reflex the stimulus should always be applied to the outer border of the sole, for an extensor response may sometimes be obtained from this region when the inner border of the sole yields a flexor response. Oppenheim's reflex, namely dorsiflexion of the great toe evoked by firm moving pressure on the skin over the tibia, is physiologically the same as Babinski's reflex, differing only in the site of the stimulus.

It is important to remember that the normal flexor response and the full extensor response are the extreme ends of a scale. With slight degrees of corticospinal tract damage the response may be a flexor one but less vigorous and ample than normal. With a somewhat greater degree of damage the great toe may move neither downwards nor upwards. These deviations from the normal are significant.

An extensor plantar reflex is often observed during sleep and deep coma from any cause, for a short time after an epileptic convulsion, and usually in the first year of life, that is, when the corticospinal tract fibres are either functionally depressed or incompletely developed. In other circumstances it nearly always indicates an organic lesion of the corticospinal tract.

The grasp reflex

The simple patterns of acceptance or rejection are observed in infants before they become conditioned responses. These, when released from inhibition by the adult by focal brain damage, become the grasp reflex and avoiding responses. 'Frontal lobe' grasping and 'parietal lobe' avoiding are mediated through the basal ganglia.

The grasp reflex of the hand consists of tonic flexion of the thumb and fingers in respose to a moving tactile stimulus, such as the observer's fingers passing across the patient's palm and between his thumb and index finger. Once it is initiated the observer's attempt to withdraw his fingers only intensifies the patient's grasp. In the foot a similar moving stimulus applied to the plantar aspect of the toes causes them to flex and remain in tonic flexion – the foot grasp reflex.

Other primitive reflexes which may be present include sucking and pouting. In the sucking reflex, tactile contact with the lips provokes contractions of the muscles of the lips, tongue, and jaw which are involved in sucking. If the reflex is unilateral and associated with a grasp reflex on the same side it is called the 'rooting' reflex. A tap on the centre of the closed lips may provoke the type of pouting which is also called the 'snout' reflex.

Palmomental reflex

This reflex is elicited if the examiner scratches or strokes the palm of the patient there is a twitch of the mentalis muscle near the angle of the chin. This occurs with an upper motor neurone lesion above the level of the facial nucleus on the opposite side.

The bulbocavernous and anal reflexes

The bulbocavernosus reflex consists of contraction of the bulbocavernosus muscle which can be detected by palpation in response to squeezing the glans penis. The spinal segments concerned are sacral 2, 3, and 4. The anal reflex consists of contraction of the external sphincter ani in response to a scratch upon the skin in the perianal region. The spinal segments concerned are sacral 4 and 5. These reflexes may be abolished in tabes and in lesions of the conus medullaris and the cauda equina.

SENSATION

The neurologist is concerned with sensation primarily for diagnostic purposes. The contribution which sensory examination may make to diagnosis depends upon:

1. The observation that certain forms of sensation are appreciated less than normally, or not at all.

2. The demarcation of the area over which impairment of sensation is found.

3. The observation that apart from, or in addition to, impairment of sensation, the response to a sensory stimulus may be in other respects abnormal. The modes of sensibility which are tested are therefore those which are found to be of value for diagnostic purposes. They are:

(i) *Light touch,* such as a touch with a wisp of cotton wool or a camel's-hair brush.

(ii) *Pressure touch,* which may be investigated by pressing with a blunt object such as the unsharpened end of a pencil.

(iii) *Localization of touch* implies the ability of the patient in some way to identify the spot touched.

(iv) *Superficial pain* is evoked by a painful stimulus such as the prick of a pin.

(v) *Pressure pain* is the pain evoked by deep pressure upon a muscle or by squeezing a tendon.

(vi) *Temperature* comprises the appreciation of hot and cold stimuli.

(vii) *Postural sensibility* or sense of position implies the ability to describe or imitate on the opposite side of the body with the eyes closed the position in which a limb has been placed.

(viii) *Passive movement* is normally appreciated when a segment of a limb is passively moved at a joint.

(ix) *Vibration* is a tingling sensation felt when a vibrating tuning fork is applied to the skin, especially over an underlying bone.

(x) *Tactile discrimination* is the ability to recognize as double two compass points simultaneously applied to the skin.

(xi) *Appreciation of form* is tested by asking the patient, with his eyes closed, to recognize common objects placed in his hand.

Some of the sensory tests employed by the neurologist involve simple sensory stimuli, but others are concerned with more complex perceptual experiences. The application and interpretation of these tests are considered below.

Anatomy and physiology

The sensory fibres in the peripheral nerves are the axons of the ganglion cells of the spinal dorsal root ganglia or the corresponding ganglia of the sensory cranial nerves. Sensory fibres in the peripheral nerves vary in size and in the rate at which they conduct nervous impulses. Touch and pressure impulses are probably conducted by the largest. The centripetal fibres of the spinal dorsal root ganglion cells enter the spinal cord, within which considerable segregation of the sensory pathways occurs. After entering the spinal cord the incoming fibres lie on the medial side of the apex of the posterior horn of grey matter, whence three groups of ascending fibres can be recognized (see Fig. 3.5).

1. The fibres which convey impulses concerned with the appreciation of posture and passive movement and of the vibration of a tuning fork pass upwards in the posterior columns of the same side, moving gradually towards the middle line as they do so, so that those derived from the lower limb occupy the fasciculus gracilis (column of Goll) and those from the upper limb are found in the fasciculus cuneatus (column of Burdach), and both terminate in the medulla in the nuclei gracilis and cuneatus (Fig. 3.6). It is probable that some fibres concerned with the sensation of light touch also pass up in the posterior column.

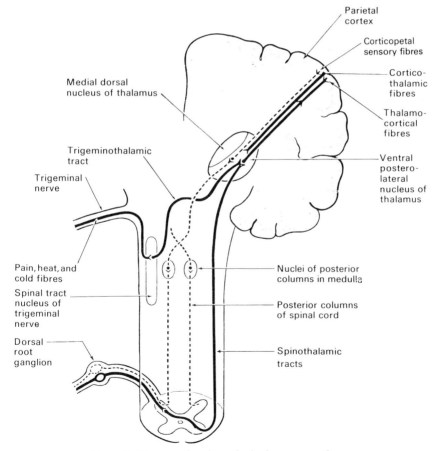

Fig. 3.6. Diagram showing principal sensory pathways.

2. The remaining fibres concerned in the appreciation of light touch also pass up in the posterior column of the same side for a considerable distance, but ultimately enter the posterior horn of grey matter round the cells in which they terminate. From these cells further fibres take origin and cross the middle line in the grey and anterior white commissures to reach the opposite anterior column. There they turn upwards to constitute the ventral spinothalamic tract (Figs. 3.5 and 3.6).

3. The fibres which conduct impulses concerned with the appreciation of pain, heat, and cold ascend in the spinal cord for the shortest distance before terminating among the cells of the posterior horn. These distances range from three to five segments in the lowest part of the cord to one to two segments in the upper cervical region. From the cells of the posterior horn of grey matter fibres of the second relay take origin and, crossing the middle line like those of the previous group, enter the anterolateral column more posteriorly, and turning upwards constitute the dorsal spinothalamic tract. There is considerable intermingling of the fibres for pain, heat, and cold in this tract, but on the whole those which underlie pain lie dorsal to those concerned with temperature. Some fibres also run to the central reticular formation.

Within the brainstem some reorganization of the sensory pathways occurs. The fibres of the posterior columns of the spinal cord have already been traced to their termination in the nuclei gracilis and cuneatus in the posterior part of the medulla. From these nuclei the second fibres of this sensory path take origin and cross to the opposite side of the sensory decussation, after which they occupy a position on either side of the middle line as the medial lemniscus, and so pass upwards through the brainstem to reach the optic thalamus. The medial lemniscus is joined in the pons by fibres from the principal sensory nucleus of the trigeminal nerve which are concerned in the appreciation of light touch, pressure, and postural sensibility within the trigeminal area.

It will be recalled that the fibres from the trigeminal nerve concerned with the appreciation of pain, heat, and cold enter the spinal tract and nucleus of that nerve. From this nucleus relay fibres cross the middle line to the opposite side of the medulla as the trigeminothalamic tract, which comes to be associated with the spinothalamic tract in the pons (Fig. 3.6). All these sensory pathways pass upwards through the tegmentum of the pons and midbrain to the thalamus. Here they end in the posterior part of the ventral nucleus (Fig. 3.6). There is evidence that the thalamus is the end-station for impulses concerned with the qualitative element in the appreciation of pain, heat, and cold, and the affective element, that is the pleasant or unpleasant character, of other forms of stimuli.

From the posterior part of the ventral nucleus of the thalamus a sensory pathway runs through the white matter of the corona radiata to the cerebral cortex of the postcentral gyrus (Fig. 3.7), and also to part of the precentral gyrus. The sensory functions of the cortex concern the appreciation of posture and passive movement on the opposite side of the body, the recognition of light

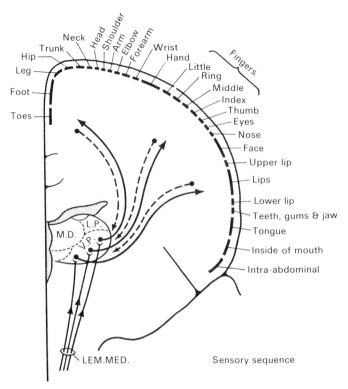

Fig. 3.7. Somatic sensation. Cross-section of the left hemisphere along the plane of the postcentral gyrus. The afferent pathway for discriminative somatic sensation is indicated by the unbroken lines coming up, through the medial lemniscus, to the postcentral gyrus.

touch and its accurate localization, tactile discrimination, the discrimination of different degrees of heat and cold and the appreciation of size, shape, form, roughness, and texture.

Recent evidence suggests that pain perception is modulated by the peptide substance P in the substantia gelatinosa and enkephalins at opiate receptors in the brainstem.

SENSORY DISTURBANCES IN RELATION TO THE SITE OF THE LESION

The diagnostic value of sensory examination depends upon the knowledge of how sensation is likely to be disturbed both qualitatively and in distribution in relation to the site of the lesion. We shall now consider, therefore, the characteristics of sensory disturbances resulting from lesions at different anatomical levels.

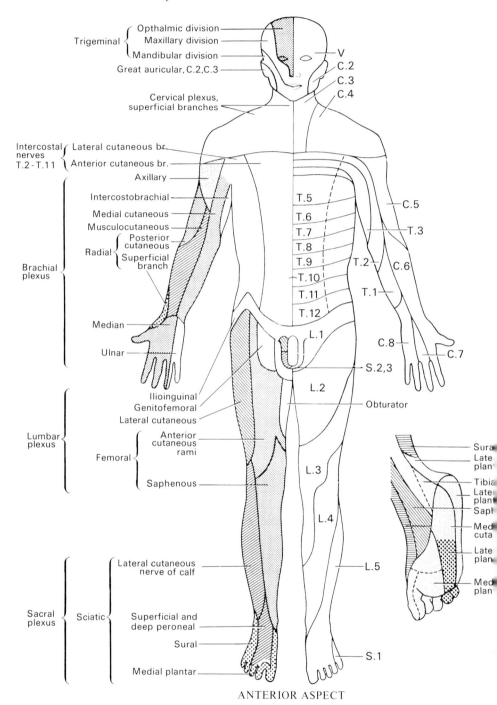

Trigeminal
- Opthalmic division
- Maxillary division
- Mandibular division

Great auricular, C.2,C.3

V
C.2
C.3
C.4

Cervical plexus, superficial branches

Intercostal nerves T.2-T.11
- Lateral cutaneous br.
- Anterior cutaneous br.

Axillary

Intercostobrachial
Medial cutaneous
Musculocutaneous

Radial
- Posterior cutaneous
- Superficial branch

Brachial plexus

Median

Ulnar

Ilioinguinal
Genitofemoral
Lateral cutaneous

Lumbar plexus

Femoral
- Anterior cutaneous rami
- Saphenous

Sacral plexus

Sciatic
- Lateral cutaneous nerve of calf
- Superficial and deep peroneal
- Sural
- Medial plantar

T.5
T.6
T.7
T.8
T.9
T.10
T.11
T.12
L.1

C.5
T.3
T.2
C.6
T.1
L.2
Obturator
L.3
L.4
C.8
C.7
S.2,3
L.5
S.1

Sura
Late plan
Tibia
Late plant
Saph
Med cuta
Late plan
Med plan

ANTERIOR ASPECT

Fig. 3.8. (a) Cutaneous areas of distribution of spinal segments and the peripheral nerves.

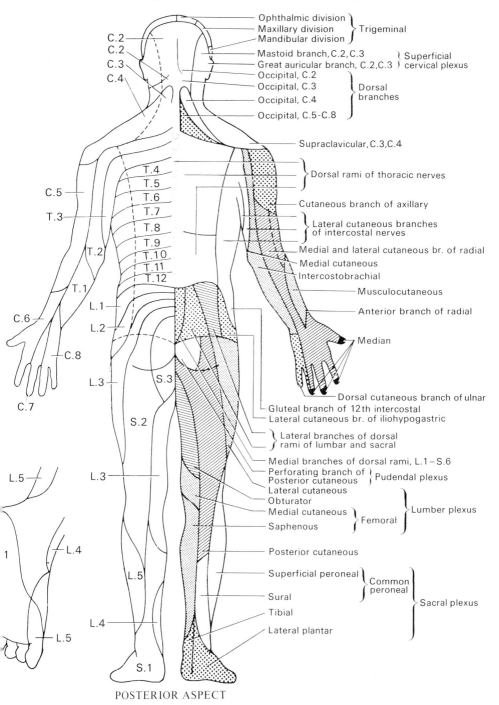

POSTERIOR ASPECT

b) Cutaneous areas of distribution of spinal segments and the peripheral nerves.

Lesions of peripheral nerves

Lesions of individual peripheral nerves cause sensory symptoms which have a distribution corresponding to the cutaneous area exclusively supplied by the nerve affected (see 3.8 (a) and (b)). In the case of incomplete lesions, which are commonly encountered in medical neurology, dysaesthesiae such as numbness and tingling are commonly experienced in the distribution of the affected nerve. All forms of cutaneous sensibility are impaired, and pin-prick may have a diffusely unpleasant character, though the threshold for this stimulus is raised: this is termed hyperpathia. The more distal the lesion the less likely is appreciation of passive movement to be affected. Unless the nerve affected is purely sensory, sensory symptoms will be accompanied by those of a lower motor neurone lesion in the muscles innervated by that nerve.

When the peripheral nerves are diffusely affected in polyneuritis, all forms of sensibility are diffusely impaired in the distal parts of the limb – 'glove and stocking anaesthesia'. On moving a stimulus upwards from the periphery the transition from abnormal to normal sensation is a gradual one. Hyperpathia of both skin and muscles is common.

Lesions of spinal nerve roots

Each spinal dorsal nerve root innervates a certain limited area of skin, known as a spinal segmental area or dermatome, as well as certain deeper structures, namely bones, joints and muscles. The characteristic of a root lesion therefore is that its symptoms are referred to the anatomical area of its distribution (Fig. 3.8 (a) and (b)). The positive symptom of root irritation is the root pain, usually lancinating in character and possessing the characteristic distribution of the affected root, and frequently made worse by coughing and sneezing and by changes in the position of the relevant area of the spine. The affected dermatome may be hyperaesthetic and hyperalgesic or anaesthetic and analgesic. Appreciation of passive movement is usually unimpaired after a single root lesion.

Lesions of the spinal cord

Several types of sensory disturbance are encountered as the result of lesions of the spinal cord. A lesion limited to one-half of the spinal cord causes *Brown-Séquard's syndrome*. (Brown-Séquard was born in Mauritius and was appointed physician to the National Hospital, Queen Square, in 1860. He later held a chair at Harvard and finally succeeded Claude Bernard in Paris.) In the syndrome bearing his name destruction of the posterior columns causes loss of appreciation of posture and passive movement of the joints, of the vibration of a tuning fork, and of tactile discrimination below the level of the lesion. Destruction of the lateral spinothalamic tract causes analgesia and thermo-anaesthesia on the opposite side of the body. Since fibres entering this tract do not cross the cord for several segments, the upper level of this sensory loss is likely to be a few segments below the level of the lesion. Conversely, the fibres entering the cord just below the lesion may be caught before they cross, causing a narrow zone of similar analgesia and thermo-anaesthesia immediately below the lesion on the same side. Owing to the double route of fibres for light touch and tactile localization, partly crossed and partly uncrossed, there is rarely any loss of these forms of sensibility after a unilateral lesion of the cord. Hemisection of the cord of course interrupts descending as well as ascending tracts, and the clinical picture therefore includes the signs of a corticospinal tract defect below the lesion, and destruction of the anterior horn causes a lower motor neurone lesion with a segmental distribution corresponding to the level of the lesion.

Degeneration of the posterior columns alone, such as occurs in *tabes dorsalis* and *subacute combined degeneration*, leads to loss of appreciation of posture, passive movement, tactile discrimination and vibration below the level of the lesion. Damage to one fasciculus cuneatus above the level of the cervical enlargement such as sometimes occurs in *multiple sclerosis* causes these symptoms in the ipsilateral upper limb. A lesion of one spinothalamic tract due either to disease or to surgical division causes loss of appreciation of pain, heat and cold on the opposite side of the body, with an upper level two or three segments below that at which the lesion has occurred.

A lesion limited to the central part of the spinal cord causes the characteristic '*dissociated sensory loss*' in which appreciation of pain, heat and cold is lost bilaterally over the dermatomes, sensory fibres from which are decussating at the level of the lesion, all other forms of sensation being preserved. This is the usual type of sensory loss encountered in syringomyelia.

Lesions of the brainstem

Lesions involving the lateral part of the tegmentum of the brainstem, such as thrombosis of the posterior inferior cerebellar artery, are likely to cause hemianalgesia and thermo-anaesthesia on the opposite side of the body, leaving postural sensibility and appreciation of passive movement and tactile discrimination intact. When the lesion is situated in the medulla, below the point at which the spinothalamic tract has been joined by the trigeminothalamic tract, analgesia and thermo-anaesthesia involve the opposite side of the body below the face only, while similar sensory loss is likely to occur on the face of the side of the lesion, owing to damage to the spinal tract and nucleus of the trigeminal nerve. Deeply seated lesions may involve the medial lemniscus without the spinothalamic tract, thus producing loss of postural sensibility, of appreciation of passive movement and of tactile discrimination on one or both sides of the body, but leaving appreciation of pain, heat, and cold unimpaired. Massive lesions, such as tumours, are likely to involve all forms of sensibility, though often to a varying extent.

Lesions of the thalamus

A severe and extensive lesion of the thalamus may cause gross impairment of all forms of sensibility on the opposite side of the body, as the result of damage to the ventral nuclei. Less severe lesions may cause less serious sensory disturbance, but appreciation of posture and passive movement usually suffer severely. The threshold for pain may be normal, but is frequently raised, even when painful stimuli cause an exaggerated response. This is known as *thalamic over-reaction*. It is generally agreed that damage to the lateral nucleus is necessary for this to occur. Pain of central origin which may be extremely severe may be referred to the opposite side of the body. Although the threshold to sensory stimuli is usually raised on the affected half of the body, such stimuli when they are effective excite sensations of a peculiarly unpleasant character – a form of hyperpathia. Extremes of heat and cold similarly excite a feeling of great discomfort on the affected side, and the same is true of such stimuli as scraping, tickling, and a vibrating tuning fork. Thalamic over-reaction is most often seen after vascular lesions.

Lesions of the sensory cortex

An epileptic discharging lesion of the sensory cortex usually causes a feeling of numbness or tingling in the corresponding area of the body. Sometimes this part feels as though it has disappeared. Destructive lesions cause loss of those sensory modalities which are mediated by the cortex, namely appreciation of light touch and its localization, the discrimination of two compass points, of posture and passive movement, and of size, shape and form in three dimensions. The power of discrimination of sensory stimuli, including their intensity, is also impaired. The inability to recognize an object by feeling it, without seeing it, is called *astereognosis*. One striking feature of a lesion of the sensory cortex is the extreme variability of the patient's response to sensory stimuli, and the difficulty or impossibility of obtaining a threshold. Owing to the wide extent of the sensory cortex a lesion of it is likely to cause sensory loss of the cortical type over only a limited part of the opposite side of the body. Such loss is likely to be chiefly distal in either the upper or the lower limb according to the site of the lesion.

In addition to testing for astereognosis, other aspects of cortical sensory function should be investigated by tests for proposagnosia (the recognition of faces of famous people) and other visuospatial tests. In these the patient may be asked to draw a house, a bicycle, a cross, a star, and to bisect a line. They may also be asked to place numbers on a clock face, or place major towns on a map of their country.

Sensory inattention

Sensory inattention, extinction, or suppression is a symptom of a lesion of the parietal lobe. A sensation is experienced when light touch or pin-prick is applied to the opposite side of the body alone, but not when the corresponding spot on the side of the lesion is simultaneously stimulated. The same phenomenon demonstrated by stimuli in opposite halves of the visual field is known as visual inattention and this group of disturbances has been called simultanagnosia.

Hysterical sensory loss

We cannot at present attribute hysterical sensory loss to any localized cerebral lesion, but it is no doubt the outcome of a disorder of cerebral function which we do not at present understand. The characteristic features of hysterical sensory loss are that its distribution corresponds to the patient's idea of a part of the body rather than to the anatomical supply of any part of the nervous system, that hysterical anaesthesia and analgesia are found in areas with sharp lines of demarcation from adjacent normal sensibility, that they tend to vary in response to suggestions made by the examiner, and that they do not in themselves lead to the disability which results from corresponding sensory loss of organic origin; for example, a patient with hysterical loss of appreciation of posture and passive movement in a limb may be able to find it without difficulty with the eyes closed and, if it is not paralysed, to use it without inco-ordination.

TROPHIC LESIONS

Trophic lesions are lesions of tissues other than the muscles – chiefly the skin and joints – which occur as a direct or indirect result of lesions of the nervous system. Their pathogenesis is not completely understood, but the chief causal factor seems to be analgesia which not only allows injuries to the skin and joints to pass unnoticed, but is associated with an impairment of the normal tissue reactions to injury.

The skin

The commonest cause of trophic lesions of the skin in the upper limb is syringomyelia. The syringomyelic patient often fails to notice cuts and burns, which may become acutely infected or lead to ulceration. Similar lesions may occur after damage to a peripheral nerve, and are sometimes seen in cases of compression of the median nerve in the carpal tunnel. Swelling of the hand sometimes occurs in hemiplegia and in other conditions causing prolonged immobility.

In the lower limbs the chief causes of trophic lesions of the skin are tabes dorsalis, congenital malformations of the lumbosacral region of the spinal cord such as those which may be associated with spina bifida occulta, and diabetes mellitus. The commonest such lesion is a perforating ulcer, which begins as a localized thickening of the epidermis on the sole, usually overlying the head of one of the metatarsals. The centre of this breaks down into a chronic ulcer, which carries infection to the underlying tissues, including sometimes the bones and joints. As in the upper limb, trophic skin lesions may also follow nerve injury, in this case of the sciatic nerve. Cyanosis and a tendency to chilblains may occur in the lower limbs after poliomyelitis.

The joints

Arthropathy – Charcot's joint – is seen chiefly in syringomyelia, tabes dorsalis, and diabetes mellitus. An arthropathic joint is usually painless and swollen, the swelling being due either to osteophyte formation or effusion or both. In advanced cases there is pathological mobility of the joint and crepitus. X-rays show severe erosion of the articular surfaces, often with much proliferation of osteophytes from the joint margins. Any joint may be the site of arthropathy: in syringomyelia those of the upper limb are most affected, in tabes dorsalis and diabetes mellitus those of the lower limb. Some syringomyelics show arthropathy of the cervical spine, while the lower dorsal and lumbar spine suffers most in tabes dorsalis, and sometimes in diabetes mellitus.

A joint lesion which may sometimes be reasonably regarded as arthropathic is the 'frozen shoulder', the chief causes of which are pain in the neighbourhood of the joint and immobilization. The former is the chief factor when frozen shoulder complicates cervical spondylosis, the latter when it occurs in a patient with hemiplegia or Parkinsonism. It may sometimes be associated with referred pain of cardiac origin. Pain and swelling of the joints on the affected side are sometimes a troublesome complication of hemiplegia.

STANDING AND WALKING

Anatomy and physiology

Normal standing requires sufficient power in the muscles of the lower limbs and trunk to maintain the body erect, normal postural sensibility to convey information concerning their position, normal impulses from the labyrinth to convey information concerning the position of the body in space and in relation to gravity, a central co-ordinating mechanism, the chief part in which is played by the vermis of the cerebellum, and, finally, the activity of higher centres concerned in the willed maintenance of posture. Walking employs the same neuromuscular mechanisms, with the addition of those required for the appropriate movements of the lower limbs. It follows that standing and walking will be disordered by lesions which interfere with the mechanisms concerned at any point.

Disorders of standing

A patient with severe weakness of the lower limbs whether due to upper or lower motor neurone lesions or a disorder of the muscles themselves will be unable to stand. A severe lesion of the cerebellum, especially if it involves the vermis, also may make standing impossible. Here the difficulty arises from the swaying movements of the trunk which make it impossible to maintain the erect position. In milder cases of cerebellar lesion the patient may be able to stand with the feet widely separated but not when they are together. A somewhat similar effect is produced by severe vertigo, when the patient tends to reel or sway, but in such cases the posture of the body as a whole is affected, whereas in cerebellar disease the defect is equally noticeable in the adjustment of the parts to one another. Severe loss of postural sensibility in the lower limbs also interferes with standing, but except in cases in which the loss develops very acutely the patient can usually stand if he compensates for his sensory deficit by vision. He is, however, unable to stand with the eyes closed. This point may be brought out by asking him to stand with the feet together and the eyes open and then to close the eyes, when he will sway – *Romberg's sign.* Inability to stand due to hysteria is distinguished by the absence of any adequate organic cause for the difficulty and by the fact that whereas the patient who has difficulty in standing owing to organic disease usually does his best to help those who are supporting him, the hysterical patient tends to throw himself about in such a way as to add to their difficulties. Inability to stand is sometimes known as astasia.

Disorders of walking

Most patients with hemiplegia are able to walk, but walking is impeded by the stiffness of the affected lower limb and the plantar flexion of the foot produced by the spastic calf muscles. The patient seeks to overcome this difficulty by circumducting the leg at the hip while swinging it forward. There is a tendency for the toe to catch the ground and the sole of the shoe becomes worn at the tip. The gait in paraplegia or spastic diplegia is the result of the bilateral extensor spasticity and weakness with the addition that spasm of the adductors of the hips tends to make it difficult to separate the legs and in congenital diplegia the adductor spasm may be so severe as to lead to the legs crossing in front of one another, the so-called 'scissor gait'.

In parkinsonism the generalized muscular rigidity and slowness of movement cause a slow shuffling gait and the flexed attitude of the trunk may cause the patient to exhibit propulsion, a tendency to move forwards which he finds difficult to control. At times in severe cases he may be temporarily immobilized. Normal arm-swinging is lost in parkinsonism, a conspicuous feature when the symptoms are unilateral.

The *marche à petits pas* is a shuffling gait consisting of very small steps and seen characteristically in double hemiplegia due to cerebral vascular disease.

An ataxic gait may be the result of cerebellar disease, due to a combination of inco-ordination of movements of the individual lower limbs and unsteady balancing of the trunk. In disseminated sclerosis there is often a combination of spastic weakness with ataxia. In tabes dorsalis the ataxia is due mainly to loss of postural sensibility in the lower limbs. The gait is broad-based, the feet are lifted too high and then brought down in a stamping fashion.

'Steppage gait' is the term applied to the gait which results from foot-drop caused by lesions of the lower motor neurones to the peronei and tibialis anterior, or diseases of these muscles themselves. The commonest causes are polyneuritis and the myopathies. The feet are lifted high in order to clear the ground and when lifted droop flaccidly at the ankles under the influence of gravity. A waddling gait associated with lordosis of the lumbar spine is characteristic of the myopathies and may be associated with a steppage gait.

Hysterical gaits are varied and bizarre in character and do not resemble any kind of abnormal gait produced by organic nervous disease.

AUTONOMIC NERVOUS FUNCTION

It is now possible to test autonomic function in a variety of different organs and these tests throw some light on the site of involvement of autonomic pathways (Figs. 3.9 and 3.10).

In testing pupils use is made of Cannon's law of denervation of supersensitivity. An effector organ after peripheral or postganglionic denervation becomes hypersensitive to its particular transmitter. The sympathetic denervated pupil, in for example Horner's syndrome, dilates to 1 per cent noradrena-

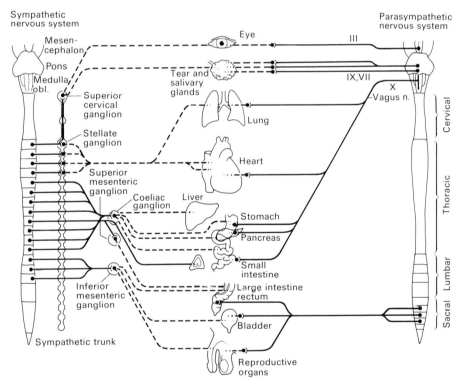

Fig. 3.9. Peripheral autonomic nervous system. The sympathetic innervation of vessels, sweat glands, and piloerector muscles is not shown. Solid lines, preganglionic axons; dashed lines, postganglionic axons.

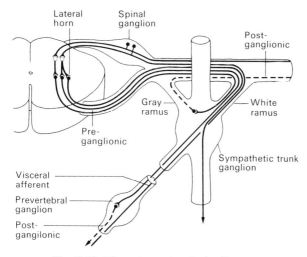

Fig. 3.10. The autonomic spinal reflex arc.

line which does not affect a normal pupil. The normal pupil will, however, respond to cocaine which blocks the reuptake of noradrenaline and so potentiates its effect. With a complete sympathetic lesion, especially if postganglionic, no transmitter is released and so cocaine is without effect. 1 per cent hydroxy-amphetamine which releases noradrenaline from normal sympathetic endings will not cause any dilatation in the sympathetically denervated pupils. A similar principle applies to the parasympathetic innervation of the pupils. The normal pupil will not constrict in response to ocular instillation of 2.5 per cent methacholine but the denervated pupil will, as in Adie's syndrome, and constricts promptly. Tear secretion may be tested by Schirmer's test by which one end of a strip of filter paper is inserted into the lower end of the conjunctival sac and the length of the moistened area is measured.

Symptoms which suggest the probability of autonomic defects are postural hypotension, loss of sweating, or bladder or sphincter disturbances. The investigation of postural hypotension requires the assessment of both cardiac and peripheral autonomic function. The sympathetic control of the heart can be tested by the blood pressure and pulse rise on emotional stress (mental artithmetic) or painful stimuli (the ice-cold water pressor test) or by supersensitivity to infusion of isoprenaline. The basic defect in peripheral sympathetic activity which leads to postural hypotension is a loss of sympathetic vasoconstriction in muscle and splanchnic blood vessels leading to pooling of blood in the extremities. The useful overall test of sympathetic function, albeit a cholinergic function, is that of the sweat response throughout the body in response to raising central body temperature by a heat cradle. If absent in patients with postural hypotension it can be assumed that the postural hypotension is the result of a sympathetic efferent lesion. Normal cardiac parasympathetic control of the heart can be deduced by the presence of a normal sinus arrhythmia on deep breathing. If an arterial pressure recording can be taken then it is simple to test cardiac and peripheral cardiovascular responses by means of the Valsalva manoeuvre in which there is an obstruction to venous return by a rise of intrathoracic pressure caused by blowing up a column of mercury. The blood pressure falls initially but as a result of the compensatory tachycardia and peripheral sympathetic vasoconstriction recovery of blood pressure occurs after about 5 seconds. At the end of 10 seconds blowing, the positive intrathoracic pressure is released and there is an overshoot of blood pressure which stimulates the carotid baroreceptors, thus leading to vagally induced bradycardia and reduction of peripheral and splanchnic sympathetic vascular tone, the homeostatic mechanisms (Fig. 3.11).

Cutaneous autonomic responses can be tested by means of an intracutaneous injection of 1:1000 histamine. The full triple response consists of a central wheal and red areola and an extensive erythematous flare. The flare depends on the axon reflex in sensory fibres by antidromic transmission and is absent in the congenital autonomic disorder familial dysautonomia, as well as in peripheral neuropathies with involvement of sympathetic fibres.

Partial or complete failure of the autonomic system may be the result of diseases affecting different levels of the autonomic nervous system, from the

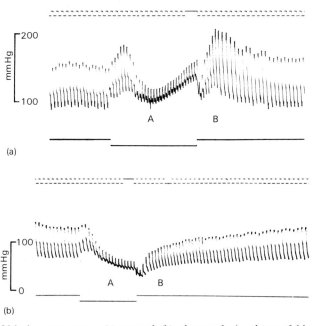

Fig. 3.11. Valsalva manoeuvre (a) normal (b) abnormal. A: phase of blood-pressure fall; B: phase of blood-pressure overshoot. Upper trace: time in seconds; Lower trace: event marker, indicates raised thoracic pressure.

hypothalamus to the periphery, though peripheral involvement is commoner. Rarely the autonomic neuropathy has an acute or subacute onset, possibly viral in nature but more often it is chronic, some of the commoner causes being diabetes, nutritional deficiencies associated with alcoholism, a distant carcinoma, and amyloid. Autonomic fibres which are unmyelinated are often involved as part of the more generalized neuropathy affecting motor and sensory fibres as in the Guillain–Barré syndrome (see p. 421). Autonomic failure may also be the result of interruption of autonomic reflex arcs more centrally in a neuronal degeneration which affects the brainstem pigmented nuclei, particularly the vagal nuclei, and also the intermediolateral columns, in the syndrome of progressive autonomic failure, also known as idiopathic orthostatic hypotension. In this syndrome the predominant symptoms are due to defective control of blood pressure though detailed testing reveals more widespread abnormalities. Progressive autonomic failure may also be part of the disturbance of basal ganglia and brainstem function called multiple system atrophy (the Shy–Drager syndrome). Autonomic failure also occurs in association with Parkinson's disease. Rarely it also results from a central lesion in the genetically determined disease congenital insensitivity to pain and in the disorder of familial dysautonomia in children, in which though nerve biopsy has shown a loss of peripheral unmyelinated fibres, there are central defects in addition.

The management of the main disabling symptom of autonomic failure, postural hypotension, is difficult. Two principles used are increasing the extracellular fluid volume by head-up tilt at night and increasing the response of partially denervated sympathetic endings to small amounts of noradrenaline which can still be released. This can be achieved by means of fludrocortisone in a small dose. In a larger dose fludrocortisone will of course also increase extracellular fluid volume.

ANATOMY OF BLADDER AND SEXUAL FUNCTION

The bladder wall consists mainly of the unstriated detrusor muscle innervated by parasympathetic nerves (S2–4 segments) via the nervi erigenti, stimulation of which also relaxes the internal sphincter (Fig. 3.12). Afferent fibres also travel with these nerves and record the degree of bladder distension and at a certain level initiate rhythmical contractions of the bladder wall. Initiation of normal micturition requires intact pathways from the superior frontal gyrus, the midbrain, and the pons. Descending pathways lie in the lateral columns of the spinal cord. Relaxation of the voluntary external sphincter, which consists of striped muscle innervated by the pudendal nerve, precedes relaxation of the involuntary internal sphincter and the act of micturition.

Bladder function is tested by cystometrography in which the intravesical pressure is raised slowly by the infusion of sterile saline. The intravesical pressure is recorded during spontaneous bladder contraction and also during

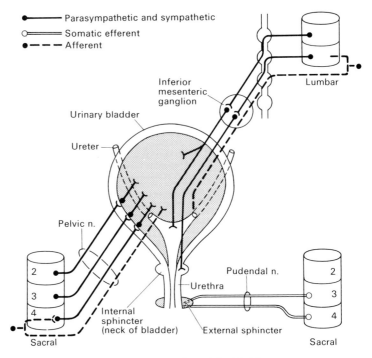

Fig. 3.12. Innervation of the bladder.

voluntary attempts at micturition during which the flow rates and function of the internal and external sphincter can be assessed.

The function of the bladder and urethral sphincter is closely related to the control of sexual function in the male. The parasympathetic nerves produce erection and later ejaculation and the sympathetic pathways from L2 and 3 are responsible for emission of semen into the urethra. Bladder dysfunction is considered further on pages 360, 385, and 488.

If impotence is associated with urinary symptoms there should be suspicion of involvement of the autonomic fibres as in diabetes, tabes dorsalis, or autonomic neuropathy. Impotence due to posterior nerve root involvement occurs in cauda equina lesions. The pathways concerning sexual and bladder function ascend and descend in the lateral column of the spinal cord and may be involved in traumatic paraplegia, disseminated sclerosis, tabes dorsalis, syringomyelia, Freidreich's ataxia, and spinal cord tumours. Lesions of the hypothalamus and hypophyseal region may cause impotence and particularly important in this respect is the prolactinoma. There may not be other obvious features to suggest an endocrine disturbance. Finally lesions of the temporal lobe may cause impotence, for example following temporal lobectomy for epilepsy or very rarely, if irritative, hypersexuality.

REFERENCES

Bannister, R. (ed.) (1983). *Autonomic failure.* Oxford University Press.

Critchley, M. (1953). *The parietal lobes.* Arnold, London.

Davidoff, R.A. (1978). Pharmacology of spasticity. *Neurology, Minneap.* **28** Suppl., 46–51.

Gijn, J. Van (1975). Babinski response; stimulus and effector. *J. Neurol. Neurosurg. Psychiat.* **38**, 180–6.

Head, H. (1920). *Studies in neurology,* Vols. 1 and 2. Oxford University Press, London.

Lance, J.W. and McLeod, J.G. (1981). *A physiological approach to clinical neurology,* 3rd edn. Butterworth, London.

Marsden, C.D., Merton, P.A., and Morton, H.B. (1976). Servoaction in the human thumb. *J. Physiol., Lond.* **257**, 1–44.

Matthews, P.B.C. (1972). *Mammalian muscle receptors and their central actions.* Arnold, London.

Walshe, F.M.R. (1942). The anatomy and physiology of cutaneous sensibility. A critical review. *Brain* **65**, 48–112.

Williams, A., Goodenberger, D., and Calne, D.B. (1978). Palatal myoclonus following herpes zoster ameliorated by 5-hydroxytryptophan and carbidopa. *Neurology, Minneap.* **28**, 358–9.

Young, R.R. and Delwaide, P.J. (1981). Drug therapy: spasticity. *New Engl. J. Med.* **304**, 28–33, 96–9.

4 Speech and its disorders

The nature of speech

Speech is a mode of communication by means of sounds which stand for something which may be called their meaning. The object of communication may be, amongst other things, to convey an idea, a feeling, or a command. Speech therefore involves in its expressive aspect the production of the appropriate movements of the lips, tongue, palate, vocal cords, and respiratory muscles to cause the appropriate sounds. In its receptive aspect it implies the auditory discrimination of these sounds. Between the two, as it were, exist the psychological functions concerned with the meanings of the sounds heard or uttered. Speech having been acquired by the individual, reading and writing involve a superstructure whereby words are represented by means of visual symbols.

Physiological and anatomical considerations

At the psychological level the meaning of a written or a spoken word is the outcome of the association of the visual or auditory sensations which constitute the word with other forms of sensation or ideas in the past. For example, initially the word dog acquires its meaning by the association of the sounds of which it is composed with the visual sensations involved in seeing dogs when speech is being learned. At the physiological and anatomical levels the basis of such meanings is presumably a linkage of neurones. Visual impulses reach the cerebral cortex in the regions of the calcarine sulcus of the occipital lobes (Fig. 4.1); auditory impulses in the posterior part of the superior temporal gyri (Wernicke's area). Kinaesthetic impulses from the muscles of articulation terminate in the lower half of the postcentral gyrus. It is to be expected therefore that the anatomical linkages of neurones upon which verbal meanings depend will join together these regions of the cerebral cortex. It has been shown that there is in fact an anatomical difference between the dominant and non-dominant hemispheres, namely a larger planum temporale on the superior surface of the temporal lobe on the dominant side.

Handedness

More precise evidence of cerebral dominance for language has been provided by the effect of unilateral electroconvulsive therapy and also from pre-operative intracarotid amylobarbitone used to establish the dominant hemisphere for speech. About 95 per cent of persons are right-handed, and in these the left cerebral hemisphere plays the predominant role in speech, and the associational

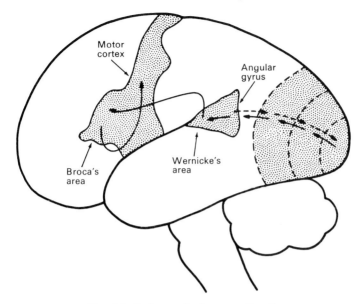

Fig. 4.1. Pathways for language function.

paths just described are situated in the left hemisphere in right-handed people. The posterior half of the left cerebral hemisphere in right-handed people is thus the site of the neural organization which underlies the comprehension of heard and written speech. By comparison nearly 60 per cent of left handers, without any evidence of left hemisphere damage, show speech representation on the left, 20 per cent on the right and 20 per cent bilaterally. In a group of left-handed patients with evidence of left hemisphere damage as opposed to 'genetic' left handedness, speech function was much less often in the left hemisphere. Women appear to have less functional brain asymmetry, including language specialization, than men.

Articulation involves movements of the jaw, lips, tongue, palate, larynx, and respiratory muscles which are represented in the lowest part of the precentral gyrus (Broca's area). If meanings are to gain articulate expression, the posterior half of the left cerebral hemisphere must therefore be linked to the lowest part of the precentral gyrus. An important part in this association is played by the external capsule, the tracts of white matter lying outside the lentiform nucleus. Speech, however, requires co-ordinate bilateral movements of the muscles of articulation, and this co-ordination is effected by fibres passing from the lower part of the left frontal lobe to the corresponding region of the right hemisphere by the corpus callosum. From the lower part of the precentral gyri the motor fibres concerned in articulation pass downwards in the corticospinal tracts to end in the relevant motor nuclei and spinal anterior horn cells. As in the case of other motor activities, the cerebellum exercises a co-ordinating and regulating influence upon articulation.

The distinction between dysphasia and dysarthria

It is now possible to draw a distinction between dysphasia and dysarthria. Dysphasia is the term applied to a disorder of the symbolic function of speech; that is, the comprehension and expression of meanings by means of words. Dysarthria is a disorder of articulation, the motor function whereby words, having been formulated, are converted into sounds. It therefore does not involve any disturbance of the proper construction and use of words.

DYSARTHRIA

From what has been said above it will be clear that articulation may be disordered as the result of lesions of the upper or lower motor neurones concerned, of auxiliary extrapyramidal or cerebellar pathways, or of the muscles themselves.

Upper motor neurone lesions

A unilateral corticospinal tract lesion does not cause permanent dysarthria. After bilateral corticospinal tract lesions, however, as for example in congenital diplegia, motor neurone disease, and bilateral vascular lesions, the articulatory muscles are weak and spastic. Hence the speech is slurred, the production of consonants, especially labials and dentals, being especially affected.

Lesions of the corpus striatum

With lesions of the corpus striatum articulation is impaired partly at least as a result of muscular rigidity. Thus in Parkinsonism articulation is slow and slurred owing to immobility of the lips and tongue, and the pitch of the voice is monotonous. In severe cases speech may be unintelligible.

Disorders of co-ordination

The co-ordination of articulation suffers severely when the vermis of the cerebellum is damaged, and also when lesions involve the cerebellar connections in the brainstem. Syllables tend to be slurred and unduly separated – scanning or syllabic speech. In severe cases speech is explosive and associated with violent grimaces. Ataxic dysarthria of this kind is commonly seen in disseminated sclerosis and the hereditary ataxias. It also occurs in chorea and athetosis.

Lower motor neurone lesions

Lower motor neurone lesions cause wasting and weakness of the muscles of articulation. In the early stages the pronunciation of labials suffers most. Later, progressive weakness of the tongue impairs the production of dentals and gutturals, and weakness of the soft palate gives the voice a nasal quality. To this may be added impairment of phonation, and finally speech becomes completely impossible. Progressive bulbar palsy due to motor neurone disease is the commonest example of this. It may also occur in the bulbar form of polio-myelitis.

Combinations of these varieties of dysarthria are common, for example in disseminated sclerosis the articulatory muscles may be both spastic and ataxic, and in motor neurone disease a combination of upper and lower motor neurone lesions may be present.

Myopathies

Disease of the muscles such as occurs in myasthenia gravis and in some myopathic conditions leads to dysarthria similar to that resulting from lesions of the lower motor neurones. In myasthenia fatigability may cause increasing slurring of speech if the patient is asked to count.

Other non-dysphasic disorders of speech

Mutism is the term applied to complete loss of speech in a conscious patient in the absence of both aphasia and anarthria. It is usually a symptom of a psychological disorder, either a psychosis or hysteria. In hysterical mutism other hysterical symptoms, such as convulsions, rigidity, or anaesthesia are often present. Lesions in the neighbourhood of the third ventricle may cause akinetic mutism (p. 175).

In *aphonia* phonation is lost, but articulation is preserved; hence the patient talks in a whisper. Aphonia may be the result of organic disease causing bilateral paralysis of the adductors of the vocal cords, or of disease of the larynx. It is most commonly a symptom of hysteria, in which case the patient, though unable to phonate when speaking, can do so when coughing.

Palilalia is a rare disorder of speech usually associated with Parkinsonism and characterized by repetition of a phrase which the patient reiterates with increasing rapidity.

DYSPHASIA

As stated above, dysphasia is a disorder of the symbolic function of speech involved in the comprehension and expression of meanings by means of words. The nature of dysphasia has been discussed for a century and agreement on the subject is still lacking. These discussions, though interesting and important in themselves, have on the whole little clinical significance, since it is striking that most clinicians are agreed in distinguishing a limited number of varieties of dysphasia even though they call them by different names and interpret them in different ways. A general distinction can be made between sensory aphasias, disorders of comprehension of the spoken word, and motor aphasias, disorders of the production of speech. But in attempts to localize defects of function it is necessary to consider the effects of isolation of different areas concerned with speech and language function as well as the disordered functioning of the remaining brain. The following are the principal forms of dysphasia.

1. Broca's aphasia (expressive or motor aphasia)

This is due either to a lesion of Broca's area (see Fig. 4.1) or a subcortical lesion cutting off Broca's area. Expression both in speech and writing is severely affected. In extreme cases non-fluency reaches the point at which the patient can say nothing and write nothing, his utterance being reduced to mere grunts. A slightly less severely affected patient may say 'yes' or 'no'. In mild cases there is a noticeable defect in the formation of words and the structure of sentences. Consonants tend to be slurred and the smaller words indicating relationships omitted (telegram style). Words which are not available other- wise may be provoked by strong emotion, for example, in swearing. Though the patient speaks with difficulty, facial movements are usually normal for other forms of expression; often the patient can sing reasonably well. Faults of speech are grammatical, with laboured, slow and impaired articulation. The same errors as occur in speech occur in writing. Broca's aphasia is non-fluent but makes sense because only speech production is disturbed. The patient has a full understanding of the spoken and written language. Not infrequently there is an associated right hemiparesis.

2. Wernicke's aphasia (receptive, central, or sensory aphasia)

Wernicke's aphasia is due to a disorder of the central organization upon which speech is based, namely that concerned with the recognition of words. It thus leads to a disorder of both comprehension and expression of meaning by words, both spoken and written, and of the meanings conveyed by their grammatical relationship in sentences. The same kind of defect is present in expression, which is hampered by errors in syntax and grammar and by the use of wrong words or even non-existent words. Speech is fluent because Broca's area is intact but speech nevertheless often becomes unintelligible and the patient is unaware of his mistakes and, indeed, of the fact that he is talking nonsense – so called jargon aphasia. Speech may be fluent with the recogniz- able structure of sentences and may be phonetically and grammatically fairly normal but the meaning, if any, is only conveyed in a roundabout way, with 'paraphasias', whether phonetic or verbal.

3. 'Conduction' aphasia

This results from a lesion of the arcuate fasciculus connecting Broca's and Wernicke's areas. There is fluent speech which is semantically abnormal but Wernicke's area provides normal comprehension. However, there is a marked disturbance of repetition and difficulty in reading aloud; sometimes a right facial weakness may be present.

4. Lesions in the region of the angular gyrus

When the speech area is intact but isolated by surrounding lesions there may be fluent speech with excellent repetition, often associated with echolalia, which is the repetition of the last phrase of the questioner. The lesions in this region may also cause a variety of nominal dysphasia, a difficulty in naming objects, also described as amnesic dysphasia. When using the term nominal aphasia it must be appreciated that it may only reflect the result of a number of different functional impairments and has relatively poor localizing significance. In amnesic dysphasia the patient usually insists that he knows what the object is and frequently tries to convey recognition by describing its use. He will usually totally reject the wrong name if offered it and accept the right one. Writing exhibits the same nominal defect as articulated speech and there is much difficulty in comprehending spoken and written language.

5. If there is a combination of motor aphasia and a comprehension defect the term 'global' may be used to describe the aphasia.

In addition to these syndromes there are also rarer disorders in which a more restricted disability occurs. For example pure word deafness may be caused by a subcortical lesion below the superior temporal gyrus, pure word blindness with or without agraphia is due to a lesion of the visual association area and pure word dumbness is due to a subcortical lesion below Broca's area.

READING, WRITING, AND CALCULATION

Reading and writing are processes superimposed upon the utterance of speech and its comprehension, and employing visual symbols to represent words, and calculation also makes use of the visual symbols for any but its most elementary processes. Reading, writing, and calculation may thus be disorganized at two levels, as it were; at the level at which the visual symbols peculiar to their functions are organized, or, more fundamentally, as part of dysphasia when the symbolic use of words is itself disturbed. It is to disorganization at the former level that the terms dyslexia, dysgraphia, and dyscalculia, meaning a disturbance of reading, writing and calculation, are applied.

Dyslexia

Two forms of dyslexia are recognized. In pure or subcortical word-blindness, or visual dysphasia, the patient cannot recognize words, letters, or colours. He cannot copy, but can write spontaneously. The lesion is in the medial occipito-temporal (lingual) gyrus on the dominant side and involvement of the optic radiation causes an associated right homonymous hemianopia. Pure word-blindness is very rare and is commonly associated with dysgraphia, in which case it is described as visual asymbolia or cortical word-blindness. This combination of symptoms is due to a lesion of the left angular gyrus.

Dysgraphia

By dysgraphia is meant a disorder of writing unrelated to paralysis of the right hand. When that is present, therefore, it must be shown that the patient is unable to write with the left hand also. As stated above, dysgraphia may be associated with dyslexia as a symptom of visual asymbolia, but this is not always the case. Several varieties of pure dysgraphia have been described and it may be produced by a lesion in the posterior part of the middle frontal gyrus. *Paragraphia* means writing non-existent words.

Dyscalculia means a defect in the use of mathematical symbols and is commonly the result of a lesion in the left angular gyrus.

EXAMINATION OF A PATIENT WITH DYSPHASIA

Examination of a patient with dysphasia requires care and patience and should be carried out in a systematic manner. The following scheme fulfils all ordinary clinical requirements.

1. Is the patient right or left-handed, and, if the latter, did he write with the right hand? Is there any family history of left-handedness? Does he kick a ball with the right foot for preference? Does he 'take aim' using his right eye?

2. What was his stage of education as regards reading, writing, and foreign tongues?

3. Does he understand the nature and uses of objects, and can he understand pantomime and gesture, or express his wants thereby?

4. Is he deaf? If so, to what extent and on one or both sides?

5. Can he recognize ordinary sounds and noises?

6. Can he comprehend language spoken? If so, does he at once attempt to answer a question?

7. Is spontaneous speech fluent? If not, to what extent and in what manner is it impaired? Does he make use of wrong words, recurring utterances, or jargon?

8. Can he repeat words uttered in his hearing?

9. Is the sight good or bad; is there hemianopia, or papilloedema?

10. Does he recognize written or printed speech and obey a written command? If not, does he recognize single words, letters or numerals?

11. Can he write spontaneously? What mistakes occur in writing? Is there paragraphia? Can he read his own writing some time after he has written it?

12. Can he copy written words, or from printed to printing? Can he write numerals or perform simple mathematical calculations?

13. Can he read aloud?

14. Can he name at sight words, letters, numerals, and common objects?

15. Can he write from dictation?

16. Can he match an object with its name, spoken or written, when a series of objects and names are simultaneously presented?

17. Any other tests, emotional, rhythmical, or musical, which may raise the physiological level of speech centres.

18. Any other means of proving in what way he can receive and express ideas.

The anatomical diagnosis of dysphasia is one of the most difficult aspects of neurology but as a general guide, fluency points to the intactness of Broca's area whereas non-fluency implies a lesion of Broca's area itself. Paraphrasias point to posteriorly placed lesions. As has already been pointed out in considering handedness, speech functions in right-handed people are almost always localized to the left hemisphere. But in apparently genetically left-handed people, dysphasia results from the lesion of the left hemisphere in about 60 per cent of the patients (see p. 131). An extra dimension of precision in the site and extent of localization of lesions causing aphasia has been provided by the CAT brain scan. Some fascinating differences occur in the extent of the hemisphere dominance for languages in which, as a Chinese and Japanese, there is a pictorial as well as a phonetic component.

The causes of dysphasia

Dysphasia is rare in childhood and increases in frequency with increasing age. It is most frequently met with after middle life since the commonest cause is a vascular lesion, especially thrombosis, and transitory attacks of dysphasia may occur in patients suffering from cerebral atheroma and occasionally in migraine. An intracranial tumour is the commonest cause of dysphasia during the first half of adult life. It may also occur as the result of an abscess involving the left temporal lobe or of traumatic lesions. Dysphasia is also a symptom of the degenerative cortical disorders, such as Alzheimer's disease and Pick's disease.

Prognosis and treatment

The prognosis of dysphasia depends chiefly upon its cause. It is poor when there is a tumour. After an ischaemic vascular lesion the speech is likely to improve as shock passes off, and improvement may continue for a year or two. On the whole the outlook is better when the dysphasia is of the expressive type than when it is of the central or receptive types. This applies, also, to the response to treatment which requires much patience and the help of a speech therapist to re-educate the patient in the use of vowel and consonant sounds, the pronunciation of words and the association of names with pictures and their written equivalents.

Speech disorders in childhood

Delay in learning to speak may be due to *mental subnormality,* or to deafness, specially deafness to high tones. Congenital word-deafness, or congenital auditory imperception, appears to be due to an inability to appreciate the significance of sounds, although hearing is normal. It is sometimes familial. For a number of years a child may not speak at all. Sooner or later, however, most patients acquire a vocabulary of their own, known as idioglossia. These children are not usually mentally defective, but suffer from the limitations imposed by their inability to understand what they hear. *Developmental dyslexia,* sometimes known as congenital word-blindness, is much commoner than congenital word-deafness. It also is sometimes familial. Affected children have great difficulty in learning to read, to spell, and to write. They often show a tendency to mirror-writing. The frequent association of developmental dyslexia with left-handedness suggests some disorder of cerebral dominance. There is also a variety in which phonetic difficulties predominate. It has not been established whether minimal brain damage plays some part.

Children who suffer from congenital word-deafness or developmental dyslexia require training by expert teachers.

Stuttering is a disturbance of articulation not usually caused by organic nervous disease but closely linked with left-handedness and characterized by abrupt interruptions of the flow of speech or repetition of sounds or syllables. The association between stuttering and left-handedness is obscure, but there seems no doubt that stuttering may be precipitated if a naturally left-handed child is forced to use the right hand. A familial tendency is common.

The flow of speech may be broken by pauses, during which is it entirely arrested, or by the repetition of sounds or syllables. The spastic element is usually called *tonus,* and the repetitive *clonus.* Stutterers often go out of their way to avoid certain words by reconstructing sentences. How far neurosis is a cause of stuttering is undecided, but there is no doubt that stuttering itself causes embarrassment and may lead to neurotic reactions. Mild stuttering tends to disappear spontaneously, as is shown by the fact that stuttering is much less common in adult life than in childhood.

For stutterers the technique of speaking only while breathing out may unlock the spasm of the vocal cords. Some success has been obtained from treatment with delayed auditory feedback. When stuttering occurs in a left-handed child who has been made to use the right hand, a return to left-handedness often produces great improvement. Re-education of speech by a trained teacher is essential. Associated psychological difficulties will require treatment.

APRAXIA AND AGNOSIA

Apraxia

Apraxia is defined as the inability to carry out a purposive movement, the nature of which the patient understands, in the absence of severe motor paralysis, sensory loss, and ataxia. Apraxia may involve any movement normally voluntarily initiated, movements of the eyes, face, muscles of articulation, chewing and swallowing, manipulation of objects, gestures with the upper limb, walking, or sitting down.

Lesions in the left parietal lobe (normally the dominant one) are likely to produce bilateral apraxia. Lesions between this region and the left precentral gyrus may lead to apraxia of the limbs on the right side, and lesions involving the anterior part of the corpus callosum, or of the subcortical white matter on the right side, may cause left-sided apraxia. The commonest form of apraxia is that involving the lips and tongue, which is frequently encountered in association with right hemiplegia due to a lesion of the left hemisphere. The patient, when asked to protrude his tongue, is unable to do so on request, although he may carry out inappropriate movements such as opening his mouth. A moment later, he may spontaneously protrude his tongue to lick his lips. Apraxia for dressing is usually the result of a lesion of the right parietal lobe.

Constructive apraxia is the term applied to a particular disturbance of the spatial organization of movements. The patient, for example, cannot copy a simple arrangement of matches, but recognizes his mistakes.

Agnosia

In order that we may recognize an object it is necessary not only that the appropriate sensory pathways up to and including the cerebral cortex, e.g. visual, auditory, or tactile, should be intact, but that these should be able through association pathways, to arouse the appropriate sensory images, memories, and dispositions towards action. If these responses are not evoked, the object may be seen, heard, or felt, but will not be recognized. Such a failure of recognition is known as agnosia, qualified by the epithet visual, auditory, or tactile, according to the sensory medium involved.

A patient suffering from visual agnosia fails to recognize common objects which he clearly sees. This condition may result from lesions in the left parieto-occipital region in right-handed persons. Auditory agnosia implies the failure to recognize sounds in a patient who is nevertheless not deaf. A person suffering from this in a severe form will fail to appreciate not only the nature of words, but also musical tunes. This results from a lesion of the left temporal lobe in right-handed persons. In tactile agnosia the patient, though not suffering from gross sensory defect in the fingers or hands, is nevertheless unable to recognize an object placed in the hand. This may be produced by a lesion of the parietal lobe situated posteriorly to the postcentral gyrus at the level of the hand area. Agnosia usually affects the recognition of objects through one sensory channel only. Thus a patient suffering from visual agnosia, who cannot recognize a key when he sees it, can usually recognize it when it is placed in his hand. Conversely, a patient who cannot recognize objects placed in his hand recognizes them readily when he sees them.

A special form of agnosia is the failure to recognize part of the body – auto-topagnosia. A patient suffering from this may deny that his arm belongs to him. If he is hemiplegic he may deny this also. The rejection of evidence of bodily disease, e.g. hemiplegia, blindness, is known as anosognosia (Anton's syndrome). These symptoms in right-handed persons are observed after lesions of the right parietal lobe and therefore refer to the left side of the body. The disorder of awareness of the body which occurs after left parietal (angular gyrus) lesions in right-handed persons is finger-agnosia, characterized by an inability to recognize and select individual fingers when looking at both hands. This is usually associated with agraphia, acalculia, and a failure to discriminate between right and left (Gerstmann's syndrome).

DISCONNECTION SYNDROMES

Lesions of the cerebral commissures

Lesions of the interhemisphere commissures may be the result of infarction of the anterior cerebral artery in which case the anterior four-fifths of the callosum may be affected, may be due to tumours or, if total, may be caused by surgical section of the corpus callosum for intractable epilepsy. The full syndrome results in an incapacity to transfer visual or tactile information or information concerning language from one hemisphere to the other (Fig. 4.2). Thus a patient cannot match an object held in one hand with the other hand or

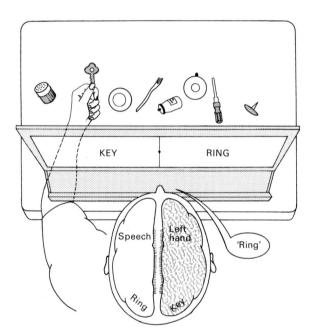

Fig. 4.2. Split-brain preparation (after Sperry). The patient sits in front of a screen on which the word 'key' is briefly presented to the right hemisphere; 'ring' to the left hemisphere. He reports that he has read the word 'ring' (by way of his 'speaking' left hemisphere) but denies that he has seen the word 'key' in the left field. He cannot name any object placed in his left hand but he can use his left hand to select the correct object, though he says he has no knowledge of the object. If asked to name the object he has selected, the 'speaking' hemisphere calls it 'ring'.

match an object seen in one visual field with an object seen in the other visual field. More complex signs result from hemisphere language specialization in the left hemisphere. The patient may carry out verbal commands correctly only with the right hand, writing correctly with the right hand and producing only an aphasic scrawl with the 'disconnected' left hand. Only objects placed in the right hand of the blindfolded patient can be named correctly. Provided non-verbal tests are used, sensation can be shown to be normal in the left hand which has its own sensory 'memory' and can select without sight an object previously felt. Reading is restricted to the right visual field. With closer study of these patients, further information has been obtained about the nature of hemisphere specialization other than that of language. The constructional apraxia of each hand differs after callosal section. In arranging blocks to form a pattern the right hand is clumsy and may fail to form any pattern at all. The left hand, however, may skilfully arrange the blocks into a square but it may not correspond to the correct pattern.

Aphasia due to intrahemisphere disconnection

The principle of disconnection is one which can be applied not only in lesions of the commissures but in any situation in which a region of cortex is partially isolated by the lesion but still linked to an effector system. It has been used to explain some forms of aphasia. The earliest example was called 'conduction' aphasia. The patient has fluent but paraphrasic speech and similar defects of writing but near normal comprehension of written and spoken speech. The striking difficulty is the repetition of test phrases. There is not usually any hemiparesis or sensory loss though sometimes there is a contralateral cortical sensory loss or pain loss. In this situation Broca's and Wernicke's areas are thought to be intact but the lesion lies in the parietal operculum where it inter-rupts the arcuate fasciculus connecting Wernicke's and Broca's areas (see Fig. 4.1).

Apraxia due to disconnection syndrome

Apraxia can be caused by a lesion involving the pathway from Wernicke's area to the premotor region and movements neither of face nor limbs on either side can be carried out to command. There is sometimes selective sparing of facial movements which may be controlled from the left side so that a patient with a callosal lesion may be able to move his face to command but not the left-sided limbs. The lack of a significant motor deficit may be shown by the capacity to imitate movements fairly well. In this form of apraxia whole body movements, even of quite a complex kind like imitating a boxer's stance, can be carried out, presumably because they are mediated by the more primitive ipsilateral non-pyramidal medial motor system descending from separate cortical centres. The holding of an object will facilitate the response of command, probably because it makes access possible to the non-pyramidal system.

INTERHEMISPHERE RELATIONSHIPS

The development of lateralization of hemisphere function is of course the hall-mark of the human brain. In right-handed persons the left hemisphere appears in general to be specialized for logical and analytical functions for which words are a good medium, though this may interfere with the overall perception or 'gestalt', for which the right hemisphere is more specialized. The right hemisphere also seems to specialize in the emotional and active responses needed for survival in relation to danger. Following surgical section of the corpus callosum it is possible for sensations and images to be presented almost exclusively to one hemisphere and so to test its verbal and non-verbal responses. When presented with information in the left visual field such patients can perform tasks with the left hand which show that the right hemisphere can perceive, remember, and learn. They have little difficulty in analysing the information coming from the outside world to either hemisphere but cannot relate the information from one hemisphere to that of the other. Each hemisphere seems to form a separate realm of experience, so that they do not have just one inner visual world but two separate and independant visual worlds. Most surprising the right and left hand can express different and contrary wills of the two hemispheres. From this it is only a small step to regard each hemisphere as having a 'consciousness' of its own. The 'mute' right hemisphere can, in this way, be shown to be more adept at solving spatial problems, the left at giving prompt verbal responses. It seems likely that in the intact brain the same event is perceived in different terms by the two hemi-spheres. The left 'dominant' hemisphere which, as it were, usually wins control of executive functions, may ignore conflicting information from the right hemisphere but it does not prevent this hemisphere from storing information which can, under certain circumstances, affect future behaviour.

There is now a realization that the non-dominant hemisphere has special functions related to language, recognition of melody, emotional tone, and humour. If there is a lesion of the non-dominant hemisphere then this causes an extensive disturbance of attention and a confusional state even though there is a single lesion, for example an infarct. The left hemisphere appears to attend to one stimulus and is easily distracted. The right hemisphere 'scans' the environ-ment and appears to decide when to shift attention to another stimulus which has become important. Clearly this concept presents a new way of looking at obvious disorders of function such as stuttering (p. 138), as well as disorders of behaviour previously explained by the psychological mechanism of 'repression' which now may have a more physiological explanation. Evoked potentials, auditory as well as visual (p. 160), may be helpful in detecting complete and incomplete dominance and may offer some hope for treatment, by means of feedback training techniques. By such techniques it has already been shown that it is possible to modify physiological functions such as those of blood pressure.

REFERENCES

Benson, F.D. (1978). Neurological correlates of aphasia and apraxia. In *Recent advances in clinical neurology* (ed. W.B. Matthews and G.H. Glaser) pp. 160–75. Churchill Livingstone, Edinburgh.

Critchley, M. (1975). *Silent language.* Butterworth, London.

Critchley, M. and Henson, R.A. (1977). *Music and the brain: studies in the neurology of music.* Heinemann, London.

Dimond, S.J. and Beaumont, J.G. (eds.) (1974). *Hemispheric function in the human brain.* Elek, London.

Geffen, G., Traub, E., and Stierman, I. (1978). Language laterality assessed by unilateral ECT and dichotic monitoring. *J. Neurol. Neurosurg. Psychiat.* **41**, 354–60.

Geschwind, N. (1974). *Selected papers on language and the brain.* Reidel, Boston.

Naeser, M.A. and Hayward, R.W. (1978). Lesion localization in aphasia with cranial computed tomography and Boston Diagnostic Aphasia Exam. *Neurology, Minneap.* **28**, 545–51.

Sasanuma, S. (1975). Kana and Kanji processing in Japanese aphasics. *Brain Lang.* **2**, 369–83.

5 Ancillary investigations

SKULL X-RAYS

Over the calvarium the skull X-rays may show osteolytic lesions, fibrous dysplasia, myeloma, or Paget's disease. Hyperostosis may occur in acromegaly or a meningioma (Fig. 5.1). Calcification within the brain substance may be due to an oligodendroglioma (Fig. 5.2), craniopharyngioma or meningioma or rarely a chronic abscess, tuberculoma, or toxoplasmosis. In hypoparathyroidism there may be calcification of the basal ganglia. Sometimes within the substance of the brain the pattern of the calcified arteriovenous malformation may be seen or an angioma associated with the Sturge–Weber syndrome. Chronic subdural haematoma tend to calcify. Calcification may also be seen in the carotid artery especially in the region of the syphon. The pituitary fossa may be enlarged with a pituitary tumour and may have a double floor (Fig. 5.3). Posterior clinoids are eroded with raised intracranial pressure of some duration. A special view (Towne's view) is needed to show the internal auditory meati to exclude a cerebellopontine angle tumour. When present, pineal calcification is a useful guide to the shift of midline structures. Basal invagination occurs when the odontoid peg of the axis projects above a line drawn back along the line of the hard palate. If congenital it suggests the Arnold–Chiari malformation in which the cerebellar tonsils are abnormally low in position and syringomyelia may occur. This may also be associated with a widened cervical canal.

THE CEREBROSPINAL FLUID

Anatomy and physiology

The cerebrospinal fluid is mainly formed by the choroid plexuses of the cerebral ventricles. That formed in the lateral ventricles passes through the interventricular foramina (of Monro) into the third ventricle. Thence the fluid flows through the cerebral aqueduct (of Sylvius) into the fourth ventricle, which it leaves by the median aperture of the fourth ventricle (foramen of Magendie) and the two lateral apertures of the fourth ventricle (foramina of Luschka) to reach the subarachnoid space, which lies between the arachnoid membrane externally and the pia mater internally, and extends superficially over the whole surface of the brain and spinal cord. It is deepest at the base of the brain and between the inferior surface of the cerebellum and the medulla, where its expansions constitute the various cisterns, the largest of which is the

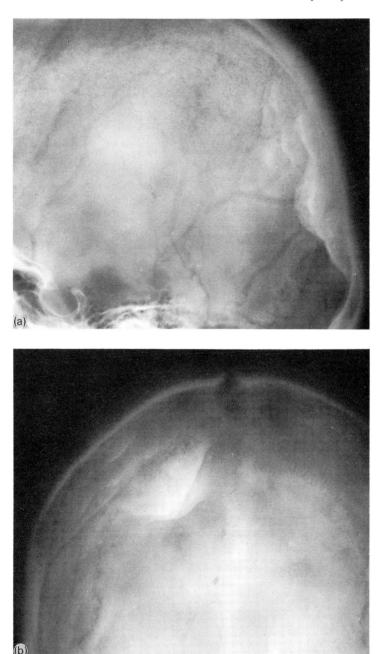

Fig. 5.1. Large internal hyperostosis associated with an occipital meningioma. Note also the increased vascular markings extending to the lesion. (a) Towne's view; (b) lateral view.

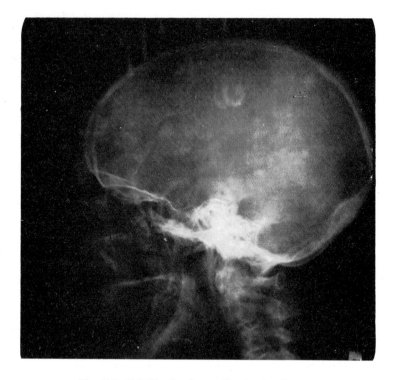

Fig. 5.2. Calcification in an oligodendroglioma.

cerebellomedullary cistern (cisterna magna) beneath the cerebellum. It is also prolonged into the substance of the nervous system by means of extensions which constitute the perivascular spaces. The cerebrospinal fluid probably receives a contribution from these, and possibly also from the lymphatics of the cranial and other peripheral nerves. After bathing the surface of the spinal cord and the base of the brain it passes upwards over the convexity of the hemispheres to be absorbed into the intracranial venous sinuses through the microscopic arachnoid villi (Fig. 0.1, p. 3).

The volume of the cerebrospinal fluid in adults is normally about 130 ml and its pressure when the patient is horizontal is about 120 mm of water. The more important of its normal constituents are: (i) protein, in the ventricular fluid 0.1 to 0.2 g/l, in the cisternal fluid 1.5 to 2.5 g/l, and in the lumbar fluid 0.2 to 0.4 g/l; (ii) glucose, 2.5 to 4.0 mmol/l; (iii) chloride (as NaCl) 115 to 125 mmol/l; (iv) cells, 1 to 3 mononuclear cells per mm^3. The c.s.f. sugar should not be estimated without obtaining a blood sugar at the same time.

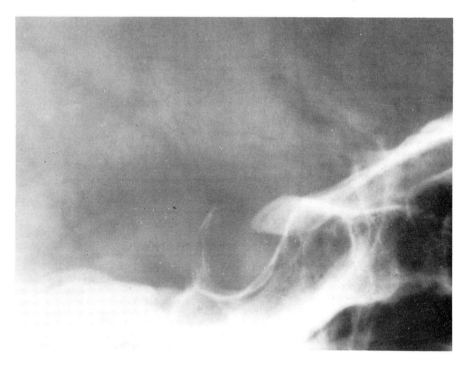

Fig. 5.3. Chromophobe adenoma showing ballooning of the sella and backward bulging of the dorsum.

LUMBAR PUNCTURE

Indications and contra-indications

Lumbar puncture is the simplest method of obtaining access to the subarachnoid space. It is now less frequently indicated with the advent of CT scanning. For example a patient with suspected intracranial bleeding whether subarachnoid or intracerebral should have a CT scan prior to examination of the cerebrospinal fluid as the examination itself may precipitate 'coning'. Where there are no contra-indications the examination is carried out for the following purposes: (i) to obtain cerebrospinal fluid for examination and to estimate its pressure; (ii) for the relief of intracranial pressure and the removal of fluid for diagnostic purposes in the various forms of encephalitis and meningitis, intracranial haemorrhage, etc. This is the only way of excluding a pyogenic meningitis which simulates subarachnoid bleeding; (iii) to introduce therapeutic substances or local anaesthetics into the subarachnoid space; (iv) to introduce air or contrast media into the subarachnoid space for radiographic purposes – encephalography and myelography; (v) lowering the pressure in benign intracranial hypertension.

There are a number of contra-indications to lumbar puncture. In the presence of greatly increased intracranial pressure, especially when there is reason to suspect a tumour in the posterior fossa, sudden withdrawal of fluid from the spinal canal may cause herniation of the medulla into the foramen magnum – the 'cerebellar pressure cone' – with fatal results. In such cases ventricle puncture is the only safe method of obtaining cerebrospinal fluid. Withdrawal of cerebrospinal fluid may aggravate the symptoms of spinal cord compression and so should only be undertaken when prompt surgical treatment is feasible. The presence of infection in the lumbar region is a contra-indication, owing to the risk of infecting the spinal canal. Marked spinal deformity may render lumbar puncture difficult or impossible.

Method of puncture

Lumbar puncture may be performed with the patient either sitting up or lying on one side. For diagnostic purposes, the puncture is usually carried out with the patient lying. An anxious patient may be given sodium amylobarbitone, 200 mg one hour beforehand. The patient usually lies on the left side with a pillow under the head. The spine should be horizontal and the plane of the iliac crests vertical. The most important point is to secure the greatest possible degree of flexion of the lumbar spine. If the patient is conscious and co-operative he should be asked to bend his legs until his knees approach his chin, and then to clasp his hands beneath his knees, or an assistant can aid flexion of the spine by applying pressure with one hand behind the neck and the other behind the knees. The skin is sterilized, and the space between the tips of the third and fourth or fourth and fifth lumbar spinous processes is found. (A line joining the highest points of the iliac crests usually passes between the third and fourth lumbar spinous processes.) A few drops of 2 per cent procain solution are injected into the skin at this point. The lumbar puncture needle is held in a sterile towel and introduced midway between the spinous processes in the selected interspace in the middle line. After its point has entered the skin, the needle is passed forwards and slightly upwards in the sagittal plane. At an average depth of about 4.5 cm the point of the needle encounters the increased resistance of the ligamentum flavum, and after penetrating a further half centimetre it should enter the subarachnoid space. The stylet is now withdrawn and laid upon a sterile towel, and if the puncture has been successful cerebrospinal fluid drips from the butt of the needle.

The next step is to measure the pressure, which is done by attaching a graduated glass manometer to the needle. The patient should be allowed to straighten his spine slightly and directed to relax his muscles and breathe quietly and regularly, as muscular tension and holding the breath raise the pressure. The pressure is measured in millimetres of cerebrospinal fluid and normally shows oscillations corresponding to respiration and finer variations synchronous with the arterial pulse.

Removal of fluid for examination

The pressure of the fluid both before and after jugular compression and its rate of rise and fall having been recorded, some fluid should be withdrawn for examination. In normal circumstances it is convenient to collect about 3 ml in one sterile test tube and a further 3 ml in another. If, as sometimes happens, the lumbar puncture has caused bleeding into the subarachnoid space, though the contents of the first tube may be bloodstained, those of the second are likely to be clear. If the inital pressure of the fluid is more than 300 mm the fluid should be withdrawn very cautiously, and the pressure should not be lowered more than 25 per cent.

After lumbar puncture the patient should be kept flat with one pillow for 24 hours to minimize the risk of headache. Postlumbar puncture headache is more likely to be due to subnormal pressure of the cerebrospinal fluid produced by continuous leakage of fluid through the puncture hole than the result of the patient's suggestibility. It is best dealt with by raising the foot of the bed and increasing the patient's intake of fluid. Lumbar puncture occasionally causes an intensification of the symptoms of the disease from which the patient is suffering, especially in cases of compression of the spinal cord.

CISTERN PUNCTURE

Indications and contra-indications

The principal indications for cistern puncture are: (i) to inject opaque media in radiographic investigation of blockage of the spinal subarachnoid space; (ii) to introduce therapeutic substances; (iii) to obtain cerebrospinal fluid; especially if for some reason lumbar puncture is impossible; (iv) to introduce air for encephalography.

Cistern puncture should not be carried out when there is reason to suspect a tumour or abscess in the posterior fossa, when the cerebellomedullary cistern is likely to be obliterated by inflammatory adhesions, when there may be a congenital abnormality in the region of the foramen magnum, or when there is a marked rise of intracranial pressure. Though safe in expert hands it should not be attempted by the inexpert.

ROUTINE EXAMINATION OF THE CEREBROSPINAL FLUID

Naked eye appearance

Turbidity

The normal cerebrospinal fluid is clear and colourless, and resembles water. Turbidity, when present, is usually due to an excess of polymorphonuclear cells. In acute meningitis these are often present in such numbers that a deposit of pus forms at the bottom of the tube, and the supernatant fluid may be yellow.

Fibrin clot

The development of a clot of fibrin in a specimen of fluid implies the presence of fibrinogen and of fresh blood. Such a clot may occur either in a fluid of which the protein content is only slightly raised, or in the highly albuminous fluids characteristic of spinal subarachnoid block, and sometimes occurring in polyneuritis. In the former case the clot forms a faint 'cobweb' which takes from 12 to 24 hours to appear. This is most frequently seen in tuberculous meningitis. The clot which forms in highly albuminous fluids may solidify the whole specimen. In such cases clotting may be precipitated by the addition of fibrin ferment in the shape of a drop of fresh blood.

Blood

Blood may be present in the cerebrospinal fluid either as an accidental result of injury to an intrathecal vein by the lumbar puncture needle, or as the product of pre-existing haemorrhage into the subarachnoid space. As already stated, in the former case after the withdrawal of 2 or 3 ml of fluid, the remainder is likely to be clear, whereas after subarachnoid haemorrhage both specimens are uniformly bloodstained. Further, if the haemorrhage is traumatic the supernatant fluid is usually colourless after the red cells have been given time to settle, whereas within a few hours of subarachnoid haemorrhage the supernatant fluid shows a yellow coloration.

Subarachnoid haemorrhage is usually due to rupture of an intracranial aneurysm or angioma into the subarachnoid space, or to the bursting of an intracerebral haemorrhage into the ventricular system. It is also commonly found after severe head injury. After subarachnoid haemorrhage the yellow coloration of the fluid appears in few hours and reaches its greatest intensity at the end of about a week. It has usually disappeared in two to three weeks. The red cells disappear from the fluid in two or three days. The presence of blood in contact with the meninges excites a cellular reaction, and the fluid may therefore contain a moderate excess of mononuclear cells.

Xanthochromia

Xanthochromia, or yellow coloration of the cerebrospinal fluid, is found, as just described, after subarachnoid haemorrhage and also when pus is present in considerable amount in the fluid. Xanthochromic fluid is also occasionally found in cases of intracranial tumour and after cerebral infarction. It is also characteristic of obstruction of the spinal subarachnoid space, as in acoustic neuromas, and occurs in some forms of polyneuritis, such as the Guillain–Barré syndrome, when the cell count is usually normal.

Correction for contamination of cerebrospinal fluid with blood

A contaminated c.s.f. tap can still provide some useful information if a correction is applied. To correct for the contamination with blood, for every thousand red cells, 0.01 g/l should be deducted from the observed protein level and one white cell from the total number of white cells per mm³.

Cytological and chemical abnormalities
Cells

The normal cerebrospinal fluid contains a small number of cells – lymphocytes or large mononuclear cells – which should not exceed 3 per mm³. In pathological states a greater variety of cells may be present, and these may occur in very large numbers. Those most frequently encountered are lympocytes, large mononuclear cells, and polymorphonuclear cells. Micro-organisms and parasitic cells may also be found, and rarely tumour cells.

The majority of cells are probably derived from the meninges, though some may come from the nerve tissue and pass into the subarachnoid space from the perivascular spaces. In general a pleocytosis, or excess of cells, in the spinal fluid indicates meningeal irritation, though this does not necessarily imply meningeal infection. Whether the cellular increase is polymorphonuclear or mononuclear depends partly upon the acuteness of the pathological process and partly upon the nature of the infecting organism. A predominantly polymorphonuclear count is usually found in acute infections and in acute exacerbations of chronic infections, while a mononuclear count is characteristic of chronic infection. But while pyogenic organisms excite a mainly polymorphonuclear leucocytosis except in their most chronic stages, a mononuclear pleocytosis is the most frequent reaction to infections with neurotropic viruses, though polymorphonuclear cells are sometimes present in such cases when the infection is most acute. We thus encounter predominantly polymorphonuclear, predominantly mononuclear, and mixed cell counts.

A predominantly polymorphonuclear pleocytosis is found in meningitis due to pyogenic organisms, when the cells are usually present in very large numbers. A mononuclear pleocytosis occurs in the acute stage of infection with many neurotropic viruses, and in some forms of acute virus meningitis the cell count may reach 1000 per mm³. Usually, however, it does not exceed 200 or 300. A mononuclear pleocytosis also occurs in many cases of neurosyphilis, in some cases of tuberculous meningitis, in poliomyelitis after the first few days of the infection, and in some cases of disseminated sclerosis during the more acute exacerbations. Cerebral abscess and subarachnoid haemorrhage may also be associated with a mononuclear pleocytosis.

The mixed type of pleocytosis, in which polymorphonuclear and mononuclear cells are present in approximately equal numbers, is found in many cases of tuberculous meningitis and in poliomyelitis during the first few days, and in some cases of virus meningitis. It may also occur in cases of cerebral abscess. In cases of brain tumour, tumour cells are sometimes found.

Protein

The total protein content of the normal cerebrospinal fluid is from 0.2 to 0.4 g/l, albumin and globulin being present in the ratio of 8 to 1. Increase in the protein is extremely common. A moderate increase, usually to below 1.0 g/l, is found in inflammatory diseases of the nervous tissue of the meninges, such as the various forms of meningitis, encephalitis, poliomyelitis, disseminated sclerosis, and syphilis of the nervous system. Intracranial tumour often causes a moderate rise in protein, and an acoustic neuroma a considerable rise in many cases. The protein content of the fluid is often raised for 2 to 3 weeks after cerebral infarction.

Great increase in the protein content of the fluid, i.e. up to 5.0 g/l or higher, when the fluid is not frankly purulent, is most likely to be due to either obstruction of the spinal subarachnoid space or acute infective polyneuritis.

The albumin–globulin ratio

A rise in the albumin content of the fluid is often associated with a relatively greater increase in the amount of globulin, which may be demonstrated by a variety of agents giving a positive result in such tests as the Lange colloidal gold test which depends on changes in the protein content of the cerebrospinal fluid. These tests are still useful if more specific techniques are not available. Globulins are now usually estimated by specific electrophoretic and immuno-chemical tests. The c.s.f. is an ultra-filtrate of serum with proteins derived from brain cells (interstitial fluid) and from cells in the c.s.f. compartment. Abnormalities of many kinds can therefore be detected by its electrophoretic study on polyacrylamide gel electrophoresis which separates proteins according to molecular size, as opposed to the measurement of IgG by immunochemical methods. With an impaired c.s.f. barrier, the c.s.f. contains increased amounts of normal serum proteins. Serum immunoglobulins can be distinguished from locally produced immunoglobulins; instead of being polyclonal immuno-globulins of varying size and charge they show restricted heterogeneity from a few B cell clones and are oligoclonal rather than strictly monoclonal. The oligo-clonal pattern is positive in 95 per cent of patients with clinically definite multiple sclerosis, a higher correlation yielded than by biochemical or neuro-physiological tests. An oligoclonal pattern, which differs from that in multiple sclerosis is found in neurosyphilis, acute polyneuropathy, subacute sclerosing panencephalitis, meningitis, encephalitis, systemic lupus erythematosis, and sarcoid.

An increase in the IgG fraction of γ globulin, measured by immunochemical techniques, with a normal total protein content is also suggestive of multiple sclerosis (p. 511).

Glucose

The normal glucose content of the cerebrospinal fluid is somewhat lower than that of blood and lies between 2.5 and 4.0 mmol/l. A marked diminution in the glucose content is characteristic of bacterial or fungal meningitis, and is parti-cularly valuable in differentiating tuberculous meningitis from virus infections which may produce a similar pleocytosis in the fluid.

Chlorides

The normal chloride content of the fluid is 115–125 mmol/l. The chloride level in the cerebrospinal fluid follows the serum level closely and the low values in purulent meningitis and tuberculous meningitis probably reflect the serum level in these grave infections.

Other investigations

Special staining techniques are needed for yeasts and for suspected carcinomatous meningitis after centrifugation of neoplastic cells. Bacteriological investigation of the cerebrospinal fluid is called for in cases of suspected meningitis.

Serological and cerebrospinal fluid tests for syphilis

The Wassermann complement fixation test was based on antigen extracted from syphilitic tissue but the active component in the extract was not treponemes but a substance called cardiolipin, present not only in treponemes but in many mammalian tissues as well. These antibodies were then given the name 'reagin'. The VDRL test is a flocculation test in which a mixture of cardiolipin, lecithin, and cholesterol reacts with the patient's serum. The biological false-positive 'reagin' test occurs in most conditions with excessive normal globulins or abnormal globulins, as well as yaws. The *Treponema pallidum* immobilization test (TPI), which was specific, has now been replaced by another highly specific test, the *T. pallidum* microhaemagglutination assay test (MHA-TP), which can be quantitive and determine recent or active infection and can follow the effect of treatment. Reference laboratories also use the more specific test now available, an IgM – fluorescent treponemal antibody absorption test (FTA-ABS test).

MYELOGRAPHY

Myelography is radiography after injection of an opaque substance into the lumbar spinal subarachnoid space, usually at the L2–3 level. Iohexol has now largely replaced Myodil because, as a soluble contrast medium, it does not have to be removed after the procedure has been completed. As iohexol does not give such good contrast, for studies of the neck region it is usually put in intracisternally by the radiologist. Iohexol and other similar substances are a marked improvement on previous soluble media such as metrizamide, which caused headaches and occasionally seizures, leading to the need for prophylactic anticonvulsants. So far there are no reports of seizures after iohexol, headaches are no more common than after lumbar puncture for other reasons and, though iohexol may cause a cellular inflammatory reaction, there is no evidence that it causes arachnoiditis. Though better soluble contrast media may be devised, iohexol comes closer than any previous substances to being an ideal medium.

CT scanning with myelography

An important advance in radiological investigation of posterior fossa and spinal lesions, from syringomyelia to lesions of the lumbosacral nerve roots and cauda equina, has been the combination of CT scanning with myelography using a water-soluble medium such as iohexol. Reconstruction techniques can be used to outline the spinal cord and nerve roots with a precision hitherto impossible.

Myelography is obviously contra-indicated if lumbar puncture is contra-indicated or, in view of the iodine content to the contrast, if the patient is allergic to iodine or if thyroid function tests are needed. Metrizamide is contra-indicated as a medium if the patient has hepatic or renal disease. Myelography should not be undertaken in a patient with progressing paraplegia, unless neurosurgical help is at hand, because of the risk of irreversible progressive spinal cord damage with a spinal tumour (see p. 364).

ELECTROENCEPHALOGRAPHY

Electroencephalography is the method of recording changes of potential in the brain. For the most part these records are made from electrodes applied to the scalp. Sometimes it is necessary to introduce a needle to make a record through the base of the skull from the temporal lobe, and the process of recording from the brain directly during operation is known as electrocorticography. Apart from the diagnosis of epilepsy, the EEG is helpful in the investigation of suspected cerebral abscess, hypoglycaemia and unexplained dementia or in assessing the recovery from an encephalitic illness. The CT scan has almost replaced the electroencephalogram in the diagnosis of focal brain lesions and the EEG is no longer in Britain regarded as necessary in contributing towards the diagnosis of brain death (see p. 180).

Berger in 1929 first showed that it was possible to record the changes when they occurred in the human brain. The first electrical rhythm described by Berger as the alpha rythm consists of an almost sinusoidal discharge with a frequency of about 10 Hz (cycles per second), and with a potential varying irregularly from 0 to about 100 μV in some subjects (Fig. 5.4). The area of the alpha discharge is usually limited to the parieto-occipital region of both hemispheres, but it may be seen elsewhere. The alpha rhythm is inhibited by visual activity and decreased or abolished when the eyes are shut or by intellectual concentration. Theta activity (4–7 Hz) is usually seen in frontal and temporal regions in children and young people and is seldom abnormal.

The applications of electroencephalography are described in the relevant sections of this book. Certain general principles, however, may be briefly stated now. Electroencephalography may reveal localized or diffuse brain damage, but in many instances CT scanning has now superseded the EEG. An area of cortical damage may be indicated by a localized area of slow waves known as delta waves, with a rhythm of less than 4 Hz (Fig. 5.5). Sometimes a particular

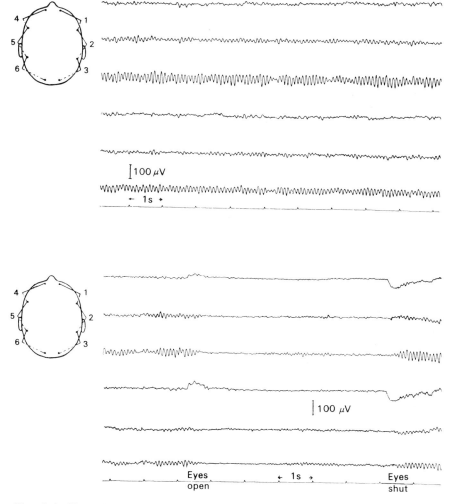

Fig. 5.4. Normal electroencephalogram. Dominant 10-Hz alpha activity in the posterocentral regions. Almost complete blocking of the dominant alpha rhythm to eye opening.

form of dysrhythmia may be associated with a particular pathological change. The other principal use of electroencephalography is in the diagnosis of epilepsy (Chapter 7). A focal epileptic attack may be correlated with a focal electrical discharge (Fig. 5.5), while characteristic abnormal rhythms symmetrically distributed may indicate epilepsy of a constitutional or central origin. In interpreting the EEG it is well to remember that 10 per cent of normal and healthy individuals have a record which is electrically 'abnormal'.

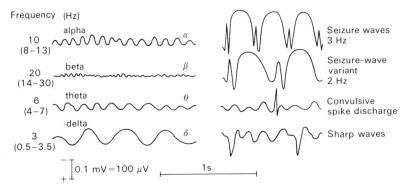

Fig. 5.5. The EEG on the left shows the different types of wave that can appear in a healthy person. On the right examples of seizure potentials as recorded primarily in epileptics. The sequence of rapid and slow phases is called a wave-and-spike complex.

COMPUTERIZED TOMOGRAPHY

Computerized tomography (CT), developed by a British physicist, Dr G.N. Hounsfield, and for which he was awarded a Nobel Prize, has provided the greatest technical aid in neurological diagnosis since the introduction of the contrast studies of air-encephalography and angiography some 50 years ago. In one large neurological department, since the introduction of tomography, the need for air-encephalography has become negligible and for angiography has been approximately halved. The CT brain scan has become virtually indispensable in major neurological and neurosurgical centres throughout the world within a few years by virtue of its speed, safety, and accuracy. In the space of some 25 minutes a series of pictures through the head is provided which reveals intracranial pathology with a higher degree of certainty than previous invasive techniques. The total dose of irradiation is not greater than for conventional full skull radiography.

The X-ray tube emits a narrow beam of radiation as it passes in a series of scanning movements through an arc of 180 degrees around the patient's head. The sensitivity is such that small variations in X-ray absorption coefficients between the normal intracranial contents can be displayed, identifying cortex, white matter, internal capsule, and corpus callosum within the brain as well as the ventricles and cortical subarachnoid spaces. Tumour tissue, intracranial calcification, blood clot, and oedema have different absorption coefficients, making it possible to identify the site and nature of many pathological processes. It has the unique capacity to distinguish between infarction and haematoma and to identify brain oedema, which was not possible with any previous special investigation. The accuracy of computerized axial tomography has been greatly increased by the use of an intravenous dose of 60 ml of sodium iothalamate (Conray) which enhances the contrast between certain tissue densities. This iodine-containing contrast medium may be present in abnormal amounts either as a result of breakdown of the blood–brain barrier or of situations where blood flow is increased.

Continuing improvements in successive generations of scanner have increased definition by altering the window control and so affecting the contrast of lesions by comparison with surrounding brain parenchyma. Current high-grade scanners can construct sections of coronal, sagittal, or oblique planes from actual planes which make clear details for example in the region of the pituitary or internal auditory meatus. Such views now make the air-encephalogram virtually superfluous. It is now also possible to use variable contrast and special resolution to concentrate on the areas of interest without increasing the radiation to the patient. Arteries may be viewed in cross-section after an intravenous angiogram on the CT scan and sometimes the patency of the carotid confirmed non-invasively.

Some of the clinical questions which this new technique is particularly helpful in answering may be listed:

1. Are the signs of papilloedema and raised intracranial pressure due to a tumour or to benign intracranial hypertension? The scan distinguishes between dilated or distorted ventricles as in the former, probably outlining the tumour, and normal ventricles as usually found in the latter.

2. Is a patient's dementia due to a frontal tumour, or to cerebral atrophy with dilated ventricles, or to communicating hydrocephalus with an obliteration of the cortical subarachnoid spaces (see Figs. 10.1; 11.2, pp. 260 and 269)? If the last, treatment by ventriculo-atrial shunting can be considered.

3. Is a stroke due to cerebral haemorrhage with haematoma or infarction? This technique gives a better basis, in conjunction with other factors, for making a decision about the use of anticoagulants if progressive thrombosis is suspected (see Fig. 14.3, p. 294).

4. What is the site and extent of the haemorrhage or oedema following a head injury?

5. What is the effect of treatment on the progress of intracranial lesions such as tumours or abscesses (see Fig. 12.1, p. 274), or the change of ventricular size after treatment of hydrocephalus by shunting?

6. What is the site of a lesion causing visual symptoms, compression of the visual pathway by a pituitary tumour or proptosis due to a meningioma (Fig. 5.6)?

7. Location and sometimes identification is also possible in a much wider range of soft tissue intracranial lesions such as focal encephalitis, leucodystrophy, and spongiform brain degenerations.

Clearly the great potential of this technique is now being realized but at the same time it is obvious that it may be used indiscriminately, uncritically, and unnecessarily for the investigation of relatively trivial neurological symptoms. Any attempts to use it to replace skilled neurological judgement can, of course, easily lead to errors of omission or commission.

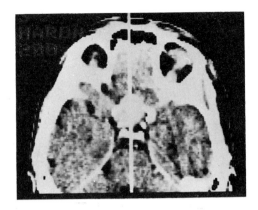

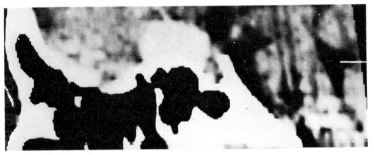

Fig. 5.6. CT scan showing meningioma: (upper) coronal view: (lower) sagittal reconstruction.

ISOTOPE ENCEPHALOGRAPHY

Radioactive isotopes are now only occasionally used for the detection and location of intracranial lesions and their importance has declined with the development of CT scanning. Isotope encephalography may provide information not shown on the CT scan in recent infarcts and isodense subdural haematomas.

NUCLEAR MAGNETIC RESONANCE (NMR) SCANNING

The NMR scan makes use of the magnetic properties of the hydrogen nucleus excited by radio-frequency radiation transmitted by a coil surrounding the head; the signals produced by the excited nuclei are detected as induced electric currents in a receiver coil lying within the transmitter coil. The inversion–recovery (IR) sequence of protons, depending on the spin–lattice relaxation time T_1, shows a high level of grey–white matter contrast. It is followed for successive projections of an axis and repeated through 180 degrees for each slice. Fat and bone marrow, with short 'relaxation' times, appear white; tissue or fluids with longer 'relaxation' times appear black (see Figs. 0.2, p. 4 and 5.7). Cortical bone which has a low concentration of hydrogen also appears black. Different modes of operation can be selected according to the nature of the scanning problem. The spin–echo (SE) sequences depend on the spin–spin relaxation time T_2, which is increased in a variety of lesions such as multiple sclerosis, encephalitis, and periventricular oedema. The NMR scan has no apparent hazard to the patient and the results are sometimes more revealing than those of the best CT scan. There is no limitation of X-ray exposure. The most obvious improvement over the CT scan is the better differentiation between grey and white matter because grey matter contains more hydrogen in the form of water than white matter and the hydrogen atoms are less bound in fat and large molecules. For example, the caudate and lentiform nuclei are visible in the basal ganglia and the pons, cerebellum, and peduncles can be seen in the posterior fossa views without the usual CT bone artefact (see Fig. 0.2). Blood can be distinguished from c.s.f. because the relaxation time constant which determines the density of the image is long for water and short for blood. The better differentiation between white and grey matter than on the CT scan makes it probable that it will be complementary to CT scanning and will particularly aid diagnosis of cerebral and cerebellar degenerations, toxic, metabolic and infective encephalopathies, meningitis, and multiple sclerosis. It is also useful when lesions are adjacent to bone as in the pituitary region and in the spinal cord.

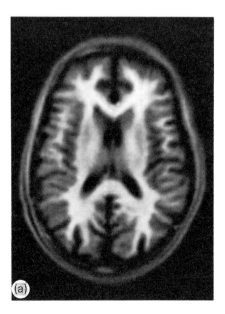 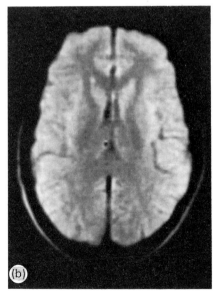

Fig. 5.7. NMR scans: (a) inversion–recovery (IR) (b) spin–echo (SE). The spin-echo scan shows much less grey–white matter contrast but shows oedema in pathological brain.

EVOKED RESPONSES

These involve artificial stimulation of pathways within the central nervous system in order to reveal, painlessly and safely, disturbances of conduction in order to confirm a diagnosis.

Visual evoked responses: The first potentials recorded were occipital cortical evoked responses to a reversing checkerboard visual pattern (Fig. 5.8). They are delayed and reduced in amplitude in 70 per cent of patients with definite multiple sclerosis even if there is no history of optic neuritis. The abnormalities are not specific for optic neuritis and are also found in local eye and optic nerve disease and conditions such as spinocerebellar degenerations and vitamin B_{12} deficiency. They are also abnormal after hemi-field stimulation in patients with chiasmatic lesions.

Auditory brainstem evoked responses to an auditory click stimulus are abnormal in many patients with multiple sclerosis and also in patients with cerebellopontine angle lesions and certain brainstem degenerations.

Somatosensory potentials can be recorded after electrical stimulation of a nerve such as the median nerve and can be recorded from the skin surface over the spinal cord or contralateral cerebral cortex. They may be abnormal in multiple sclerosis and also in degenerative conditions such as Friedreich's ataxia.

These abnormal potentials are rarely pathognomonic and should never be regarded as a routine investigation but together with the correct interpretation of the clinical features, they can be a valuable aid to diagnosis in atypical cases. For example they can be helpful if a visual defect is not recovering or if there is an apparent isolated lesion of the brainstem or spinal cord. In a patient with a spinal cord lesion causing a progressive spastic paraplegia, they may occasionally avoid the need for myelography. They represent therefore a special and at times useful extension of the clinical examination. The visual evoked response test can be helpful in the exclusion of any organic neurological lesion in a patient with visual symptoms due to hysteria; conversely they can be useful in the proof of an organic visual defect in a patient with visual symptoms which have been attributed to hysteria (Fig. 5.8). It must be remembered that hysterical symptoms may quite commonly co-exist with an underlying organic lesion. Other evoked potential techniques can be helpful in other comparable situations. A plaque of demyelination usually causes permanent changes in evoked potential response even if clinical recovery apparently occurs. Visual evoked responses may also provide a clue to a silent lesion and in a patient with one lesion elsewhere already known, therefore increase the probability of a correct diagnosis of multiple sclerosis.

POSITRON EMISSION COMPUTERIZED TOMOGRAPHY (PET)

This technique, using injected or inhaled radionuclides and scanning techniques similar to X-ray computerized tomography, is non-invasive but remains

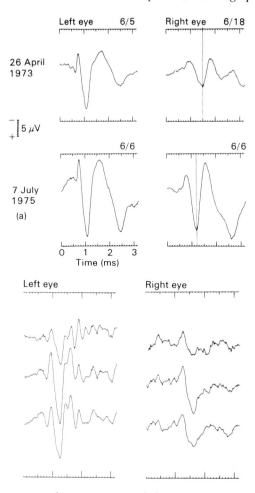

Fig. 5.8. (a) Pattern reversal responses recorded on two separate occasions from a patient with multiple sclerosis. The responses shown above were recorded at the age of 24, one month after the onset of an attack of right optic neuritis. The response from the affected eye, which still has a lowered visual acuity, is of reduced amplitude and delayed latency. The response from the unaffected left eye is within normal limits. The responses shown in the lower records were recorded two years later, by which time the visual evoked response from the right eye has not only recovered in amplitude, paralleling the improvement in visual acuity, but has regained a peak latency almost within the normal range. This is very unusual.

(b) The responses recorded from a patient who had been seen intermittently over several years with a vague history of impairment of balance and paraesthesiae. No confirmed abnormality on examination had been found in the past. She was referred again with a complaint of acute right unilateral visual loss which was thought at first to be hysterical. The optic discs were normal but there was a delay in the visual evoked response from the affected side, typical of that seen in acute optic neuritis. Her subsequent course has included a number of undoubtedly organic episodes, leading to a diagnosis of multiple sclerosis.

essentially a research investigation because the short-life isotopes are prepared by a cyclotron. The technique is most promising for metabolic studies using oxygen-15 or deoxyglucose labelled with fluorine-18. The reconstructed images can give information about regional blood flow, oxygen extraction, or utilization by glucose uptake (see Fig. 14.9, p. 299).

DOPPLER IMAGING (see p. 296)

Computer techniques have been applied to doppler imaging and in skilled hands this has an important place in the non-invasive screening for extra-cerebral stenotic vascular lesions.

DIGITAL SUBTRACTION ANGIOGRAPHY (see p. 290)

An adaptation for venous injection may replace the need for arteriography in some patients. A relatively small bolus of contrast medium is injected quickly into a peripheral vein via a catheter and a computer scans the required field of view of, for example, the carotid bifurcation. The results can be converted into a high-quality video display or film angiogram which is similar to the contrast with arterial angiography. The venous technique is ideal as a post-operative investigation following surgery to confirm the patency of cerebral vessels and as a preliminary investigation in an asymptomatic patient with, for example, a carotid bruit. It will demonstrate some 80 per cent of stenoses and 50 per cent of major carotid artery atheromatous ulcerations but will miss small ulcerations and is not usually adequate to demonstrate abnormalities of the intracranial circulation. Digital subtraction arteriography still provides the greatest resolution and there are a variety of techniques utilizing film and television techniques to increase its usefulness for particular purposes. Such techniques have to be compared with doppler ultrasound imaging, which also at present shows, without risk, 80 per cent of major stenoses and some 50 per cent of ulcerative lesions.

ELECTRODIAGNOSIS IN NEUROMUSCULAR DISORDERS

Electromyography, the recording of electrical changes present in muscles at rest or evoked by voluntary movement, is a necessary part of the investigation of neuromuscular disorders. The recording is made by introducing a concentric needle electrode into the muscle to be tested. It will be recalled that each lower motor neurone conveys impulses which cause a number of muscle fibres to contract. When a normal muscle is completely relaxed, no electrical activity can be detected in it. When a voluntary contraction is induced, the record shows the characteristic response of a motor unit which is usually biphasic, that is, shows a positive followed by a negative phase. As the contraction increases in strength,

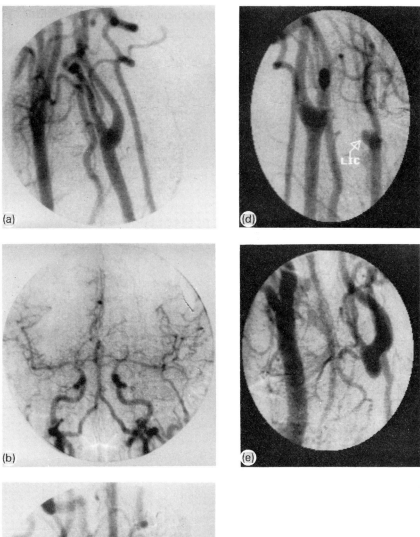

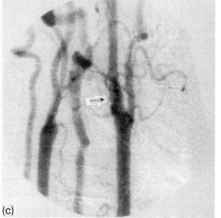

Fig. 5.9. Digital venous angiography. (a) Normal neck vessels; (b) normal vertebral circulation; (c) moderate atheromatous irregularity of the proximal left internal carotid artery; (d) left internal carotid occlusion; (e) filling of the left carotid vessels above a common carotid tie, performed for an intracranial aneurysm. It would obviously be impossible to demonstrate the left-sided anatomy by carotid catheter.

more and more motor unit contractions are added to the record (Fig. 5.10). Lesions of the lower motor neurone or muscle produce on the electromyogram the effects which might be expected.

1. *Denervation* leads to the appearance of fibrillation potentials, positive sharp waves and fasciculation potentials at rest. On activity, units are reduced in number but generally normal in appearance, though in severe chronic denervation many surviving units are increased in amplitude and duration. The characteristic finding in *motor neurone disease* is spontaneous fibrillation on mechanical stimulation by the exploring needle, a duration and amplitude of action potentials greater than normal, and even in cases of moderate weakness a marked reduction in the number of spikes on maximal contraction. The last feature is the result of the reduction in the number of motor neurones and consequently of the motor units available for contraction.

2. In *myopathy*, on the other hand, the characteristic response to voluntary movement is the occurrence of spike potentials with an abnormally short

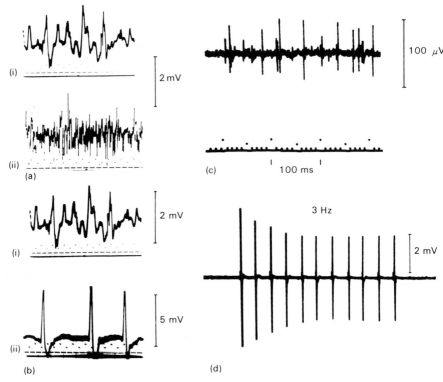

Fig. 5.10. Electromyograms. (a) Electromyogram recorded from normal muscle (i) and from muscle of a patient with muscular dystrophy (ii) on maximum effort. (b) Electromyogram recorded on maximum voluntary effort from muscle which is normal (i) and denervated (ii). Time marker: 5 ms intervals. (c) Spontaneous fibrillation recorded from denervated muscle. (d) Myasthenia gravis. Successive muscle action potentials recorded with surface electrodes over abductor digiti minimi muscle on stimulating ulnar nerve repetitively at 3 Hz. Note rapid progressive decline in amplitude.

duration, and much weaker than the normal action potential, and an increased proportion of polyphasic action potentials. Only when the weakness is severe is there a reduction in the number of action potentials.

3. In *polymyositis* the changes resemble those in myopathy but there are more polyphasic action potentials and sometimes also fibrillation potentials due to involvement of the distal part of the neurone.

4. In *myotonia* mechanical stimulation of a muscle leads to a repetitive discharge of the muscle fibres declining in frequency very rapidly, which when conducted to the electromyographic loudspeaker causes the characteristic 'dive-bomber' sound.

5. In *myasthenia gravis* various abnormalities have been described in the electromyogram, but its chief diagnostic use is to record the improvement in the response produced by an intravenous injection of edrophonium (Tensilon). In myasthenia there is a marked reduction in the electromyogram after exercise. In the myasthenic syndrome of Eaton–Lambert, though at rates of stimulation of 3 per second the amplitude declines, there is a parodoxical potentiation at high frequencies, though from a lower than normal initial amplitude.

Electromyography is thus of value in distinguishing between lesions of the lower motor neurone and of the muscle itself. Electrophysiological studies are now also an important part of the complete examination of a patient with a peripheral nerve lesion. By recording from a muscle and stimulating its nerve at two different points along its course, the velocity of conduction along the intervening segment of the nerve may be calculated. There is a greater slowing of conduction in neuropathies with demyelination than in those with degeneration (p. 419). In traumatic and compressive lesions of the peripheral nerve such as the carpal tunnel syndrome or the ulnar nerve lesion at the elbow, slowing of conduction occurs distal to the lesion (Fig. 5.11). A change may be of help in estimating the recovery of a peripheral nerve lesion. More refined techniques make it possible to record sensory action potentials from the median or ulnar nerves at the wrist after stimulating percutaneously the corresponding digital nerves in the fingers with ring electrodes. A loss of potentials may be found in a sensory neuropathy in the absence of any abnormality of motor fibres. Intensity–duration curves (I/T curves) are a supplementary method of investigating peripheral nerve function; if a muscle fails to contract on stimulation with a current pulse of less than 1 ms duration then it may be concluded that the motor nerve has ceased to function. Segmental electromyography can detect denervation and help the diagnosis of lumbar-root lesions caused by the posterior facet joint in which unlike a prolapsed disc, the plain X-rays and myelogram may be entirely normal.

MUSCLE BIOPSY

The modern investigation of neuromuscular disorders, in addition to serum enzyme studies (p. 430) and electromyography may require muscle biopsy. In addition to routine histology, enzyme histochemistry (see Plate 8) may show an

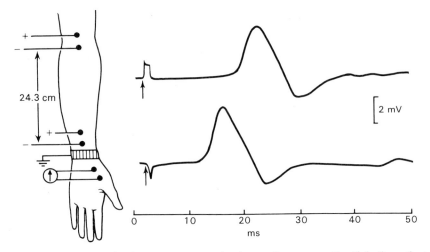

Fig. 5.11. Motor conduction measurement in the median nerve of a diabetic patient with the carpal tunnel syndrome. The latency of 10.0 ms between the stimulus at the wrist and the evoked potential is greatly prolonged. Since the latency after stimulation at the elbow is 16.0 ms and the distance between the stimulating cathodes 24.3 cm, the conduction velocity elbow to wrist is 40.4 m/s.

absence of differentiation suggesting a congenital dystrophy or a specific abnormality within the muscle fibre not apparent on routine staining (central core disease or nemaline myopathy) or absence of a particular enzyme, such as phosphorylase in McArdle's disease. It may also help to identify a neurogenic atrophy by the uniformity of enzyme activity in the reinnervated fibres.

SURAL NERVE BIOPSY

A sural nerve biopsy leaves a very small area of sensory impairment which does not inconvenience the patient. In about half the chronic neuropathies the routine investigations fail to reveal a cause. In these patients sural nerve biopsy may be justified and sometimes aids diagnosis. For example, a nerve may be infiltrated with amyloid, myeloma, or carcinoma and there may be evidence of vasculitis or sarcoid. A distinction can be made between demyelinating and axonal neuropathies (see p. 417) and a congenital hypertrophic neuropathy.

REFERENCES

Andersen, M. (1982). Nuclear magnetic resonance imaging and neurology. *Br. med. J.* **284**, 1359–60.

Bydder, G.M., Steiner, R.E., Young, I.R., Hall, A.S., Thomas, D.J., Marshall, J., Pallis, C.A., and Legg, N.J. (1982). Clinical NMR imaging of the brain *Amer. J. Radiol.* **139**, 215–36.

Chiappa, K.H. and Ropper, A.H. (1982). Evoked potentials in clinical medicine. *New Engl. J. Med.* **306**, 1140–50.

Halliday, A.M. and McDonald, W.I. (1981). Visual evoked potentials. In *Clinical neurophysiology* (ed. E. Stalberg and R.R. Young) pp. 228–58. Butterworth, London.

Lenman, J.A.R. and Ritchie, A.E. (1983). *Clinical electromyography,* 3rd edn. Pitman, London.

Kiloh, L.G., McComas, A.J., and Osselton, J.W. (1981). *Clinical electroencephalography,* 4th edn. Butterworth, London.

Swash, M. and Schwartz, M.S. (1981). *Neuromuscular diseases: a practical approach to diagnosis and management.* Springer, Berlin.

Tatler, G.L. and Mosely, I.F. (1982). The use of non-invasive techniques in neurological investigations. *Br. med. J.* **285**, 1026–8.

Weisberg, L.A. (1978). *Cerebral computed tomography: a text-atlas.* Saunders, Philadelphia.

Wise, R.J.S., Bernardi, S., Frackowiak, R.S.J., Legg, N.J., and Jones, T. (1983). Serial observations on the pathophysiology of acute stroke: the transition from ischaemia to infarction as reflected in regional oxygen extraction. *Brain* **106**, 197–222.

6 Consciousness and unconsciousness

ANATOMY AND PHYSIOLOGY

There is a broad distinction between the content of consciousness, that is, what we are at any moment conscious of, sensations, emotions, ideas, or memories, for example, and the process of consciousness itself. This is borne out by everyday clinical experience. A person may be at one moment conscious of one thing and at another moment conscious of another, but on each occasion he is equally conscious. Moreover, the content of consciousness may be impaired by disease, as when a patient loses part of a visual field or sensation over part of the body. Nevertheless, such a person remains fully conscious. On the other hand, a person may be completely unconscious, and between full consciousness and unconsciousness there are states in which he is partially conscious, that is, he has some degree of awareness of his surroundings, but it is incomplete. Hence the content of consciousness may be reduced without any alteration in consciousness as a process, or consciousness as a process may be impaired in which case none of the functions normally associated with it can be adequately carried out. Research has shown that the maintenance of consciousness depends to an important extent upon the central reticular formation.

The central reticular formation

This structure occupies a central position in the brainstem and is situated in the tegmentum of the medulla, pons and midbrain, above which it merges into the thalamic reticular system (Fig. 6.1). The reticular formation of the brainstem was originally merely an anatomical concept, referring to the reticular or net-like appearance of the central part of the brainstem, until Moruzzi and Magoun's classical paper in 1949 entitled 'Brain stem reticular formation and the activation of the EEG'. These authors appreciated that the anatomical site of the activating system they had identified physiologically was not known precisely but others have failed to keep the distinction clear by using the term reticular activating system. The 'ascending activating system' is a physiological concept and to use the 'reticular formation' as synonymous with the 'activating system' is incorrect. When referring the activating function it is appropriate to use the words 'activating system of the brainstem' which comprises the medulla, pons, and mesencephalon. It has been shown experimentally that damage to the central reticular formation which spares the lemniscal ascending sensory pathways causes persistent unconsciousness in animals, which then show the electroencephalographic changes normally associated with sleep. The

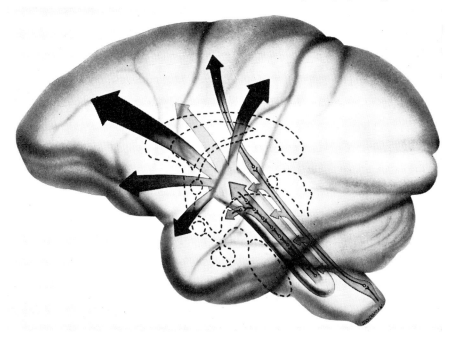

Fig. 6.1. Lateral view of the monkey's brain, showing the ascending brainstem activating system in the brainstem receiving collaterals from different afferent paths and projecting primarily to the associational areas of the hemisphere.

central reticular formation is therefore regarded as the anatomical basis of an alerting system which acts in a complex manner upon both the cerebral cortex and the afferent pathways in order to maintain the brain in a condition in which consciousness can occur. The experimental lesions just described can be paralleled in human pathology, and there is now evidence that lesions of the central reticular formation in man, even as low as the medulla, may cause loss of consciousness. Lesions of the cerebral cortex and subcortical white matter, including extensive ablations, do not cause loss of consciousness. Discharging cortical lesions, however, may do so, especially when they are situated in the temporal or frontal lobes. How loss of consciousness is produced in epileptic attacks is not fully understood, but it would appear that when a discharging lesion causes loss of consciousness it probably does so by interfering with the activity of the central reticular formation, and it has been suggested that the disturbance occurs in the upper part of the diencephalon in the neighbourhood of the thalami.

COMA

The word coma (Greek κῶμα, meaning a deep sleep) is the term used for prolonged states of unconsciousness. From what has already been said it will be clear that coma may be produced by lesions involving the central reticular formation. This may be the area of the brain primarily damaged, or it may suffer indirectly as the result of, for example, a space-occupying or vascular lesion elsewhere. It may be assumed that when coma occurs in a patient suffering from a focal lesion of the brain, it is to an important extent the result of disturbance of function of the central reticular formation. In many cases, however, coma is the result of some disorder which acts diffusely upon the nervous system, for example a toxic state, however produced. While there are some substances, for example anaesthetics, which seem to act to some extent selectively upon the central reticular formation, when a toxic substance is carried to the nervous system in the blood stream and causes coma, though the coma may be the result of its effect upon the central reticular formation, it is usually impossible to separate this from its effects upon the rest of the brain, including the cerebral cortex.

We shall first consider the causes of coma, then the examination and investigation of the comatose patient, and finally his management.

THE CAUSES OF COMA

Cerebral vascular lesions

A cerebral vascular lesion is one of the commonest causes of coma. When a cerebral vascular lesion causes coma it does so partly at least because, directly or indirectly, it interferes with the functions of the central reticular formation. This is most likely to occur after:

1. A massive subarachnoid haemorrhage.
2. A subarachnoid haemorrhage invading one cerebral hemisphere.
3. A massive intracerebral haemorrhage, or one rupturing into one cerebral ventricle.
4. An area of infarction of one cerebral hemisphere large enough to cause considerable oedema of the hemisphere.
5. Infarction of the central reticular formation itself, especially in a case of thrombosis of the basilar artery.

The symptomatology of these lesions is described elsewhere, but broadly it may be said that a vascular cause for coma is suggested by the presence of atheroma or hypertension, a sudden or relatively sudden onset, focal signs corresponding to those produced by a vascular lesion, or signs of meningeal irritation of sudden onset; and supported by the presence of red blood cells or xanthochromia and a raised protein in the cerebrospinal fluid.

Space-occupying lesions

Coma due to an *intracranial tumour* or *abscess* almost always comes on much more slowly than that due to a cerebral vascular lesion, though occasionally haemorrhage into a tumour may cause rapid loss of consciousness. A history of symptoms of increased intracranial pressure, especially headache, is usually obtainable, and papilloedema is likely to be present, and is often severe. Signs of vascular disease are usually absent, but diagnosis may be difficult when a tumour develops late in life in a patient who also suffers from hypertension or atheroma. *Subdural haematoma* is most likely to occur in the middle aged or elderly, in whom it may develop without discoverable cause or insidiously after a head injury. Headache is usually a prominent symptom, and unconsciousness when it develops often fluctuates strikingly in depth. Papilloedema and signs of focal cerebral compression are often present, but may be absent.

Head injury

When head injury is the cause of coma, there is usually a history of the injury, and there may be bruising of the scalp or signs of fracture of the vault, or of the base of the skull, such as bleeding from the ear, or bleeding or discharge of cerebrospinal fluid from the nose. It must be remembered, however, that a patient who becomes unconscious from some other cause may injure his head in falling. Sometimes a 'lucid interval' occurs between recovery from the effects of concussion and the ensuing coma resulting from brain compression by continuing arterial bleeding. Traumatic intracranial arterial haemorrhage leads to progressively deepening coma with signs of a focal lesion of one hemisphere, often beginning with convulsions and leading to hemiplegia. The classical Hutchinsonian pupil, which may be observed in such circumstances, consists of first a contraction and then a dilatation with failure to react to light of the pupil on the side of the lesion, followed later by the same sequence of events in the opposite pupil.

Meningitis and encephalitis

When meningitis is the cause of coma, the onset of symptoms is usually subacute, and the severity of the headache associated with fever, cervical rigidity, and Kernig's sign (see p. 471) indicate meningeal irritation, the cause of which is to be established by the discovery of the characteristic changes in the cerebrospinal fluid, from which it may be possible to isolate the causal organism. The onset of encephalitis is also usually subacute, and also associated with fever. The signs are those of more or less diffuse damage to the brain, and in many cases also the spinal cord, the precise distribution of which varies in relation to the cause. Signs of meningeal irritation are usually absent but may be present, and there is often, but not invariably, a pleocytosis in the cerebrospinal fluid.

Narcotic drugs

When a narcotic drug is the cause of coma there is usually evidence of this, sometimes in the patient's own statement before becoming unconscious, sometimes in the fact that he or she is known to have had a supply of such a drug. In practice the drugs most commonly taken for suicidal purposes include a wide range of hypnotics, analgesics, sedatives, and antidepressants. Self poisoning has been described as the modern epidemic disease and causes 10 per cent of acute hospital admissions in Britain. Drugs which may produce coma as the result of a therapeutic overdosage include the barbiturates, any of the drugs generally used in the treatment of epilepsy, the tranquillizers and hypnotics. When alcohol is the cause of coma this can usually be established from the history; the face is flushed, the pulse rapid and the blood pressure low. The size of the pupils varies according to the causal agent: they tend to be dilated in alcoholic coma, contracted in coma due to morphine, but in the case of other drugs intermediate in size. The reaction to light is usually sluggish, and may be lost. The tendon reflexes tend to be diminished or lost, and the plantar reflexes extensor. Respiration is shallow, and the pulse rapid and of low tension. The drug responsible should be sought in the stomach washings and its level estimated in the blood. Specimens can be sent to a drug reference laboratory for assay.

Metabolic disorders

Uraemic coma

Uraemic coma may occur in chronic nephritis and other conditions causing renal destruction. Headache, vomiting, dyspnoea, and muscular twitchings or generalized convulsions are likely to precede the coma. The raised blood urea establishes the diagnosis.

Diabetic coma

In diabetic coma the patient is usually wasted and pale. Both the rate and amplitude of the respirations are increased, and the ocular tension is very low. Reaction of the pupils to light may be lost even while the patient can still be roused. Large quantities of sugar are demonstrable, together with acetoacetic acid and acetone, in the urine, and the blood sugar is much raised.

Hypoglycaemic coma

Hypoglycaemic coma is easily recognized if it is due to an overdose of insulin which the patient is known to be taking. The presence of sugar in the urine does not exclude this, since the urine may have been excreted before the patient became hypoglycaemic. Spontaneous hypoglycaemia sufficient to cause coma is almost always the result of excessive production of insulin by a tumour composed of cells of the islets of Langerhans in the pancreas. In such cases fainting fits or convulsions or periods of mental disorder may precede the onset of coma by weeks or months. The hypoglycaemic patient sweats profusely, the pupils are dilated, the tendon reflexes increased, and the plantar reflexes may be extensor. The diagnosis can be made by examination of the blood sugar, which is found to be extremely low, in the region of 2.0 to 3.0 mmol/l, or even lower. The cerebral disturbances of hypoglycaemia are promptly relieved by intravenous injection of glucose. The diagnosis of spontaneous hypoglycaemia may be difficult and prolonged fasting may be necessary to provoke an attack. It may be necessary to provoke an attack by an intravenous injection of tolbutamide.

Hepatic coma

Hepatic coma gives rise to no difficulty when the patient is known to be suffering from liver failure. Jaundice, however, may be absent. In the earlier stages the patient usually suffers from memory defect, disorientation and hypersomnia, and may exhibit a mixture of corticospinal, extrapyramidal and cerebellar signs, especially the characteristic 'flapping tremor' or asterixis. This results from a transient inhibition of postural mechanisms. Otherwise the diagnosis rests upon the presence of the physical signs of liver disease and biochemical evidence of disturbed liver function. The blood ammonia level may be raised. The EEG is abnormal, often with repetitive bifrontal bursts of 2–4 Hz waves. It is also a sensitive method of detecting the response to treatment with neomycin.

Coma of endocrine origin

Coma of endocrine origin presents a diagnostic problem when it occurs in patients in whom the pre-existing endocrine disease has not been recognized. Coma in *hypopituitarism* may be sudden, for example if it is precipitated by an infection. The patient is usually a woman who exhibits the endocrine changes of hypopituitarism. The blood pressure and blood sugar are likely to be low and the body temperature may be subnormal or above normal. The thyroid function is likely to be significantly impaired and the plasma cortisol levels very low. The coma which may occur in *myxoedema* is likely to be associated with a slow pulse and a subnormal temperature. The appearance of the patient is characteristic. The coma of *suprarenal cortical failure* may be difficult to recognize if it occurs suddenly as the result of stress, for example surgical operation, in a patient not known to be suffering from suprarenal cortical deficiency. The low blood pressure and low serum sodium are characteristic.

Coma due to carbon dioxide intoxication

Carbon dioxide retention may occur as the result of chronic pulmonary disease or respiratory failure of neuromuscular origin in, for example, motor neurone disease, poliomyelitis, polyneuritis, myopathy, and myasthenia. It causes a fall in the pH and a rise in the H_2CO_3 in the blood. In chronic CO_2 retention the respiratory centre fails to react to the raised level of CO_2 and respiration is then maintained by the receptors which respond to oxygen lack. Administering oxygen to such patients may remove the stimulus to respiration, raise the blood CO_2 still further and precipitate coma. Milder degrees of CO_2 intoxication cause drowsiness and confusion.

Coma due to carbon monoxide intoxication

In carbon monoxide intoxication there is almost always a history of exposure to coal-gas or the exhaust fumes of a motor-car. In doubtful cases the diagnosis can be made by the spectroscopic examination of the blood.

Epilepsy

In a case of post-epileptic coma there is usually a history of epilepsy or at least of the attack which preceded the coma. In the absence of this information, scars on the face or a bitten tongue may provide a clue. Focal signs of a cerebral lesion are usually absent, but the plantar reflexes may be extensor. After a single epileptic attack the period of unconsciousness is usually short, not more than half an hour to an hour, but status epilepticus may be followed by prolonged coma.

Hysteria

In hysterical trance the patient, though apparently unconscious, usually shows some response to external stimuli. An attempt to elicit the corneal reflex often causes a vigorous contraction of the orbicularis oculi. Rigidity of the hysterical type may be present, and if so any attempt passively to overcome the rigidity excites a proportional increase in the stiffness which resists the observer's efforts. Signs of organic disease are absent.

THE INVESTIGATION OF THE UNCONSCIOUS PATIENT

When examining the unconscious patient the first point to investigate is the depth of unconsciousness. The simplest way to estimate this is to examine the patient's response to various kinds of stimuli. The most deeply unconscious patient will not respond in any way to any stimulus. A patient who is somewhat less deeply unconscious will respond to a painful stimulus, such as pressure over the supraorbital nerve, by contracting the facial muscles, but will not give any other evidence of awareness of what is happening. Patients with either of these degrees of unconsciousness are described as comatose. A patient who is still less deeply unconscious will show some awareness of his surroundings, the the extent, for example, of rousing when shaken vigorously and called by his name, but, though he may answer, he will not speak rationally, and will rapidly relapse into unconsciousness. This condition is called *stupor*. Patients suffering from encephalitis lethargica were observed to spend most of the day in a condition resembling sleep, from which they could be roused to speak in a fairly rational manner and even to take their meals, only to fall asleep again immediately afterwards. Thus all degrees of unconsciousness exist ranging from deep coma in which the patient responds to no stimulus to a condition resembling sleep from which the patient can be aroused to a state approaching normality. For postures in coma see page 90.

Reflex responses vary with the depth of unconsciousness. The plantar reflexes early become extensor: in deeper coma the corneal reflexes, the tendon reflexes and finally the pupillary reflexes are lost.

The comatose patient should be subjected to a most detailed and systematic examination, since any part of the body may provide a clue to the cause of the unconsciousness.

Apart from the general state of unconsciousness, information about the level of the brain involved and the nature of the involvement can be obtained from study of particular systems.

Persistent vegetative state, akinetic mutism, and the 'locked-in' syndrome

Some confusion surrounds the use of these different terms. During the recovery from deep coma usually after a head injury the patient may pass through a stage in which he is awake and may follow people with his eyes and respond in a limited way to primitive postural and reflex movements without any awareness of the environment or inner need. The EEG may even be normal. Jennett and Plum describe this as the *persistent vegetative state.* The precise site of the lesion in the brainstem is unknown because such patients usually recover, though in cases in which the patient has eventually died there may be no focal brainstem lesion but diffuse degeneration, often necrosis, of white matter tracts in the cerebrum with degeneration of descending tracts.

The term *akinetic mutism* was first used by Cairns to describe a reversible amnesic state in a patient with a third ventricular cyst. The patient appeared to be awake, looked around, and retained some part of consciousness but did not speak and was almost totally unresponsive. It has also come to be used with patients with bilateral frontal or cingulate lesions who lack any psychic drive or any impulse to action although the major motor and sensory tracts are intact. Both these states can be distinguished from the *'locked-in' syndrome*, a state in which the patient is fully aware or conscious but cannot make any responses. The lesion here has preserved the activating system but interrupted the cortico-bulbar and spinal pathways so that the patient cannot speak or move. Terms also used are pseudocoma, the deafferented state, or *coma vigil* (the French term). The lesion is in the ventral pons with preservation of the dorsal tegmental area. The patient is obviously both akinetic and mute but in a different sense from akinetic mutism described above. A few such patients eventually recover and may give an interesting and all too frank account of what people around them said and did during their illness.

Clearly with multiple vascular or hypoxic lesions in the forebrain, midbrain, and pons, variations of these types of lesions can be identified which are difficult to categorize. One is reminded of a comment by Penfield 'there is no room or place where consciousness dwells'. It is perhaps more important to record the patient's precise degree of wakefulness and response to a variety of stimuli. The following code suggested by Jennett and Teasdale (1974) is a useful guide in following a patients changing level of consciousness.

The Glasgow coma scale (adapted from Teasdale and Jennett (1974))

Eye opening
1. Spontaneous.
2. To speech or shouting.
3. To painful stimulation.
4. None.

Verbal response
1. Orientated to place, person, and time.
2. Confused conversation, attention held.
3. Inappropriate speech, random or shouting.
4. Incomprehensible sounds or moaning.
5. None.

Best motor response
1. Obeys commands.
2. Localizes; limb moves to prevent noxious stimulus.
3. Flexor response, hemiplegia or decorticate posturing, extensor response.
4. None.

The pattern of breathing

Periodic (Cheyne–Stokes) respiration is due to an abnormally increased ventilatory response to CO_2 followed by post-hyperventilation apnoea. It suggests bilateral cerebral lesions, or a high brainstem lesion, often with cardiac disease causing a prolonged circulation time. Sustained deep breathing occurs with certain midbrain lesions due to tumours, infarction, or compression due to herniation. Irregular breathing with clustered breaths, gasping or jerking inspiration occurs with low pontine or medullary lesions, indicating disturbance of the medullary inspiratory and expiratory neurones.

The pupils

The pupils are moderately dilated and do not respond to light with a high midbrain lesion. Unilateral dilatation with a fixed pupil suggests tentorial herniation due to increase intracranial pressure. Pontine lesions produce bilaterally small pupils by interrupting the descending sympathetic pathways.

Eye movements and vestibulo-ocular responses

Involuntary conjugate deviation of the eyes towards a normal arm after hemiparesis, indicates a hemisphere lesion, and towards the paralysed limbs a pontine lesion. The *oculocephalic* or *doll's head reflexes*, contralateral conjugate eye movement on sudden head movements, oculovestibular reflexes, and nystagmus on aural stimulation with cold water, are absent with pontine lesions.

The head

The head should be examined for evidence of injury indicated by cuts or abrasions. The skull should be palpated for a depressed fracture, and the ears and nose examined for haemorrhage and leakage of cerebrospinal fluid. The ears should also be investigated for infection of the middle ear. Scars on the face may point to injuries received in previous epileptic attacks, and the tongue should be examined to see if it has been recently bitten or is the site of similar scars.

The breath

The smell of the breath may provide a clue. In alcoholic intoxication the characteristic odour of alcohol can be detected, and that of acetone in diabetic coma. The smell of the breath in uraemia may be simulated by that present in many unconscious patients with oral infection.

The skin

Cyanosis will be present when coma is due to CO_2 intoxication, and the characteristic brown pigmentation in Addison's disease. Carbon monoxide poisoning causes a cherry-red colour. Multiple telangiectases are found in hereditary telangiectasia, in which condition a cerebral telangiectasis may give rise to cerebral haemorrhage, and spider naevi over the upper part of the body are characteristic of hepatic disease. Purpura may be associated with an intra-cranial haemorrhage in thrombocytopenic purpura, with a cerebral embolus in subacute infective endocarditis and with meningococcal meningitis. The skin is coarse in myxoedema and fine and supple in hypopituitarism. In both there may be a deficiency of scalp and body hair. The scars of injections may be present in diabetics and drug addicts.

The nervous system

Examination of the nervous system is of special importance in view of the large number of nervous disorders which give rise to coma. Special attention should be paid to the fundi where papilloedema may indicate increased intracranial pressure or be associated with hypertensive retinopathy, to signs of hemiplegia and the presence of cervical rigidity indicating meningitis or subarachnoid haemorrhage.

Other organs

The lungs may yield evidence of the cause of CO_2 retention; the cardiovascular system of hypertension, atheroma, or mitral stenosis and auricular fibrillation, a common cause of cerebral embolism. The abdomen may show the venous congestion and hepatomegaly of chronic liver disease or the renal enlargement of polycystic kidneys.

Summary of signs with lesions at different levels

If there are bilateral cortical lesions the signs may include decorticate posturing with arm flexion, Cheyne–Stokes breathing, tonic deviation of the eyes and small reactive pupils. If the midbrain is damaged there is decerebrate posturing with extension of both arms and legs, central neurogenic hyperventilation with preserved oculocephalic movements, and fixed pupils of moderate size. If the pons is damaged the posture may be decerebrate or flaccid, ventilation may be apneustic and oculocephalic reflexes are variable but the pupils are small and fixed. If the medulla is damaged, tone is flaccid and there may be respiratory ataxia or lack of breathing with absent oculocephalic reflexes and pupils of mid-size but fixed.

Laboratory investigations

The urine

The urine should be examined for sugar, albumin, bile, and porphyrins.

The blood

The blood sugar and the blood urea should always be examined if no focal cerebral cause for the coma is discovered. The blood electrolytes will need to be investigated if it is thought that the coma is the result of their disorder and also to make sure that they are maintained at a normal level in the management of the unconscious patient.

The cerebrospinal fluid

Examination of the cerebrospinal fluid is essential to establish the diagnosis of meningitis or subarachnoid haemorrhage. In general lumbar puncture is contra-indicated in states of increased intracranial pressure due to a space-occupying lesion.

Other investigations

Other investigations which may be necessary include X-rays of the skull, CT scans, angiography, electroencephalography, and electrocardiography.

THE MANAGEMENT OF THE UNCONSCIOUS PATIENT

Nursing

The unconscious patient should be nursed in the lateral position and turned every two hours. The usual attention should be paid to the care of the skin, especially the pressure areas.

The respiratory tract

The mouth and pharynx should be cleansed regularly by means of a swab held in forceps. Mucus and saliva tend to accumulate in the pharynx and should be sucked out by means of a soft rubber catheter attached to a mechanical sucker. A physiotherapist should carry out regular percussion over the lungs, especially the bases. If there are signs of pulmonary collapse the patient will require bronchoscopy in order that an obstructed bronchus may be cleared by suction. An oral airway will be required by a deeply unconscious patient. A patient with severe respiratory depression will require artificial respiration best carried out in most cases by a positive pressure mechanical respirator combined with tracheal intubation or tracheostomy. If artificial respiration is likely to be required for long periods or repeatedly, tracheostomy is necessary, and a cuffed tracheostomy tube has the advantage of preventing the aspiration of food or saliva. Penicillin should be given regularly as a prophylactic against pneumonia, but if chest infection occurs a broad-spectrum antibiotic should be substituted.

Feeding

A patient who remains unconscious for more than a few hours will require both food and drink, and since he cannot swallow this must be given by an oesophageal tube. A fluid balance chart should be kept. It must be borne in mind that this is not a complete safeguard against the aspiration of food since a feed may be regurgitated, and vomiting may occur. Unless a special diet is indicated a diet such as the following will prove satisfactory. A fortified milk mixture is made consisting of 2.5 litres of milk, 225 g of skimmed milk powder, 110 g of dextrose and one teaspoonful of yeast extract. This provides 160 g of protein as well as carbohydrate, mineral salts, and vitamins, and has a calorie value of 2880. Vitamins and a liquid preparation of iron should be added if liquid feeding has to be continued for long periods, or the necessary vitamins can be given by intramuscular injection. Complan (Glaxo) is a convenient preparation containing all dietary requirements.

The blood electrolytes

The blood electrolytes may be disordered when the unconsciousness is the result of a metabolic disturbance. This will call for special treatment. Apart from that, however, they may become abnormal as the result of the cerebral lesion, e.g. brain injury or intracranial tumour, which is causing the unconsciousness. The blood electrolytes should therefore be estimated regularly in the unconscious patient and any necessary correction carried out.

The sphincters

The unconscious patient will have retention or incontinence of urine, and this is best dealt with by use of a self-retaining catheter which should be changed every three days. Constipation is dealt with by enemas.

THE DIAGNOSIS OF BRAIN DEATH

Efficient intensive care units now make possible the resuscitation of more patients following prolonged hypotension due to myocardial infarction and other causes, and with more successful organ transplantation there is growing demand for organs, particularly kidneys, from suitable donors in whom brain death has occurred. Decisions about the degree of irreversible brain damage must be taken against a fraught emotional background. Some difficulties arise in the lay-mind from linking the presence of life with the central idea of the heart continuing to beat. The heart may, of course, continue to beat by intrinsic mechanisms after total brainstem death and after spontaneous respiration has ceased, if oxygenation is maintained with artificial respiration. It is usually possible to distinguish, by the retention of brainstem reflexes, between massive cortical damage alone and the total damage to both hemispheres and the brainstem. It is important to stress that a flat electroencephalogram (EEG), though helpful, is not an infallible index of brain death; there have been instances of flat EEGs being recorded at an interval of 24 hours but being subsequently followed by a degree of cerebral recovery which, though incomplete, was quite unexpected.

After a head injury if the patient is totally unresponsive and without any movement response even to pain after 24 hours, the prognosis for useful brain recovery is poor. In patients with lack of brainstem reflexes at the time of admission there is less than a one in 20 chance of independent recovery. There is in general no significant chance of recovery if these signs persist for three days.

Criteria for brain death were first agreed by a council of the medical Royal Colleges in the United Kingdom in 1976 and there were further guidelines issued by the Royal Colleges in 1979. The criteria are all designed to 'distinguish between those patients who retain the functional capacity to have a chance of even partial recovery and those in which no such possibility exists'. The patients will usually have suffered a head injury in a road traffic accident or will have had an intracerebral haemorrhage. The basic concept is that human death is the irreversible loss of the capacity for consciousness and the capacity to breathe. Since both functions reside in the brainstem, this leads us to replace the earlier concept of total brain death by the concept of brainstem death. The irreversible cessation of brainstem function implies death of the brain as a whole but not necessarily the death of every brain cell. It is assumed that within hours or days or brainstem death the heart will stop, causing death of any surviving cells in the brain. The criteria depend on the tests of brainstem death and diagnosis of an irreversible disorder causing coma.

The first step in the diagnosis of brainstem death is that the comatose patient is unable to breathe spontaneously and is therefore unconscious and is on a ventilator. The second step is to establish that the cause of the coma is structural and therefore irreversible and untreatable. Only from a precise diagnosis can the certainty of irreversibility be known. Exclusions are the potentially reversible comatose states due to drug intoxication, hypothermia (with a temperature of about 35°C) or a metabolic disturbance such as hypoglycaemia. Some of these can be excluded by the history, some by examination but some require special investigation. Life support must be continued until the various tests, including biochemical tests, have been completed. The greatest worry is drug overdosage which accounts for most of the cases of coma of unknown cause and blood assays should be readily available for a range of possible drugs including carbon monoxide, salicylate, barbiturate, and ethanol and for urinary phenothiazines.

The third step in establishing brainstem death is the proof that all brainstem reflexes are absent. These involve the lack of pupillary and corneal reflexes, the lack of vestibulo-ocular reflexes either by caloric responses to slow injection of cold water into the ear or lack of oculocephalic or doll's head eye movements. There must also be the lack of facial response to pain and of the gag and coughing reflexes to larnygeal suction. Finally there is the lack of spontaneous breathing when the patient has been taken off the respirator after having been ventilated with 100 per cent oxygen for 10 minutes and then 95 per cent oxygen and 5 per cent CO_2 for five minutes which if gas analysis is available to confirm this, should give a pCO_2 in arterial blood of 50 mm of CO_2. The patient is then disconnected with 100 per cent oxygen attached to the airway for 10 minutes. This would ensure that at the end of that time the pCO_2 would rise to around 60 mm of pCO_2, an adequate hypercapnic stimulus to respiration.

There is an almost infinite variety of other special tests but in the United Kingdom these are regarded as unnecessary. In particular an isoelectric EEG cannot increase the criteria's reliability because an isoelectric EEG is occasionally found in patients who recover and an EEG has been recorded in patients diagnosed clinically as brain dead who ultimately died.

The neurologist in charge has a responsibility to the patient and his family. Organ donation from the brain-dead patient must be an entirely separate issue. Incidentally since only 14 per cent of a series of patients involved in organ donation were ventilated for less than 24 hours the application of these rules should not greatly affect the availability of donors.

In 1979 further guidelines from the conference of medical Royal Colleges included the recommendation that the diagnosis of brain death should be made by two medical practitioners who have expertise in this field 'who should assure themselves that the preconditions as to the cause of the coma have been met before testing is carried out'. The length of time before the preconditions can be satisfied as to irreversibility will vary. It might be as long as 24 hours but occasionally may extend even longer. The tests showing brainstem death should always be repeated though the interval between the two sets of testing is a matter for clinical judgement. If the criteria are followed then there should never be a diagnosis of brainstem death in a patient who might survive. A recent survey of 609 patients from three neurosurgical centres in the United

Kingdom provided reassurance that the British criteria properly applied after the onset of a coma with double examination at 12 to 24 hours are free from any significant risk of error.

SLEEP AND ITS DISORDERS

Anatomy and physiology

Sleep is characterized by a state of cortical inactivity reflected in an electro-encephalogram characterized by slow random waves. The production of this state physiologically depends upon a complex interplay between the cerebral cortex and the central reticular formation in which the alerting influence of the central reticular formation upon the cortex temporarily falls into abeyance. A 'sleep centre' has been postulated on the ground that electrical stimulation of an area of the hypothalamus can induce sleep, but to localize sleep in this way is to take too simple a view. As we have seen, destruction of the central reticular formation produces unconsciousness accompanied by cortical electro-encephalographic changes similar to those observable in sleep. On falling asleep muscles relax and the EEG shows low-amplitude, fast-frequency waves, stage 1 of non-rapid eye movement sleep (NREM) sleep. As sleep becomes deeper and arousal becomes more difficult the EEG changes to spindles at 12–16 Hz waves (stage II) and then to higher amplitude slow waves (stages III and IV). After about 90 minutes of NREM sleep the first episodes of rapid eye movement (REM) sleep occurs with darting eye movements and changes of blood pressure and respiration and pulse. If awakened at this stage the sleeper describes the occurence of vivid dreaming. From infancy to old age the proportion of time spent in REM sleep declines.

Insomnia

Individual sleep patterns vary enormously but poor sleepers spend less time in REM sleep. Many drugs used to treat insomnia are not helpful in the long term and with the further disturbance in stopping the drug a dependance on a hypnotic can often be created. Flurazipam (Dalmane) is less disruptive than other drugs to the normal sleep pattern but the basic approach to insomnia should be to seek an underlying psychological disturbance rather than prescribe hypnotics.

Parasomnia

The term hypersomnia has been used for states resembling prolonged sleep from which the patient can be aroused. The most striking examples of this were observed in patients suffering from encephalitis lethargica. In most if not all such cases, however, the patient is not normally alert and orientated when aroused, in which respect the state differs from normal sleep. Parasomnia is therefore a better term to use. Parasomnia may be regarded as a variety of stupor. It is commonly the result of a lesion involving the central reticular formation at the level of the upper part of the brainstem.

Hypersomnia

Hypersomnia is, unlike narcolepsy, a tendency to sleep which is resistible. There are a number of causes which include the periodic respiratory insufficiency due to obesity (the Pickwickian syndrome described by Dickens) and the Klein–Levine periodic syndrome in young boys in which it is associated with excessive appetite and behavioural and memory changes. No pathological basis for this syndrome is known.

Sleep apnoea

REM sleep is characterized by regular breathing during which apnoea up to 15 seconds may occur. In some people apnoeas are much more frequent and prolonged (up to 120 seconds) and are described as the sleep apnoea syndromes. There are two basic types. In the first there is a lesion in the brainstem, probably a vascular lesion, causing a disturbance of the central respiratory generating mechanism leading to hypoxia. The second type, which may also be due to a central lesion, is associated with upper airways obstruction and is accompanied by snoring and noisy breathing. There is selective failure of the muscles which control the pharynx and tongue so that the tongue and pharyngeal wall fall inwards during the inspiratory effort and cause apnoea. The hypoxia may lead to secondary pulmonary and systemic hypertension, cardiac arrhythmia, and even death. It may be associated with obesity, tonsillar hypertrophy or in rarer cases acromegaly or myxoedema. Occasionally it may be the presenting symptoms of a rare neuronal degeneration of multiple system atrophy associated with progressive autonomic failure (the Shy–Drager syndrome, see page 127). Sleep apnoea from whatever cause leads to transient hypertension both systolic and pulmonary and if severe may require treatment, by means of tracheostomy.

Narcolepsy

Narcolepsy is the term applied to attacks of falling asleep in a manner which is abnormal because its onset is irresistible though the circumstances may be inappropriate and excessive fatigue is absent. The patient can be roused from a narcoleptic attack as from normal sleep. Narcolepsy is described as symptomatic, when it is usually the result of a lesion in the neighbourhood of the third ventricle. The relationship between narcolepsy and epilepsy has been much discussed. In most cases narcolepsy is probably merely an undue propensity for sleep: in a minority of cases, however, it may be the only symptom of an epileptic discharging lesion. The EEG in narcolepsy is usually normal in the intervals between the attacks, while during an attack the rhythm characteristic of sleep is found. The patient with symptomatic narcolepsy may show the signs of the causative lesion in the neighbourhood of the hypophysis and hypothalamus.

Cataplexy

In a cataplectic attack the patient suddenly loses all power of movement and of maintaining posture, but consciousness is preserved. In a severe attack the patient sinks limply to the ground with the eyes closed, but in a milder attack he merely sags at the knees or simply feels weak. Cataplectic attacks usually last less than a minute and recovery is rapid. They are commonly precipitated by strong emotion, pleasurable or otherwise, especially by laughter, and the patient may be unable to move until he has controlled his emotion.

The narcolepsy-cataplexy syndrome

In patients without any underlying brain lesion narcolepsy is frequently associated with cataplexy. The addition to narcolepsy and cataplexy of sleep paralysis and vivid hallucinations just before falling asleep constitutes the full tetrad of the narcolepsy–cataplexy syndrome. This disorder is accompanied by reversal of the two stages of sleep, REM rather than NREM occurring at the onset of the sleep attacks and also in their normal sleep. This makes the hypnogogic hallucinations (a form of dreaming) and sleep-onset paralysis, more explicable. The sleep latency, the time between trying to fall asleep, and the onset of EEG sleep pattern, is reduced in narcoleptics, pointing to a generalized disorder of sleep–waking function in the narcolepsy–cataplexy syndrome. Patients with narcolepsy are at risk as car drivers and this is not allowed until treatment has been proved to be effective. Amphetamine (5 mg three times a day or as a spansule to slow absorption) can be legitimately prescribed in Britain. However, it is preferable to attempt treatment first with other drugs increasing arousal such as methylphenidate (Ritalin 10 mg three times a day initially), clomipramine (Anafranil 25 mg three times a day initially) or protriptyline (Concordin 5 mg three times a day initially). While treatment along these lines may give considerable symptomatic relief, the liability to the attacks is likely to continue indefinitely, although occasionally they cease spontaneously.

Other forms of sleep disturbance

Sleep paralysis is the term applied to a state through which the subject passes while falling asleep or awakening. Though fully conscious, he is unable to move a muscle. He usually imagines the paralysis to last for many minutes but the actual paralysis is in fact much briefer. This sometimes occurs in a patient who suffers from narcolepsy or some other sleep disturbance, but it is not rare in people otherwise normal. It is described as predormital or postdormital according to whether it occurs at the onset of sleep or on awakening. *Hypnagogic hallucinations*, that is visual or auditory hallucinations occurring during the phase of falling asleep are also not uncommon in normal persons, but may be particularly vivid in patients suffering from narcolepsy. Hallucinatory states also sometimes occur when the subject awakens during the night. The night terrors of childhood are probably a similar form of sleep dissociation. *Somnambulism,* or sleep-walking, is a form of automatic behaviour in which complex activities may occur although the patient is not fully aware of them at the time and does not remember them afterwards.

Sleep-walking and *enuresis* occur during stage IV NREM sleep, not during REM sleep. Amitriptyline at night may stop these disturbances by reducing the depth of sleep. Night terrors, for which children subsequently have no memory, also occur during stage IV NREM sleep. Nightmares are normal frightening dreams occuring during normal REM sleep for which there is good recall.

REFERENCES

Diagnosis of brain death. Statement issued by the Honorary Secretary of the Conference of Royal Medical Colleges and their Faculties in the United Kingdom on 11 October 1976. *Br. med. J.* **ii**, 1187–8 (1976).

Diagnosis of death. Memorandum issued by the Honorary Secretary of the Conference of Medical Royal Colleges and their Faculties in the United Kingdom on 15 January 1979. *Br. med. J.* **i**, 332 (1979).

Diagnosis of death. *Lancet* **i**, 261–2 (1979).

Jennett, B., Gleave, J.R.W., and Wilson, P. (1981) Brain death in three neurosurgical units. *Br. med. J.* **282**, 533–9.

Levy, D., Bates, D., Caronna, J.J., Cartlidge, N.E.F., Knill-Jones, R.P., Lapinski, R.H., Singer, B.H., Shaw, D.A., and Plum, F. (1981). Prognosis in non-traumatic coma. *Ann. intern. Med.* **94**, 293–301.

Moruzzi, G. and Magoun, H.W. (1949). Brain stem reticular formation and activation of the EEG. *Electroenceph. clin. Neurophysiol.* **1**, 455–73.

Parkes, J.D. and Marsden, C.D. (1974). Narcolepsy. *Br. J. hosp. Med.* **12**, 325–34.

Pallis, C. (1982). *ABC of brainstem death.* British Medical Journal, London.

Plum, F. and Posner, J.B. (1980). *The diagnosis of stupor and coma,* 3rd edn. Davis, Philadelphia.

Richardson, G.S. (1978). Excessive day time sleepiness in man. Multiple sleep latency measurement in narcoleptic and control subjects. *Electroenceph. clin. Neurophysiol.* **45**, 621.

Teasdale, G. and Jennett, B. (1974). Assessment of coma and impaired consciousness: a practical scale. *Lancet* **ii**, 81–4.

7 Epilepsy

THE NATURE OF EPILEPSY

What is epilepsy? Hughlings Jackson described it as 'an occasional, and excessive and a disorderly discharge of nerve tissue'. This description could only be a speculation until Burger in 1929 discovered a method of recording the electrical rhythms of the brain known as electroencephalography. This showed that different varieties of epileptic attack are associated with abnormal electrical rhythms recorded from the surface of the head, and differing in their characteristics and localization, and led to the description of epilepsy as a cerebral dysrhythmia. This was a great step forward, but it still leaves some questions unanswered, for we do not yet understand the physiological relationship between the dysrhythmia and the epileptic attack or the nature of the physicochemical disturbance which causes the dysrhythmia. There seems no doubt, however, that whatever its immediate or remote cause, an epileptic attack is the manifestation of a paroxysmal discharge of abnormal electrical rhythms in some part of the brain. If one adds that such discharges are likely to be repetitive, one has defined the cardinal features of epilepsy. It will be noted that loss of consciousness is not an essential feature of the epileptic attack. Loss or impairment of consciousness frequently occurs in association with an attack, but a paroxysmal electrical discharge may involve certain limited areas of the brain without interfering with consciousness.

NEUROPHYSIOLOGY OF EPILEPSY

The experimental epileptic neurone is not merely an uninhibited neurone. A group of cells may become epileptic as a result of glial proliferation or isolation of areas of cortex once the original abnormality has occurred. An epileptic focus may trigger a 'minor' focus in the contralateral hemisphere, probably by so called 'kindling' of a focus by repetitive excitation of anatomically linked regions.

Cortical surface potentials are generated by postsynaptic activity of dendrites and cell bodies in the form of excitatory and inhibitory postsynaptic potentials (EPSPs and IPSPs) by partial depolarization or hyperpolarization respectively. These synaptic potentials have relatively large fields and generate EEG potentials when synchronously discharged in vertically orientated neurones – up to eight pyramidal cells in a hundred micrometre cube. The characteristic potential of a single neurone is a paroxysmal depolarization shift (PDS) in a epileptiform EEG spike discharge shown by intracellular recordings in animals with experimental epilepsy. The PDS arises in the dendrite and has a much larger amplitude and greater duration than an EPSP. This appears to be an intrinsic property of epileptic neurones. The dendrites are negative relative to the cell body and so current flows from the cell body to the dendrite, recorded from the scalp as a negative spike during the PDS. Both spikes and waves can arise from the cortex without the intervention of thalamus or reticular formation. It appears that spike and wave discharges may also arise either from midline structures or diffusely in the cortex if the reticular 'activating system' (RAS) which usually desynchronizes the cortex is suppressed. Thalamic stimulation has long been known to cause immobility associated with a prolonged 'absence' associated with a 3 Hz wave-and-spike recording, though higher amplitude stimulation may cause a grand mal seizure.

Current research into epilepsy is directed towards understanding the molecular mechanisms which control the stability of neuronal circuits. Interest has centred on defects in the GABA inhibitory system for which there are specific binding sites. There may also be specific receptors for anticonvulsant drugs such as benzodiazepines and phenytoin. Isotopically labelled benzodiazepines show high-affinity binding sites in the cerebellum and hippocampus and the binding is enhanced by the presence of GABA and GABA-adenylase. There is a close interaction between the sites recognizing benzodiazepine and the sites recognizing GABA. Benzodiazepine antagonists that compete with specific binding sites also block the anticonvulsant action of benzodiazepines in experimental epilepsy. Part of the anticonvulsant action of barbiturates and hydantoins is related to enhancing inhibitory transmission through action at a site closely related to the chloride ionophore, thereby stabilizing the resting membrane potential.

CLINICAL VARIETIES OF EPILEPTIC ATTACK

Many classifications of epilepsy have been proposed but the following serves to combine practical clinical features with what is known broadly about the pathophysiological basis of epilepsy.

Generalized seizures
Absences (petit mal)
Clonic-tonic (grand mal)
Atonic-myoclonic, tonic or myoclonic

Partial seizures
Simple motor (Jacksonian)
Simple sensory
Complex, with temporal lobe and psychomotor features (special sensory, autonomic psychic, and memory disturbances)
Partial seizures secondarily becoming generalized

Special types of epilepsy
Reflex and self induced
Epilepsy partialis continua
Automatism with epilepsy

Epileptic status
Febrile convulsions
Epilepsy related to menstruation

Absences (petit mal epilepsy)

The term petit mal should be restricted to recurrent brief attacks of loss of consciousness usually associated with a characteristic EEG abnormality, namely a 3 Hz wave-and-spike dysrhythmia synchronous over both frontal lobes (Fig. 7.1). Petit mal attacks start in infancy or childhood and may cease or be replaced by grand mal seizures in adolescence. The clinical features of petit mal consist of a brief loss of consciousness lasting for only a few seconds. The patient has a somewhat dazed appearance and his eyes may stare, and there is often facial pallor. He pauses in what he is doing, but does not fall and there is no convulsion. As soon as the attack has passed he goes on as if nothing had happened. In very slight attacks the patient may not be completely unconscious, but is aware of feeling abnormal, a state often described as a 'sensation'. Petit mal attacks may be few or frequent and sometimes occur many times a day. The EEG may record wave-and-spike disturbances which are not associated with any detectable change in the patient – subclinical attacks, but frequent subclinical attacks impair his mental efficiency.

The wave-and-spike dysrhythmia is not observed as the result of acquired lesions of the brain. It is therefore a constitutional disturbance, a manifestation

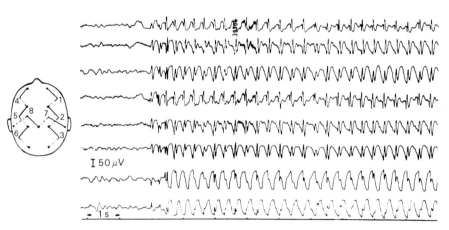

Fig. 7.1. Male, aged 18. Generalized, bilaterally synchronous and symmetrical 3 Hz wave-and-spike discharges during petit mal attack.

of idiopathic epilepsy. The site of origin of the discharge has been speculatively placed in the diencephalon.

Tonic-clonic epilepsy (grand mal epilepsy)

A major epileptic attack is the most dramatic manifestation of the disorder. It begins in about three-fifths of all cases with an aura, or warning of the attack. This is a symptom produced by the beginning of the epileptic discharge and perceived by the patient before consciousness is lost. In the remaining cases the patient experiences no warning, but becomes unconscious at the onset of the attack. Since the focus of origin of the attack may be situated in a variety of localities within the brain there is a corresponding variety of auras, which may take the form of a complex mental state, an emotion, such as fear, or a hallucination in the sphere of one of the senses, such as smell, taste, vision or hearing, or an abnormal feeling referred to some part of the body – often the epigastrium. The aura may consist of an inability to speak, or the attack may begin with a movement of some part of the body.

The convulsion proper may begin with a loud cry, but this is more often absent than present. Consciousness is lost either immediately after the aura or at the very beginning of the attack, and the patient falls to the ground, in the course of which he may injure himself. The first motor manifestation of the convulsion is a phase of tonic spasm of the muscles which is for the most part symmetrical on the two sides of the body, though it is not uncommon for the head and eyes to be turned, and for the mouth to be drawn, to one side. The upper limbs are usually adducted at the shoulders and flexed at the other joints. The lower limbs are usually extended with the feet inverted. Owing to spasm of the respiratory muscles, breathing ceases during the tonic phase, which usually lasts from a few seconds to not more than half a minute. It is succeeded by the clonic phase, in which the sustained tonic contraction of the muscles gives place to sharp, short, interrupted jerks. In this phase the tongue may be bitten, and foaming at the mouth may occur. The patient is often incontinent of urine, less frequently of faeces. Progressive cyanosis occurs during the arrest of respiration in the tonic phase, but this passes off when respiration is re-established. A severe epileptic convulsion may give rise to subconjunctival or cutaneous petechial haemorrhages.

Towards the end of the clonic phase the intervals between the muscular contractions become longer and the jerks finally cease. The patient remains unconscious for a variable time, usually from a few minutes to half an hour, and on recovering consciousness often sleeps for several hours. Headache is common after an attack, and for a short time the tendon reflexes may be abolished and the plantar reflexes extensor.

The EEG abnormality characteristic of grand mal consists of multiple high-voltage spikes which are usually widespread and synchronous in both hemispheres. This has been interpreted as meaning that the underlying dysrhythmia originates at some central diencephalic site which, however, must differ from that responsible for a petit mal attack, since the EEG is different, and the tonic and clonic phenomena of grand mal are likely to be the result of rapid spread of the disturbance to brainstem centres concerned with posture and tonus. Like petit mal, grand mal may be constitutional in origin, a manifestation of idiopathic epilepsy; but, unlike petit mal, grand mal may also be symptomatic of a cerebral lesion situated in any lobe of the brain but most frequently in one frontal or temporal lobe. In such cases it must be supposed that a discharging lesion in the affected lobe rapidly spreads to the central mechanism responsible for the loss of consciousness and the generalized convulsion.

Simple motor epilepsy (Jacksonian epilepsy)

Jacksonian epilepsy, described by Hughlings Jackson, is a convulsion originating in the precentral motor cortex. It begins as a rule with clonic movements, rarely with tonic spasm, of a small part of the opposite side of the body, usually the thumb and index finger, the angle of the mouth, or the great toe. As the convulsion becomes more severe the initial movement becomes more violent, and the movement spreads, in the case of a limb, centripetally, involving the flexor muscles predominantly. A convulsion beginning in a limb then spreads to the other limb on the same side centrifugally, and to the face, and finally may become bilateral, when consciousness is usually lost. Up to a point it is true to say that the spread of the convulsion corresponds to the representation of movements in the motor cortex, but the cortical march must be interpreted in physiological and not in purely anatomical terms. A Jacksonian epileptic attack is often followed by transitory weakness of the muscles involved in the convulsion, which may last for from a few hours to a day or two, and is known as Todd's paralysis. The EEG is likely to show a focal discharge (Fig. 7.2). It is of interest that Hughlings Jackson in 1873, long before any direct measurement of electrical activity in the brain was possible, defined epilepsy as 'sudden,

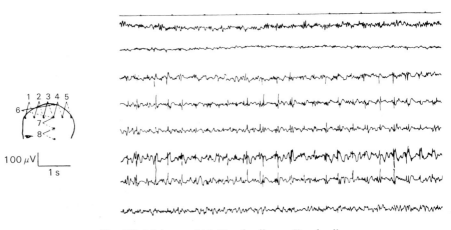

Fig. 7.2. Male, aged 14. Focal epilepsy. Focal spikes.

excessive and rapid discharge of grey matter of some part of the brain; it is a local discharge'.

Simple sensory epilepsy

This term is applied to attacks ushered in by some form of sensory hallucination which may involve any sensory modality. One of the commonest is a feeling of numbness or tingling experienced in some part of the body, which may spread in a manner similar to the motor convulsion in a Jacksonian attack. Such an attack usually originates in the opposite parietal lobe in the neighbourhood of the postcentral gyrus, and may develop into a motor Jacksonian attack or a generalized convulsion.

Complex partial epilepsy (temporal lobe epilepsy)

It is convenient to group together those epileptic attacks which result from a discharging lesion in or near one temporal lobe. The cause is often a small benign lesion in the medial temporal lobe, probably caused by perinatal hypoxia or prolonged seizures in childhood. Their most constant feature is a disturbance of the content of consciousness, which may take many forms, e.g. sensory hallucinations, especially of smell or taste, or of a more elaborate kind such as a remembered visual scene or musical tune; disordered awareness of the external world involving especially the size or distance of objects seen, or of the patient's own body, i.e. perceptual illusions; the *déjà vu* phenomenon – a feeling as though what is happening at the time has happened before; a vivid revival of past memories; and abnormal emotional experiences of an unpleasant kind, especially states of fear or depression. The motor accompaniments of temporal lobe epilepsy are equally varied. The patient looks dazed and does not respond, or respond adequately, when addressed. Attacks which begin with an olfactory or gustatory aura sometimes lead to automatic movements of chewing, tasting, or smacking the lips – these are known as uncinate attacks. The patient may carry out unconsciously some motor activity of a highly organized kind, such as undressing. Aggressive behaviour sometimes occurs. The term psychomotor epilepsy is sometimes applied to the combination of a disordered mental state with complex motor activity. Dysphasia may occur if the dominant temporal lobe is involved. In some cases the attack ends in a generalized convulsion.

The EEG characteristic of temporal lobe epilepsy is a discharge consisting of sharp spikes detectable in this region either on the surface of the skull or by the use of sphenoidal leads from the under surface (Fig. 7.3).

Reflex epilepsy

It sometimes happens that a convulsion is excited by some form of external stimulation such as a touch on the skin, or a sudden loud noise – acoustico-motor epilepsy, or music – musicogenic epilepsy, or a visual (photic) stimulus, e.g. looking at television. Reflex inhibition of an attack is an allied

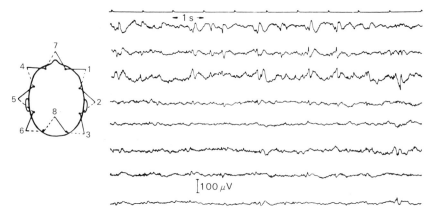

Fig. 7.3. Male, aged 30. Temporal lobe epilepsy. Focal sharp and slow waves in the right temporal region.

phenomenon. When a convulsion has a focal onset, and begins with movement, for example, of one limb, a strong stimulus, such as a firm grip, rubbing, or passive movement applied to the limb will often abort an attack if it is begun immediately after the onset. In patients with 'television' epilepsy, the tendency can often be confirmed during electroencephalography by the photoconvulsive response to a flickering light. Patients should be advised against adjusting a flickering television set or sitting too close to the screen. Now a further type of photoconvulsive epilepsy has been reported due to electronic video games!

Self-induced epilepsy

Some patients induce their attacks, usually by looking at the sun and pasing the hand with the fingers separated to-and-fro before their eyes.

Akinetic epilepsy

In akinetic epilepsy the patient suddenly falls to the ground without warning, sometimes with sufficient violence to break a bone. The only evidence for loss of consciousness is unawareness of the fall itself, and the victim is usually able to get up again at once. These are known as 'drop attacks'. A 'drop attack' may have other causes. Many patients suffering from these attacks are middle-aged obese women without any history of epilepsy or of similar attacks previously. This condition rarely leads to serious incapacity. There is often associated evidence of cervical osteoarthritis and such attacks are commonly presumed to be a result of brainstem ischaemia, possibly aggravated by compression of the vertebral arteries by cervical osteophytes.

Epilepsia partialis continua

This is a rare form of focal convulsion in which persistent clonic movements occur confined to a limited part of the body, for example flexion of the thumb and one or more digits. These movements continue for long periods, often for days and sometimes for months, without stopping. They are the result of a focal lesion involving the corresponding area of the opposite motor cortex.

Tonic epilepsy

A convulsion may consist of an attack of muscular rigidity associated with loss of consciousness but not followed by clonic movements. In the usual form of tonic convulsion the head is extended, the upper limbs are thrown out in front of the patient, extended at the elbows, internally rotated and hyperpronated, with the fingers somewhat flexed. The lower limbs are extended. These attacks are usually the result of organic disease of the brain producing temporary decerebration, but they occasionally occur in idiopathic epilepsy.

Myoclonus in epilepsy

Myoclonus may be associated with epilepsy in various ways. Sufferers from idiopathic major epilepsy sometimes exhibit repeated myoclonic jerks, symmetrically affecting particularly the flexors of the upper limbs and occurring especially in the early morning (Fig. 7.4). Such jerks may subside spontaneously or be followed by a generalized convulsion. Occasionally brief myoclonic jerks accompany an attack of petit mal. Epilepsia partialis continua is a variety of localized myoclonic epilepsy. There are also inherited forms of epilepsy in which myoclonus is a prominent feature. These include inherited myoclonic epilepsy with dementia, myoclonus associated with lipidoses and also with other rare diffuse cerebral degenerations.

Automatism associated with epilepsy

Automatism is the term applied to the behaviour of a patient who carries out a series of more or less complex acts without being normally conscious at the time

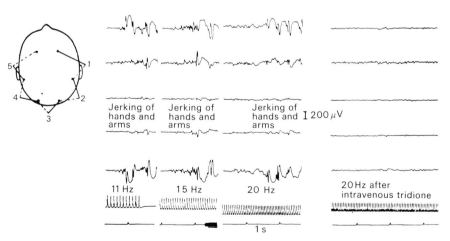

Fig. 7.4. Female, aged 19. Epilepsy, myoclonic. Photomyoclonic response at various flash frequencies and subsequent effect of intravenous tridione.

and without having any subsequent recollection of them. We are seldom in a position to say how far automatism is itself a manifestation of an epileptic discharge and how far it reflects the ill-adjusted activity of lower centres in the nervous system temporarily removed by the attack from their normal higher control. Automatism is most frequently seen as a manifestation of temporal lobe epilepsy, but sometimes follows an attack of grand mal or petit mal.

Status epilepticus

An epileptic patient may have a succession of convulsions with recovery of consciousness between the attacks – serial epilepsy. Sometimes, however, one follows another without any intervening period of consciousness – status epilepticus. Unless the convulsions can be arrested, coma deepens, and pyrexia or even hyperpyrexia develops and death occurs. Some patients exhibit a special tendency to develop status epilepticus, and do so on many occasions. It is, however, an exceptional occurrence. Status epilepticus may be precipitated by the sudden withdrawal of anticonvulsant drugs, especially the barbiturates. It must be remembered that in barbiturate addicts there may be no history of treatment with drugs. The fits following barbiturate withdrawal may occur several days after the withdrawal of the drugs.

THE TIME-RELATIONSHIP OF ATTACKS

Individuals differ greatly in regard to the frequency of their attacks. There are three common modes of onset. A patient may have petit mal for years before having a major attack; or the first attack may be generalized and major attacks, with or without minor ones, may occur thereafter at short intervals; or there may be major attacks separated by months or even years. Probably three-quarters of all epileptics have more than one attack a month. Some children with petit mal have dozens in a day. About one-third of epileptics have attacks both by day and by night. Among the remainder twice as many have diurnal attacks only as nocturnal only. Nocturnal fits are most likely to occur shortly after going to sleep or between 4 and 5 a.m.; and the commonest time for diurnal attacks is soon after awakening. Many women have attacks just before the menstrual period, less frequently during or after it. Some patients have attacks in bouts with intervals of freedom which sometimes last many months.

CONCLUSIONS ON THE NATURE OF EPILEPSY

From what has been said it will be clear that epilepsy is a symptom of a discharging lesion, which may be situated in many different areas of the brain and be due to many different causes. Since, however, the same causes operating in different individuals do not always lead to epilepsy, it is probable that the liability to develop epileptic attacks varies from one person to another, depending on constitutional, environmental, and hereditary factors. The term 'epileptic' implies a person who has a recurring liability to epileptic seizures, rather than a person who has merely had a single isolated attack, perhaps under special provoking circumstances which are unlikely to be repeated. Electroencephalography and other diagnostic advances have enabled us to recognize and localize focal lesions responsible for the attacks in many patients who would previously have been regarded as suffering from idiopathic epilepsy. Nevertheless, the broad distinction between symptomatic and idiopathic epilepsy remains. In idiopathic epilepsy there is a constitutional predisposition to epileptic attacks of the petit mal or grand mal variety, or both, which is sometimes inherited, and which is sufficient to cause the attacks in the absence of any focal cerebral lesion. In symptomatic epilepsy, on the other hand, such a focal lesion is present.

The incidence of epilepsy may be gauged from a recent survey of general practices in Britain in which it was found that 5 per cent of a sample of the population gave a history of having had an epileptic attack at some time during their lives. On the other hand a recurring tendency to epileptic seizures occurred in only four persons per thousand.

THE DIAGNOSIS OF EPILEPSY

When a patient presents himself suffering from paroxysmal cerebral disturbances with or without loss of consciousness, they should arouse the suspicion of epilepsy, and the doctor then has to take two steps in diagnosis. The first is to establish that the patient is suffering from epilepsy and not from some other paroxysmal disturbance, and, when that is established, the second step is to decide, if possible, the cause of the epilepsy. The main part of the first step is to distinguish an epileptic attack characterized by loss of consciousness from other disorders which may be confused with it. The distinction between 'fits' and 'faints' is one of the commonest, yet most important, problems a doctor faces. Upon it may depend the social and occupational future, as well as the medical future, of the patient.

Syncope

Syncope may be defined as a sudden loss of consciousness due to temporary failure of the cerebral circulation. This may be the result of:

1. Loss of blood in haemorrhage.

2. Inadequate venous return to the heart. This is the common cause of syncope in adolescents and soldiers on parade. Heat and immobility tend to cause pooling of blood in the lower part of the body. Disturbance of reflex control of the circulation may produce the same effect in a patient who has had splanchnic sympathectomy, or is taking ganglion-blocking drugs, or who has a lesion of the spinal cord at the cervical level and whose posture is suddenly changed from the horizontal to the vertical, and in tabes dorsalis and some forms of polyneuropathy. Interference with the return of venous blood to the heart also causes fainting in the Valsalva manoeuvre and in some elderly men on violent coughing – *cough*

syncope, or 'laryngeal epilepsy', but these patients usually also have some cerebral arteriosclerosis. *Micturition syncope* is the form which occurs in men after getting out of bed in the night and emptying a full bladder.

3. The circulatory system itself may be primarily at fault, when fainting occurs in Stokes–Adams attacks resulting from heart block, and in disturbances of cardiac rate or rhythm such as paroxysmal tachycardia and auricular flutter. Ambulatory cardiac monitoring may be necessary to exclude an arrhythmia. Some, such as the sick sinus syndrome, may require a cardiac pacemaker.

4. Carotid-sinus syncope. In a few susceptible individuals pressure on the carotid sinus causes loss of consciousness, usually by producing slowing of the heart rate and a fall of blood pressure, though in some cases an effect upon the cerebrum itself cannot be excluded. If anticholinergic drugs fail to stop the attacks, denervation of the carotid sinus may be necessary.

5. Reflex causes of syncope include a variety of minor surgical procedures such as venepuncture, pleural puncture, and even cistern puncture. Accidental bodily trauma may operate in the same way.

6. Syncope may follow emotional stress, such as a sudden emotional shock, extreme fear, or merely the sight of blood. Emotional stress, however caused, provokes syncope by causing a sudden reversal of the normal arteriolar vasocon-striction and tachycardia which maintain blood pressure on standing, thus leading to vasodilatation of muscle arterioles and bradycardia. Fairly rapid loss of consciousness by fainting is the result and the enforced recumbency which this causes at any rate ensures a rapid restoration of the cerebral circulation. The teleological value of this mechanism to man during emotional conflicts is uncertain.

7. Syncope may be a presenting symptom of postural hypotension. The autonomic vascular reflexes which protect against the effects of pooling of blood in the legs on standing may be defective in the elderly or those taking a variety of drugs which block autonomic transmission. Postural hypotension occasionally results from a rare degenerative disease affecting the autonomic nervous system (idiopathic orthostatic hypotension), sometimes associated with multisystem atrophy (Shy–Drager syndrome) (see p. 127).

The principal features which distinguish syncope from epilepsy are the existence of an adequate cause for a faint, operating in one of the ways just described, and the fact that both the onset of and recovery from a faint are gradual. Thus the recovery is slower than that from petit mal but more rapid than that from grand mal. During a faint the patient becomes pale and limp, the respiration is usually sighing, the pulse is generally slow, and its tension low. Occasionally a convulsion and even urinary incontinence occur, hence neither of these symptoms is pathognomonic of an epileptic attack. The important fact to establish is whether prodromal symptoms of syncope preceded the epileptic seizure. If they did, investigation from the point of view of epilepsy is usually unnecessary.

Other paroxysmal disorders

In *narcolepsy* consciousness is lost, but convulsive movements are absent, and the patient, unlike the epileptic, can be immediately aroused, and when aroused is normal. In *cataplexy* voluntary power is lost but consciousness is retained.

Hysterical convulsions are usually easily distinguished from epileptic attacks if the patient is seen when convulsed. Their onset is gradual, and they occur only in the presence of an audience. Consciousness is not completely lost, for the patient can usually be aroused by forcible measures, and an attempt to elicit the corneal reflex usually evokes a vigorous contraction of the orbicularis oculi. If the patient cries out during the attack he usually articulates words or phrases, and laughing and crying may occur. The movements which constitute a hysterical convulsion are not clonic jerks as in epilepsy, but such as can be carried out voluntarily, for example, clutching at objects in the neighbourhood. The tongue is not bitten, nor does incontinence of urine occur.

Anxiety attacks are occasionally confused with epilepsy. In these consciousness is not lost, but the predominant symptom is an intense sense of anxiety which is often associated with a feeling of giddiness, and with palpitation and sweating. Anxiety may be associated with hyperventilation. The loss of carbon dioxide leads to alkalosis, reduction of ionized calcium in the blood, and tetany. This may be confused with hypocalcaemia due to hypoparathyroidism.

Under the term *vasovagal attacks* Gowers described 'prolonged seizures, the symptoms of which consists chiefly in disturbance of some of the functions of the pneumogastric'. The patient complains of gastric, respiratory, or cardiac discomfort, and these symptoms are often associated with vasoconstriction and coldness of the extremities, and sometimes with *angor animi* (a sense of impending death). The pulse rate is usually abnormally slow and may be irregular, and the volume of the radial pulse is often subnormal. The face may be pale or flushed. Women are more subject to these paroxysms than men. They are distinguished from epilepsy by their gradual onset and longer duration, lasting from a few minutes to half an hour, as a rule, and by the usual absence of loss of consciousness.

Migraine is a paroxysmal disturbance which may simulate epilepsy. The onset of an attack of migraine, however, is gradual and though visual disturbances sometimes constitute the aura of an epileptic attack, their march is much more rapid than the slow progression of migrainous teichopsia. Consciousness is only rarely lost in migraine, and headache usually occurs. *Aural vertigo* is sometimes confused with epilepsy, since giddiness may be the aura of an epileptic attack. In vertigo of aural origin, however, consciousness is retained and other symptoms of aural disease, such as tinnitus and deafness, are usually present. Though an attack of aural vertigo may be brief, it usually lasts longer than the aura of an epileptic attack and passes away more gradually. Occasionally, however, aural vertigo may merge into an attack of epilepsy, *vestibulogenic epilepsy.*

Hypoglycaemia must be considered among the metabolic disturbances which may cause alteration of consciousness resembling epilepsy. In addition to attacks of loss of consciousness there may be intermittent confusional states as well as transient focal neurological disturbances.

THE DIAGNOSIS OF THE CAUSE OF EPILEPSY

When it is established that the patient is suffering from epilepsy, the next step in diagnosis is to try to establish its cause. This differs so much in relation to the age of the patient that it is best considered at three ages: (i) in infancy; (ii) in childhood; and (iii) in adult life.

In infancy

In the neonatal period birth injury, associated with cerebral anoxia, hypoglycaemia or hypocalcaemia, may lead to convulsions. If, however, these are not rapidly corrected, permanent damage may be done to the brain which may lead to the continuance of the attacks, so that the child becomes a permanent sufferer from epilepsy. Convulsions may also occur in infancy as a result of metabolic disturbances acting upon the immature brain which has a lower 'convulsive threshold' than the adult brain. Febrile illness such as pertussis, measles, and chickenpox may be associated with isolated epileptic seizures.

Apart from these, the causes of epilepsy in infancy fall into two main groups, non-progressive, and progressive disorders.

1. The non-progressive but serious disorders which may cause major epileptic fits at this age include hydrocephalus; congenital diplegia, hemiplegia, or generalized cerebral damage from birth injury; more rarely hereditary forms of mental defect such as epiloia, in which epilepsy is associated with mental defect and adenoma sebaceum. Epilepsy at this age is an occasional sequel of meningitis.

2. Progressive neurological disorders in infants are often associated with massive myoclonic jerks affecting the whole body, usually called 'lightning spasms' or if they are slower 'salaam attacks'. These may also occur without obvious cause or may follow a wide variety of pre-, peri-, or postnatal disorders which include epiloia, meningitis, metabolic defects such as phenylketonuria, birth injury with anoxia or hypoglycaemia, prenatal toxoplasmosis and cytomegalic inclusion disease or rare 'allergic' disorders such as occasionally follow immunization, for example, by triple vaccine. Mental defect is common and the electroencephalogram often shows irregularly occurring spikes in all leads interspersed with many high voltage slow waves. This pattern is termed hypsarrhythmia. It is important to recognize this condition because the spasms can often be stopped, at any rate for a time, by the administration of steroids, seemingly irrespective of the aetiology. Other progressive disorders associated with epilepsy for which no treatment is possible include rare degenerative diseases such as amaurotic family idiocy.

In childhood

Epilepsy developing in childhood after the first year of life may be due to any of the congenital or acquired lesions just mentioned. In addition, constitutional or idiopathic epilepsy accounts for a proportion of cases, and the attacks are sometimes associated with lesions of one temporal lobe which can be localized only electroencephalographically. Diffuse sclerosis and subacute inclusion encephalitis are rare causes.

In adult life

In adult life idiopathic epilepsy rarely begins after the age of 25.

Epilepsy is a common symptom of intracranial tumour, but tumour probably accounts for less than one-third of the cases of epilepsy beginning in adult life. After the age of 50, epilepsy is most often due to cerebral athero-sclerosis. Other causes which need to be borne in mind are heart block leading to Stokes–Adams attacks, and spontaneous hypoglycaemia due to a tumour of the islet cells of Langerhans of the pancreas. Neurosyphilis is a cause, varying infrequency according to the incidence of syphilis in any particular country. Head injury is followed by epilepsy in some 20 per cent of cases of penetrating injury involving the meninges, but is rare after closed head injuries. Withdrawal of alcohol in an alcoholic should not be forgotten as a cause of epilepsy. Cysticercosis may cause epilepsy in patients who have been exposed to the infestation by tropical residence. The attacks begin on average about eight years after the acquisition of the parasite. At that stage the cysts in the muscles are usually found to be calcified but rarely those in the brain.

THE VALUE OF ELECTROENCEPHALOGRAPHY IN DIAGNOSIS

What are the value and limitations of electroencephalography in the diagnosis of epilepsy?

1. Electroencephalography is only an aid to diagnosis, and is valuable only when its results are considered in relation to the history and clinical examination of the patient.

2. In a patient known to be epileptic, the EEG demonstration of bilateral synchronous wave-and-spike 3-Hz dysrhythmia (Fig. 7.1), and to a less extent of diffuse multiple high-voltage spikes, indicates that the cause is genetically determined.

3. When the diagnosis is doubtful, the presence of such abnormal rhythms in the intervals between attacks suggests that the attacks are epileptic.

4. Focal spike discharges (Fig. 7.2) suggest a focal origin for the attack. When this is in the temporal lobe (Fig. 7.3), the discharges may be only or better demonstrated by the use of a sphenoidal lead.

5. An area of delta waves indicates an area of organic brain damage (Fig. 9.7, p. 243).

6. Diffuse degenerative disorders associated with epilepsy are likely to show widespread areas of grossly abnormal rhythms.

7. Abnormal rhythms commonly associated with epilepsy may persist indefinitely even for years after the patient has ceased to have attacks.

8. In patients with 'television epilepsy' the EEG may show a photoconvulsive response to flickering light.

9. It is not uncommon for abnormalities usually seen in association with epilepsy to be present in patients suffering from brain damage or from immature or psychopathic personalities, but who have never had an epileptic attack.

THE INVESTIGATION OF A CASE OF EPILEPSY

The object of investigating a case of epilepsy is to see whether there is a causal lesion present which may need treatment other than the symptomatic treatment of the epilepsy. The initial question is whether either clinical examination or electroencephalography provides evidence of a focal lesion or generalized abnormality. Plain X-rays of the skull may also provide useful information on this, more often in adult life than in childhood. If none of these provides evidence of a focal lesion, it is unlikely that at that stage further investigations will do so. If, however, there is evidence of a focal lesion, its probable diagnosis will determine the next step in the investigation. In any patient with epilepsy of late onset, whether or not there are focal seizures or a focal abnormality in the EEG, a CT scan is necessary as operable tumours such as meningiomas occur in about 20 per cent of such patients. If it is thought to be neoplastic, angiomatous malformations being included among neoplasms, a CT scan may be followed by angiography, also necessary to exclude atheromatous narrowing of a major cerebral vessel. Ancillary investigations in appropriate cases include serological tests for syphilis, electrocardiography to exclude heart block, blood sugar tests to exclude an islet-cell tumour, and X-rays of the muscles if there is a suspicion of cysticercosis.

PROGNOSIS

The risk that death will occur during an epileptic fit is slight, except in status epilepticus, in which condition the patient's life is always threatened until consciousness returns, and death may occur even after recovery of consciousness. When death occurs as the result of a fit it is usually the accidental result of the loss of consciousness.

The prognosis of epilepsy is obviously correlated with that of the causal condition. Leaving that on one side, however, there is a large group of patients who suffer either from constitutional epilepsy or from epilepsy as a symptom of some stationary brain lesion, and the prognosis of epilepsy in such cases means the prospect that the attacks will respond to treatment. The term recovery in this connection means the cessation of the attacks, but even when this has been achieved and the patient remains free from attacks without treatment, there is usually some risk, even if only a slight one, of a recurrence at some future date. To achieve recovery it is necessary to abolish the attacks by means of treatment for long enough for the patient to lose the epileptic habit. Persevering and thorough treatment is therefore essential, and must be continued for at least three years after the attacks have ceased. In some cases it is a wise policy to continue with a mild dose of anticonvulsants indefinitely. The sooner the treatment can be begun after the first attack, the better the outlook, and the prognosis for idiopathic epilepsy is best in those in whom the attacks begin after the age of 20. A family history of the disease is not necessarily an adverse factor in prognosis, and patients with an epileptic heredity often do better than those without. Individuals suffering from frequent severe fits are least likely to be completely cured. Frequent minor attacks in children sometimes cease spontaneously. Marked mental deterioration and severe cerebral damage make the outlook worse. Thus few patients in institutions become free from attacks and the death rate among institutional epileptics is four times that of the general population. Probably about 30 per cent of non-institutional epileptics are cured, in the sense of remaining free from attacks indefinitely. The incidence of schizophrenia in chronic epileptics appears to be higher than can be explained by chance. Schizophrenia occurs most commonly in temporal lobe epileptics and it has been suggested that the schizophrenia and epilepsy are in some way causally related.

TREATMENT

General management

There are many irrational lay fears about epilepsy and, having made the diagnosis, the physician must seek to eradicate these and help the patient to adjust to his disability. It is desirable that an epileptic patient should as far as possible lead a normal life. Minor attacks, unless very frequent, usually do not prevent a child from attending school. Adults, if not otherwise handicapped, should be able to carry on an occupation, though certain trades will necessarily be ruled out. Occupations involving working at heights, or near machinery or water, or driving vehicles, are obviously unsuitable, and sufferers from epilepsy are now precluded by law from obtaining a motor driver's licence in Great Britain. The risks of everyday life must be explained to the patient and his friends, but it is difficult, if not impossible, to guard against them all. Institutional treatment may be necessary for mentally defective patients and those having severe and frequent attacks, if adequate home care is not available. Those in whom the disorder renders an ordinary occupation impossible often do well at an epileptic colony.

There is no evidence that marriage affects the tendency to attacks either beneficially or adversely, except during the honeymoon period when the normal sleep pattern may be disturbed and a tendency to epilepsy may be first revealed. Pregnancy may make the attacks worse and add to the risks of a fall. The likelihood of transmitting the disorder to the children must be individually assessed in each case. This risk is greatest when there is a family history of epilepsy, and least when a focal lesion of the brain can be held partly responsible for the attacks. Even when the epileptic tendency is hereditary, it is exceptional for a patient to transmit the disorder in the direct line.

Moderate exercise is desirable, but violent exertion sometimes precipitates attacks. Alcohol and the consumption of large quantities of fluids should be avoided, as should long periods without food or sleep.

Treatment with drugs (see Table 7.1)

Certain drugs have been found to diminish the severity and frequency of epileptic attacks, and in favourable cases to abolish them completely. The object of drug treatment is to secure an abolition of the attacks for a sufficient length of time to enable the patient to lose the epileptic habit. When the attacks occur fairly regularly at the same hour of the day or period of the month, the doses are timed correspondingly so as to produce their maximal effect when the attack is expected. Thus when the attacks are nocturnal a single dose at bedtime may be sufficient. When they occur only at the monthly periods, the dose should be increased just before and during those times. When the attacks are irregular, the dose must be taken several times a day according to the rate of absorption and metabolism of the drug. Perseverance in treatment is essential, and the patient must continue to take the effective drug for at least three years after the attacks cease, if a relapse is to be avoided. It is insufficient, however, to persevere with an inadequate dose: the dose, therefore, must be kept under review.

There are two aspects of the drug control of epilepsy, first the inhibition of the discharge of abnormal neurones and, second, the prevention of spread of the discharge, probably by suppression of post-tetanic potentiation. In this respect any drugs which stabilize the normal neuronal membrane can be expected to be of benefit and includes drugs which increase the concentration of the inhibitory transmitter GABA, phenytoin (Epanutin), or sodium valproate (Epilim).

There is an interaction between different anticonvulsants used together and between anticonvulsants and other drugs. Alcohol, antituberculous drugs, analgesics, antibiotics, and antirheumatic drugs may increase the plasma levels of anticonvulsants, particularly phenytoin. On the other hand anticonvulsants can reduce the effectiveness of the contraceptive pill, anticoagulants, steroid hormones, and antidepressant drugs such as mianserin and nomifensine.

It is better to be familiar with the pharmacokinetic side-effects of a few drugs than to resort to polypharmacy. It has been shown that a high proportion of

Table 7.1. *Pharmacological data of common anticonvulsants (adapted from Laidlaw and Richens 1982)*

	Time to peak after single oral dose (h)	Adult minimum elimination half-life (h)	Minimum dose (frequency/day)	Therapeutic levels (µmol/l)	Adult-range maintenance dose (mg/day)	Child-range maintenance dose (mg/kg per day)
Phenytoin	4–12	24	1	up to 80	150–600	5–15
Carbamazepine	4–24	12	2	up to 50	400–1800	10–30
Phenobarbitone	1–6	96	1	up to 170	30–240	2–6
Valproate	1–4	10	2	up to 700	600–3000	20–50
Primidone	2–5	18	1	*	250–1500	15–30
Ethosuximide	1–4	36	1	up to 700	500–1500	10–25
Clonazepam	1–3	19	1	†	1–10	0.01–0.02

*Monitor phenobarbitone as metabolite if necessary.

†Not generally available.

epileptic patients can be maintained free of seizures on a single drug, provided blood drug level is carefully controlled.

Sudden withdrawal from any anticonvulsant drug may cause an aggravation of the attacks. If it is necessary to reduce the dose or switch to another drug this should be done gradually and withdrawal covered by giving another anticonvulsant. In the treatment of petit mal there is some evidence that giving a major antiepileptic drug to a teenager may reduce the risk of developing grand mal seizure.

The following are the most generally useful drugs and the doses are given for adults:

1. Phenytoin, a hydantoinate, appears to inhibit the spread of seizure discharges rather than prevent their initiation. It is probably the best drug of first choice for all the epilepsies except petit mal and myoclonic epilepsy. It has a high therapeutic ratio which means that the toxic dose is close to the therapeutic dose because its metabolism is saturable. It has a fairly long half-life so that the blood level is likely to reflect the mean drug level. The drug need only be given in a total dose of 300 mg once a day or at the most twice a day for adults.

2. Carbamazepine is chemically related to the tricyclic antidepressant imipramine. Its pharmacological properties are similar to phenytoin. It is the drug of first choice for complex partial seizures and temporal lobe epilepsy. It does not produce hirsutism and so may be preferred in treating young women with epilepsy. It has sedative properties and should be started in a low dose and increased over two months. It causes water retention and rarely water intoxication. If used with phenytoin the plasma level of carbamazepine falls but the level of its active metabolite carbamazepine epoxide remains unaltered. It also has the unusual features of stimulating its own metabolism so that over the first two months the dose must be increased to maintain the same blood level. The usual adult dose is 200 mg three times a day.

3. Sodium valproate is an inhibitor of enzymes which metabolize the inhibitory transmitter GABA and so produces an anti-epileptic effect. It is a second choice drug for generalized epilepsy of all types, particularly petit mal and myoclonic seizures, but may have toxic effects on the liver. A usual adult dose is 200 mg four times a day.

4. Phenobarbitone is a safe anticonvulsant acting as a depressant both for the cortex and reticular formation and is effective in all forms of epilepsy including partial epilepsies, febrile convulsions, and sometimes myoclonic seizures. Its relegation to second choice is because of its sedative effects, though in children it may cause irritability and restlessness and in temporal lobe epilepsy aggravation of psychic disturbances. It should not be combined with primidone which is metabolized to phenobarbitone. A usual adult dose is 60 mg twice daily.

5. Primidone has all the advantages and disadvantages of phenobarbitone to which it is metabolized. A usual adult dose is 0.25 g three times a day but a trial

dose of half a tablet should be given as severe drowsiness may be caused initially.

6. Ethosuximide was devised particularly for the treatment of petit mal. It does not control grand mal seizures and so another anticonvulsant should be given to control these, especially as puberty approaches when as many as half the patients with petit mal may develop grand mal epilepsy.

7. Clonazepam, like diazepam, is a benzodiazepine which raises the after discharge threshold of the thalamus but not of the cortex. It has the broadest spectrum of action of any anticonvulsants including an action on myoclonic epilepsy.

Treatment of epilepsy in children

For most seizures in children phenobarbitone in a dose of 4 to 6 mg per kg per day is the drug of choice unless irritability or other side-effects prevent its use, when sodium valproate 20 to 30 mg per kg per day in two divided doses is preferable. Valproate has more serious side-effects but is preferable for epilepsy in children in the presence of developmental or other neurological abnormalities. For phenobarbitone the blood drug levels can be checked and for valproate salivary fluid estimation is possible. For a child with myoclonic epilepsy clonazepam or nitrazepam can be given in increasing doses until drowsiness is produced. If control of seizures is not achieved valproate should then be substituted.

Blood drug levels (see Table 7.1)

The concept of the therapeutic range of an anticonvulsant drug may be misleading. There is a minimum drug level compatible with control of the patient's epilepsy and an upper level which if exceeded causes unacceptable toxicity. These levels differ from patient to patient according to genetic factors and the degree of plasma protein binding and receptor binding. Other factors include the presence of other drugs or hepatic, gastrointestinal or renal diseases which may affect the metabolism of the drug. It must not be forgotten that it is the patient who is being treated not the reported blood drug level but it must also be stressed that blood drug levels particularly for phenytoin, carbamazepine, phenobarbitone, and primidone can ensure that there are not idiosyncratic metabolic factors upsetting the control of fits with standard doses of single drugs. Use of blood drug levels can also ensure compliance which is by no means as total as we might wish to believe, and can help to confirm the suspicion that clinical signs of toxicity have appeared. Blood drug levels can help the adjustment of the drug in pregnancy when blood therapeutic levels may fall because of the increase in blood volume, and when it is particularly important to try to avoid seizures. Blood drug levels are particularly useful in children whose variable metabolism and growth rate can cause problems. The blood drug levels are not very useful for valproate because of the short half-life of this drug and a wide range between the therapeutic and toxic dose.

In what clinical circumstances does the drug level help particularly? On starting a drug like phenytoin it will, after a month, ensure that there are no idiosyncratic factors upsetting an optimum drug level. It is useful in relation to phenytoin and carbamazepine because both have a low therapeutic ratio, that is the toxic dose is close to the therapeutic dose, in the case of phenytoin because its metabolism is saturable. Also both drugs have a fairly long half-life so that the blood level reflects the likely mean drug level. These drugs also interact with other drugs so affecting the expected blood levels. Carbamazepine stimulates its own metabolism over the first one to two months so that the dose must be gradually increased to produce the same blood level. There is also the special risk of water intoxication to be considered with carbamazepine. In contrast to these two drugs, valproate levels are not very useful because of the short half-life and the higher therapeutic ratio.

If it is necessary to give another drug because the fits do not respond despite a standard dose, the blood drug level will ensure knowledge of the effective interaction between the two drugs. A blood drug level is also helpful if intoxication is suspected especially if there is an unusual neuropsychiatric syndrome. The blood drug level is also useful if there is an increased frequency in fits in a previously well-controlled patient and it must not be forgotten that an increase in the dose of phenytoin or carbamazepine to toxic levels can sometimes actually increase the frequency of seizures. Finally if non-compliance is suspected serum levels are virtually the only way to prove it.

The concept of a therapeutic range is to some extent artificial and can be misleading unless it is properly understood. For each individual patient a minimal drug level compatible with control of a patient's fits must be found as well as an upper limit which if exceeded may cause unacceptable toxicity. These levels differ from patient to patient according to genetic factors which probably affect protein binding and receptor sensitivity. The quoted range may be too high for one patient with mild epilepsy and too low for a patient with severe epilepsy. In fact it is probably better only to give an upper toxic range but to remember that this can vary. For example, in one patient toxic symptoms may be at a level below the quoted upper range but increasing the level in another patient may successfully control seizures without increasing side-effects. It would be wrong to reduce the level in the latter patient merely because it was above the quoted range for the laboratory. Laboratory errors are also not unknown. However, with these provisos if we remember we are treating the patient not his serum levels, the added information levels provide in answering precise questions has much improved the management of epileptic patients. This in turn may release more of the physician's time and energy to analyse epileptic precipitating factors and the psychosocial problems in epileptic patients which are also of great importance.

Toxic effects of drug treatment

The toxic effects may be grouped according to the system involved. Most anti-convulsant drugs if given in excess produce toxic effects on the nervous system, particularly ataxia, slurred speech, extensor plantar responses, confusion, and stupor. Haemopoietic defects include a megaloblastic aneamia which responds to folic acid and is probably the basis of the neuropathy caused by anticonvulsant drugs. It has recently been shown that chronic epileptics taking anticonvulsants may also develop a vitamin B_{12} deficiency as well as a folic acid deficiency even though they are not anaemic. There are also defects of coagulation caused by vitamin K deficiency. Agranulocytosis occurs and occasionally immunosuppression. The poor diet of chronic epileptics in institutions may be one factor contributing to the anaemia. Epileptic patients with B_{12} deficiency occasionally develop a dementia with cerebellar signs and nystagmus and occasionally a neuropathy. Though the mental state of such patients improves after treatment of the B_{12} or folic acid deficiency the frequency of seizures may temporarily increase, suggesting that these drugs reverse both the anti-epileptic and the retarding effects of the anticonvulsants. Dermatological side-effects include erythematous or morbiliform rashes. Such rashes usually disappear rapidly on discontinuing the drug, which can usually be restarted without the rash coming back. Hirsutism occurs and this may be a reason for using another anticonvulsant, particularly in young women. Acne is a further dermatological side-effect. Connective tissue may be affected in that gum hypertrophy is usual with phenytoin. Bone metabolism may be deranged causing osteomalacia due to vitamin D deficiency and malabsorption of calcium. Endocrine defects include alteration of hypothalamic control.

There is now an increasing awareness of the potential hazards of prolonged drug treatment. Some patients may not complain because they have never known life without drug therapy and this applies particularly to mental retardation. Now that serum drug levels are available it is easier to control reversible or permanent toxic effects. Any patient developing new neurological or psychiatric symptoms should have the serum anticonvulsant level measured.

Phenytoin and other anticonvulsant drugs carry a teratogenic risk but it does not justify discouraging a woman who needs anticonvulsant treatment from having a child or require changing her drugs when her epilepsy is well controlled on them.

Treatment of convulsions during febrile illnesses in children

Febrile fits occur in 5 per cent of the population of infants and in approximately an equal percentage of these seizures may continue into adult life. Febrile convulsions may be defined as fits lasting for less than 15 minutes, without focal features, in a child under the age of 5, during a fever and without evidence of central nervous system infection or metabolic cause. It is advisable to admit a child to hospital after a first epileptic seizure in order to exclude the diagnosis of meningitis. If an electroencephalogram after the first attack shows an abnormality then phenobarbitone 4–6 mg/kg per day may reduce the risk of further epileptic attacks during subsequent febrile illnesses. If an EEG is not easily available then anticonvulsant treatment can be started following a second febrile convulsion.

Practical management of a patient with grand mal epilepsy

In a patient with idiopathic grand mal epilepsy and normal investigations except for an abnormal electroencephalogram a single seizure is not usually an indication for starting drug treatment straight away. If further attacks occur and the decision is made to treat them it is best to start with a dose of phenytoin, 200 mg at night for an adult and to increase the dose gradually guided as necessary by serum levels. If a patient on the optimum dose of one drug is still not controlled then it is probably better to substitute a different drug such as carbamazepine before deciding to use two drugs together. The difference in response between two individuals means that one individual may be better suited to a second drug. Some patients after having a trial of two different drugs are still not controlled and it may then be necessary to use two drugs together. Before adding a third drug because of poor control it must be remembered that some patients have epileptic fits with an optimum dose of two drugs and yet may not be improved by adding a third drug. It is better to avoid polypharmacy in the first place than to attempt to withdraw drugs later.

It is unwise to make frequent changes in the anticonvulsants if the attacks are not responding. On reflection it may be apparent that a focal cause for the attacks exists, or psychological and environmental factors may be responsible for the poor control. If emotional factors are important then a tranquillizer such as diazepam (Valium) may be helpful, though it is important not to give any tranquillizer, such as chlorpromazine, which may have a convulsant action.

Treatment of epileptic status

The mortality may be up to 20 per cent. Apart from the immediate mortality damage to the temporal lobes particularly in status in children can lead to Ammon's horn sclerosis and chronic temporal lobe epilepsy. The initial drug treatment of choice is diazepam 10 mg given intravenously over two minutes as a bolus and not added to an intravenous infusion because it precipitates in plastic tubing. Next a maintenance dose of longer-term anticonvulsants is given, usually 0.3 g phenobarbitone intravenously and up to 500 mg of phenytoin given by stomach tube and continued daily in appropriate doses. If the fits do not cease then the intravenous injection of diazepam (10 mg) should be repeated every 15 minutes until 40 mg have been given or the seizures have ceased, though a maximum dose of 100 mg of diazepam over 24 hours may be needed.

At the same time as the drug treatment is started but between the seizures a pharyngeal airway should be inserted though attempts to do so during seizures are likely to result in broken teeth. If the seizures have not been brought under control within half an hour then the patient should be anaesthetized and an endotracheal tube should be inserted to ensure satisfactory ventilation. All the longer-term measures needed for the treatment of a patient in coma are also necessary with the maintenance of fluid balance and correction of hyperpyrexia.

If diazepam fails over the course of an hour then phenytoin is the next drug of choice, given slowly intravenously in doses up to 50 mg per minute for 5 minutes and then repeated hourly for 4 hours. Phenytoin cannot be given by intramuscular injection as it causes muscle necrosis.

In the unlikely event of failure of diazepam and phenytoin other possibilities remain. They may still be replaced with the old-fashioned drug paraldehyde 5–10 ml injected intramuscularly, taking care to avoid nerves and being aware of the fact that it may erode some types of plastic syringes. Clonazepam, in one-tenth of the dose of diazepam has been reputed to be effective but there is as yet insufficient experience of its use. Chlormethiazole (Heminevrin) has also been reported to be effective in an 0.8 per cent solution by continuous intravenous infusion up to a total dose of 800 mg. In children diazepam in appropriately scaled down doses is suitable or failing this paraldehyde. Ethosuximide may be used for petit mal status.

SURGERY FOR EPILEPSY

The scope of surgery in the treatment of epilepsy is limited. If fits fail to respond to medical treatment, and electroencephalography has shown a consistently occurring focus of epileptic spikes in the frontal or temporal lobes, then excision of the site of the focus may be considered. The best results have occurred in selected patients with temporal lobe seizures, in whom an area of gliosis, or a vascular anomaly, has been found within the temporal lobe. The extent to which removal of a focus in the temporal lobe is possible depends in part on the certainty of the hemisphere which is dominant for speech. Temporal lobectomy in selected cases has resulted in the abolition of seizures in 50 per cent of cases and considerable improvement in 25 per cent of cases. Stereotactic surgery may also be used to produce focal lesions in subcortical structures of the temporal lobes in some patients where there is no clearly resectable lesion demonstrated on the CAT scan. Occasionally, in children with uncontrollable epilepsy, temper tantrums, mental retardation and a hemiplegia present from birth, the whole of the abnormal hemisphere has been excised and improvement has been reported. Not surprisingly the operation has a considerable mortality and is only seldom performed. Section of the corpus callosum has also been performed in the hope of preventing seizures becoming generalized. This is still an experimental treatment but has caused interest in relation to the disconnection syndromes which result (see p. 140).

EPILEPSY AND DRIVING

There are clearly different laws for each country but in Britain new regulations came into force in 1982. These new regulations make no mention of whether or not the patient is taking anticonvulsant drugs and recognize the existence of the controlled epileptic and the epileptic with consistently nocturnal attacks.

An applicant for a licence in Britain, suffering from epilepsy, should satisfy the conditions that:

1. He should have been free from any epileptic attack during the two years immediately preceding the date when the licence is to have effect.

2. In the case of an applicant who has had such fits whilst asleep during that period, he shall have had such attacks only whilst during asleep during a period of at least three years immediately preceding the date when the licence is to have effect.

3. The driving of a vehicle by him is not likely to be a source of danger to the public.

Printed on each British driving licence is the sentence 'you are required by law to inform DVLC (Drivers and Vehicles Licensing Centre), Swansea, at once if you have any disability which is or may become likely to effect your fitness as a driver unless you do not expect it to last for more than three months'.

If there is uncertainty about eligibility to drive the patient's case can be referred in Britain to the Medical Advisor to the Vehicles Licensing Authority.

It is worth quoting from a recent memorandum sent by the Ministry of Transport to the Registration and Licensing Authorities: 'Epilepsy should be regarded as a continuing liability to recurrent epileptic attacks. It follows that a person who has in the past had one or more attacks of convulsions or of disturbance of consciousness, in circumstances which are unlikely to recur, need not necessarily be regarded as suffering from epilepsy. Certain people who may think they have, or may have been regarded as having, suffered from epilepsy, may therefore in fact not be suffering from epilepsy. In order to determine whether this is so it is appropriate to take into account such matters as the frequency of attacks in the past and the duration of freedom from attacks since any treatment ceased.'

The holders of a driving licence who have had epilepsy must accept that driving is allowed only while effective treatment continues unchanged and they should stop driving if a fit occurs or if treatment is changed for whatever reason. If a driver who has been an epileptic stops treatment on his own account or on medical advice, he should not drive again until an additional fit-free period of some twelve months has elapsed on the reduced drug regime, for there is added uncertainty as to whether the attacks will recur under these circumstances. If a fit does occur after more than two fit-free years then driving should not be allowed until another two years have elapsed without a fit.

Special consideration should be given in cases of television epilepsy or where some specific provoking factor, which is unlikely to recur, has been associated. A suitable restriction of the right to drive under these circumstances might reasonably be six months. A single fit with a clinically clear-cut EEG abnormality or some other evidence of an intermittent persistent brain disorder should be regarded as constituting the disease of epilepsy. A single fit, secondary to some systemic disorder or to stress or some toxic state which is not likely to recur, need not, however, lead to a diagnosis of epilepsy. A single unexplained fit with negative EEG could reasonably debar a person from driving only for some twelve months. However, employment as a driver in any capacity should never be permitted thereafter. Anyone suffering from an epileptic fit after the age of five should be barred from holding a heavy goods or public service vehicle licence.

There is reasonably some worry, now that in Britain driving licences may be held until the patient reaches the age of 70, that those applying merely for a renewal of their annual road fund licence may not observe the law which states that they should notify the driving authority if there is any change in their health which might make them ineligible to hold a continuing driving licence.

REFERENCES

Cloyd, J.C., Gumnit, R.J., and McLain, L.W. (1980). Status epilepticus; the role of intravenous phenytoin. *J. Am. med. J.* **244**, 1479–81.

Critchley, E.M.R. and Wright, J.C. (1983). Evaluation of syncope. *Br. med. J.* **256**, 500–1.

Davidson, S. and Falconer, M.A. (1975). Outcome of surgery in 40 children with temporal-lobe epilepsy. *Lancet* **ii**, 1260–3.

Egger, J. and Brett, E.M. (1981). Effect of sodium valproate in 100 children with special reference to weight. *Br. med. J.* **283**, 577–81.

Harvey, P. and Hopkins, A. (1983). Views of British neurologists on epilepsy, driving and the law. *Lancet* **i**, 401–4.

Laidlaw, J. and Richens, A. (1982). *A textbook of epilepsy,* 2nd edn. Churchill Livingstone, Edinburgh.

Meldrum, B.S. (1982). Epilepsy. In *Disorders of neurohumoral transmission* (ed. T.J. Crow) pp. 183–254. Academic Press, London.

Montouris, G.D., Fenichel, G.M., and McLain, L.W. (1979). The pregnant epileptic: a review and recommendations. *Archs Neurol.* **36**, 601–3.

Nelson, K.B. and Ellenberg, J.H. (1976). Predictors of epilepsy in children who have experienced febrile seizures. *New Engl. J. Med.* **295**, 1029–33.

Polkey, C.E. (1981). Surgery for epilepsy. *Br. J. hosp. Med.* **25**, 48–57.

Reynolds, E.H. (1980). Serum levels of anticonvulsant drugs: interpretation and clinical value. *Pharmac. Ther.* **81**, 217–35.

Shorvon, S.D. and Reynolds, E.H. (1979). Reduction in polypharmacy for epilepsy. *Br. med. J.* **iii**, 1023–5.

Statutory Instrument (1982). No. 423 Road Traffic Act (Driving Licences) Regulations (United Kingdom).

Spero, L. (1982). Neurotransmitters and CNS disease. Epilepsy. *Lancet* **ii**, 1319–22.

Wolf, S.M. (1979). Controversies in the treatment of febrile convulsions. *Neurology, Minneap.* **29**, 287–90.

8 Headache and migraine

HEADACHE

There are many causes of pain in the head, but comparatively few ways in which it can be produced. The principal pain-sensitive structures within the skull are the large blood vessels, and there is abundant evidence that many of the common causes of headache produce it through their effect upon the intracranial vessels. The extracranial branches of the external carotid artery are also pain-sensitive and contribute to some forms of headache. The other important pain-sensitive structures in the head are the sensory nerves and nerve roots, and they are responsible for the pain associated with the various forms of neuritis, neuralgia, and radiculitis. Pain in the head may be referred, either from some structure within the head itself, chiefly the eye, nasal sinuses, temporomandibular joint, or teeth, or occasionally from one of the thoracic or even abdominal viscera. Finally, and probably overall most commonly, pain in the head may be psychogenic. The mode of production of headache will now be considered in relation to its commoner causes.

Space-occupying lesions

It has been established that space-occupying lesions cause headache by exerting traction upon the intracranial blood vessels, especially perhaps those at the base. The characteristics of this type of headache are described elsewhere (p. 229).

Meningeal irritation

Irritation of the meninges either by inflammatory exudate in meningitis or by extravasated blood in subarachnoid haemorrhage causes severe headache. The features of this are described elsewhere (pp. 312 and 471). There are probably two factors in the causation of these headaches, displacement of blood vessels, and dilatation and irritation of the vessel walls by the products of inflammation.

Toxic headache

Many forms of toxaemia give rise to headache, probably as the result of dilatation of the cerebral vessels, an effect strikingly produced by histamine.

Headache in hypertension

Benign hypertension does not usually cause headache, though a patient who knows that he has hypertension may complain of headache. Headache, however, is a striking feature of malignant hypertension. These headaches are characteristically worst in the early hours of the morning. They are certainly vascular in origin, but their precise mode of production is unsettled. The extra- as well as the intracranial vessels may be involved, though whether the pain is due to dilatation or contraction of the vessels is uncertain. During treatment of depression with monoamine oxidase inhibitors such as phenelzine (Nardil), or tranylcypromine (Parnate), the eating of foods, especially cheese, Bovril, Marmite, and bananas, which contain tyramine cause attacks of severe head-ache, flushing, sweating, and hypertension. Tyramine is a pressor amine and the headaches probably result from a blocking of its normal oxidation by these drugs.

Traumatic headache

There may be more than one factor in the causation of headache following head injury. Although it might be expected that chronic changes within the skull, for example meningeal adhesions, would play an important part in causing headache after head injury, similar headaches are rare after operations on the brain and meninges. Extracranial structures may therefore by a more important source of headache, especially the muscles and joints of the upper part of the neck and the upper cervical sensory nerves. Psychological stress also plays an important part in the maintenance of headache in some cases of head injury.

Cranial arteritis

Severe headache may be experienced by a patient with cranial arteritis, the pain originating in the inflamed vessels of the scalp which are thickened and tender and show diminished pulsation. This disease was first recognized by Jonathan Hutchinson who in 1890 examined an aged man with 'red streaks on his head' which prevented him from wearing his hat. Hutchinson described the loss of pulsation in the painful swollen temporal arteries (Fig. 8.1). This disorder, which occurs only in the elderly, may affect any intra- or extracranial cerebral vessels and is therefore better called *cranial* than *temporal arteritis*, though it may be a part of an even more generalized arteritis. The affected vessels show the changes of granulomatous arteritis; there is cellular infiltration with mononuclear, plasma, and giant cells into the media. This process leads to a gradual arterial occlusion, affecting the temporal, occipital, or facial branches of the external carotid artery and particularly the ophthalmic branch of the internal carotid artery. Apart from headache, sudden blindness is one of the more frequent presenting symptoms and cranial arteritis is one of the commoner causes of sudden blindness in the elderly due to involvement of the ciliary arteries supplying the optic nerve and retina. Other symptoms include facial pain, particularly 'claudication' on chewing. Usually, though not always, there is a preceding headache and even earlier vague generalized symptoms of aches in the joints and limbs and anorexia. The diagnosis is established by a

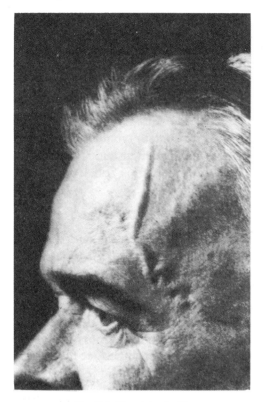

Fig. 8.1. Cranial arteritis.

greatly raised sedimentation rate and, if necessary, can be proved by biopsy of an affected extracranial artery. Cranial arteritis should be regarded as a medical emergency and steroid therapy (60 mg of prednisone daily) should be started when the diagnosis is made and should be continued for up to a year or more with a gradual reduction in dosage after one month according to the symptoms and sedimentation rate. Alternate-day steroids are ineffective. If vision is already impaired steroid therapy may not prevent the loss of sight but may prevent involvement of the other eye.

Neuritis and neuralgia

Pain due to these causes is usually paroxysmal and possesses the distribution characteristic of the nerves involved, which are tender on pressure. Cutaneous hyperalgesia of similar distribution may be present. A not uncommon cause of occipital headache in the elderly is cervical spondylosis, especially when it involves the upper part of the cervical spine. This type of headache is probably due chiefly to involvement of sensory nerve roots, but changes in the calibre of the vertebral arteries may play a part.

Referred pain

Pain referred from a viscus is experienced at a site more or less remote from its origin, though the viscus itself of course may also be painful. Dental disease as a source of pain in the head is perhaps the form of referred pain of the most practical importance. When pain is referred from the eye or nasal sinuses the local cause is usually obvious.

Cough headache

This is a very distinctive, brief but often severe bursting kind of pain experienced after coughing, usually by a middle-aged man. Its mechanism is obscure. In most cases it is benign, and disappears spontaneously; rarely it is a symptom of an intracranial tumour.

Headache following lumbar puncture

When a persistently low pressure of the cerebrospinal fluid follows lumbar puncture, it is apt to cause headache because lack of support to the brain causes a shift in relative positions, which exerts a painful traction on the intracranial vessels.

Psychogenic headache

It is remarkable how many varieties of painful sensations in the head are the subject of complaint by patients who show no evidence of any organic basis for them. Some psychogenic headaches are simply explained as by-products of the tension in the muscles of the scalp and neck which reflects the patient's mental tension. Others can only be regarded as abnormal states of the patient's mind. Psychogenic headache varies from a constant sense of pressure at the vertex to the classical symptom of a sensation 'like a nail or wedge being driven into the skull'. It is occasionally difficult to decide whether a pain in the head is psychogenic or is the result of some organic lesion involving the central pain mechanism. This doubt may arise in some cases of intractable facial pain occurring chiefly in middle-aged or elderly women in whom no local cause can be found and the complaint sometimes becomes a dominant feature of their personality. It is sometimes a symptom of underlying anxiety or depression and responds to treatment by means of reassurance, tranquillizers, or antidepressants.

MIGRAINE

Definition

The cardinal feature of migraine, derived from the term hemicrania, is a paroxysmal headache, commonly but not invariably unilateral, recurring at irregular intervals, and often associated with visual disturbances and other disorders of cerebral function, and vomiting. Migraine is one of the commonest neurological disorders. Some 5 per cent of the population are estimated to have suffered from it at some time in their lives and there can be few who have not on some occasion experienced a headache which has some of the features of migraine.

Aetiology and pathology

The disease affects intra- and extracranial vessels and stress, genetic, hormonal, and biochemical factors, including drugs, probably alter the threshold of a central, possibly hypothalamic trigger mechanism. Cerebral blood flow studies in hemiplegic migraine show that hypoperfusion of the brain starts in the posterior part of the cortex before any focal symptoms and then spreads anteriorly, persisting after the focal symptoms have disappeared. The focal symptoms may therefore be the result of a primary neuronal disturbance and not merely a consequence of reduced blood flow.

There is abundant evidence that the headache in migraine is due chiefly to stretching, by dilatation, of the branches of the external carotid artery and possibly to a lesser extent of the internal carotid artery. Constriction, possibly due to sympathetic overactivity, of one of the vessels supplying an area of cerebral cortex seems the most likely explanation of the visual and other cerebral symptoms to be described below. A vasoactive peptide such as histamine or serotonin may be released following ischaemia with the coincident release of ATP. Heredity seems the most important causal factor. Those who suffer from migraine often have a conscientious or obsessional personality. In the predisposed individual an attack may be precipitated by emotional stress, by eating some particular article of diet, by alcohol, or by menstruation. Eyestrain may also play a part, at least as a precipitant. Allergy in the patient or his family is not uncommon. There is an association between migraine and the cyclical vomiting of childhood, and car-sickness. Migraine usually begins at or shortly after puberty, much less frequently in middle life or later, though an onset at about the menopause is not very uncommon. Women are more subject to migraine than men and usually suffer more severely.

Any theory must explain a number of facts. During the prodromal phase of an attack arterial constriction occurs and has been shown by arteriography; it parallels the reduced blood flow which has been demonstrated by isotope studies. There is a transient rise in plasma serotonin, which has vasoconstrictor effects, at the onset of an attack, followed by a fall during the headache phase. Reserpine (Serpasil), which lowers the level of plasma serotonin (but also lowers the levels of noradrenaline and dopamine), will perpetuate an attack. However, plasma serotonin, possibly released from platelets, whose aggregation is increased in many patients with migraine, is unlikely to be the only factor, because fluid taken from the walls of distended temporal vessels in migraine has shown the presence of a polypeptide which when injected into the region of an artery causes pain and a sterile inflammation. Swelling of the superficial cranial vessels, which is observed during the headache phase of an attack, may explain why ischaemic symptoms indicating inadequate flow may occur despite an enlarged vessel. In the case of the carotid this swelling may cause compression of the cervical sympathetic coat surrounding the artery and hence a partial Horner's syndrome.

Symptoms

A classical attack of migraine begins in about a quarter of patients with a visual disturbance which occurs within one pair of homonymous half-fields, indicating ischaemia of one occipital cortex. For example, the patient notices that he cannot see clearly in a small area to one side of the fixation point. This area of defective vision may be described as misty or shimmering, and it may have an irregular and scintillating and sometimes coloured outline, known as teichopsia, or fortification spectra. This area of disturbed vision tends to move slowly in the course of 15–30 minutes from the central part to the peripheral part of the half-fields. As it moves vision in the central part is restored to normal, while the fortification spectra tend to become larger and more dazzling as they reach the periphery. The visual symptoms may be accompanied or followed by a similar slow development and spread of cutaneous symptoms, numbness and tingling most frequently involving the lips and tongue, and the hand, much less frequently the lower limb, and there may be transitory dysphasia or, rarely, hemiparesis.

The headache usually begins as the visual manifestations are passing off, as a boring pain in a localized area on one side, often the temple, and gradually spreads to the whole of the affected side of the head – and sometimes the other side as well is involved. It gradually increases in intensity and acquires a throbbing character, being intensified by stooping and all forms of exertion, and by light. The superficial temporal artery on the affected side is dilated and exhibits vigorous pulsation, compression of which may at first reduce the pain. There may be congestion of the nasal mucosa and conjunctiva on the affected side. In milder cases the headache lasts for several hours but passes away if the patient can sleep, or after a night's rest. In more severe cases it persists for days.

Nausea is usually present during the stage of headache and vomiting may or may not occur.

Though a classical attack of migraine has been described, there are many variants. Frequently headache occurs without any cerebral symptoms, the patient often awakening with it in the morning. Sometimes the visual disturbances are not followed by a headache.

Ophthalmoplegic migraine is the term applied to recurrent attacks of headache associated with paralysis of one or more oculomotor nerves, which persists for days or weeks after the attack, and tends to become permanent. Some cases so described in the past, but not all, have probably been examples of intracranial aneurysm.

Basilar artery migraine is the term applied to attacks in which the premonitory symptoms point to a disturbance of brainstem rather than hemisphere function. Giddiness, ataxia, dysarthria and even loss of consciousness may occur. The syndrome is commoner in adolescent girls and young women. It seems probable that in such patients the territory of the basilar artery is affected by a migrainous disturbance.

Course and prognosis

The frequency of attacks of migraine varies considerably in different patients. Often the disorder seems to possess a rhythm which is little influenced by outside factors, the attacks occurring once a week, once a fortnight, or once a month, with great regularity. Apart from treatment, attacks tend to grow less frequent and less severe as the patient grows older, but may be exacerbated by the approach of the menopause. They usually cease spontaneously in middle life, but some patients continue to suffer from migraine into old age.

Migraine does not shorten life, but in severe cases in women a state of chronic exhaustion may occur. Very rarely, persistent cerebral symptoms remain after an attack of migraine, suggesting that some irreversible vascular change has occurred.

Diagnosis

If all the classical features of migraine are present, it is unlikely to be confused with any other condition. It may, however, occasionally be simulated by an angioma in one parieto-occipital region. In such a case, however, the visual symptoms would always be referred to one side, that is the side opposite to the tumour, whereas in migraine they occur on either side indiscriminately. An early onset is important, since migraine usually begins at puberty, whereas most organic conditions with which it may be confused are encountered in adult life. A short history of headaches of progressive intensity may call for investigations to exclude a space-occupying lesion. Migraine is occasionally confused with epilepsy, but in migraine the progress of the attack is slow, whereas in epilepsy it is rapid, and the retention of consciousness in the former should put the diagnosis beyond doubt. When migrainous headache occurs without other symptoms it must be distinguished from pain in the head due to other causes. Psychogenic headaches sometimes closely simulate migraine.

Treatment

There are three aspects of treatment of migraine. First general health measures, second prophylactic treatment to reduce the likelihood of attacks, and third the treatment of the attacks themselves. Sufferers from migraine should try as far as possible to avoid those circumstances, including mental stress, which experience shows precipitate the attacks. Refractive errors, if present, should be corrected. Diet is important but individual idiosyncrases are marked. Some patients benefit from a diet in which animal fat is restricted and other foods likely to precipitate attacks include eggs, chocolate, and raw fruit, especially apples and oranges, mushrooms, cheese, and beef products. Alcohol should be curtailed or stopped completely. The effect of oral contraceptive drugs is variable. In some women particularly on days when the contraceptive pill has not been taken the migraine is more likely to occur. If attacks of migraine occur for the first time when a woman starts the contraceptive pill this should of course be stopped to abolish the migraine and to avoid the slightly increased risk of cerebral thrombosis during attacks.

The large number of drugs used in the attempted prophylaxis of migraine is a testimony to the fact that when personality and genetic factors predominate treatment with drugs is extremely difficult. Most of the drugs which have been shown to have an effect exert blocking actions on sympathetic or serotonergic function or affect platelet aggregation. A first attempt at treatment is the use of soluble Aspirin 600 mg each morning with a further dose at the onset of the headache. Propranolol (Inderal) 20 mg up to three times per day is usually helpful and is unlikely to cause postural hypotension. Pizotifen (Sanomigran) is a serotonin antagonist which also inhibits histamine, tryptamine, acetylcholine, and bradykinin. It can be given in an initial dose of 0.5 mg three times a day but should not be used with patients with glaucoma. Cyproheptadine (Periactin) in a dose of 2 mg three times a day also acts similarly. Methysergide (Deseril) is best avoided because of the risk of retroperitoneal fibroplasia.

For the acute attack in which nausea is a prominent feature, metoclopramide (Maxolon) in a small dose of 10 mg may be followed by two or three soluble Aspirin tablets which have the effect of discouraging platelet aggregation. This treatment coupled with the opportunity to sleep may be all that is necessary. Domperidone (Motilium) in a dose of 60 mg daily is a peripheral dopamine receptor agonist with antiemetic properties and if the patient has clear-cut physical or psychic warning of the impending attack it may be also given prophylactically.

Ergotamine has a long established place in the treatment of severe migraine. It has complex effects but by blocking alpha noradrenergic and serotonergic receptors may act mainly as a partial agonist so constricting smooth muscle and reducing the stretching of the branches of the external carotid artery which are the site of the severe pain. It may be given by mouth as ergotamine tartrate in 1–2 mg tablets, best allowed to dissolve under the tongue. No more than 10 mg should be given in any week. There are several preparations of oral ergotamine combined with caffeine or an antihistamine.

Does the administration of ergotamine tartrate involve any risks? Ergotamine overdose can itself cause headaches. Ergotamine should not be given to patients with generalized arterial disease or during pregnancy and in any case the possibility of some cumulative disturbance of the peripheral circulation should always be borne in mind. Some patients take the drug without any apparent ill-effect on a regular basis for years but the risk of ergotism with prolonged treatment cannot be ignored. Exceptionally a single dose will cause thrombophlebitis presumably as a result of venous spasm and very rarely peripheral gangrene occurs. The use of ergotamine can be supported by diuretics especially in migraine occurring at the time of menstrual period in women, or with mild tranquillizers such as diazepam (Valium) or anti-depressants such as amitryptiline in a dose of 20–50 mg at night, even if the patient is not overtly depressed.

MIGRAINOUS NEURALGIA

Migrainous neuralgia is a highly distinctive form of headache also known as cluster headache. It is much commoner in men. It consists of paroxysms of severe pain usually in the frontotemporal region and the eye, occurring several times in the twenty-four hours and lasting for from half an hour to two hours. At the height of the attack there may be lacrimation and nasal discharge, more marked on the same side as the headache. It possesses its own rhythm, each bout tending to last a few weeks and then being followed by a free interval of months or even a year or more, when the same series of events is repeated. No associated abnormality is to be found, and the pathogenesis of the condition is unknown.

Oral ergotamine usually has a highly specific effect and can be taken by mouth prophylactically at the time attack is expected during the day. Since the attacks sometimes wake the patient regularly in the early hours of the morning, the ergotamine may be given as a suppository containing 2 mg before the patient goes to bed. If the patient fails to respond to ergotamine then lithium carbonate in a dose of 800 mg at night with control of plasma levels has been shown to be effective in many patients. Very rarely it may be justifiable to permit subcutaneous injections of 0.25–0.5 mg of ergotamine at appropriate intervals, which the patient can learn to give himself. By omitting a dose of ergotamine, either oral or by injection, he can ascertain whether the disorder has entered a remission.

REFERENCES

Aring, C.D. (1972). The migrainous scintillating scotoma. *J. Am. med. Ass.* **220**, 519–22.

Dalessio, D.J. (ed.) (1980). *Wolff's headache and other head pain,* 4th edn. Oxford University Press, New York.

Graham, E., Holland, A., Avery, A., and Ross Russell, R.W. (1981). Prognosis in giant cell arteritis. *Br. med. J.* **282**, 269–71.

Kudrow, L. (1980). *Cluster headache: mechanisms and management.* Oxford University Press.

Part II
Disorders of anatomical regions

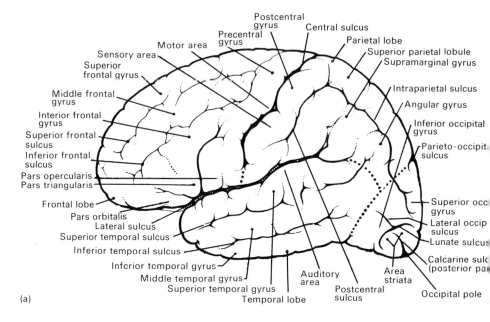

(a)

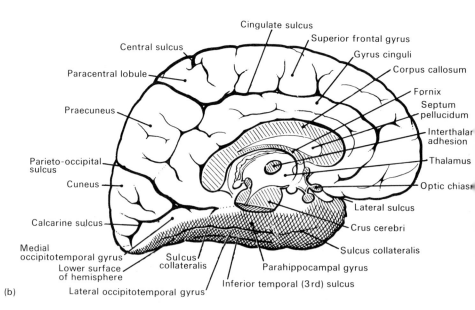

(b)

Fig. 9.0. Left cerebral hemisphere: (a) external (lateral) aspect; (b) internal (medial) aspect.

9 Intracranial tumour

The term intracranial tumour, though primarily applied to neoplasms, is extended a little loosely to include other space-occupying lesions of slow growth such as a tuberculoma. Other inflammatory conditions such as an abscess may sometimes produce a clinical picture indistinguishable from that of a neoplasm, and the same is true of some parasitic cysts. Intracranial neoplasm may also be simulated by certain forms of hydrocephalus, and by a subdural haematoma. Since intracranial neoplasm, however, is by far the commonest cause of increased intracranial pressure, that condition will first be considered in relation to its pathological physiology and symptomatology, and the other conditions which may be confused with it will be dealt with later, more particularly in relation to diagnosis and treatment.

AETIOLOGY AND PATHOLOGY

Gliomas

The gliomas are the commonest form of intracranial neoplasm. They are derived from cells which form the glia, the supporting tissue of the nervous system. The classification of the gliomas is still the subject of controversy. It is not always easy to identify anaplastic cells in a tumour, and tumours derived from the same type of cell may behave differently in different situations. With the exception of the ependymoma the gliomas are all infiltrative tumours, which explains the great difficulty of complete surgical removal, and the liability to recurrence after operation. The following are the commonest gliomas. The *astrocytoma* is a white infiltrating growth which may occur at any age and in either the cerebral or the cerebellar hemispheres. Astrocytomas grow slowly and are relatively benign and are particularly liable to undergo cystic transformation. Microscopically they exhibit abundant astrocytes (Fig. 9.1). The *glioblastoma multiforme* is an extremely malignant glioma arising in middle life and almost invariably found in the cerebral hemispheres. It is a reddish, highly vascular tumour which tends to infiltrate the brain extensively (Fig. 9.2), and microscopically consists of relatively undifferentiated round or oval cells. The *medulloblastoma* is a rapidly growing tumour, most frequently encountered in the cerebellum in children. It is composed of round undifferentiated cells, and shows a tendency to become disseminated through the subarachnoid space. The *oligodendroglioma* is a rare, slowly growing, relatively benign tumour occurring in the cerebral hemispheres of young adults,

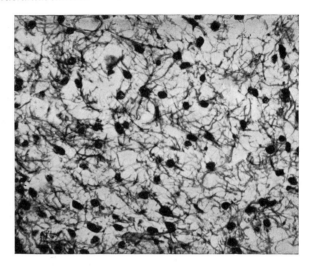

Fig. 9.1. Astrocytoma.

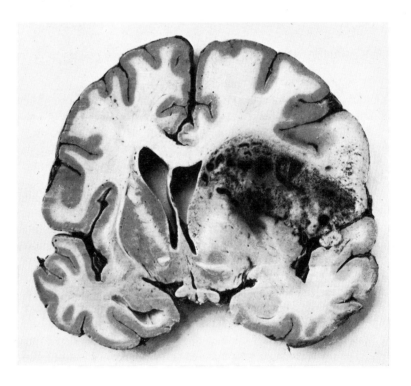

Fig. 9.2. Glioblastoma multiforme. Note haemorrhagic areas and displacement of ventricular system.

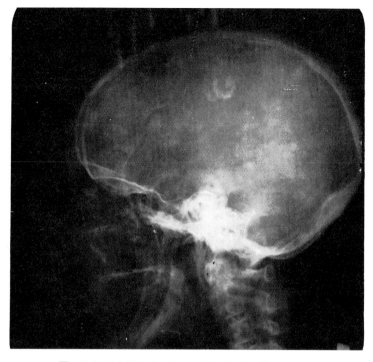

Fig. 9.3. Calcification in an oligodendroglioma.

which shows a marked tendency to calcification (Fig. 9.3). The *ependymoma* is a firm whitish tumour, sometimes papilliferous, arising from the ependyma, frequently in the roof of the fourth ventricle.

Meningioma

The meningioma is an extracerebral tumour believed to arise from the arachnoid cells of the arachnoid villi. It is composed of specialized connective tissue cells characteristically arranged in columns or whorls (Fig. 9.4). The meningioma is a single large more-or-less irregularly lobulated growth, frequently arising in close relationship to the skull, and tending to invade the overlying bone in which it provokes a characteristic hyperostosis. Since the meningiomas arise from the cells of the arachnoid villi, they are commonly found along the course of the intracranial venous sinuses, and their sites of greatest predilection are the superior sagittal sinus – parasagittal meningiomas – the sphenoidal ridge, the convexity of the hemispheres, and the suprasellar region (Fig. 9.5). They are rare below the tentorium.

Blood-vessel tumours

The two principal types of blood-vessel tumour are the *angioblastomas* and the *angiomas*. The angioblastomas are true neoplasms composed of angioblasts, and

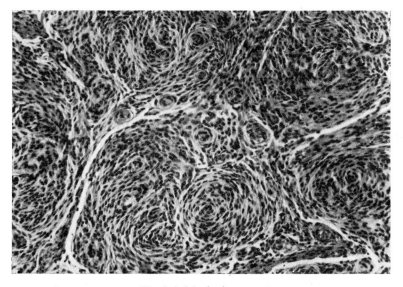

Fig. 9.4. Meningioma.

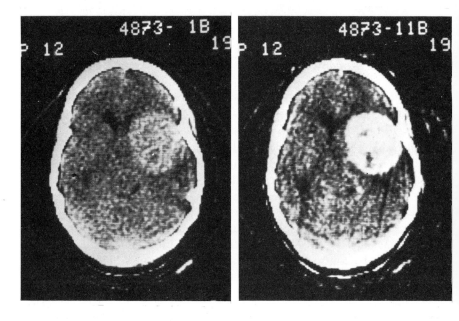

Fig. 9.5. Meningioma, arising from the right sphenoidal wing, showing high-density well-circumscribed mass, enhanced (right).

they exhibit a marked tendency to form cysts in the surrounding nerve tissue, the cysts containing xanthochromic fluid. They are almost invariably subtentorial tumours, chiefly involving the cerebellum. The patient may also have an angioblastoma of the retina.

Angiomas are regarded as congenital abnormalities, capillary, venous or arteriovenous malformations (see Fig. 9.15). They consist of a mass of enlarged and tortuous cortical vessels, supplied by one or more large arteries, and drained by one or more large veins. They are most frequently met with in the field of the middle cerebral artery. The Sturge–Weber syndrome is capillary-venous malformation in one hemisphere associated with a facial naevus.

Tumours related to the hypophysis and third ventricle

The common tumours arising in the hypophysis itself are adenomas. The commonest of these are the *chromophobe adenoma* and the *prolactinoma*, composed of cells which stain poorly (see Fig. 9.10). The *chromophil* or *acidophil adenoma* is composed of cells which resemble the acidophil cells of the normal gland. It gives rise to symptoms of hyperpituitarism – gigantism and acromegaly. The *craniopharyngioma,* also known as the hypophysial epidermoid tumour, or the tumour of Rathke's pouch, is derived from an embryonic remnant of the craniopharyngeal pouch which comes to lie above the sella turcica. Tumours of this type contain cells resembling those of the buccal epithelium of the embryo, and are very liable to undergo cystic degeneration and calcification.

Colloid cysts of the third ventricle are rounded cystic tumours measuring from 1 to 3 cm in diameter and arising from the choroid plexus of the third ventricle (see Fig. 9.16). Owing to their position they readily cause hydrocephalus.

Pineal tumours are rare and of several pathological varieties, one of which is thought to be a teratoma.

Acoustic neuroma

Acoustic neuromas are usually unilateral, and consist of elongated cells like spindle fibroblasts with much collagen and reticulum. Since they are believed to be derived from Schwann cells, they are known as schwannomas (see Fig. 9.9).

Metastatic tumours

About 1 in 5 cerebral neoplasms is secondary to a primary growth elsewhere, usually in the lung, breast, stomach, prostate, thyroid, or kidney. Secondary cerebral tumours are usually multiple and rapidly growing. They are pinkish, rounded, and well defined from the surrounding brain tissue (see Fig. 9.10).

Tumours of infective origin

The invasion of the brain by an infecting organism occasionally causes a space-occupying lesion, the commonest of which is a tuberculoma. Cerebral gumma is rare. A pyogenic abscess also comes into this category, and so may sarcoidosis. The parasitic cysts which may give rise to increased intracranial pressure include hydatid and cysticercus.

PATHOLOGICAL PHYSIOLOGY

The functions of the brain depend upon the maintenance of the circulation of the blood and the cerebrospinal fluid at their appropriate pressures. The brain is unique among the viscera in being confined within a rigid box, the cranium. It follows that the total volume of the intracranial contents, the brain and its coverings, the blood vessels and the blood, and the cerebrospinal fluid is constant, and that an increase in the volume of any of them can only occur at the expense of the others. The intracranial contents react in complicated ways to changes in their volume or pressure. An intracranial tumour usually increases the mass of the brain, though in the case of certain slowly growing infiltrating tumours the increase in mass may be very slight, with the result that symptoms of increased intracranial pressure are for a long time slight or absent. The effect of a tumour upon the circulation in its neighbourhood tends to cause oedema of adjacent areas of brain and so add to the local rise of pressure. Tumours may cause a rise in the pressure of the cerebrospinal fluid in various ways. Direct obstruction of the ventricular system may occur in the third ventricle, the cerebral aqueduct, or the fourth ventricle. The upward passage of the fluid may be interfered with at the level of the tentorium, and its absorption may be impaired by a rise of pressure in the cerebral venous sinuses (see Plate 7(a)). Mechanical displacements of brain tissue may occur, leading in the case of a supratentorial tumour to herniation of the parahippocampal gyrus through the tentorial opening, or in the case of tumour in the posterior fossa, to the cerebellar 'pressure cone' formed by downward displacement of the cerebellar tonsils into the foramen magnum.

SYMPTOMS

Mode of onset

The mode of onset of symptoms of a cerebral tumour is extremely variable, depending upon the nature and site of the tumour. It is important to remember that neurological symptoms, particularly epilepsy, often precede those of increased intracranial pressure, sometimes by many years. On the whole, the history tends to be long in the case of astrocytomas, oligodendrogliomas, meningiomas, acoustic neuromas, and hypophysial adenomas, and shortest – from a few months to a year – in glioblastoma multiforme and secondary carcinoma. The commonest modes of onset are:

1. Progressive focal symptoms, e.g. focal epilepsy, monoplegia, hemiplegia, aphasia, cerebellar deficiency, associated with symptoms of increased intracranial pressure.

2. Symptoms of increased intracranial pressure alone.

3. Progressive focal symptoms alone, e.g. visual failure, unilateral deafness, dementia.

4. Generalized epileptic attacks preceding other symptoms perhaps by many years.

5. An epileptic onset with loss of consciousness and perhaps hemiplegia.

6. A personality change may be the first sign of a cerebral tumour, particularly if the frontal lobes are involved.

Symptoms of increased intracranial pressure

The symptoms of a cerebral tumour are conveniently divided into those attributable to increased intracranial pressure, focal symptoms which are due to local effects of the growth, and certain false localizing signs (p. 230). Headache, vomiting, and papilloedema have long been regarded as the classical triad of symptoms of increased intracranial pressure.

Headache

The headache of intracranial tumour is probably mainly due to abnormal states of tension in the cerebral blood vessels. It is at first paroxysmal, tending to occur chiefly during the night and in the early morning. As the growth increases in size, headaches become more prolonged and may ultimately be continuous. They are intensified by any activities which raise the intracranial pressure. The headache is not of much localizing value, but in the early stages of a tumour of one cerebral hemisphere it tends to predominate on the affected side. A tumour in the posterior fossa tends to cause occipital headache radiating down the neck, while the headache of hydrocephalus is diffuse and also radiates down the neck.

Vomiting

Vomiting usually occurs during the night or in the early morning when the headache is especially severe. Though sometimes, especially in children, preceded by little nausea, vomiting of cerebral origin is not always precipitate.

Papilloedema

The pathogenesis and appearance of the papilloedema are described on page 39. Its incidence varies according to the situation of the tumour. It is usually present when the tumour is in the cerebellum, fourth ventricle or temporal lobe, but is absent in half the cases of pontine and subcortical tumours, and is often late in developing when the tumour is prefrontal. The changes in the visual fields due to papilloedema consist of enlargement of the blind spot with concentric constriction at the periphery of the field. Visual acuity deteriorates, and, if the condition progresses, optic atrophy and complete blindness are likely to result. Patients with papilloedema sometimes have brief transitory attacks of blindness which are probably due to a temporary increase in the obstruction of the blood supply of the retina.

Mental symptoms and the state of consciousness

The progressive growth of a cerebral tumour, if unrelieved, ultimately leads to loss of consciousness. This may occur rapidly, for example after a haemorrhage into the tumour, or gradually, in which case the patient passes through a phase of mental confusion with disorientation in space and time, somnolence, and stupor to coma. Apart from that, a chronic rise of intracranial pressure, as the result for example of the hydrocephalus produced by a tumour in the posterior fossa, may lead to progressive dementia.

Disturbances of pulse rate and respiration

An acute or subacute rise of intracranial pressure usually causes slowing of the pulse rate to between 50 and 60 beats a minute. If the pressure continues to rise, the pulse becomes extremely rapid and often irregular. A gradual rise of sufficient rapidity and severity to cause loss of consciousness usually leads at first to slow and deep respirations. Later the respiratory rate may become irregular, e.g. of the Cheyne–Stokes type, and in the terminal stages the respirations are rapid and shallow.

Hypopituitarism

Hydrocephalus resulting from increased intracranial pressure may lead to symptoms of hypopituitarism, namely adiposity and genital atrophy, espeically in children. This is due to downward pressure of the floor of the distended third ventricle upon the hypothalamus and hypophysis.

Changes due to local brain compression with raised intracranial pressure

With hemisphere lesions there may be cingulate herniation in which the cingulate gyrus herniates under the falx causing compression of the anterior cerebral arteries with infarction of the region of the paracentral lobules. With a temporal lobe tumour uncal herniation may occur with the uncus of the temporal lobe becoming compressed at the free edge of the tentorium cerebelli. This causes a unilateral dilated pupil and lateral deviation of the eyes as oculomotor nerve fibres are paralysed. It may be followed by progressive brainstem compression. Posterior fossa lesions may produce herniation of the cerebellar tonsils through the foramen magnum. This leads to flexion of the head towards the side of the herniation and cardiac and respiratory arrest due to compression of the medulla (see p. 90).

False localizing signs

A cerebral tumour, as described above, may produce mechanical displacements and distortions of structures remote from it within the cranium. These have been termed false localizing signs. The most important of these are a sixth nerve palsy on one or both sides, bilateral extensor plantar reflexes or bilateral grasp reflexes resulting from interference with the function of the cerebral hemispheres by distension of the ventricles in hydrocephalus; an extensor plantar response occurring on the same side in a tumour of one cerebral hemisphere, produced by compression of the opposite cerebral peduncle against the tentorium; cerebellar symptoms resulting from tumours of the frontal lobe, and midbrain symptoms produced by a tumour of the cerebellar vermis.

Epilepsy as a symptom of cerebral tumour

In addition to focal epilepsy, described below, generalized epileptiform convulsions are a common symptom of cerebral tumour and may precede all others by many years. Epilepsy occurs in some 30 per cent of cases of cerebral tumour, and is the first symptom in about two-thirds of the cases of astrocytoma and meningioma, and about half of the cases of glioblastoma. It is most frequently encountered when the tumour is in the frontal or the temporal lobe, but it may be a symptom of a tumour in any part of the cerebral hemisphere.

FOCAL SYMPTOMS

Frontal lobe

Prefrontal tumours

By prefrontal tumours are meant tumours confined to that part of the frontal lobe lying in front of the precentral gyrus. Tumours in this region are often hard to localize. Headache as a rule occurs early, but papilloedema and vomiting usually develop late. Mental symptoms, especially a progressive dementia, have long been held to be characteristic of a frontal lobe lesion, but they are often inconspicuous. Generalized convulsions occur in about 50 per cent of cases. Expressive dysphasia may occur when the tumour involves the posterior part of the dominant inferior frontal gyrus – Broca's area. The unilateral *grasp reflex* is pathognomonic of a frontal lobe lesion. It is most frequently observed in the opposite hand, but may be found only in the foot when the tumour is in the superior part of the lobe. Pressure upon neighbouring corticospinal tract fibres may lead to weakness upon the opposite side of the body, usually most marked in the face and tongue. Pressure upon the olfactory nerve, lying upon the floor of the anterior fossa, may lead to anosmia on the side of the lesion. This is most likely to occur in the case of a meningioma arising from the olfactory groove.

Precentral tumours

These are perhaps the easiest to localize on account of the early development of symptoms of excitation and destruction of the corticospinal fibres. Corticospinal excitation in the precentral or motor cortex leads to a *focal convulsion*, in typical cases a Jacksonian attack (p. 190). Partial Jacksonian attacks may occur, in which the convulsion is limited to a small part of one side of the body, without loss of consciousness. Motor weakness is the result of the destruction of the corticospinal tract fibres by the tumour, and exhibits a regional distribution corresponding to the representation of parts of the body in the precentral gyrus. Owing to the large surface extent of the pyramidal cells on the cortex, even a large cortical tumour is likely to cause weakness of only a part of the opposite side of the body, that is a monoplegia. With inferiorly placed tumours there is weakness, often accompanied by apraxia, of the face and tongue on the opposite side, and weakness of movements of the thumb, which is represented in the adjacent area. If the tumour is at a higher level the thumb may escape, though the fingers and arm are affected, while a tumour involving principally the medial aspect of the hemisphere is likely to cause a monoplegia involving only the foot or the whole lower limb. The usual reflex changes associated with a corticospinal tract lesion are found, and these may be limited to the paretic part.

A tumour of the falx in the region of the paracentral lobule is likely to produce weakness of both lower limbs, beginning in the feet, and retention of urine may occur. When the sensory area of the paracentral lobule is involved there will be impairment of postural sensibility in the toes.

Jacksonian convulsions are usually associated with permanent weakness of the part of the body which is the focus of the fit, but after each convulsion there is often a temporary increase in both its severity and extent (Todd's paralysis).

Temporal lobe

The focal symptoms of temporal lobe tumours are often slight, especially when the tumour is on the right side. One characteristic group of symptoms of a discharging lesion in this situation is the variety of attacks known as temporal lobe epilepsy described on page 191. Generalized convulsions may also occur when a tumour involves the temporal lobe. Visual field defect may be produced. The lower fibres of the optic radiation are likely to be caught in their path around the tip of the descending horn of the ventricle. The characteristic defect is therefore a crossed upper quadrantic hemianopia, the loss being usually more extensive in the ipsilateral field. Temporal lobe tumours may cause tinnitus or auditory hallucinations. Left-sided temporal lobe tumours cause aphasia in about 50 per cent of cases. This may consist merely of a defect in naming objects. In more severe cases central dysphasia, with or without word-deafness, is present. The patient is unable to understand spoken words, and this disability may extend to written words also. When speech is even more severely disordered the patient speaks jargon, his speech consisting of a voluble outpouring of meaningless phrases and words of his own construction.

Neighbourhood symptoms include signs of a corticospinal tract lesion on the opposite side, especially weakness of the face, and occasionally a third nerve palsy.

Parietal lobe

The parietal lobe is the principal sensory area of the cerebral cortex. Sensory disturbances therefore constitute a prominent part of the symptoms of tumours of this region. The postcentral gyrus is the part most concerned with sensation. Parts of the body are here represented for purposes of sensation in a manner similar to their motor representation in the precentral gyrus (p. 115). Irritation of the postcentral gyrus causes sensory Jacksonian fits which consist usually of paraesthesiae, such as tingling or a sensation of electric shock which begin in that part of the opposite side of the body corresponding to the focus of excitation. The paraesthesiae then spread to other parts in the order of their representation in the gyrus, and this may be followed by a similar spreading motor discharge due to the extension of the excitation to the precentral gyrus.

A destructive lesion of the postcentral gyrus leads to sensory loss, the extent of which corresponds in distribution to the extent of the cortical lesion. The sensory loss is the cortical type, that is, it involves the spatial and discriminative aspects of sensation, especially postural sensibility and tactile discrimination, while the crude appreciation of pain, heat, and cold is left intact. As the result of this sensory loss the patient may be unable to recognize objects placed in his affected hand – astereognosis.

Postcentral lesions lead also to hypotonia and wasting of the affected parts – parietal wasting, and to both static and kinetic ataxia, the latter resulting from sensory loss.

Parietal tumours reaching deep into the white matter may lead to thalamic over-reaction, an exaggerated response to unpleasant stimuli on the opposite side of the body. Involvement of the fibres of the optic radiation causes a crossed homonymous defect of the visual field, and since the upper fibres are the more likely to be caught, the field defect may be confined to the lower quadrant.

The posterior part of the parietal lobe constitutes a 'watershed' between the three great cortical sensory areas, the optic, auditory, and somatic. A left-sided lesion of this area may therefore be expected to cause considerable disturbance of speech on its receptive side. Lesions of the left angular gyrus usually cause dyslexia and dysgraphia with which may be associated finger-agnosia and dyscalculia. Lesions of the same area on the right side cause disturbances of awareness of the opposite side of the body, and the left half of space. Parietal lobe lesions may cause sensory and visual inattention.

Occipital lobe

Tumours of the occipital lobe are comparatively rare. Epileptiform convulsions occur in a considerable proportion of cases. They may be preceded by a visual aura, such as flashes of light moving from one side towards the middle line, but this is not constant. Such attacks may begin with turning of the eyes to the opposite side. The characteristic focal sign of an occipital tumour is a visual field defect. This may consist of a crossed homonymous hemianopia extending up to the fixation point, or of a crossed homonymous quadrantic defect. Hemianopia may have been discovered by the patient owing to his collisions with people on his blind side.

Lesions of the left occipital lobe cause visual object agnosia and agnosia for colours. Neighbourhood symptoms may be present due to extension of the tumour into the parietal or temporal lobes. Occasionally symptoms of cerebellar deficiency occur as a result of pressure transmitted through the tentorium to the cerebellum.

Corpus callosum

Tumours of the corpus callosum are not common, but yield a distinctive clinical picture. Mental symptoms are prominent and are often the first to be noticed. It is said that mental changes are more frequently observed in cases of tumour of the corpus callosum than when the tumour is situated in any other part of the brain, including the frontal lobe. Apathy, drowsiness, and defect of memory are the commonest mental disturbances, but depression and anxiety may occur. There may be epileptiform convulsions.

The situation of the tumour in the middle line extending laterally to the central white matter on both sides leads to early damage to the corticospinal tracts, often asymmetrical in the early stages. Anteriorly placed tumours extending into the frontal lobes may cause a grasp reflex on one or both sides. Apraxia may be present, sometimes on the left side only, owing to interruption of the fibres linking the left supramarginal gyrus with the right corticospinal tract. Signs of increased intracranial pressure are often late in developing. The protein content of the cerebrospinal fluid is likely to be high.

Central hemisphere tumours

Tumours situated deeply in one or other cerebral hemisphere may cause little disturbance of the intracranial pressure at first, but they usually lead to motor or sensory symptoms early. Owing to the concentration of fibres near the internal capsule the whole of the opposite side of the body is likely to be affected. Anteriorly placed tumours cause a progressive spastic hemiplegia. When the tumour is situated more posteriorly the presenting symptoms are sensory, and all forms of sensibility are usually impaired on the opposite side, sensory ataxia being present. A crossed hemianopia may be added if the optic radiation is involved. Somnolence indicates extension of the pressure to the central reticular formation, and pressure upon the upper part of the midbrain may lead to pupillary abnormalities and ophthalmoplegia.

Third ventricle

The third ventricle may be the primary site of the tumour, e.g. a colloid cyst (see Fig. 9.16), or it may be invaded by a tumour arising in its neighbourhood. A tumour in the third ventricle is likely to cause hydrocephalus, which may be acute, subacute, intermittent, or chronic. Severe paroxysmal headaches are common, and may be influenced by changes in the position of the head. Headache and papilloedema may be the only symptoms. Progressive dementia may occur, or coma may suddenly develop.

Midbrain

Tumours arising in the midbrain usually cause internal hydrocephalus early owing to obstruction of the cerebral aqueduct and hence lead to headache, papilloedema, and vomiting. Ocular abnormalities are prominent. Lesions of the upper part usually cause weakness of conjugate deviation upwards. Lesions of the lower part lead to weakness of conjugate deviation downwards, with which ptosis and weakness of convergence may be combined. The pupils are often unequal and tend to be dilated. The reactions both to light and on convergence-accommodation may be lost, or the latter may be preserved when the former is lost. Asymmetrical nuclear ophthalmoplegia may occur. The corticospinal tracts are usually involved on both sides though often asymmetrically. Tremor is common, and nystagmus and ataxia result from injury to the cerebellar connections. Sensory changes are due to damage to the long ascending sensory pathways, and compression of the lateral lemniscus may lead to unilateral or bilateral deafness. Tonic convulsions characterized by opisthotonus with extension of all four limbs, and loss of consciousness may occur.

Pineal body

Pineal tumours are rare. They usually give rise to signs of increased intracranial pressure, and of pressure upon the midbrain, and in exceptional cases disturbances of growth and development, which are found only in certain cases when the tumour develops in young boys. They consist of abnormal growth of the skeleton and premature sexual development.

Tumours in the neighbourhood of the hypophysis

The three types of tumour which commonly occur in the small region at the base of the brain in and around the hypophysis and the optic chiasma are: (i) tumours of the hypophysis itself; (ii) craniopharyngiomas; and (iii) suprasellar meningiomas.

Hypophysial tumours

As already stated, the two types of hypophysial adenoma which may cause neurological symptoms are the chromophobe and the chromophil tumours. The basophil usually produces endocrine changes only. The symptoms of these two tumours may be divided into: (i) pressure symptoms and (ii) endocrine disturbances.

The common pressure symptoms are headache, usually with a bitemporal distribution, and visual disturbances. Since the optic chiasma lies above the sella turcica, visual field defects are an important and early symptom of hypophysial tumour. Usually the tumour, as it enlarges upwards, first compresses the decussating fibres of the chiasma, hence bitemporal hemianopia is the field defect most frequently encountered. This is as a rule symmetrical, the defect beginning on one side before the other and, as the tumour grows, the nasal field of the eye first affected is encroached upon, so the patient may reach a stage of complete blindness in one eye with a temporal hemianopia of the opposite side. Later, if the pressure is not relieved, the second eye becomes blind.

Cushing's syndrome is usually due to pituitary-dependent bilateral adrenoplasia associated with a pituitary hyperplasia or tumour and does not cause pressure symptoms.

Compression of the optic chiasma causes primary optic atrophy, which is often more advanced in one eye than in the other. In the later stages the tumour may expand beyond the sella to involve the base of the brain or the cranial nerves in the wall of the cavernous sinus (Plate 7(b)).

X-ray evidence of the pressure is to be found in a uniform expansion of the sella turcica with thinning of its walls (see Fig. 5.2). The latest CT scanners can provide computer reconstructed views of the pituitary region replacing the need for air encephalography, but angiography may be necessary.

The endocrine changes characteristic of the *chromophobe adenoma* were usually attributed to hypopituitarism, and consist of a depression of sexual function, which in women takes the form of amenorrhoea. There is a loss of hair over the limbs and trunk, and a man no longer needs to shave as often as he did. The skin becomes soft and pliable, and the metabolic changes of hypopituitarism are likely to be present, including depression of function of the suprarenal cortex and the thyroid (see p. 173).

Acromegaly

The chromophil adenoma leads to the endocrine symptoms of hyperpituitarism, especially in the sphere of the growth hormone. When the tumour arises before the growth has ceased, gigantism occurs. When, as more frequently happens, the tumour begins during adult life, acromegaly is the result (Fig. 9.6). This is characterized by slow changes in the skin and subcutaneous tissues, bones, viscera, general metabolism, and sexual activity. The skin and subcutaneous tissues, especially of the fingers, lips, ears, and tongue, exhibit a fibrous hyperplasia. Overgrowth of the bones is most evident in the skull, face, mandible, and at the periphery of the extremities. The calvarium is thickened, the malar bones enlarged, and as the result of overgrowth of the mandible the lower jaw becomes prognathous and separation of the teeth occurs. The hands become broad and spade-like, and hyperostoses may develop on the terminal phalanges ('tufting'). Similar changes occur in the feet, and the patient frequently notices that he requires a larger size in gloves and shoes. Kyphosis in the upper thoracic spine is common, and enlargement of many of the viscera

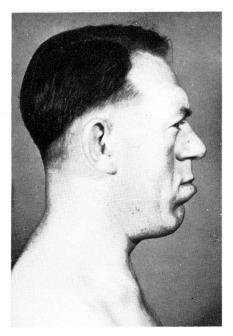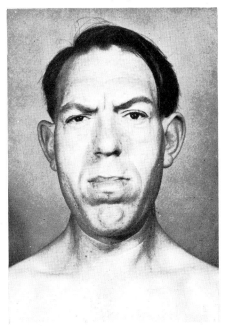

Fig. 9.6. Acromegaly.

has been described. Carbohydrate metabolism is often disturbed, leading to hyperglycaemia and glycosuria. The metabolic rate is usually increased. Impairment of sexual function occurs in both gigantism and acromegaly.

The plasma growth hormone levels in acromegaly before treatment are always raised but the concentration does not correspond closely with the other features of acromegaly. Various methods of treatment are used, sometimes in combination; for example transphenoidal or transfrontal hypophysectomy and removal or craniotomy and removal or cryosurgery and external irradiation (by proton beam where available) or radioactive implants. Medical treatment with bromocriptine, which lowers the level of growth hormone in many patients with acromegaly, has been disappointing and is no more than an adjuvent to surgical treatment and irradiation.

Prolactin-secreting tumours

The concept of the so-called 'chromophobe' adenoma is changing in that it is likely that many of these may be prolactin-secreting tumours. Prolactin-secreting pituitary tumours in women, without evidence of associated acromegaly or Cushing's disease, may present with amenorrhoea. Galactor-rhoea may not be present since other factors including high levels of oestrogen are necessary for galactorrhoea to occur. Prolactin levels should therefore be measured in any patient with amenorrhoea and may be raised in some 20 per cent of patients with secondary amenorrhoea and nearly all these patients have pituitary adenomas, even if plain X-rays of the skull are normal. Tumours secreting prolactin are often small and laterally placed giving an expanded border in the sella and sometimes a double contour to the floor. It may be some 10–20 years after the onset of the amenorrhoea before the tumour increases in size sufficiently to be radiologically apparent or cause pressure symptoms. In men prolactinomas often present later than in women, with impotence, loss of libido, and symptoms suggesting raised intracranial pressure. Investigation, after endocrine assays, and plain skull films which may be normal, is by high-grade CT brain scanning if necessary aided by intrathecal iohexol. Angiography may be necessary to exclude an aneurysm but air encephalography is hardly ever needed.

The management of such tumours depends on the fact that prolactin secretion is controlled by an inhibitory factor secreted by the hypothalamus (unlike the other hypothalamic 'releasing' factors). The prolactin inhibitory factor is probably dopamine and can also be released in response to thyroid releasing hormone. Excessive prolactin secretion in patients with such tumours can be readily suppressed by giving the ergot derived dopamine agonist drug bromocriptine (Parlodil), and surgery postponed or sometimes avoided. The complication which may arise is that such women then become highly fertile and these tumours often enlarge rapidly during pregnancy, then threatening the visual fields. Therefore it is wise to irradiate the pituitary before pregnancy is made possible by treatment with bromocriptine. The CT scanning techniques can be used to follow the response to medical treatment. If vision is threatened and the suprasellar extension is very large, a transfrontal surgical approach may be needed but surgery is now almost always by the transphenoidal route, using the operating microscope. However, the majority of prolactinomas are now treated medically in the first instance with the prolactin inhibitor bromocriptine by monitoring carefully the symptoms and serum prolactin level. Prolactinomas often decrease in size with bromocriptine so that even so some large tumours can be approached transphenoidally. After surgery it is equally important to repeat the serum prolactin measurement as reproductive difficulties after hypophysectomy are more likely to be due to persisting hyperprolactinaemia than to pituitary deficiency, and are therefore reversible by secondary treatment with bromocriptine.

Craniopharyngioma

The pathology of these tumours has already been described. Since they depend upon abnormalities of development, symptoms usually appear at an early age, i.e. in childhood or adolescence. They may, however, cause no symptoms until middle life.

Endocrine disturbances

They may produce a large variety of disturbances of growth and metabolism. In Cushing's words, 'The patient may show extreme degrees of adiposity or emaciation, of polyuria or the reverse, of dwarfism, of sexual infantilism, or of premature physical senility'.

Pressure symptoms

Symptoms of increased intracranial pressure are usually conspicuous. When the tumour arises in childhood the skull may be enlarged, and the sutures separated. Headache and vomiting may be severe and papilloedema is rather commoner than optic atrophy. The tumour may compress the optic nerves, chiasma, or tracts, leading to corresponding visual field defects. The frontal lobes, temporal lobes, and cerebral peduncles may also be compressed.

Radiographic appearances

These consist of: (i) general signs of increased intracranial pressure, such as convolutional thinning; (ii) erosion of the clinoid processes and flattening of the sella turcica; and (iii) signs of calcification within the tumour which is present in about 75 per cent of cases, and varies from a few faint opaque flecks to a considerable mass lying above the sella turcica.

Empty sella syndrome

Patients are occasionally encountered with no signs of visual failure or endocrine disturbance, but an enlarged sella and thinned dorsum sellae are found on skull X-ray. The patients are usually obese females, sometimes hypertensive and frequently complain of headaches. It has been concluded from post-mortem studies that this condition probably arises as a result of a congenital deficiency of the diaphragma sellae or a previous episode of transient raised intracranial pressure. The normal pulsations of c.s.f. remodel the sella and so causing the 'empty sella' syndrome. High-grade CT scanning will exclude a co-existent adenoma (see Fig. 9.12).

Cerebellum

The cerebellum is a common site of tumour, especially in childhood. Medulloblastomas arise in the region of the roof of the fourth ventricle, usually during the first decade of life. Astrocytomas may also occur in the cerebellum in childhood, and angioblastomas are almost exclusively cerebellar tumours.

When a cerebellar tumour arises in the middle line, the history is usually short. Symptoms of increased intracranial pressure occur early. Symptoms of cerebellar deficiency are usually most marked on standing and walking, and there may be little or no ataxia of the upper limbs. The patient tends to fall backwards, or sometimes forwards. The gait tends to be ataxic, especially on turning. Nystagmus is often absent. Compression of the midbrain may lead to tonic convulsions (p. 90) and the pupils are occasionally dilated and exhibit sluggish reactions. There is, as a rule, little weakness of the limbs, though an extensor plantar response on one or both sides may be found.

A tumour involving mainly the lateral lobe of the cerebellum also usually gives rise to symptoms of increased intracranial pressure early, but a cystic angioblastoma may grow to a large size without causing conspicuous symptoms (see Fig. 9.15). Nystagmus is usually marked and most evident on conjugate lateral ocular deviation to the side of the lesion. It may be horizontal or rotary, the quick phase being directed towards the periphery and the slow phase towards the centre. Other signs of cerebellar deficiency are most marked in, and often confined to, the limbs on the side of the lesion, and consist of hypotonia, swaying of the outstretched upper limb, ataxia of limb movements, and dysdiadochokinesia. The gait is unsteady, the leg on the affected side being ataxic. The patient tends to walk with a wide base and deviate to the affected side, and is liable to fall to the affected side when standing with the feet together and the eyes closed. The head may be flexed to the side of the lesion, and rotated so that the occiput is directed to that shoulder.

Neighbourhood symptoms are usually more conspicuous with lateral cerebellar tumours than when the tumour is in the middle line. Forward pressure by the growth may cause a disturbance of function of any of the cranial nerves from the fifth to the twelfth, the fifth, sixth, and seventh being most frequently affected. Pressure upon the ipsilateral half of the pons and medulla is likely to lead to signs of corticospinal tract defect on the opposite side of the body.

Fourth ventricle

Tumours arising in the fourth ventricle are usually ependymomas, though the ventricle may be invaded by tumours arising in the vermis of the cerebellum or in the pons. In the early stages the symptoms are those of hydrocephalus, and vomiting is often conspicuous. Headache tends to radiate to the neck and even to the shoulders and arms. Sometimes there are disturbances of the visceral functions of the medulla, and invasion of the cerebellar vermis may produce a picture indistinguishable from that of a midline tumour of the cerebellum described above.

Pons and medulla

The commonest tumour of the brainstem is the pontine glioma of childhood. This tumour usually gives rise to localizing signs and symptoms early, and probably for this reason signs of increased intracranial pressure are often slight when a patient first comes under observation. Diplopia is usually the first symptom. At first the signs may point to a lesion limited to one half of the pons, but they soon become bilateral. Weakness of the lateral rectus on one or both sides develops early and may be followed by paresis of conjugate ocular deviation. Crossed paralysis is often seen at an early stage, the precise combination of ipsilateral paralysis of the cranial nerves and crossed hemiplegia depending upon the level of the tumour in the pons or medulla. Nystagmus and some degree of ataxia of the limbs are common, even though the cerebellum is not itself invaded. A medullary tumour may cause hiccup, and disturbances of the cardiac and respiratory rate and rhythm. In the later stages bilateral paralysis of the bulbar muscles and limbs usually develops.

Eighth nerve

Eighth nerve tumours, acoustic neuromas, are usually unilateral. They rarely give rise to symptoms before the third decade of life, and most commonly during the fifth decade. They are tumours of slow growth, and focal symptons commonly exist for years before there is increased intracranial pressure. Owing to the situation of the tumour the first symptoms are those of a disturbance of function of the eighth nerve. Tinnitus is followed by progressive deafness, though sometimes giddiness precedes disturbances of hearing. Not uncommonly a patient when he first comes under observation has been completely deaf in the affected ear for years.

Headache at first is usually occipital and tends to radiate from back to front through the mastoid region. In the late stages it becomes general, and characteristic of a space-occupying lesion in the posterior fossa. Neighbourhood symptoms include paraesthesiae referred to the face, attacks of facial spasm, and double vision.

On examination, hearing is much reduced and may be completely lost, and there is often loss of all response to caloric tests of labyrinthine function on the affected side. Other signs result from pressure by the tumour upon neighbouring cranial nerves. There is usually some facial weakness on the affected side, though this may be slight. Sensory loss may occur in the trigeminal distribution, but reduction or loss of the corneal reflex may be the only sign of involvement of the fifth nerve. Weakness of the lateral rectus may be present. Compression of the ipsilateral cerebellar hemisphere causes symptoms of cerebellar deficiency on the side of the tumour. Crossed hemiparesis and hemianaesthesia may occur as the result of compression of the long descending and ascending tracts in the brainstem. Occasionally the clinical picture is atypical and presents with the signs of brainstem involvement, hydrocephalus, or even dementia.

A valuable X-ray sign is erosion of the petrous portion of the temporal bone or the internal acoustic meatus by the tumour.

Basal meninges

Neoplastic infiltration of the basal meninges leads to a distinctive clinical picture. This condition may be due to metastases from extracranial neoplasms or to extension within the cranial cavity of a primary carcinoma or other growth arising in the nasopharynx. It leads to progressive cranial nerve palsies which are usually bilateral but often asymmetrical. Papilloedema may be present or absent, and there may be symptoms of invasion of the hypothalamus or the brainstem.

THE INVESTIGATION OF A CEREBRAL TUMOUR SUSPECT

When the clinical investigation of a patient suspected of having a cerebral tumour is complete, the question of further investigations arises. The object of these is first to confirm the presence of the tumour when this is not already established on clinical grounds, and secondly to throw light upon its situation and nature.

Examination of the head

Inspection and palpation of the scalp and skull may reveal arterial or venous congestion, or a bony boss, usually indicating a meningioma. A bruit on auscultation is suggestive of an angioma.

Lumbar puncture

A lumbar puncture should not be carried out in a patient suspected of having a cerebral tumour if there are clinical grounds for thinking that the pressure of the cerebrospinal fluid will be high. The risk is greatest with a tumour in the posterior fossa, for then the withdrawal of fluid from the lumbar sac may precipitate herniation of the cerebellar tonsils into the foramen magnum, possibly with fatal results. Similarly, if there is a large tumour of one cerebral hemisphere, lumbar puncture may increase the pressure on the brainstem. The safest general rule is not to lumbar-puncture a patient suspected of having a cerebral tumour who has papilloedema.

In most cases of cerebral tumour the pressure of the cerebrospinal fluid will be high, on the average from 180 to 300 mm of water. Pressures as high or higher, however, are encountered in the benign forms of hydrocephalus.

The protein of the fluid may be normal, but is often somewhat raised. The highest protein levels are met with in cases of eighth nerve tumour and tumour of the corpus callosum, when the level may reach 2.0 or 3.0 g/l.

The cell content of the fluid is usually normal. Sometimes there is a small excess of mononuclear cells. The presence of more than a few of these should suggest the possibility of an inflammatory lesion, such as abscess, tuberculoma, or parasitic cyst. Tumour cells may be present.

Electroencephalography

The chief value of electroencephalography is to localize an area of abnormal brain tissue, especially an area of delta waves (Fig. 9.7). Sometimes it is possible to go further and say that the abnormality found is likely to be due to tumour or, on the other hand, to cerebral vascular disease. The EEG may also localize a discharging area associated with epileptic attacks. A diffuse EEG abnormality may be produced by a tumour of the midbrain or in the posterior fossa. The EEG is negative in 20 per cent of patients with epilepsy due to cerebral tumour.

Plain X-rays

Plain X-rays of the skull may be of value in several ways. If the pineal is calcified, as it is in 60 per cent of adults, it may be displaced to the opposite side by a tumour of one cerebral hemisphere. Changes in the bones of the skull may

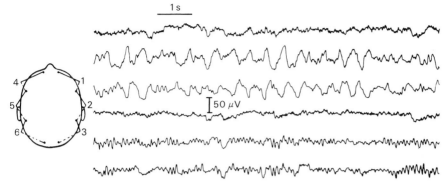

Fig. 9.7. Female, aged 13. Right posterior temporal glioma (grade 1). Reduced alpha activity on the right side and focal slow activity, mainly at delta frequency and occasionally at theta frequency (4–7 Hz) in the right posterior temporal area.

be diffuse – convolutional thinning owing to increased intracranial pressure – or localized due to erosion by a meningioma, often with reactive new bone formation, or by a metastatic tumour. The petrous portion of the temporal bone may be eroded by an eighth nerve tumour which may cause unilateral enlargement of the internal acoustic meatus.

Hypophysial tumours cause a uniform expansion of the sella turcica, with thinning of its walls. The ballooned sella projects downwards and forwards into the sphenoidal sinuses and the upward pressure of the growth may erode the clinoid processes. Finally, calcification may occur in a tumour, and is most often seen in a craniopharyngioma lying above the sella turcica, or in a glioma of one hemisphere (Figs. 9.4 and 9.5).

Computerized tomography (Figs. 9.8–16)

Computerized tomography has largely superseded other special investigations for cerebral tumour and will show up to 95 per cent of all cerebral tumours. On computerized tomography (see Fig. 9.5) meningiomas show up as homogeneous high-density lesions which enhance uniformly and markedly with Conray, showing their actual size (Fig. 9.5). Gliomas (Fig. 9.8) show several different patterns. Low density is a feature of rapidly growing tumours or surrounding oedema. Enhancement with Conray will then outline the boundary between the tumour and oedema, although associated calcification is not of course enhanced. Metastases, sometimes multiple (Fig. 9.9), often show themselves by greater surrounding oedema than is present with gliomas.

Posterior fossa lesions may be identified as extra-axial, that is outside the brain, if the brain is displaced inwards away from the inner tablet with a widening of the subarachnoid systerns and sometimes bone erosion. Acoustic neuromas are usually lucent to isodense, enhance greatly with Conray, are centred on the internal auditory canal and are not calcified. NMR scanning may be necessary, especially for brainstem or posterior fossa lesions (Fig. 9.17).

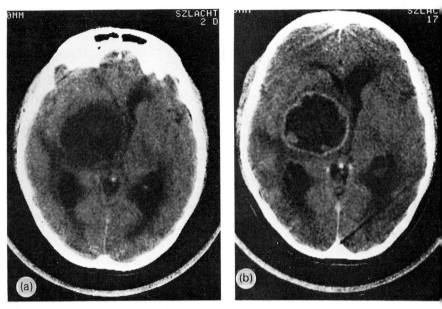

Fig. 9.8. CT scan, cystic glioma, left hemisphere, with distorted and enlarged ventricles unenhanced (a), and contrast-enhanced (b).

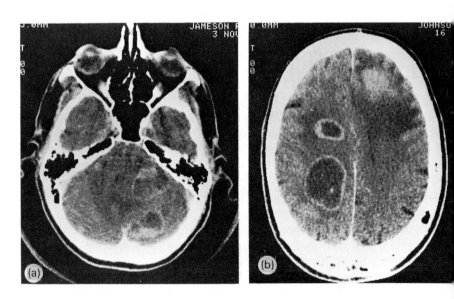

Fig. 9.9. (a) CT scan, cerebral metastases in posterior fossa, contrast-enhanced; (b) CT scan, cerebral metastases, cystic in left hemisphere, solid in right hemisphere, with oedema, contrast-enhanced.

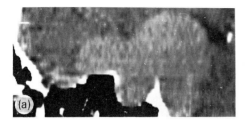

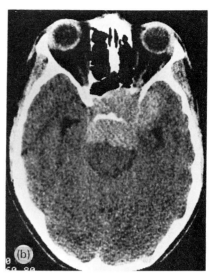

Fig. 9.10. CT scan, large pituitary tumour, chromophobe adenoma, with (a) sagittal reconstruction, left anterior; (b) suprasellar extension.

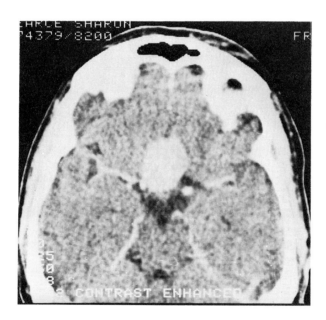

Fig. 9.11. CT scan, meningioma, anterior pituitary region, contrast-enhanced.

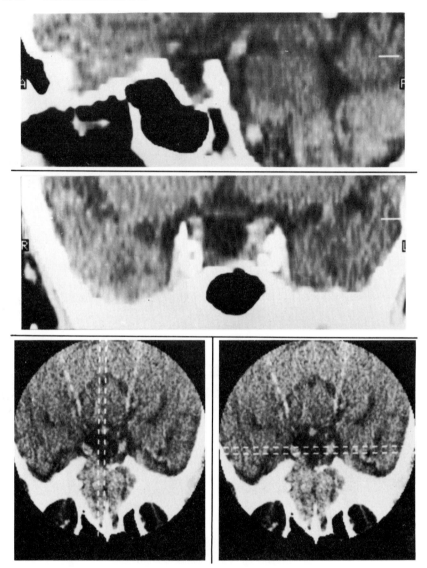

Fig. 9.12. CT scan, empty sella, sagittal reconstruction (above) coronal reconstruction (below); bottom, dotted lines show planes of reconstruction.

Nuclear magnetic resonance imaging

This is proving to have distinct advantages over CT scanning, as discussed previously (see p. 158). A selection of NMR scans compared with the CT scans is shown in Figs. 9.17–20.

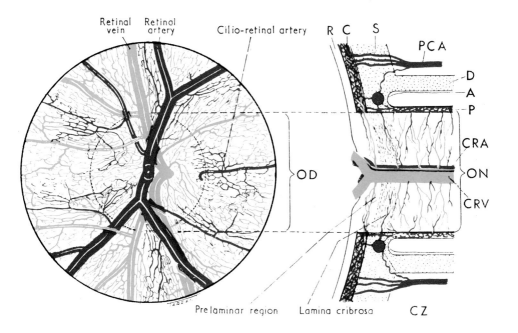

Plate 1 Diagrammatic representation of blood supply of optic nerve head

A	Arachnoid	OD	Optic disc
C	Choroid	ON	Optic nerve
CRA	Central retinal artery	P	Pia
CRV	Central retinal vein	PCA	Posterior ciliary arteries
CZ	Circle of Zinn and Haller	R	Retina
D	Dura	S	Sclera

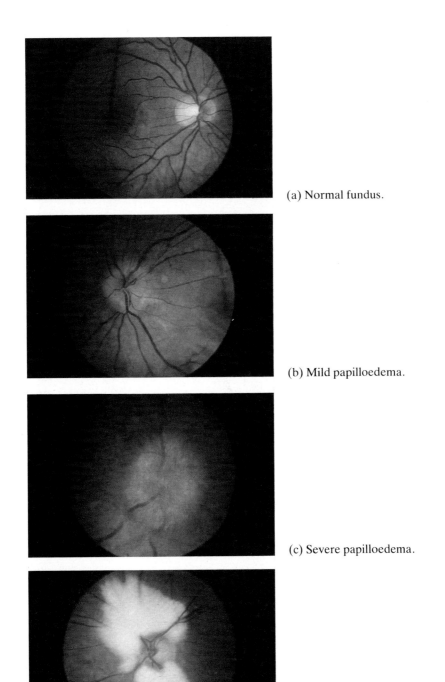

(a) Normal fundus.

(b) Mild papilloedema.

(c) Severe papilloedema.

(d) Medullated nerve fibres.

Plate 2

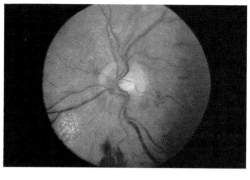

(a) Hypertensive retinopathy with swollen disc, haemorrhages, and exudates.

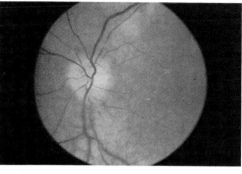

(b) Ischaemic optic neuritis showing pale swollen disc, narrow arteries, and exudates.

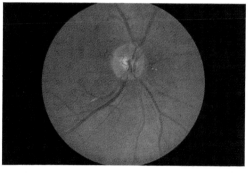

(c) Refractile cholesterol-containing embolus in artery.

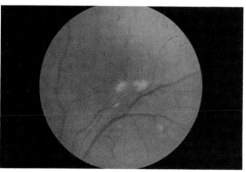

(d) Embolus with retinal ischaemia.

Plate 3

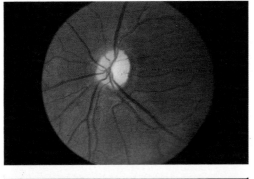

(a) Primary optic atrophy.

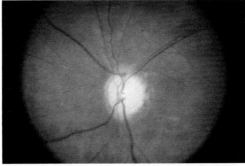

(b) Consecutive optic atrophy.

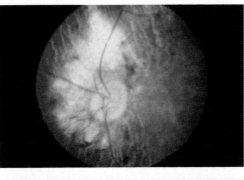

(c) Retinitis pigmentosa.

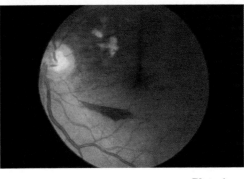

(d) 'Boat-shaped' subhyaloid haemorrhage after sub-arachnoid haemorrhage.

Plate 4

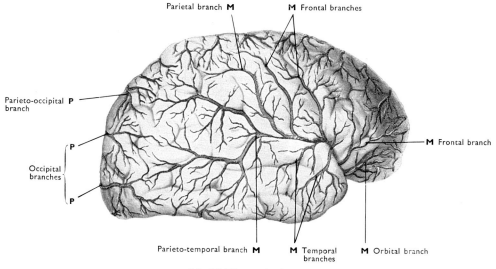

Distribution of cerebral arteries on the supero-lateral surface of the right cerebral hemisphere.

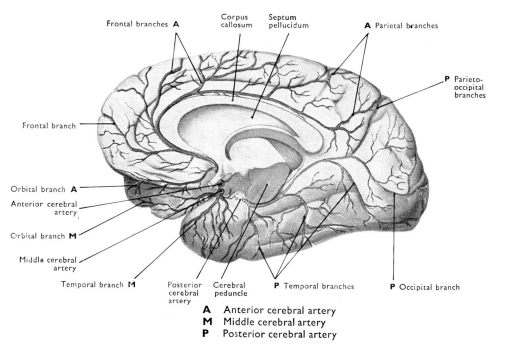

Distribution of cerebral arteries on the medial and tentorial surfaces of the right cerebral hemisphere.

Plate 5

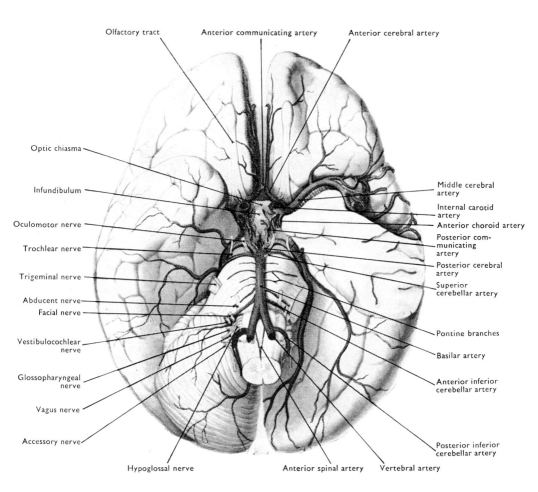

Olfactory tract

Anterior communicating artery

Anterior cerebral artery

Optic chiasma

Infundibulum

Oculomotor nerve

Trochlear nerve

Trigeminal nerve

Abducent nerve

Facial nerve

Vestibulocochlear nerve

Glossopharyngeal nerve

Vagus nerve

Accessory nerve

Middle cerebral artery

Internal carotid artery

Anterior choroid artery

Posterior communicating artery

Posterior cerebral artery

Superior cerebellar artery

Pontine branches

Basilar artery

Anterior inferior cerebellar artery

Posterior inferior cerebellar artery

Hypoglossal nerve

Anterior spinal artery

Vertebral artery

Plate 6 Arteries of the base of the brain.

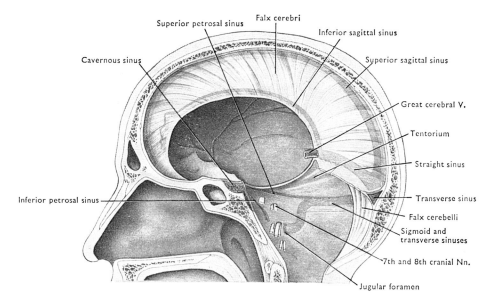

(a) Sagittal section through the skull to show the falx cerebri and cerebral sinuses.

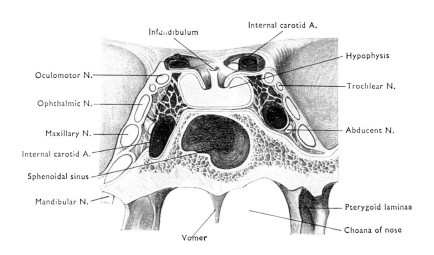

(b) Coronal section through the cavernous sinus.

Plate 7

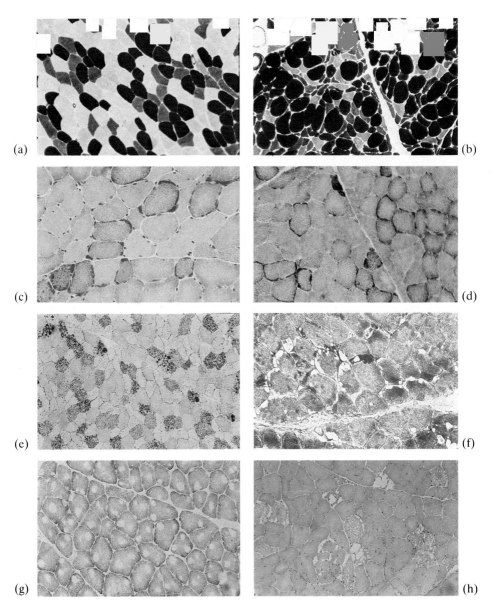

Plate 8 (a) Normal muscle to show the three histochemical fibre types. Type 1 fibres dark; type 2a fibres light and type 2b fibres intermediate. ATPase reaction at pH 4.6. (b) Atrophy of the 2a and 2b fibres in steroid myopathy. ATPase reaction at pH 4.6. (c) Mitochondrial myopathy to show typical ragged red fibres. Gomori trichrome stain. (d) Mitochondrial myopathy to show increased succinic dehydrogenase activity. (e) Lipid storage myopathy due to carnitine deficiency. Oil red O stain. (f) McArdle's syndrome to show multiple peripheral vacuoles, some of which are filled with PAS positive material. (g) Central core disease. NADH tetrazolium reductase reaction. (h) Vacuolar myopathy due to acid maltase deficiency. Gomori trichrome stain.

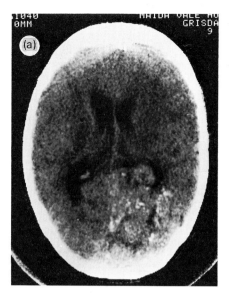 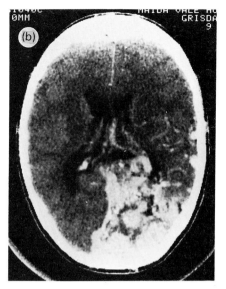

Fig. 9.13. CT scan, angioma with calcification, right parieto-occipital region, (a) unenhanced, (b) contrast-enhanced.

Angiography

Carotid angiography may be indicated after CT scanning when the patient has a large tumour involving one cerebral hemisphere. The angiogram then is likely to show displacement of the anterior cerebral artery on the same side across the middle line, with a convexity towards the opposite side (Fig. 9.21). The middle cerebral artery may also be displaced in accordance with the position of the tumour, and a vascular flush may show the position of the tumour itself (see Fig. 9.14). Carotid angiography is valuable in the diagnosis and localization of vascular abnormalities, especially angiomas of one cerebral hemisphere where some uncertainty remains as to the nature of the tumour or the source of its blood supply. Vertebral angiography is useful to demonstrate vascular abnormalities in the posterior fossa and in doubtful cases of posterior fossa tumour it may be helpful by showing displacement of the vertebrobasilar system.

DIAGNOSIS

The conditions most likely to be confused with cerebral tumour are: (i) other disorders giving rise to increased intracranial pressure; and (ii) disorders producing progressive or recurrent symptoms of a kind commonly produced by a cerebral tumour.

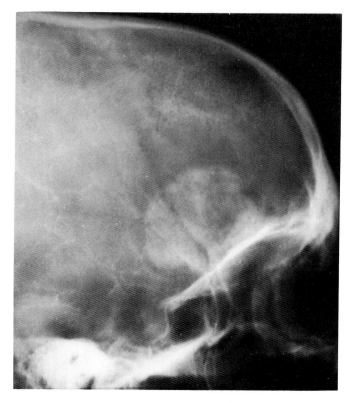

Fig. 9.14. CT scan, meningioma showing typical 'blush' or smear in venous phase. The tumour is growing from the floor of the anterior fossa.

Other conditions causing increased intracranial pressure

Intracranial abscess

In most cases intracranial abscess is readily distinguished from tumour, since its development is usually acute or subacute, and a primary focus of infection is almost always to be found either in the neighbourhood of the brain or elsewhere. Rarely, however, a chronic abscess may arise, its source of infection being latent or having disappeared. In such cases the diagnosis from tumour may be impossible, and the nature of the lesion is unsuspected until operation. Points in favour of abscess are a sudden or apoplectiform onset and a considerably raised protein in the cerebrospinal fluid, accompanied by a pleocytosis, usually lymphocytic, rarely polymorphonuclear.

Hydrocephalus

The benign forms of hydrocephalus may simulate cerebral tumour by causing papilloedema together with signs, usually slight, of involvement of the nervous

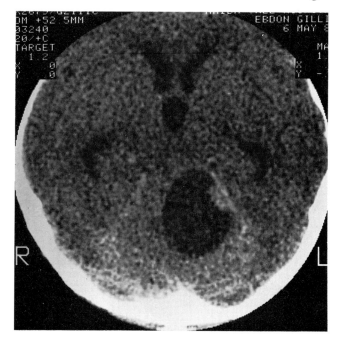

Fig. 9.15. CT scan, cerebellar haemangioblastoma with opacification of nodule in wall.

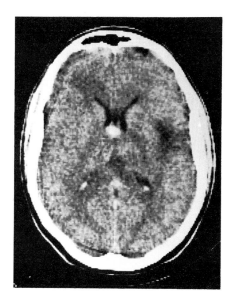

Fig. 9.16. CT scan, colloid cyst of third ventricle. Unenhanced scan shows high-density fluid.

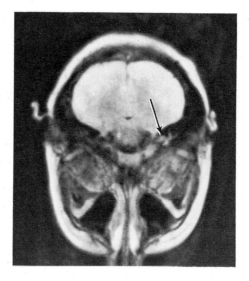

Fig. 9.17. Intracanalicular acoustic neuroma: NMR(SE) scan. The tumour appears as an expansion of the acoustic nerve (arrow).

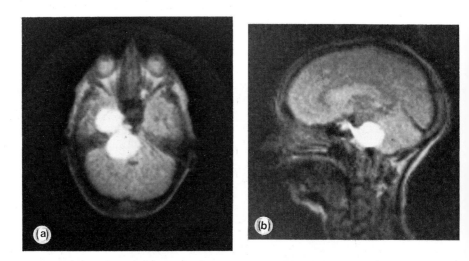

Fig. 9.18. Chrondroma: (a) Transverse NMR(SE) and (b) sagittal NMR(SE) scans. The tumour is calcified on the CT scan but its extent is better shown on the SE scans.

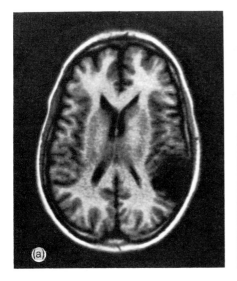
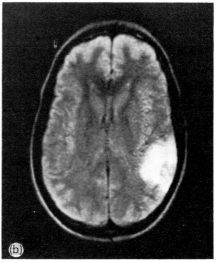

Fig. 9.19. Astrocytoma: (a) NMR(IR) (b) NMR(SE) scans. Although the tumour is well seen differentation between tumour and peritumoural oedema may be difficult.

system. In such cases, though papilloedema may be severe, headache is usually slight and sometimes absent. In doubtful cases ventriculography may be necessary to exclude a space-occupying lesion, and in most such cases the ventricles are not enlarged. The Arnold–Chiari malformation (see p. 374) may behave like a tumour in the region of the foramen magnum.

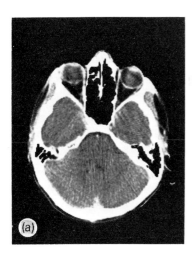
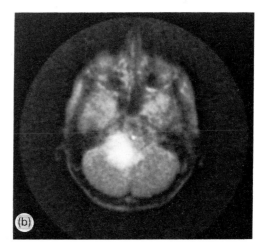

Fig. 9.20. Pontine glioma: (a) CT and (b) NMR(SE) scans. The abnormality is better seen on the NMR scans.

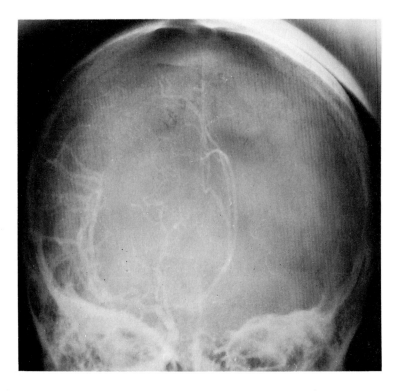

Fig. 9.21. Carotid angiogram showing deviation of anterior cerebral vessels across midline due to tumour.

Subdural haematoma

Subdural haematoma is a space-occupying lesion chiefly found in the middle-aged or elderly. Headache is a prominent symptom, and in the later stages it is associated with intermittent drowsiness. Papilloedema may be absent, and focal signs are generally slight; the pressure of the cerebrospinal fluid may not be raised, but the protein content often is.

Hypertension

Hypertension may give rise to difficulty by causing papilloedema and headaches accompanied by signs of a focal lesion of the nervous system. Hypertensive retinopathy differs in appearance from the retinal changes associated with increased intracranial pressure in that the degree of papill-oedema is usually slight compared with the severity and diffuseness of the exudative changes. Electroencephalography may be helpful by demonstrating diffuse cerebral abnormalities, but CT scanning is more useful and may show direct evidence of previous infarction.

Optic neuritis

Though this is not a symptom of increased intracranial pressure it may be conveniently considered here because it may cause papilloedema with impairment of vision. It is distinguished, however, by the acute onset, and by the fact that the visual loss is disproportionately great compared with the papilloedema. Moreover the field defect is central, whereas in papilloedema due to increased intracranial pressure it is peripheral at first.

Disorders causing progressive or recurrent symptoms

Cerebral atheroma

Progressive ischaemia of the brain due to cerebral atheroma may cause symptoms which are both focal and progressive. In general, headache is not a prominent symptom of such lesions and papilloedema is absent. After a CT scan carotid angiography may be necessary in order to decide between an ischaemic and a space-occupying lesion. Exceptionally, difficulty may arise after thrombosis of one internal carotid artery because the oedematous cerebral hemisphere resulting from a large area of infarction may behave as a space-occupying lesion and cause papilloedema. Here again angiography may be necessary to settle the diagnosis.

Epilepsy

Since epileptiform convulsions are a common symptom of cerebral tumour, the differential diagnosis of tumour from other causes of epilepsy frequently arises. Convulsions beginning after the age of 25 should always suggest the possibility of tumour, though in late middle life and old age cerebral arteriosclerosis is the commonest cause. In doubtful cases the ancillary methods of investigation may be called for to decide whether the epilepsy is a symptom of tumour.

Migraine

Headache, vomiting, visual hallucinations, and visual field defects are common both to migraine and tumours in the neighbourhood of the visual cortex, especially angioma. Migraine usually begins at puberty, and there is often a family history of the disorder. The symptoms of migraine are transitory, and visual field defects or paraesthesiae may occur on either side of the body. Signs of increased intracranial pressure are absent.

PROGNOSIS

The prognosis of intracranial tumour is influenced by the nature of the growth, and its accessibility to the surgeon. In the absence of surgical interference almost all intracranial tumours increase in size, their rate of growth depending upon their nature. The resulting increase in intracranial pressure and destruction of brain tissue ultimately prove fatal. When papilloedema is severe, death may be preceded by blindness. The more malignant gliomas, such as the medulloblastomas and the glioblastomas, grow rapidly and usually prove fatal within a year or so. The slowly growing astrocytomas and meningiomas may cause symptoms for many years before leading to a marked increase in intracranial pressure.

In the best hands, the immediate mortality of operations for the removal of intracranial tumour is under 10 per cent. Extracerebral tumours can frequently be removed without damage to the underlying brain, though the adjacent structures may be damaged, as for example the seventh nerve in removal of an acoustic neuroma. Removal of an intracerebral tumour, on the other hand, necessitates considerable cerebral trauma, with the risk of residual symptoms. The more malignant the tumour, the greater the likelihood of its recurrence after its attempted removal. Even meningiomas may recur. The prognosis is naturally bad in a case of metastatic tumours, which are frequently multiple.

TREATMENT

The treatment of election of a cerebral tumour is its surgical removal, but this is not always practicable. Where a tumour is surgically inaccessible, the operation of decompression, by abolishing the rigidity of the skull, lowers the intracranial pressure and relieves headache and papilloedema. Obstruction of the cerebral aqueduct (of Sylvius) may be relieved by by-passing it with a tube from the lateral ventricle into the cerebellomedullary cistern (Torkildsen's operation) or the peritoneal cavity.

The scope of radiotherapy in the treatment of intracranial tumour is as yet undefined. X-ray irradiation may retard the growth of a hypophysial adenoma and of some gliomas, especially medulloblastoma of the cerebellum. It often causes temporary regression in glioblastoma and also in microgliomas which are beta-lymphocyte tumours associated with immunosuppression.

Chemotherapy of cerebral tumours

The average survival for highly malignant tumours of three months after resection is often doubled by postoperative radiotherapy and is further increased if nitrosoureas such as carmustine are given in combination with vincristine.

Steroids are very effective in lowering intracranial pressure, either as a life-saving procedure or in order to reduce the risks of investigation by means of angiography. The potent glucocorticoid dexamethasone (Decadron) may be given in a dose of 10 mg intravenously and then 4 mg intramuscularly six hourly until the maximal response, usually after three to four days, is achieved. The dose may then be reduced. Dehydration is also of value for the temporary reduction of increased intracranial pressure. A simple and usually a completely effective method of lowering the intracranial pressure is to give glycerin, 15 ml three times a day by mouth (see p. 19).

REFERENCES

Franks, S., Nabarro, J.D.N., and Jacobs, H.S. (1977). Prevalence and presentation of hyperprolactinaemia in patients with 'functionless' pituitary tumours. *Lancet* **i**, 778–80.

Jordan, R.M., Kendall, J.W., and Kerber, C.W. (1977). The primary empty sella syndrome. *Am. J. Med.* **62**, 569–80.

Prescott, R.W.G., Kendall-Taylor, P., and Hall, K. (1982). Hyperprolactinaemia in men – response to bromocriptine therapy. *Lancet* **i**, 245–8.

Thomas, J.P. (1983). Treatment of acromegaly. *Br. med. J.* **286**, 330–2.

Wass, J.A., Williams, J., and Charlesworth, M. (1982). Bromocriptine in the management of large pituitary tumours. *Br. med. J.* **284**, 1980–11.

Wong, M.L. and Brackmann, D.E. (1981). Computed cranial tomography in acoustic tumour diagnosis. *J. Am. med. Ass.* **245**, 2497–500.

10 Higher cerebral function and dementia

The principal difference between the human and the subhuman brain consists in the greater development of the cerebral cortex in man. The function of the cerebral cortex, as Head pointed out in relation to sensation, is primarily discriminative, and through his cerebral cortex man has enormously enlarged the scope of his comprehension of the world and his power to act upon it. There is far less difference between man and the lower animals in respect of the thalamus and hypothalamus – which are intimately concerned with the emotional and instinctive life – and the regulation of metabolic and endocrine function. The cerebral cortex and these basal structures therefore interact with one another, and the inhibitory functions of the cortex are among its most important.

Emotion

The fact that epileptic attacks originating in the temporal lobe may lead to emotional experiences is clinical evidence that the temporal lobe is part of the anatomical basis of emotion. Papez suggests that this depends on a pathway originating in the hippocampus and thence transferred to the mammillary body, from which it reaches the anterior thalamic nucleus and irradiates to the cortex of the cingulate gyrus.

Memory

From a study of focal lesions it has been deduced that the initial retention of information is a hippocampal function and a lesion of this region can cause a pure amnesic syndrome, whereas a retrieval-scanning defect occurs with bilateral subcortical and frontal lesions, including those of the mammillary bodies. There is a defect of 'indexation' with a prefrontal lesion. It has been observed that confabulation may occur with anterior mammillary lesions without an associated memory defect.

The biochemical basis of memory

The limbic system, which has a well-established relationship with memory storage, has a major cholinergic input. The cholinergic antagonist scopolomine has been given subcutaneously and reported to reduce the capacity of human subjects to store new information and also reduces the retrieval from the store of old memories. It lowers the performance IQ but does not affect verbal IQ. Tests with cholinergic agonists such as physostigmine which cross the blood–brain barrier and arecholine, a cholinergic muscarine agonist and a choline precursor of acetylcholine, have not yet shown statistical improvement in normal subjects but this suggests that the system may already be functioning at an optimal level. Physostigmine and choline have been used in trials of treatment of Alzheimer's disease without apparent benefit.

There is also clinical evidence that the temporal lobe plays an important part in memory, for the power to retain the memory of recent events may be severely impaired by the removal of the medial aspect of even one temporal lobe, and still more by bilateral damage to the hippocampal region.

Korsakoff's psychosis is a syndrome characterized by gross defect of memory for recent events, often associated with disorientation in space and time. The patient fills the gaps in his memory by confabulating, that is by giving imaginary accounts of his activities. Korsakoff's pyschosis is most frequently due to chronic alcoholism, but may also occur in other toxic and degenerative cerebral conditions. The essential lesion is said to lie in the medial thalamus and hippocampus.

The role of the frontal lobe

Studies of frontal lobe function, which have sprung particularly from investigations of the operation of prefrontal leucotomy or lobotomy, suggest that the frontal lobe is not concerned with the intellectual functions of analysis, synthesis, and selectivity, but rather with the adjustment of the personality as a whole to future contingencies in the light of past experience. The prefrontal regions in man are therefore concerned with foresight, imagination, and the apperception of the self, and these psychological functions are invested with emotion by way of the association fibres which link the hippocampus and cingulate gyrus with the prefrontal region on the one hand and with the thalamus and hypothalamus on the other.

DEMENTIA

Dementia is the term applied to a diffuse deterioration in the mental functions manifesting itself primarily in thought and memory and secondarily in feeling and conduct. It may be produced by a large number of pathological agencies, and the clinical picture varies somewhat according to the previous temperament of the patient, the age of onset, localization, rate of progress, and nature of the causal disorder.

In the United Kingdom by 1985 there will be three million people over the age of 75, nearly 20 per cent of them with dementia, and approximately 10 per cent of people over the age of 65 have dementia. In most surveys of dementia about 10 per cent of patients have proved to have treatable or reversible causes of dementia. Some 70 per cent of patients with dementia have Alzheimer's disease. The terms presenile or senile are used according to whether the patient is above or below the age of 65 but do not have any particular pathological significance.

Symptoms

The earliest disability is an impairment of the highest intellectual functions of judgement and reasoning, manifesting itself in a failure to grasp the meaning of a complex situation. At this stage a man's business judgement begins to fail, though in the semi-automatic activities of life no defect may be noticed. Memory becomes impaired, especially for recent events, and this may later lead to disorientation in space and time. In some patients the emotional life is little disturbed, but in others impairment of higher control leads to emotional instability which finds expression in irritability and impulsive conduct, which may be out of keeping with the patient's previous standards. Delusions are not an integral part of the clinical picture of dementia, but are sometimes present as a result of the impairment of judgement and defective appreciation of reality. In the later stages of dementia the patient becomes careless in dress and in personal cleanliness, and finally incontinent. Speech undergoes a progressive disintegration and becomes increasingly meaningless and jargon-like. There is usually a general physical deterioration with loss of weight.

Investigation

The commonest potentially overlooked causes of possible treatable dementia are hypothyroidism, normal pressure hydrocephalus, anaemia, metabolic and deficiency diseases, occasionally a removable cerebral tumour such as a meningioma and infections such as neurosyphilis. The critical investigation in the diagnosis of dementia is the CT brain scan which usually, but not always, shows ventricular dilation and sulcal atrophy in cases of Alzheimer's disease. A normal CT brain scan in dementia should lead to a more intensive search for a cause other than atrophy or vascular disease. Full investigation would include haemoglobin level, white count, sedimentation rate, blood urea, serum glutamic transaminase, serum calcium, phosphorus, serum electrolytes, serum creatinine kinase, serum B_{12} and folic acid, VDRL test for syphilis, electrophoresis and immunophoresis of the plasma proteins, a tri-idothyronine and thyroxine level, and chest and skull X-rays.

Aetiology

There are as many causes of dementia as there are causes of diffuse cerebral damage. In clinical neurology dementia presents either as the irremediable sequel of past disease, such as head injury, meningitis, and encephalitis, or occasionally in association with epilepsy; or as a diagnostic problem, usually in a middle-aged patient.

Some patients with dementia due to Alzheimer's disease have a normal brain scan. Conversely some patients with atrophy on the CT scan are not obviously demented. Conray enhancement is indicated where a focal lesion is seen on the plain CT scan. Up to 30 per cent of patients with cerebral tumours may present with no symptoms other than dementia, though the majority of cerebral tumours are gliomas and therefore, effectively, are untreatable, except by palliative treatment. The clinical picture of dementia is a relatively poor guide to the eventual pathology. Cerebrovascular disease and Alzheimer's disease are so common that the two conditions may co-exist co-incidentally, without presupposing any causal relationship between them.

Some commoner causes of dementia

Alzheimer's disease
Cerebrovascular disease and multi-infarct dementia (see p. 263)
Parkinson's disease (see p. 339)
Metabolic and deficiency diseases including alcoholism and hypothyroidism (see p. 493)
Cerebral tumours (see p. 223)
Normal pressure hydrocephalus (see p. 269)

Some rare causes of dementia

Neurosyphilis (see p. 479)
Huntington's chorea (see p. 349)
Creutzfeldt–Jakob disease (see p. 455)
Wilson's disease (see p. 346)

ALZHEIMER'S DISEASE

Senile dementia of the Alzheimer type is occasionally inherited as a simple dominant mechanism or a dominant with increased penetrance. Usually there is no family history.

Clinical features

The downward course is usually more steadily progressive and sometimes more rapid than in atherosclerotic dementia. Early memory loss is rather characteristic. A profound disintegration of personality develops, with complete disorientation, deterioration in speech, and often restlessness. The critical investigation is the CT brain scan which shows both ventricular dilation and sulcal atrophy (Fig. 10.1). Similar changes are seen on air encephalography (Fig. 10.2).

Pathology

The neuropathological changes in Alzheimer's disease include neurofibrillary tangles of paired helical filaments within the perkayon which are argyrophilic and react similarly to amyloid. These are present throughout the cerebral cortex

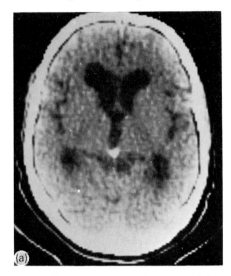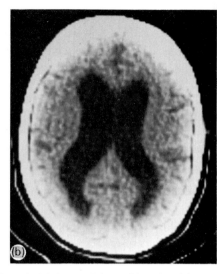

Fig. 10.1. CT scans showing dilated lateral and third ventricles, widened sylvian fissures and cortical sulci.

but particularly in the temporal neocortex, the hippocampus, and the amygdala (Fig. 10.3). The senile plaque is a mass of extracellular amyloid in the cortical neuropil, surrounded by a halo of enlarged abnormal neurites which seems to be predominantly presynaptic terminals. Both these abnormalities are seen occasionally in intellectually normal old people but are then almost confined to the hypothalamus. Astrocytes and microglia are present in Alzheimer's disease at the periphery of the plaques.

Neurochemistry of Alzheimer's disease

There is a marked diminution of choline acetyl-transferase (ChAT), the biosynthetic enzyme for acetylcholine. This loss is selective for certain regions which correspond to those in which senile plaques and neurofibrillary tangles are found, mainly the temporal neocortex, hippocampus, and amygdala. The loss of ChAT is from the nerve terminals of an ascending projection system from the septal nuclei and nucleus basalis where there is actual cell loss, and not from intrinsic cholinergic neurones in the cortex. In addition there is in some cases a defect in noradrenergic terminals arising from degenerate pigmented noradrenergic cells in the locus coeruleus in the dorsal region of the brainstem. There are also reports of loss of serotonin (5HT) in the hippocampus.

From animal experiments it has been shown that the ascending cholinergic system has a specific role in cognitive function. There is a strong suspicion that the loss of cholinergic innervation in the cortex may lead to the evolution of senile plaques but this has not been proven. Noradrenaline may also be involved in cortical arousal and cognitive function. Acetylcholine and

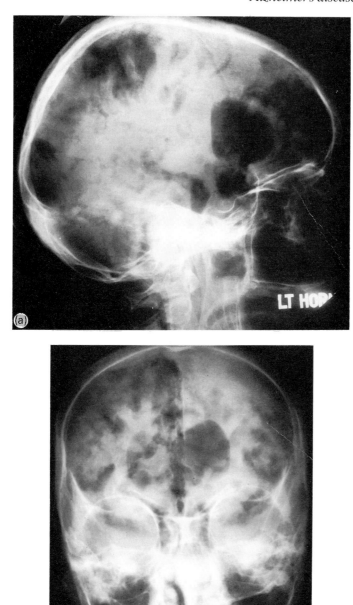

Fig. 10.2. Air encephalograms of Alzheimer's disease: (a) lateral; (b) antero-posterior, showing marked ventricular and cortical sulcal dilation.

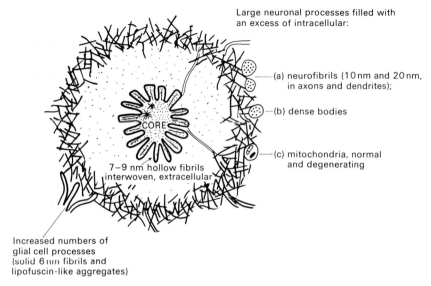

Large neuronal processes filled with
an excess of intracellular:

(a) neurofibrils (10 nm and 20 nm,
in axons and dendrites);

(b) dense bodies

(c) mitochondria, normal
and degenerating

CORE

7–9 nm hollow fibrils
interwoven, extracellular

Increased numbers of
glial cell processes
(solid 6 nm fibrils and
lipofuscin-like aggregates)

Fig. 10.3. Schematic representation of a senile plaque. The rim of the plaque is made up of large neuronal processes filled with an excess of intracellular neurofibrils, dense bodies and mitochondria. The rim also contains increased numbers of glial cell processes containing fibrils and lipofuscin aggregates. In contrast, the central core lies extracellularly. It is composed of hollow fibrils which are interwoven like those of conventional amyloid.

noradrenaline are transmitters with a diffuse modulatory role rather than a point-to-point role in transmission. This fact makes it hopeful that eventually some way may be found of finding effective direct agonists resembling arecoline rather than the precursors of acetylcholine (choline and lecithin) which, although they enter the brain, rely on the presence of a residual population of cholinergic neurones. Attempts to restore catecholaminergic and dopaminergic defects by means of levodopa have so far not improved these patients.

There are a number of other progressive degenerative disorders in which dementia may also occur. In Parkinson's disease, Huntington's chorea, and progressive supranuclear palsy there are prominent changes in the basal ganglia and these can be described as the group of subcortical dementias. Some patients with Parkinson's disease and dementia have cortical ChAT defects which may contribute the dementia. Loss of GABA and dopamine in the basal ganglia may also play a part in the cognitive impairment. Moreover the noradrenergic projection from the locus coeruleus is affected and so this provides a further clue to some degree of overlap between Alzheimer's disease and Parkinson's disease.

PICK'S DISEASE

This can be regarded as a rare variety of dementia, clinically indistinguishable from Alzheimer's disease. The diagnosis can only be made pathologically at post mortem from the predominant atrophy of the frontal and temporal lobes, in which there are a argyrophilic inclusion bodies (Pick bodies) in addition to the neuronal loss and gliosis

MULTI-INFARCT DEMENTIA (see also p. 293)

This is frequently shown by the CT scan revealing multiple bilateral infarcts in patients in whom formerly investigation by EEG or angiography would have been negative. Patients are frequently hypertensive and may have evidence of extracranial cerebrovascular disease rather than cerebral atherosclerosis which implies disease of small intracerebral vessels. Small infarcts may be lacunar or in the 'water-shed' areas between the territory of major cerebral arteries.

BINSWANGER'S DISEASE (progressive subcortical encephalopathy)

This occurs in hypertensives and is a rare disease in which the vascular damage causes white matter loss of myelin and patchy gliosis. CT and NMR scans show a characteristic diffuse subcortical loss of attenuation (Fig. 10.4). The treatment is control of the blood pressure.

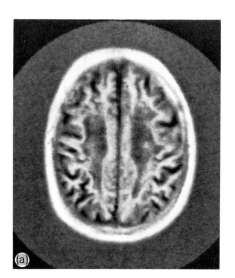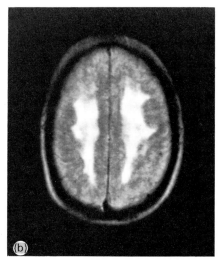

Fig. 10.4. Binswanger's disease (progressive subcortical encephalopathy): (a) NMR(IR) and (b) NMR(SE) scans. Confluent abnormal areas are seen within the centrum semi-ovale.

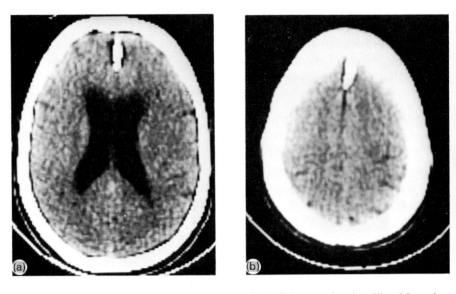

Fig. 10.5. Communicating hydrocephalus: (a) and (b) CT scans showing dilated lateral ventricles and normal cortical sulci.

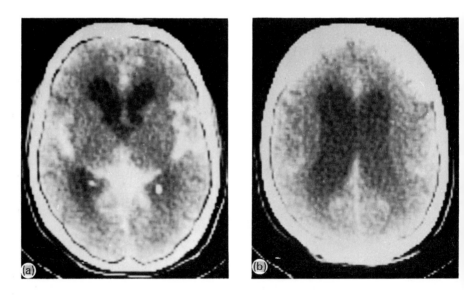

Fig. 10.6. CT scan with metrizamide in Alzheimer's disease showing ventricular dilation with metrizamide filling of the fourth ventricle (a) but not the lateral ventricles (b).

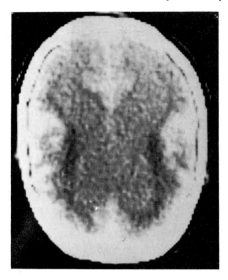

Fig. 10.7. CT scan with metrizamide of normal pressure hydrocephalus showing ventricular filling with metrizamide and low-attenuation areas around the ventricle suggesting absorption of cerebral spinal fluid without metrizamide.

METABOLIC AND DEFICIENCY DISEASES

Chronic alcoholism as a cause of dementia does not usually give rise to difficulty in diagnosis. The CT brain scan often shows cerebral atrophy. Cerebral deterioration is occasionally the presenting symptom in B_{12} neuropathy (see p. 496.

INTRACRANIAL TUMOUR

This gives rise to no difficulty when signs of intracranial pressure are present. Occasionally, however, these are absent, for example when a slowly growing meningioma or glioma produces dementia, usually subfrontal in site and involving the corpus callosum. There may be abnormalities on the skull X-rays and a CT brain scan will usually establish the diagnosis.

NORMAL PRESSURE HYDROCEPHALUS (see also p. 269)

The CT scan often shows periventricular translucencies due to oedema of white matter which are a useful sign indicating a likely successful outcome of ventricular shunting (Figs. 10.5–7). CT scanning with iohexol has now largely replaced isotope encephalography by the lumbar root in the investigation of normal pressure hydrocephalus. Normal pressure hydrocephalus must be distinguished from degenerative cerebral atrophy in that it responds to ventriculo-atrial or ventri-culo-peritoneal shunting whereas degenerative cerebral atrophy at present has no treatment (p. 257).

REFERENCES

Bradshaw, J.R., Thomson, J.L.G., and Campbell, M.J. (1983). Computed tomo-graphy in the investigation of dementia. *Br. med. J.* **286,** 277–80.

Bowen, D.M., Smith, C.B., and Davison, A.N. (1973). Molecular changes in senile dementia. *Brain* **96,** 849–56.

Cragg, B.G. (1973). The density of synapses and neurones in normal, mentally defective and ageing human brains. *Brain* **98,** 81–90.

Pearce, J. and Miller, E. (1973). *Clinical aspects of dementia.* Baillière Tindall, London.

Rossor, M.N. (1982). Neurotransmitters and CNS disease. Dementia. *Lancet* **ii,** 1200–4.

Rossor, M.N., Garrett, N.J., Johnson, A.L., Mountjoy, C.Q., Roth, M., and Iversen, L.L. (1982). A post-mortem study of the cholinergic and GABA systems in senile dementia. *Brain* **105,** 313–30.

Smith, J.S. and Kiloh, L.G. (1981). The investigation of dementia: results in 200 consecutive admissions. *Lancet* **i,** 824–7.

Wells, C.E. (ed.) (1977). *Dementia,* 2nd edn. Davis, Philadelphia.

11 Hydrocephalus

Aetiology and pathology

The term hydrocephalus means an excess of cerebrospinal fluid. This necessarily occurs in all conditions in which there is a diffuse atrophy of the brain, as in cerebral arteriosclerosis, general paresis, and the presenile dementias. The hydrocephalus is then compensatory and is of no clinical significance. Hydrocephalus produces symptoms when the cerebrospinal fluid is under increased pressure. Two varieties of this are recognized. In one, the raised pressure of the fluid is due to an obstruction at some point in its course between its formation by the choroid plexuses and its exit from the fourth ventricle by the median and lateral apertures of the fourth ventricle. This type of hydrocephalus is called *obstructive.* When there is no obstruction within or to the outflow from the ventricular system, and the cerebrospinal fluid freely reaches the spinal sub-arachnoid space and is found there to be under increased pressure, the condition is known as *communicating* hydrocephalus.

Congenital hydrocephalus

Congenital hydrocephalus is usually due to a congenital malformation which interferes with the circulation of the cerebrospinal fluid at several points and may be associated with spina bifida. The cerebral aqueduct may be narrowed or absent, or there may be an Arnold–Chiari malformation in which a tongue of the cerebellum protrudes into the foramen magnum, with obstruction to the outflow from the fourth ventricle. This abnormality is often associated with syringomyelia and lumbosacral spina bifida. In other cases the fluid may leave the ventricles and circulate freely over the spinal cord, but there is an obstruction to its upward passage above the tentorium. Adhesions following haemorrhage due to birth trauma have been blamed for this form of hydrocephalus, which is not congenital but infantile.

Acquired hydrocephalus

Acquired hydrocephalus may be due to a tumour in the third or fourth ventricle or in the midbrain where the cerebral aqueduct may be narrowed also by ependymitis (Fig. 11.1). Adhesions following meningitis or arachnoiditis may occlude the outlet from the fourth ventricle, or obliterate the cerebrospinal channels in the cisterns above the tentorium. Parasitic cysts may cause obstruction at any of these sites. Thrombosis of the superior sagittal sinus may impair the absorption of fluid. When this is secondary to otitis it is known as otitic hydrocephalus.

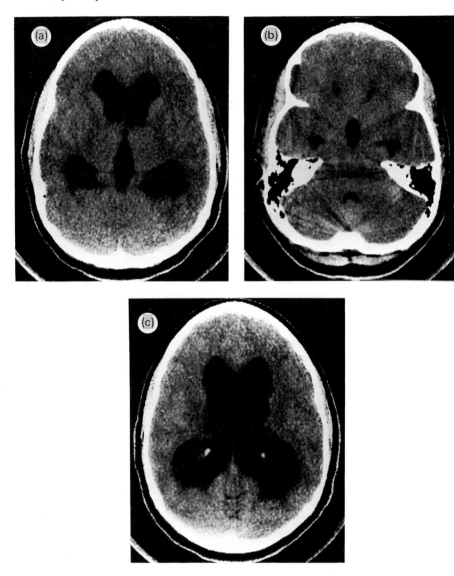

Fig. 11.1. CT scan, aqueduct stenosis, (a) dilated lateral and third ventricles; (b) normal fourth ventricle; (c) dilated lateral ventricles.

There remains a group of cases of hydrocephalus of obscure origin described as *benign intracranial hypertension,* sometimes known as toxic hydrocephalus or pseudotumour cerebri. The essential feature is an unexplained rise in the pressure of the cerebrospinal fluid, unaccompanied by any obstruction to its circulation, with ventricles of normal size.

The term *'normal pressure' hydrocephalus* has been given to a group of patients with communicating hydrocephalus. The patients usually have insidious progressive dementia with memory loss, and a clumsy gait and mild bilateral pyramidal signs. On investigation by CT or NMR scan the ventricles are enlarged and the cortical sulci are normal, though the cerebrospinal fluid pressure on lumbar puncture is within the normal range (Fig. 11.2). Such patients show a defective absorption of the cerebrospinal fluid in that there is a lack of filling of the cortical subarachnoid channels on air encephalography and an abnormal circulation of cerebrospinal fluid on isotope or iohexol encephalography. It is difficult to escape the conclusion that the pressure was at some stage raised. In some of these cases there is a history of subarachnoid haemorrhage, head injury or meningitis. In others there is no known preceding cause.

In *obstructive hydrocephalus* distension of the cerebral ventricles is the most conspicuous feature, its extent depending upon the point at which the obstruction occurs. Ventricular distension causes thinning of the cerebral hemispheres which in severe cases may be extreme and associated with some atrophy of the cortical ganglion cells. Pressure upon the bones of the skull causes them to become thin, especially where they overlie the cerebral convolutions. Separation of the sutures occurs when hydrocephalus develops early in life, but is not as a rule seen after the age of 18. The olfactory tracts and optic nerves may be atrophic.

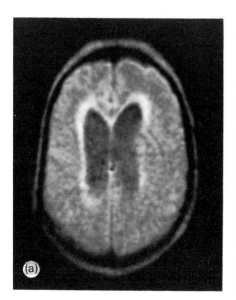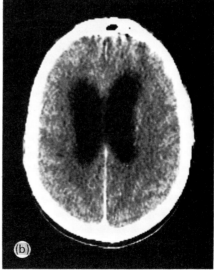

Fig. 11.2. Post-traumatic hydrocephalus in an adult. (a) CT scan and (b) NMR(SE) scan, which highlights the periventricular oedema.

Symptoms

Enlargement of the head is a conspicuous symptom of hydrocephalus occurring before birth or in early infancy (Fig. 11.3). It may occur before birth and obstruct labour, but is usually noticed first during the first few months of life. In most cases it is slowly progressive, and the head may become a huge size with a circumference of 30 inches or even more. The cranial sutures are widely separated, and the anterior fontanelle is much enlarged. In extreme cases the head may be translucent and yield a fluid thrill on percussion. Enlargement occurs in all diameters.

Children with hydrocephalus of any severity are mentally defective but there are a few striking exceptions. There is often optic atrophy. The limbs are under-developed and they usually exhibit spastic diplegia, of varying severity.

The clinical picture of acquired hydrocephalus varies somewhat with its cause. In obstructive hydrocephalus symptoms of increased intracranial pressure are conspicuous. Headache, at first paroxysmal, later becomes constant, often with intense exacerbations in which it radiates down the neck. These pains may be associated with head retraction and even opisthotonos, vomiting, and impairment of consciousness. Papilloedema is usually present. Enlargement of the head is less conspicuous than in the congenital and infantile varieties, but before the age of 18 there is often slight separation of the cranial sutures, yielding a cracked-pot sound on percussion. Cranial nerve palsies may occur. There may be slight weakness and incoordination of the limbs, and the

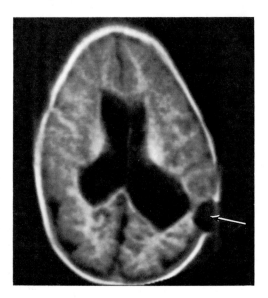

Fig. 11.3. Hydrocephalus and delayed myelination in a child of 30 months. NMR(IR) scan. The ventricular system is dilated. A shunt artefact is noted (arrow). There is also less myelination evident than in the normal infant of 20 months (see also Fig. 15.1 (b)).

plantar reflexes are often extensor. The tendon jerks may be exaggerated or diminished. Signs of hypopituitarism may be present.

In benign intracranial hypertension the initial symptom may be visual failure due to papilloedema. Headache is not as a rule severe, and may be absent, as also may vomiting. Neurological abnormalities are often slight and fleeting.

The pressure of the cerebrospinal fluid is increased in communicating hydrocephalus, and in benign intracranial hypertension may reach as high as 400 mm of water. The pressure, however, may be normal or even diminished in obstructive hydrocephalus. The fluid is usually normal in composition. Radiographs of the skull may show enlargement of the calvarium with thinning and exaggeration of the convolutional markings and sometimes separation of the sutures. CT scans will show enormous dilatation of the ventricular system except in benign intracranial hypertension in which the ventricles may be normal in size (see Fig. 11.1).

Diagnosis

Owing to the large head, congenital and infantile hydrocephalus is usually easy to diagnose. Later in life hydrocephalus usually presents with the symptoms of increased intracranial pressure with little or no localizing evidence as to the cause. The investigation calls initially for a CT scan (see Fig. 11.2).

Prognosis

In untreated cases congenital hydrocephalus often proves fatal during the first four years of life. Exceptionally the disorder becomes arrested and a state of equilibrium is reached between the formation and absorption of the cerebrospinal fluid. In patients who survive, mental deficiency, epilepsy, and blindness are common. The prognosis of acquired hydrocephalus depends upon its cause and how far this is amenable to treatment.

Treatment

When hydrocephalus is due to an obstruction to the circulation of the cerebrospinal fluid at some point, successful treatment consists in either removing the obstruction if that is possible, or by-passing it (Fig. 11.4). Aqueduct stenosis may be treated by Torkildsen's operation. Congenital hydrocephalus and 'normal pressure' hydrocephalus can now sometimes be treated by draining the cerebrospinal fluid into the peritoneal cavity or, by means of a Pudenz or Spitz–Holter valve, into one jugular vein. In acquired hydrocephalus the obstruction can sometimes be completely removed or bypassed as a palliative measure. When benign intracranial hypertension has been diagnosed, lumbar puncture should be carried out in order to reduce the pressure of the cerebrospinal fluid. Corticosteroids, acetazolamide, or hypertonic drugs which lower intracranial pressure should also be given. The process is usually self-limiting but if increased intracranial pressure threatens vision ventriculoperitoneal shunting may be necessary.

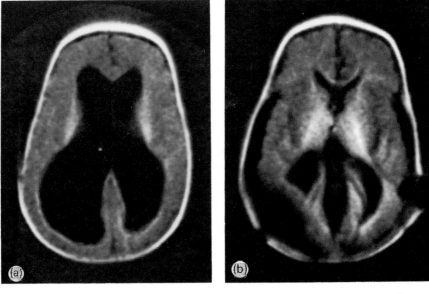

Fig. 11.4. Hydrocephalus: NMR(IR) scans (a) before and (b) after shunting in an infant of 17 months. There is a considerable decrease in the size of the hydrocephalus.

REFERENCES

Donaldson, J.O. (1981). Pathogenesis of pseudotumor cerebri syndromes. *Neurology, Minneap.* **31**, 877–80.

Jacobs, L. and Kinkel, N. (1976). Computerized axial transverse tomography in normal pressure hydrocephalus. *Neurology, Minneap.* **26**, 501–7.

Ostertag, C.B. and Mundinger, R. (1978). Diagnosis of normal pressure hydrocephalus using CT with CSF enhancement. *Neuroradiology* **16**, 216–19.

12 Intracranial abscess

Aetiology and pathology

Intracranial abscess is the result of the extension of a pyogenic infection to the brain. This is usually due to a direct spread from an air-containing structure having a connection with the upper respiratory passages, i.e. one of the nasal sinuses, the middle ear, or the mastoid. Less frequently the infection of the brain is haematogenous, the source often being intrathoracic suppuration. Congenital heart disease is a predisposing cause. Sometimes a fracture of the base of the skull offers a portal of entry. Any of the common pyogenic cocci may be the infecting agent; *Escherichia coli* is also found. Actinomycotic and amoebic abscesses of the brain occur.

Abscesses secondary to otitis are usually situated in the middle or posterior part of the temporal lobe, or in the cerebellum, the former about twice as often as the latter. The anterior part of the frontal lobe is the seat of abscess following frontal sinusitis. The first stage of an abscess is an acute encephalitis without visible pus formation. Pus then appears and a definite wall is formed, localizing the abscess. Microscopically the wall consists of an inner layer of pus cells, outside which is a layer of granulation tissue, and outside that again a layer of glial reaction. Inflammatory reactions are present in the overlying meninges.

Symptoms

The onset of the symptoms of cerebral abscess may be subacute or insidious. It is usually the former after a fracture of the skull, and in some cases in which it is secondary to suppurative otitis, but in these it is sometimes insidious, as it may be also in haematogenous cases. Sometimes, however, there is no acute disturbance of health corresponding to the lodgement of the infected embolus in the brain.

Headache is usually present, and in the more acute cases may be persistent and very severe. Papilloedema is a late sign and is often absent or slight. When present it is usually more marked on the side of the lesion. Slowing of the pulse is commoner in abscess than in tumour. In severe cases, delirium, somnolence, stupor, and coma develop.

The focal symptoms depend upon the site of the abscess. A temporo-sphenoidal abscess, if situated on the left side in a right-handed individual, may cause aphasia, usually of the nominal type. Abscess on either side may produce a defect of the visual fields, usually a homonymous upper quadrantic defect on

273

the opposite side, due to involvement of the lower fibres of the optic radiation. Damage to the corticospinal tract is usually slight, and weakness is most marked in the face and tongue.

Headache in cerebellar abscess is often predominantly suboccipital, tending to radiate down the neck and associated with some cervical rigidity. Symptoms of cerebellar deficiency vary in severity and may be slight. In general, the symptoms are similar to those of a cerebellar tumour (p. 229).

When the abscess is in the frontal lobe, headache, drowsiness, apathy, and impairment of memory and attention are usually conspicuous, but focal signs are often lacking.

The first special investigation is a CT brain scan which is likely to show an area of loss of density possibly surrounded by an area of increased Conray uptake (see Fig. 12.1). An intracranial tuberculoma presenting as a space-occupying lesion can usually be recognized on a CT scan. If it is then thought safe, the cerebrospinal fluid may be examined and changes are usually found. The pressure is likely to be raised, as is the protein also, up to perhaps 2.0 g/l, and there is usually an excess of cells, though not often more than 100 per cubic millimetre, the majority of which are lymphocytes, the remaining being polymorpho-nuclear. Organisms are not usually present.

Diagnosis

When the intracranial condition is known to be infective, the problem is to diagnose an abscess from other suppurative conditions, especially lateral sinus

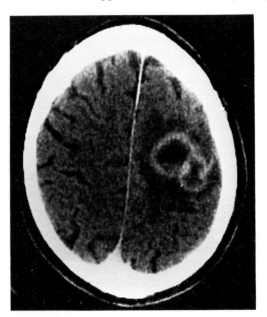

Fig. 12.1. CT scan, cerebral abscess, right hemisphere, biloculated, contrast-enhanced.

thrombosis and meningitis, with either of which it may co-exist. *Meningitis* is distinguished by the prominence of signs of meningeal irritation, cervical rigidity, in severe cases head retraction, Kernig's sign, and the characteristic changes in the cerebrospinal fluid. Persistent signs of a focal cerebral or cerebellar lesion, however, should suggest that the meningitis may be a complication of cerebral abscess. *Lateral sinus thrombosis* alone usually causes little cerebral disturbance, though the resulting congestion may lead to slight papilloedema, more marked on the affected side, and there may be slight signs of corticospinal tract defect on the opposite side.

When the symptoms of cerebral abscess are primarily those of a space-occupying lesion, it has to be distinguished from those conditions with which other space-occupying lesions may be confused (p. 248).

Prognosis

Very rarely an intracranial abscess becomes quiescent, but in general it should be regarded as uniformly fatal in the absence of surgical interference. Even with the modern surgical methods and the advantage of antibiotics, the mortality rate remains about 25 per cent. In those who survive, epilepsy is a common sequel.

Treatment

An abscess should not be approached surgically until it seems likely that the infection has been reasonably confined by appropriate systemic antibiotic therapy (p. 474). The choice then lies between primary excision, and repeated aspiration followed by the instillation of antibiotics – with secondary excision in reserve if this treatment fails.

REFERENCE

Beller, A.J., Sahar, A., and Praiss, I. (1973). Brain abscess. *J. Neurol. Neurosurg. Psychiat.* **36,** 757.

13 Injuries of the brain

THE IMMEDIATE EFFECTS OF HEAD INJURY

Aetiology with pathology

In civil life most head injuries are due to direct violence resulting from motor and industrial accidents. It is estimated that a hundred thousand cases of head injury are admitted to hospitals in this country each year, and of these some four hundred injuries cause unconsciousness lasting more than a month. Of the survivors with permanent brain damage, half are not able to work again. Less frequently they are produced by indirect violence after falls. Penetrating wounds are comparatively rare. The brain may be extensively damaged without the skull's having been fractured, and on the other hand fracture of the skull may occur without severe brain injury. Compound factures of the skull, especially those involving the base, are liable to lead to infection of the intracranial contents and thus to cause meningitis or intracranial abscess. Apart from this risk, however, the crucial question after head injury is the state of the brain rather than the state of the skull, and this alone will be considered here.

Concussion, mild or severe, and caused by diffuse cerebral injury, is now regarded as the most important disturbance after a head injury. In addition there may be added complications caused by more focal vascular lesions grouped under the terms contusion, laceration or compression. Clearly in any injury the type of focal complication may differ in different parts of the brain.

Concussion

Concussion has been defined by Trotter as 'a condition of widespread paralysis of the functions of the brain which comes on as an immediate consequence of a blow on the head, has a strong tendency to spontaneous recovery, and is not necessarily associated with any gross organic change in the brain substance'. It is thought to be due to direct injury to nerve cells, without necessarily any bruising or vascular lesions, which in milder cases is reversible, but may be permanent. It is now known that in severe cases of concussion there is widespread damage both to the brainstem and hemispheres and this may be followed by diffuse demyelination. Serial air studies have shown progressive dilatation of the ventricles within weeks, presumably due to destruction of cerebral tissue. These changes may occur without any evidence of cerebral compression, though particularly in children, diffuse cerebral oedema may complicate the acute stage of severe concussion.

Cerebral contusion

Cerebral contusion is a more or less diffuse disturbance to the brain following head injury and characterized by oedema and capillary haemorrhages, which are most frequently present at the poles of the hemispheres.

Cerebral laceration

Cerebral laceration is the term used when a cerebral contusion is sufficiently severe to cause a visible breach in the continuity of the brain substance.

Cerebral compression

Cerebral compression occurs when the injury is followed by intracranial haemorrhage which may be either extradural, subdural, or intracerebral.

Symptoms

Concussion

After a slight head injury the patient may be merely dazed or unconscious for a few seconds only, but his higher mental functions may subsequently be impaired for a period lasting up to several hours, during which he may carry out complicated activities of which he afterwards remembers nothing. This is the period of *post-traumatic amnesia,* which is best measured from the injury to the time of the beginning of continuous consciousness. The loss of memory may also extend to incidents which occurred before the accident, and is then known as *retrograde amnesia.* For example, the patient who has been injured in a motor accident may have forgotten the incidents of a long drive which preceded it. The retrograde amnesia usually lasts for a matter of seconds whereas post-traumatic amnesia may last for minutes to weeks depending on the severity of the injury. Retrograde amnesia is occasionally prolonged when there is selective bitemporal brain damage.

In cases of more severe injury, unconsciousness is more prolonged, and in addition the patient exhibits impairment of the functions of the brainstem, especially the medulla. Recovery from concussion is manifested first in an improvement of visceral function; the pulse pressure increases, respiration becomes deeper, and the pupils again react to light if they have failed to do so. Vomiting is common at this stage. On recovering consciousness the patient may be confused, restless, and irritable, and almost always complains of headache. In cases of uncomplicated concussion, however, these symptoms, with the exception possibly of headache, usually disappear within 48 hours after the injury. In the chronic post-traumatic syndrome with headaches and giddiness, the usual view that psychological factors often arising out of uncertain legal claims are a prominent factor, has been challenged.

Cerebral contusion

Slight cerebral contusion may occur without concussion. In most cases, however, the patient is rendered unconscious by the injury. In the more severe cases the depth of coma steadily increases and the patient dies from medullary paralysis within a few hours of the injury. In less severe cases the patient after recovering from concussion passes into a state of stupor or mental confusion. He is drowsy, and presents the picture long known as 'cerebral irritation' but better described as traumatic delirium, lying in a flexed attitude, resenting interference, confused and disorientated when aroused, and at times noisy and violent. This condition may last for days or even weeks, and in favourable cases gradually passes away. Sometimes, however, it persists indefinitely. Symptoms of a focal lesion of the brain are usually absent, but there may be signs of injury to the cortex or midbrain.

Acute traumatic cerebral compression

Cerebral compression leads to progressively deepening unconsciousness. Hutchinson's sign may be present (p. 48), and there are frequently symptoms of a progressive lesion of one cerebral hemisphere, for example focal convulsions and progressive flaccid paralysis of the limbs on one side. In the later stages medullary symptoms are prominent, and are those of progressive cerebral compression (p. 229).

Cranial nerve palsies

Cranial nerve palsies caused at the time of the injury are sometimes not obvious until the patient has recovered consciousness. They may be due to injury of the brainstem or of the nerves themselves in their intracranial or extracranial course. The seventh, eighth, and sixth are the most commonly affected; anosmia may be the result of damage to the olfactory nerves without fracture in the anterior fossa.

Cerebrospinal fluid

Lumbar puncture is not without risk after head injury. In all severe cases red blood cells are likely to be present, but it is doubtful whether examination of the cerebrospinal fluid often yields information of diagnostic value which cannot be obtained in other ways.

Other investigations

Inspection and palpation of the scalp and skull should be carried out, the presence of haematomas being noted, and the bone carefully examined for depressed fracture. Bleeding from the nasopharynx and ears may be an important symptom of fracture of the base of the skull, and inquiry should always be made as to the discharge of cerebrospinal fluid, which may be recognized by its sugar content. Metabolic disturbances are considered under treatment. Good-quality X-rays of the skull are needed to exclude a fracture of the skull and if a fracture is found it is always wise to admit the patient for 24 hours (Fig. 13.1). Routine X-rays are often taken for medico-legal reasons but few skull fractures would be missed if X-rays of the skull were restricted to patients

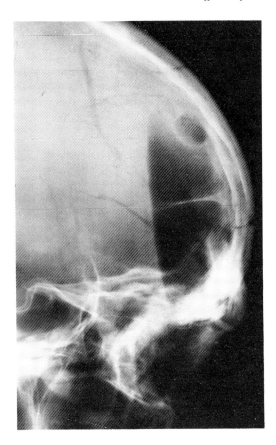

Fig. 13.1. Skull X-ray, brow-up film showing pneumocephalus following frontal fractures. Note the air-fluid level.

with skull signs or neurological signs. A CT brain scan will reveal any significant haemorrhage or contusion. In a very severe head injury the scan will eventually show massive widespread white matter lesions, of the kind described at post mortem which contribute to the dementia following severe head injury.

Diagnosis

Although in most cases the injury to the head is clearly the cause of the patient's symptoms, it is necessary to bear in mind the possibility that a pre-existing illness, especially a cerebral vascular lesion, may have led to the accident in which the head has been injured. When this has been excluded, the next step is to form an estimate of the nature of the brain injury and in particular whether there is a continuing haemorrhage. The onset of meningitis is to be suspected when the patient develops cervical rigidity or Kernig's sign, and is confirmed by the presence of a polymorphonuclear leucocytosis with or without pyogenic organisms in the cerebrospinal fluid.

Prognosis

Concussion is rarely fatal, and is usually followed by complete recovery within a few days. Contusion, when severe, may prove fatal, usually within a few hours or days, but modern methods of treatment have made it possible for patients to survive indefinitely even after severe brain damage. Acute traumatic cerebral compression is fatal in the majority of cases, and patients who recover usually have severe permanent brain damage. Diffuse demyelination occurs throughout the cerebral hemispheres and there are ischaemic lesions of the brainstem, both of which are in part due to pathophysiological changes occurring after the head injury and which can be reduced by expert intensive care unit management.

Sequels of head injury

Although a patient may recover rapidly and completely from cerebral contusion, persistent disabling symptoms are extremely common. The three cardinal late symptoms are headache, giddiness, and mental disturbances, and they usually develop out of the symptoms of the acute stage. Headache tends to be severe and to occur in paroxysms which may last for several hours, often against a background of continuous pain. It is brought on or exacerbated by physical exertion and excitement. The giddiness is not usually a sense of rotation but a feeling of instability. The commonest mental symptoms are inability to concentrate, fatigability, impairment of memory, together with nervousness and anxiety. It is often difficult, especially in cases where compensation or a pension is at stake, to distinguish between organic and psychogenic symptoms, but to some extent this distinction is artificial, and it is increasingly recognized that some symptoms often regarded as psychogenic are those of mild dementia of traumatic origin. In assessing the significance of head injuries for medico-legal purposes, the accepted view that concussion with brief retrograde amnesia causes no permanent brain injury is probably not justifiable. Recent evidence has shown that patients with more than one concussive injury took significantly longer to recover memory function than those with a single injury. The strong implication is that such concussive injuries produce some permanent brain damage though it is difficult to devise effective means of detecting this.

After a severe injury there may be profound dementia. This clinical picture may be complicated by the signs of focal damage to the brain or cranial nerves. CT scanning will usually show focal or general cerebral atrophy or communicating hydrocephalus and brain damage may be reflected in the EEG.

'Punch-drunkenness'

This is a chronic traumatic encephalopathy which may occur in professional boxers. It leads to deterioration of the personality, impairment of memory, dysarthria, cerebellar tremor, and ataxia. CT scans from boxers have shown small areas of haemorrhage after amateur as well as professional bouts.

Treatment

The correct treatment of head injury during the acute stage may not only save life but minimize the severity of the sequelae. If the patient is unconscious he will require the appropriate treatment (p. 178), but the following special points should be borne in mind. Respiratory embarrassment will call for suction of the nasopharynx and may require tracheostomy. Oxygen, if necessary, should be administered by nasal tube or tracheal catheter. Respiratory failure of central origin will need to be treated by positive pressure artificial respiration. Hyperpyrexia will call for induced hypothermia. Head injury may derange the metabolism in various ways. It is necessary, therefore, to estimate the urinary sugar, sodium, potassium, chloride, and nitrogen, and the blood sugar, sodium, potassium, chloride, and urea. If convulsions cannot be otherwise controlled, intravenous thiopentone should be given. A broad-spectrum antibiotic should be given as a prophylactic against meningitis and pneumonia. Surgery will be required to deal promptly with extradural haemorrhage from a ruptured middle meningeal artery or a subdural haematoma. At a later stage surgical treatment may be occasionally necessary for persistent cerebrospinal rhinorrhoea.

How long the patient is kept in bed depends upon the severity and duration of the acute stage. Physical and mental rehabilitation may begin in bed, and, after getting up, these are gradually increased. Throughout convalescence the patient's personality must be kept constantly in mind, and psychological tests are of value for discovering specific disabilities, for which special treatment may be required.

For traumatic epilepsy and its treatment see pages 201 and 208.

SUBDURAL HAEMATOMA

Aetiology and pathology

Subdural haematoma may occur at any age, but is most commonly seen in the elderly. It sometimes occurs in infancy. Males are affected more often than females. Trauma is the commonest cause, but a history of this may be unobtainable. Alcoholism is a common predisposing cause, perhaps because it predisposes to trauma. Subdural haematoma may also occur in patients suffering from the haemorrhagic diseases and after treatment with anticoagulants.

Blood slowly accumulates in the subdural space, possibly derived from the rupture of a vein. It usually lies over the frontal and parietal lobes, encysted between an outer wall consisting of a layer of highly vascularized granulation tissue adherent to the dura, and a thinner, inner wall of fibrous tissue. It is frequently bilateral.

Symptoms

The symptoms of subdural haematoma may follow an injury immediately, but more frequently there is a latent interval lasting weeks or months. There is a gradual onset of headache, drowsiness, and often confusion, but these symptoms tend to fluctuate greatly in severity. Focal cerebral symptoms may be slight or lacking. When present, they are likely to consist of hemiparesis with aphasia when the lesion is left-sided. Papilloedema is often absent. The pupils are frequently unequal, the larger, accompanied by slight ptosis, being found on the side of the haematoma. The cerebrospinal fluid may be normal, but the protein may be increased and the fluid may be xanthochromic. The pressure is usually raised, but may be subnormal.

A plain X-ray of the skull may show a displaced calcified pineal. A CT brain scan (Fig. 13.2) will show any ventricular displacement and, if recent, a hyperdense lesion which as it liquifies becomes a chronic isodense lesion unless outlined by intravenous contrast medium or a radio-isotope. If isodense a subdural may be missed, making angiography necessary or, if available, an NMR scan (Fig. 13.3). This is one of the few remaining neurological indications for a gamma isotope scan.

Diagnosis

The diagnosis of subdural haematoma usually offers little difficulty when there is a clear history of recent head injury. In the absence of this, the signs of a

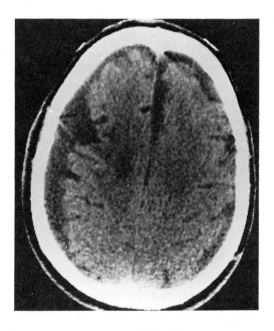

Fig. 13.2. CT scan, subdural haematoma.

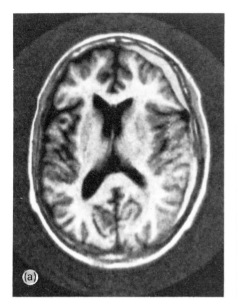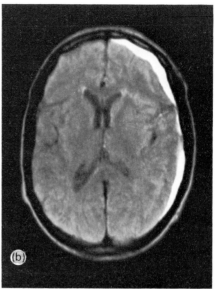

Fig. 13.3. Subdural haematoma: (a) NMR(IR), and (b) NMR(SE) scans. The haematoma has a light appearance on the IR scan and is highlighted in the SE scan.

progressive focal lesion may simulate an intracranial tumour, or the symptoms may be attributed to cerebral arteriosclerosis. Chronic alcoholism in its later stages may lead to confusion and drowsiness. In doubtful cases the ancillary methods of investigation should be used, and it may be necessary to make a burr hole on either side to explore the subdural space.

Prognosis

Provided the diagnosis is made sufficiently early, most patients make a good recovery after surgical treatment. Exceptionally, however, in spite of this, progressive deterioration occurs and the condition ends fatally.

Treatment

Treatment consists of surgical evacuation of the blood clot. The fact that the haematoma is bilateral in a substantial proportion of cases must be borne in mind.

REFERENCES

Adams, J.H., Graham, D.I., Scott, G., Parker, L.S., and Doyle, D. (1980). Brain damage in fatal non-missile head injury. *J. clin. Path.* **33**, 1132–45.
Jennett, B. and Teasdale, G. (1981). *Management of head injuries.* Davis, Philadelphia.
Jennett, B., Teasdale, G., Braakman, R., Minderhoud, J., Heiden, J., and Kurze, T. (1979). Prognosis of patients with severe head injury. *Neurosurgery* **4**, 283–9.

Jennett, B., Teather, D., and Bennie, S. (1973). Epilepsy after head injury: residual risk after varying fit-free intervals since injury. *Lancet* **ii,** 652–3.

Kaste, M., Kuurne, T., Viekki, J., Katevuo, K., Sainio, K., and Meurala, H. (1982). Is chronic brain damage in boxing a hazard of the past? *Lancet* **ii,** 1186–8.

Levin, H.S. and Grossman, R.G. (1978). Behavioural sequelae of closed head injury: a quantitative study. *Archs Neurol.* **35,** 720–7.

Plum, F. and Posner, J.B. (eds.) (1980). *Diagnosis of stupor and coma,* 3rd edn. Davis, Philadelphia.

Snoek, J., Jennett, B., Adam, J.H., Graham, D.I., and Doyle, D. (1979). Computerized tomography after recent severe head injury in patients without acute intracranial haematoma. *J. Neurol. Neurosurg. Psychiat.* **42,** 215–5.

Teasdale, G. and Jennett, B. (1974). Assessment of coma and impaired consciousness: a practical scale. *Lancet* **ii,** 81–4.

Zimmerman, R.A., Bilaniu, L.T., Genneralli, T., Bruce, D., Dolinskas, C., and Uzzel, B. (1978). Cranial computed tomography in diagnosis and management of acute head injury. *Am. J. Radiol.* **131,** 27–34.

14 Disorders of the cerebral circulation

ANATOMY AND PHYSIOLOGY

A knowledge of the anatomy and physiology of the cerebral circulation is essential in order to understand how symptoms and signs are produced by its disorders, and the principles upon which treatment must be based.

The blood supply of the brain

The brain receives its blood from four arteries, the two internal carotids and the two vertebrals. The right internal carotid springs from the right common carotid, a branch of the brachiocephalic trunk, the left from the common carotid which springs from the aorta. The vertebral arteries are derived from the subclavians. The vertebral arteries unite to form the basilar, which subsequently bifurcates into the two posterior cerebral arteries. The circle of Willis is formed as follows. The posterior communicating artery on either side joins the internal carotid to the posterior cerebral and the circle is completed in front by the anterior communicating artery which unites the two anterior cerebrals, branches of the internal carotid (Fig. 14.1).

The course and distribution of the *internal carotid artery* are shown in the normal angiogram and in Plate 4. The principal branches of the internal carotid

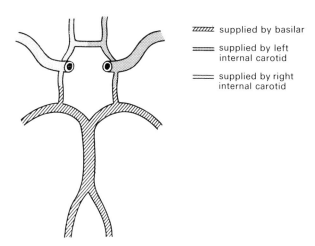

	supplied by basilar
	supplied by left internal carotid
	supplied by right internal carotid

Fig. 14.1. The circle of Willis showing normal distribution of blood through the individual arteries.

artery are: (i) the *ophthalmic artery* from which the central artery of the retina is derived; (ii) the *posterior communicating artery* described above; (iii) the *anterior choroidal artery*; (iv) the *anterior cerebral artery*; and (v) the *middle cerebral artery*.

The intracranial course of the *vertebral arteries* and the *basilar artery* are shown in Plate 4. The *vertebral arteries* run upwards in a bony canal in the cervical spine. They fuse at the level of the junction between the pons and the medulla to form the basilar artery (Plate 4). Before entering the skull each vertebral artery gives off branches which form the single anterior spinal artery and the two posterior spinal arteries. Within the skull each vertebral artery supplies with blood its own half of the medulla and sends a contribution to the cerebellum. Its largest and clinically most important branch is the *posterior inferior cerebellar artery*. The site of origin of this vessel is variable, but it usually arises from the vertebral artery a little distance below the lower border of the pons. It then passes outwards and backwards around the medulla, giving branches which supply a wedge-shaped area of the lateral aspect of the medulla, and the lower part of the inferior cerebellar peduncle. The main trunk supplies the inferior vermis and lower surface of the cerebellar hemisphere.

The *basilar artery* terminates at the upper border of the pons by dividing into the two posterior cerebrals. It supplies with blood the pons and part of the midbrain and through the *superior cerebellar* and *anterior inferior cerebellar arteries* that part of the cerebellum not supplied by the vertebral arteries.

The physiology of the cerebral circulation

The brain possesses, to a high degree, the property of autoregulation by which the blood flow and hence the oxygen concentration are maintained within narrow limits despite wide fluctuations in systemic pressure. Two factors are principally responsible. First, there is the response of the arteriolar walls to changes in the intraluminal pressure so that the arterioles constrict with a raised intraluminal pressure and dilate with a fall. Second, biochemical factors, mainly a rise in carbon dioxide, lead to arteriolar and capillary dilatation but at low levels hypoxia also causes dilatation, possibly by release of lactic acid as anaerobic glycolysis occurs. It is possible to measure the cerebral blood flow in patients, by the intracarotid injection or inhalation of radioactive krypton or xenon. The normal cerebral blood flow is 50–60 ml per 100 g of brain per minute and remains nearly constant as a result of the fluctuation of cerebro-vascular resistance by autoregulation until the mean arteriolar pressure falls to 50 mm. Autoregulation also aids the survival of a locally ischaemic region of the brain, by increasing the diameter of vessels adjoining the area and so by means of collaterals compensates for the lack of blood in the ischaemic region. Young, healthy persons can therefore compensate for moderate artificial stenosis of a carotid artery but the cerebral blood flow falls if there are multiple stenotic lesions or if there is impairment of vascular reactivity as a result of atheroma or hypertension.

The physiological importance of the circle of Willis lies in the anastomotic circulation which it provides. It has been shown that the internal carotid artery and the basilar artery share the blood supply to each cerebral hemisphere in such a way that there is normally no interchange of blood between them. The opposing streams of the two arteries meet in the posterior communicating artery at a 'dead point', at which the pressure of the two is equal. Consequently they do not mix. Similarly the territories of the two internal carotid arteries meet at a 'dead point' in the middle of the anterior communicating artery (Fig. 14.1). If, however, both internal carotids or both vertebral arteries are occluded, blood passes forwards or backwards respectively from the pair where are still patent. There is then a functioning anteroposterior anastomosis in each posterior communicating artery. Similarly, occlusion of one internal carotid artery leads to its territory being invaded by the basilar supply through the posterior communicating artery, and from the opposite internal carotid through the anterior communicating artery. The latter can readily be demonstrated in the course of angiography, for when the opaque medium is injected into one carotid, and the opposite one is compressed, it normally crosses the middle line through the anterior communicating artery, but this does not occur if normal flow through the uninjected carotid is allowed to continue.

There is a further anastomotic circulation in the brain, namely the distal anastomoses which exist between the three major cerebral arteries at the periphery of their cortical fields of supply. No cerebral artery becomes an end-artery until it has entered the brain substance, but once within the brain no artery appears ever to join another.

CEREBRAL ISCHAEMIA

Aetiology, pathology, and pathological physiology

There is a group of disorders in which the symptoms are due to insufficiency of the blood supply to the brain. The commonest of these is atheroma of the arteries supplying the brain. The pathology of atheroma is the same in the cerebral vessels as in other parts of the body. As elsewhere, for example in the coronary circulation, infarction of the brain may occur as the result of narrowing of an artery by atheroma without its complete occlusion, or as the result of its occlusion by thrombosis or embolism. The vessel affected may be large or small and the larger vessels may be affected at any point between their intrathoracic origin and their intracranial course. Moreover, the symptoms may be due predominantly to narrowing of one vessel or the result of diffuse changes involving a number of small vessels. The presence of atheroma in collateral channels often plays an important part in influencing the effects of a more advanced degree of atheroma in a single large vessel.

The pathological effects of cerebral ischaemia due to atheroma therefore range from a massive area of cerebral infarction produced by obstruction of one internal carotid or one middle cerebral artery to small areas in the cerebral cortex or white matter due to an impaired circulation through the smaller arteries and arterioles. Following occlusion of a cerebral artery there may be zones of over-perfusion and under-perfusion, determined by the degree of damage to autoregulatory function in adjacent regions of the circulation. After an acute ischaemic infarct, causing cerebral vasomotor paralysis, flow is profuse and, if pressure is maintained, is in excess of metabolic demand – so-called 'luxury' profusion. The use of vasodilator drugs can precipitate a 'steal' by adjacent areas, whereas vasoconstrictors may cause an inverse 'steal' effect. In a large area of infarction there is widespread destruction of nerve cells, nerve fibres, and the glial tissues except the microglia. The cortex presents a haemorrhagic appearance and the white matter, which is pale, undergoes ischaemic necrosis. Infarction of a large area of one cerebral hemisphere may cause so much swelling that it leads to symptoms of increased intracranial pressure.

Generalized atheroma without occlusion of any single large vessel leads to diffuse atrophy of the brain with multiple small patches of softening of various ages.

Lacunar infarcts are among the commonest cerebrovascular lesions recognized at post-mortem and represent healed ischaemic infarctions after occlusion caused by a lipohyaline change in small vessels. There are small cavities about 5–10 mm in diameter most commonly in the deep nuclei of the brain, especially the putamen. Because of their small size many are not recognized clinically but the larger ones may be shown on CT or NMR scans (see Fig. 14.2). Other rare syndromes of ischaemic brain disease are white matter lesions in hypertensives (Binswanger's disease or progressive subcortical encephalopathy) and infarctions in border zones of arterial territories, often bilaterally, following hypotension, especially in the parietal cortex where the territories of the anterior, middle, and posterior cerebral arteries meet.

What has been said above about the anatomy and physiology of the cerebral circulation explains the complexity of the factors which determine whether, and in what circumstances, atheroma of a cerebral vessel will give rise to symptoms. If the occlusion of the vessel is very slow and the collateral circulation is adequate, there may be no symptoms; for example, in a case of atheroma of the internal carotid artery just above the bifurcation of the common carotid in an individual in early middle life with a good collateral circulation. Conversely, atheroma of the opposite internal carotid artery, or of the vertebrobasilar system, or both, increases the likelihood of symptoms. Frequently a patient with atheromatous narrowing of one internal carotid artery suffers from paroxysmal symptoms of varying duration. These have not as yet been fully explained. Since the cerebral circulation depends directly upon the adequacy of the blood pressure, *a fall of blood pressure* from any cause, especially myocardial infarction or paroxysmal arrhythmia, may render temporarily inadequate the circulation through a narrowed atheromatous vessel which may become adequate when the blood pressure rises again. Local *vascular*

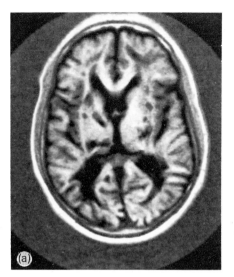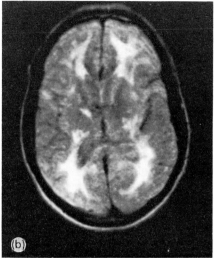

Fig. 14.2. Lacunar infarction: (a) NMR(IR) and (b) NMR(SE) scans. Multiple small dark lesions are seen within the central white matter and periventricular areas in (a) and these are also seen in (b).

spasm, associated with hypertension, is another possible cause of temporary ischaemic symptoms. Small *emboli* probably arising from atheromatous plaques on the walls of extracerebral vessels may pass into the cerebral circulation and cause ischaemic symptoms. These emboli, which are occasionally seen in the retinal circulation, are sometimes highly refractile and contain cholesterol material (see Plate 3(d)). More fragile emboli composed of fibrin-platelet material which traverse the retinal vessels are far less often seen but may also cause ischaemic symptoms. It has been shown that rotation of the head may cause temporary ischaemia of the brainstem in subjects who have both cervical spondylosis and atheroma of the vertebral arteries. Pathology shows that atheroma of a large vessel such as the internal carotid artery may cause only comparatively small areas of infarction within the area of its distribution. A haemotocrit of 50 per cent or more is associated with increased infarct size, presumably because the increased viscosity associated with a low cerebral blood flow adversely affects collateral flow.

Other forms of cerebral vascular disease which may lead to cerebral ischaemia include endarteritis due to meningovascular or tuberculous meningitis, and three rare disorders, thrombo-angiitis, polyarteritis nodosa, and giant-celled arteritis (cranial arteritis). Cerebral embolism (p. 305) is also a cause of cerebral ischaemia. There is a threefold risk of cerebral thrombosis in women taking oral contraceptives, particularly a high dose oestrogen–progesterone combination.

Symptoms

A patient who is suffering from atheromatous ischaemia is likely to be middle-aged or older. The onset of symptoms may be sudden, and not uncommonly occurs during sleep so that the patient awakens in the morning to discover his disability. On the other hand, prodromal transitory disturbances of cerebral function of vascular origin are common. The symptoms may increase in severity for 24 or 48 hours after the onset. They will sometimes present a clear-cut picture of obstruction of one particular cerebral artery, or there may be an incomplete picture of this, the lesion falling within the domain of a single vessel but not involving the whole area of its supply. Frequently consciousness is preserved, or there is merely some confusion. Profound loss of consciousness is rare except when there is a large area of infarction or the lesion involves the brainstem.

The internal carotid artery

This vessel may be completely occluded without causing symptoms. Progressive obliteration of the lumen, however, often causes recurrent transitory disturbances due to localized cerebral ischaemia, for example aphasia, mental confusion, or contralateral hemiparesis or paraesthesia – a clinical picture which has been described as 'stuttering hemiplegia'. Transitory amblyopia of the eye on the same side is not uncommon, but permanent blindness of that eye is rare. Focal or generalized epilepsy may occur. After a series of such recurrent ischaemic episodes, which may extend over months or even a year or two, there may be a sudden stroke due to extensive infarction of the affected hemisphere. Symptoms of this may include crossed homonymous hemianopia (usually transitory), hemiplegia, and loss of spatial and discriminative sensibility on the opposite side of the body, and, when the lesion is on the left side, aphasia, both receptive and expressive. Other modes of onset include a stroke of this kind occurring without preliminary warning, from which, on the one hand, a good degree of recovery may occur, or, on the other hand, no recovery at all.

It may be possible to demonstrate by palpation diminished pulsation of the affected vessel in the neck, or to hear a bruit over it. Bruits arising in the carotid artery are unlikely if the stenosis is less than one-third of the lumen. A reduction of pressure and flow beyond the stenosis is reflected by a fall in ophthalmic artery pressure which can be measured by oculoplethysmography. This has a 90 per cent success rate in diagnosing stenosis greater than 60 per cent. It is reasonable to use only non-invasive methods to investigate asymptomatic patients with carotid bruits and with an asymptomatic carotid bruit it is reasonable to treat the patient with aspirin until a transient ischaemic attack occurs. The improved non-invasive techniques such as intravenous digital subtraction angiography (see p. 162) will increase the precision of diagnosis of carotid stenosis in asymptomatic patients.

The middle cerebral artery

As far as the motor, sensory, and speech functions are concerned the symptoms of occlusion of the middle cerebral artery are indistinguishable from those of occlusion of the internal carotid artery. In doubtful cases the daignosis can be made only by angiography.

The anterior cerebral artery

A number of clinical pictures have been described as resulting from occlusion of this vessel at various sites. The main point to bear in mind is that it supplies the paracentral lobule containing the cortical centres for movements of the lower limb. Obstruction of the anterior cerebral artery, therefore, may result in a spastic monoplegia, with or without sensory loss of the cortical type, in the opposite lower limb. Other symptoms may include a grasp reflex in the opposite upper limb, and, when the lesion is on the left side, some apraxia on that side.

The posterior cerebral artery

Since this artery supplies the visual cortex of the occipital lobe its occlusion causes crossed homonymous hemianopia. The macular region of the blind fields usually escapes – macular sparing – owing to a shift of the fixation point a few degrees into the seeing half of the visual field. Visual agnosia may result from ischaemia of the left occipital lobe and impairment of memory from damage to the medial aspect of the temporal lobe.

The vertebrobasilar circulation

Since the vertebral and basilar arteries supply all the structures in the posterior fossa, and through the posterior cerebral arteries the visual cortex on both sides, atheromatous narrowing of these vessels may give rise to a very varied clinical picture. Transitory attacks of hemianopia or complete cortical blindness, either of which may become permanent, may occur, or positive visual phenomena. There may be ophthalmoplegia leading to diplopia, vertigo, nystagmus, symptoms and signs of involvement of one or both corticospinal tracts and of the long ascending sensory pathways on one or both sides. Cerebellar symptoms may occur. Paroxysmal symptoms, which may be precipitated by head movements, include vertigo, drop attacks, and syncope. Large lesions cause coma.

The subclavian 'steal' syndrome

Symptoms of vertebrobasilar insufficiency, sometimes provoked by arm exercise, may be due to the diversion of blood from the vertebral artery to the brachial artery – the subclavian 'steal' syndrome. A history of brainstem symptoms, with the finding of reduced blood pressure in one arm and a bruit at the root of the neck on the same side, should raise the suspicion of this syndrome. Angiographic investigation may then reveal stenosis or occlusion of the subclavian or innominate arteries proximal to the origin of the vertebral artery. Under these circumstances the flow of blood in the vertebral artery is reversed and the upper extremity 'steals' blood from the brainstem. If the stenosis or occlusion can be corrected surgically the symptoms may be abolished.

Transient global amnesia

Middle aged or elderly patients may suddenly develop severe but reversible memory loss spontaneously or occasionally after unaccustomed exercise such as swimming in cold water. Complete recovery usually occurs within minutes or hours. Electroencephalography in such patients may show medial temporal lobe spike discharges suggesting vertebrobasilar ischaemia affecting the posterior cerebral arterial circulation of the medial temporal lobes bilaterally and simultaneously.

The lateral medullary syndrome

There is a characteristic clinical picture which results from infarction of a wedge-shaped area of the lateral aspect of the medulla and the inferior surface of the cerebellum. This is sometimes due to thrombosis of the posterior inferior cerebellar artery, but probably more often of one vertebral artery. The onset is associated with severe vertigo, and vomiting may occur. There is dysphagia and, in some cases, pain or paraesthesiae, such as a sensation of hot water running over the face, may be referred to the trigeminal area on the affected side. There is some degree of cerebellar deficiency, with nystagmus, hypotonia, and incoordination on the side of the lesion. Ipsilateral paralysis of the soft palate, pharynx, and vocal cord results from involvement of the nucleus ambigus. Horner's syndrome – miosis and ptosis – is present on the affected side. Dissociated sensory loss occurs, though its distribution is somewhat variable. Usually analgesia and thermo-anaesthesia are present on the face on the same side as the lesion and on the trunk and limbs on the opposite side, as the result of involvement of the spinal tract and nucleus of the trigeminal nerve and of the spinothalamic tract respectively. The sensory loss on the face, however, may be confined to the first, or to the first and second, divisions of the nerve, since the regions are represented in the lowest part of the spinal nucleus, which may alone be supplied by the posterior inferior cerebellar artery. Persistent neuralgic pain in the face, on the side of the lesion, and sometimes of the limbs and trunk on the opposite side, may be troublesome sequels of this vascular lesion.

Diffuse cerebral ischaemia (lacunar infarction, see also p. 288)

The syndromes described above are those which result from narrowing of a single large cerebral artery. There are, however, patients who without developing gross focal lesions present the symptoms of a diffuse cerebral ischaemia due to atheroma, but no hard and fast line can be drawn between the two, since the diffuse picture may include the symptoms of small focal lesions. Mental symptoms are common in such cases and consist of general reduction in intellectual capacity with impairment of memory, especially for recent events and names, and emotional instability. There may be attacks of confusion, which are apt to be precipitated by removal from home and by operations. Still greater mental deterioration leads to a profound dementia. Epileptiform attacks may occur, and various forms of aphasia, agnosia, and apraxia are met with. Corticospinal tract lesions are common, and the grasp reflex may be encountered. In walking there is a tendency to take short shuffling steps. Arteriosclerotic parkinsonism also occurs.

The onset of such symptoms is often insidious, but a slow deterioration extending over several years may be punctuated by sudden slight exacerbations due to small strokes. A special form of diffuse vascular disease causing dementia is known as Binswanger's disease (progressive subcortical encephalopathy; see Fig. 10.4, p. 263.)

The general clinical picture

Patients with cerebral ischaemia may or may not have hypertension. There is often evidence of generalized atheroma, seen, for example, in the retinal arteries. There may be a history of previous myocardial infarction, or electrocardiographic evidence of this. A proportion are diabetic. Deep venous thrombosis is a not uncommon complication. There may be a cardiac rhythm disturbance or source of emboli such as a prolapsing mitral valve.

Investigations

The usual serological investigations would exclude syphilis and the blood cholesterol should be estimated. A raised erythrocyte sedimentation rate should suggest the possibility of one of the rarer forms of arteritis. A haemoglobin estimation may suggest polycythaemia or anaemia which, though rare causes of cerebral ischaemia, are easily treated.

The haematocrit

The haematocrit is the main determinent of whole blood viscosity. In polycythaemia rubra vera the high haematocrit is due to the elevated red cell mass. There are also many patients with cerebrovascular disease, principally cigarette smokers and patients with hypoxic lung disease, with relative polycythaemia. In this group as well as in true polycythaemics, there is an increased incidence of cerebrovascular disease. The patients with a high haematocrit (above 0.50) should be venesected until the haematocrit falls below 0.45. As blood haematocrit falls the oxygen content of the blood falls and it is not yet clear how much this contributes to the increase in cerebral blood flow.

A cardiac arrhythmia can be investigated by ECG and if necessary ambulatory cardiac monitoring. The extent and site of the damage to the brain may be demonstrated by computerized axial tomography.

CT and NMR scanning in cerebrovascular disease

It may not yet be possible to perform a CT scan in all patients with transient ischaemic attacks but in all patients thought to have had an infarct on clinical grounds the CT scan within 24 hours is almost certain to show the site of the lesion. A cerebral haemorrhage up to half a centimetre in diameter will be apparent immediately whereas a small cerebral infarct may not be obvious until two or three days. A CT scan largely obviates the need for examination of the cerebrospinal fluid in patients with strokes. Serial CT scanning will show the evolution of an infarct eventually to a homogeneous area of loss of density with distinct borders. The shape of the early infarct follows the pattern of known blood supply of the involved arterial territory. Often there is grey matter enhancement. The CT scan of a cerebral infarct is more likely to be positive if it is undertaken with and without contrast, taking account of the risk of the use of contrast which may leak excessively through damaged vessels. Serial studies will make clear the distinction which is sometimes difficult between an infarct and a tumour or cerebrovascular malformation. After cerebral infarction changes are usually found in the cerebrospinal fluid. The protein tends to be raised up to 1.0 to 2.0 g/l and the fluid may be yellow, and may contain a pleocytosis including a moderate excess of polymorphonuclear cells.

Nuclear magnetic resonance scanning has some advantages over the CT scan, in particular in demonstrating lesions in the posterior fossa, as discussed previously (see p. 158). A selection of NMR scans compared with CT scans are shown in Figs. 14.2–5.

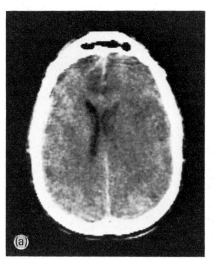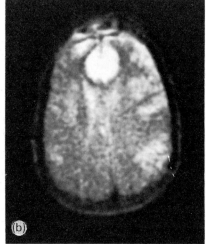

Fig. 14.3. Right hemisphere infarction after subarachnoid haemorrhage. (a) CT and (b) NMR(SE) scans: (a) shows subarachnoid blood and hemisphere swelling due to oedema and shift of ventricles to the left. Features of infarction are shown on both scans but are more extensive on the NMR scan.

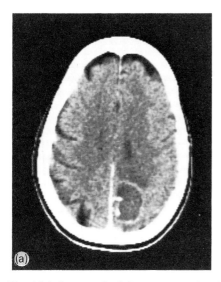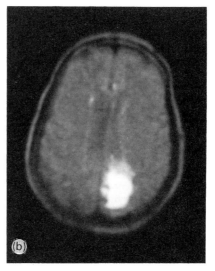

Fig. 14.4. Intracerebral haematoma. (a) Contrast-enhanced CT and (b) NMR(SE) scans. The haematoma from which blood was aspirated is seen as a ring-enhancing lesion on the CT scan.

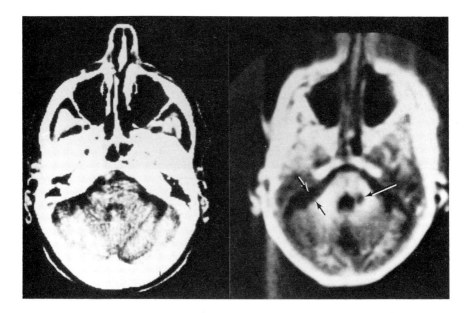

Fig. 14.5. Brainstem infarct and cerebellar atrophy, (left) CT scan and (right) NMR(IR). The area of infarction appears dark in (NMR) (long arrow). Significant c.s.f. is seen between the petrous bone and anterior margin of cerebellum, possibly related to cerebellar hemisphere atrophy (short arrows).

Angiography

Angiography may be necessary in establishing the diagnosis and demonstrating the site of the obstruction if the possibility of surgery is likely, but it is a good general rule that no method of investigation should be employed unless it may yield information which will be of value in treatment. Since it is important to visualize the total proximal cerebral circulation if surgery is contemplated, the most helpful angiographic test is usually arch-aortography by catheterization of the brachial or femoral arteries (Figs. 14.6 and 14.7). In skilled hands this carries no more risk than direct puncture of a single carotid artery, which itself may be necessary to outline more precisely a high lesion (Fig. 14.8) or the intracranial circulation. The risks of vertebral angiography by the method of direct puncture in atheromatous subjects are significantly greater, one rare complication being transient blindness. The current hope is that non-invasive techniques, such as isotope imaging of the carotid and Doppler studies measuring turbulence caused by stenosis will obviate the 0.5–2.5 per cent morbidity of angiography. Recently

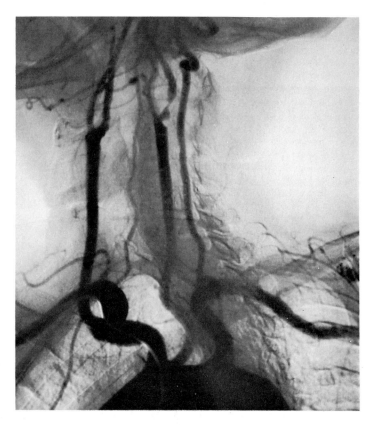

Fig. 14.6. Arch angiogram (subtraction technique) showing stenosis at the left carotid bifurcation and of the left internal carotid artery, just above the bifurcation.

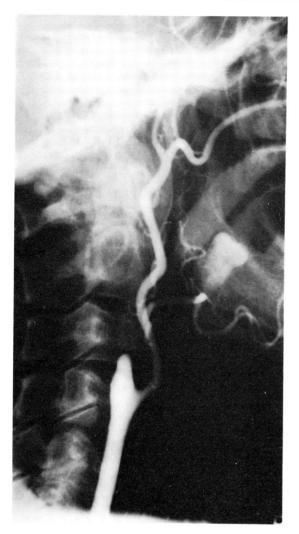

Fig. 14.7. Arch angiogram (subtraction technique) showing right and left common carotid occlusion and left subclavian stenosis. The patient was surviving from a good vertebral arterial supply.

the promising new technique of digital intravenous angiography has been introduced using video techniques and computer subtraction to give much better angiograms (see Fig. 5.9, p. 163). The PET (positive emission tomography) scan is used for research purposes and has taught us much about the pathophysiology of infarction (Fig. 14.9). ^{15}O and $C^{15}O_2$ studies will reveal areas of critical hypoperfusion which may be reversed (see p. 160).

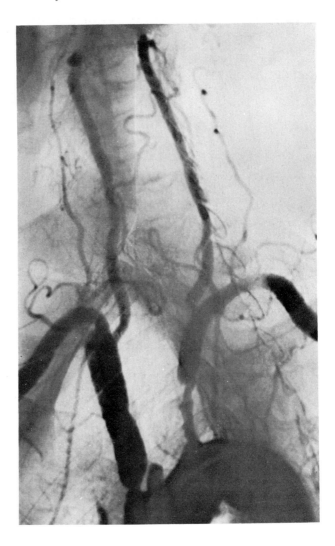

Fig. 14.8. Carotid angiogram showing internal carotid occlusion.

Diagnosis

See page 322.

Prognosis

The prognosis of cerebral ischaemia due to atheroma depends upon a number of factors, some of which cannot be accurately estimated. Chief among these are the age of the patient, the adequacy of the collateral circulation, the diffuseness of the atheromatous degeneration within the brain, the condition of the

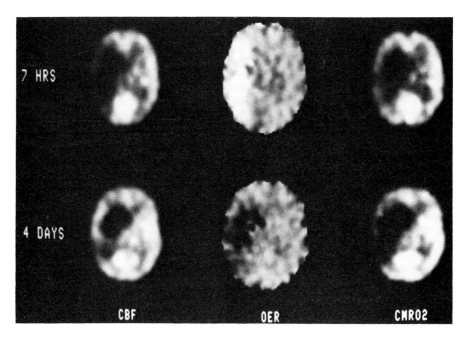

Fig. 14.9. Positron emission tomographic images of acute cerebral infarction. Serial transaxial images of cerebral blood flow (CBF), oxygen extraction ratio (OER), and oxygen metabolism (CMRO$_2$) in a patient seven hours and four days after the onset of aphasia and right hemiplegia. OER expresses the fraction of oxygen extracted from the available arterial blood (normally about 35 per cent). At seven hours CMRO$_2$ in left hemisphere cortex was partially preserved by means of maximal extraction of oxygen (high OER) from the trickle of residual blood flow. By four days there had been natural, partial reflow into the left hemisphere cortex but without recovery of CMRO$_2$ – at this time oxygen supply (CBF) was greatly in excess of demand (CMRO$_2$) and OER was low. Uncoupling of CBF and CMRO$_2$ in ischaemic or infarcted brain means that CBF does not correlate with tissue function under these circumstances. It remains to be established whether CMRO$_2$ at any particular time after the onset of symptoms reflects potential viability of the tissue.

circulation as a whole, the presence or absence of other metabolic disturbances such as diabetes, renal disease, etc.

It may be difficult to assess the prognosis of a focal ischaemic lesion during the first two or three days after the onset. When the lesion is within the territory of the internal carotid artery, however, the greater the extent of the area of cerebral damage the worse the outlook. Unconsciousness, and the association of sensory loss with hemiplegia are bad prognostic signs. A small focal lesion in any part of the brain, however, is a less serious affair than evidence of narrowing of one of the main vessels. An elderly patient may live for years after a small focal lesion with little disability and no recurrence. The clinical picture of diffuse cerebral ischaemia is insidiously progressive over a period of several years.

Treatment

This requires a knowledge of its natural history. Angiography may be contra-indicated because a patient is over 60 with coronary disease or diabetes and in other patients it is reasonable to consider if surgery would be undertaken if a lesion were demonstrated before embarking on angiography. Large surveys have shown that approximately one-half of strokes are the result of atheromatous thrombosis, one-third the result of embolism and one-sixth are associated with intracerebral haemorrhage. Strokes account for 80 000 deaths a year in the United Kingdom.

Transient ischaemic attacks

Since the aim of treatment in cerebrovascular disease is the prevention of a major stroke, the management of the transient ischaemic attack may be considered first. Transient ischaemic attacks are brief episodes of neurological dysfunction with recovery, but with a tendency to recur. They might be distinguished from other brief attacks due, for example, to migraine or epilepsy, They may be due to inadequate flow, emboli or spasm, or a combination of these factors (p. 286).

Approximately one-third of patients with transient ischaemic attacks can be expected to suffer a major stroke over the subsequent four years. This is approximately 6 per cent per year compared with a 3 per cent rate per year for matched control patients. The incidence of a major stroke is greatest in the first month after the first transient ischaemic attack. Investigation of patients with transient ischaemic attacks shows that one-third have clinical signs of extra-cranial carotid disease and a half have carotid stenosis or occlusion on investigation, as opposed to 5 per cent of control patients. Carotid stenosis produces its effect by distal infarction or microembolization (see p. 289), the latter possibly being commoner.

The incidence of carotid stenosis and atheroma varies in different surveys. In one series nearly 80 per cent of patients with symptoms of carotid stenosis and a neck bruit were proved to have carotid atheroma. In another series an operable lesion was present in one-third of patients who presented with amaurosis fugax, and hemisphere ischaemic symptoms, two of the commonest symptoms of carotid atheromatous stenosis.

The assessment of each patient is an individual matter but to illustrate the principles of management, patients may be considered in four groups according to the results of their preliminary investigations.

1. Patients with a general medical abnormality which may have contributed to the cerebral ischaemia. This may range from a haematological disorder, such as anaemia or polycythaemia; a source of emboli, such as subacute bacterial endocarditis; a cardiac rhythm disorder; a disease affecting blood vessels, such

as cranial arteritis; a collagen disorder; to a cause for insufficiency, such as cervical osteophytes distorting or compressing the vertebral arteries. These patients should in the first instance be treated for any abnormality found. For patients with cervical osteo-arthritis restriction of neck movement with a collar may be helpful if surgical treatment is not possible.

2. In a second group of patients with transient ischaemic attacks, the blood pressure may be abnormally high and it should be lowered cautiously with diuretic and hypotensive drugs until the diastolic pressure is in the upper part of the normal range for a person of the same age. Less often a patient may have an abnormally low blood pressure; the cause for this should be established and if possible treated. In a middle-aged patient hypotension due to a silent coronary thrombosis is sometimes overlooked as the cause of acute cerebral ischaemic symptoms. In the elderly, hypotension may result from pooling of blood in the legs on standing, caused by defective vascular reflexes. A variety of modern tranquillizing drugs, apart from the over-enthusiastic use of hypotensive drugs, may also lead to postural hypotension. Control of the blood pressure in such patients should be established before any further investigations are undertaken.

3. The few remaining patients are likely to be suitable for consideration of surgical treatment of the extracranial vessels. This constitutes the patients suffering from continuing recurrent transient ischaemic attacks. Symptoms may be classified according to whether they arise in the territory of the carotid or vertebral arteries, as this will influence the technique of angiography used. A smaller percentage of brainstem than carotid transient ischaemic attacks progress to completed strokes. Since vertebral angiography is both more hazardous and, except in the case of suspected brainstem 'steal' syndrome, is less likely to reveal surgically operable lesions, it is less imperative than carotid angiography. Provided the patients are neither too old nor infirm, arch-angiography should be considered, particularly if there is any clinical evidence from reduced pulsation or bruits to point to stenotic disease of the cerebral vessels in the neck. The demonstration of a stenotic lesion will naturally lead to the question of surgery (p. 303).

4. A final group comprises patients with continuing transient ischaemic attacks but in whom angiography has failed to demonstrate any stenotic disease of the great vessels. It represents only a small percentage of patients with transient ischaemic attacks. Patients may be included in this group from the beginning, either because no other causal factors have been found, or possibly because their attacks continued despite the correction of anaemia or control of their blood pressure, or because angiography excluded surgically treatable stenotic disease. At this stage the distinction between transient ischaemic attacks affecting the hemisphere and the brainstem is relevant because the former have a greater liability to major strokes. If the attacks persist it is probably justifiable to give drugs which inhibit either platelet adhesiveness or blood coagulation.

Medical treatment

Aspirin (600 mg twice daily) inhibits platelet aggregation and reduces thromboxane (A2) a vasoconstricting prostaglandin, and also prostacyclin, a vasodilating prostaglandin. Dipyridamole (50 mg eight-hourly) acts by inhibiting platelet phosphorodiesterase so that cyclic AMP is not metabolized and sulphinpyrazole (Ataran 200–400 mg daily) is believed to inhibit platelet adherence to endothelial cells. All these medical treatments have yet to be subjected to a satisfactory controlled trial. There is uncertainty whether Aspirin 600 mg twice a day is a significant improvement over 300 mg daily. For males in this group the therapeutic benefit of Aspirin in a dose of 300 mg four times a day has been proven to be better than in control subjects, though not for the females. Anticoagulants are justified if there is an undoubted cerebral embolic event and the CT scan has excluded a cerebral haemorrhage. Heparin 100 000 units every six hours in saline can be given in intravenous infusion, or 5000 units subcutaneously six hours. Warfarin can be started in a dose of 325 mg daily as soon as the diagnosis has been made and heparin can be discontinued after 48 hours.

The usual anticoagulant is the coumarin derivative warfarin. If, despite a prothrombin time two and a half to three times the control value maintained for a month, the attacks continue, there seems little point in persisting with this therapy in view of its known serious hazards, and the drug should then be gradually withdrawn. However, even if the attacks are controlled it is probably wise to attempt to withdraw the anticoagulants slowly after a number of months, since the liability to such attacks, however caused, may then have subsided. If this can be done the risk of further ischaemic attacks is probably less than the risk of haemorrhage while the patient is having long-term anticoagulant therapy. Efficient control of the anticoagulants is of course important but is no guarantee against these hazards. The final place of anticoagulants is still uncertain though earlier optimism for this form of treatment has now waned. The best hope for the future lies in the discovery of some method of prevention of arteriosclerosis.

The ingravescent stroke

This is the term given to a neurological deficit, usually a hemiplegia, which, though mild at onset, appears to be progressing. When the neurological symptoms are stepwise or progressive over less than 12 hours the diagnosis of cerebral infarction may reasonably be accepted without the necessity for specialist neurological investigation. Progression over a longer period raises the possibility of a cerebral tumour. The management is similar to that of the transient ischaemic attack though investigation is a matter of urgency and treatment with heparin may sometimes be justified in the hope of arresting the spread of thrombosis. Salicylates block platelet adenosine diphosphate release and hence may reduce the thrombosis formation on intima damaged by atheroma.

The completed stroke

In the completed stroke angiography may be necessary to exclude other than vascular causes but demonstration of a stenosis or occlusion and surgical treatment of it will be too late to benefit the patient's acute disabling symptoms. A group of patients in whom a CT scan is particularly indicated is those in whom the stroke is complete in less than two hours and intracerebral bleeding may have occurred. There is no evidence that dexamethasone or other drugs to reduce oedema significantly improve the prognosis after a complete stroke.

Surgical treatment

A knowledge of the natural history of the type of vascular disease and of the current surgical risks is necessary in order to advise management. Current evidence suggests that at a good centre with a combined morbidity and mortality for unilateral carotid endarterectomy at less than 4 per cent, surgery may be preferable to medical treatment for proven significant carotid stenosis. The studies have shown that without surgery the risk of a stroke is approximately 6 per annum and the best surgical results halve this percentage, once the immediate surgical risks are past. Though early predictions for the place of surgery were over-optimistic, there are a number of carefully selected patients who can be helped. The ideal case is a patient with marked stenosis of one carotid artery with transient ischaemic attacks but no severe neurological deficit. Less severe degrees of stenosis may justify surgery because they offer a site for the origin of emboli. The functional reserve of cerebral blood flow is reduced by stenotic disease in many middle-aged patients without cerebrovascular symptoms and so the significance of multiple stenotic lesions from a haemodynamic point of view is sometimes difficult to assess. However, the removal of an atheromatous stenotic lesion in the proximal part of the relevant cerebral vessel may well result in the abolition of symptoms. It may also remove a potential site for the formation of emboli. The problem often arises that patients' symptoms sometimes seem too mild to justify angiographic investigation, which non-invasive techniques have not yet fully replaced (but see Fig. 5.9 (a), (b), (c), and (d), p. 163), and yet if investigation is postponed and a complete stroke occurs, surgical reconstruction will then be too late to have any effect on the patient's neurological state. Each patient requires the most careful individual clinical assessment.

After a completed stroke the aim of extracranial–intracranial bypass surgery is to prevent further vascular episodes but a month must be allowed after a recent stroke for recovery of damaged cerebral vessels. If there are bilateral carotid lesions, the side appropriate to the symptoms should be treated surgically irrespective of the degree of stenosis. If there are vertebrobasilar symptoms with signs of carotid stenosis it is reasonable to operate on the carotid lesion in order to increase flow through the circle of Willis.

Extracranial–intracranial bypass surgery

There is now growing experience of the extracranial–intracranial bypass anastomosis from the superficial temporal artery to a cortical branch of the middle cerebral artery. This has a small place in the treatment of patients with transient ischaemic attacks in whom there is a complete occlusion of the internal carotid artery or a lesion of the syphon or middle cerebral artery not amenable to direct surgery. Before surgery the neurological deficit should be stable but its potential reversibility after anastomosis may be assessed in special centres by the effect of hyperbaric oxygen on the deficit and also the affect of increasing systolic pressure on somatosensory evoked potentials. If positron emission tomography is available (p. 160), it is also possible to match the ^{15}O and the $C^{15}O_2$ scan, the ^{15}O scan reflecting extraction rates and so regional cerebral metabolism and a $C^{15}O_2$ scan reflecting regional cerebral blood flow. An area of high oxygen extraction with a low carbon dioxide extraction may be regarded as an indication of potentially reversible ischaemia (see Fig. 14.9).

HYPERTENSIVE ENCEPHALOPATHY

Aetiology, pathology, and pathological physiology

The term hypertensive encephalopathy is used to describe a form of cerebral disturbance occurring in disorders which differ in their pathology but possess a common tendency to cause arterial hypertension. This, and the fact that the onset of the encephalopathy is not uncommonly preceded by a rapid rise in the blood pressure, suggest that the disturbance of function is closely related to the hypertension. Experimental work suggests that the additional rise of blood pressure occurring in a patient already hypertensive in many cases results in focal arterial spasm, with anoxic damage to neurones and to the capillary walls. The commonest pathological finding is oedema of the brain, but this is not always present and seems likely to be a by-product of the pathological process and not the cause of the symptoms.

In hypertensives the lower level of autoregulation or maintenance of un-changed flow is reset from 60 mm Hg to 110 or higher, causing a higher threshold at which ischaemic symptoms occur on lowering blood pressure. In severe hypertension CBF may paradoxically increase, thus suggesting that the symptoms in malignant hypertension may be due to over-distension of vessels rather than spasm. After a stroke CBF studies have shown ischaemic foci, hyperaemic foci, and sometimes global loss of autoregulation, in different parts of the lesion. The rate of resolution of these changes suggests that resolving obstruction by thrombolysis is present in many cases of transient ischaemic attacks rather than haemodynamic crises as formerly assumed. During an epileptic seizure the CBF is increased up to threefold. In coma the cerebral blood flow may become immeasurably small, though without irrecoverable brain damage necessarily having occurred.

The age-incidence of hypertensive encephalopathy is that of the causal disorders. Acute glomerulonephritis is commonest in childhood, adolescence, and early adult life; chronic glomerulonephritis in the second and third decades; eclampsia during the early part of the child-bearing period; and malignant hypertension in the thirties and forties, though it may occur in childhood or late middle age. Lead encephalopathy in some respects resembles hypertensive encephalopathy.

Symptoms

The onset is usually subacute, the patient complaining of headaches of increasing severity, which are often associated with vomiting of a cerebral type. Epileptiform convulsions are common, and may be followed either by mental confusion or coma. Impairment of vision, or even complete blindness, may occur. Other focal cerebral disturbances include aphasia and hemiparesis.

Arterial hypertension is present in every case, but the blood pressure may not be greatly raised in acute nephritis and eclampsia. The retinae may be normal, or there may be bilateral papilloedema, with or without the exudative changes of hypertensive retinopathy, depending upon the causal condition. Both renal function and the composition of the urine may be normal, except when the encephalopathy complicates acute or chronic renal damage. The pressure of the cerebrospinal fluid is often increased, and it may be normal in composition or show a raised protein content.

Diagnosis

See page 322.

Prognosis

Alarming though the symptoms are, the outlook is on the whole good as to recovery from the cerebral disturbance, though the ultimate outlook depends upon the underlying cause. Most patients recover from encephalopathy complicating acute nephritis and from eclampsia. Even in malignant hypertension the patient may recover from the encephalopathy. Severe and frequent convulsions are a bad sign. Recovery from the amaurosis, aphasia, and other focal symptoms is usually complete in a few days.

Treatment

Since the arteriolar spasm upon which the symptoms depend is secondary to the hypertension, the object of treatment is in general to lower the hypertension, and for this purpose hypotensive drugs such as sodium nitroprusside under close control are used. Too rapid a reduction has led to blindness. Morphine may also be given, and barbiturates and diazepam if convulsions occur. If necessary cerebral oedema can be dealt with by administering hypertonic solutions (p. 18).

CEREBRAL EMBOLISM

Aetiology and pathology

Cerebral embolism is a variety of ischaemic cerebral disease in which the ischaemia develops acutely as the result of some substance, usually blood clot, being carried in the circulation to lodge in one or more of the cerebral vessels. Embolization from atheroma of extracranial vessels has already been discussed (p. 288). A now much rarer cause of cerebral embolism is mitral stenosis, and in most cases there is atrial fibrillation, the clot coming from the paralysed atrium. A clot may form on the mural endocardium after myocardial infarction or in association with the brady-tachycardia syndrome or a prolapsing mitral valve. Clots may also form in the heart after operation on one of the valves. Infected vegetations may become detached from the aortic or mitral valve in subacute bacterial endocarditis. Sterile emboli occur in 'marantic' endocarditis in severe debilitating diseases. The source of a thrombus may be in the lung. Infected emboli from the lungs are the cause of cerebral abscess complicating pulmonary infection, and tumour cells may pass in the same way from the lung to the brain.

The arteries of the left side of the brain are the site of embolism more frequently than those of the right, and the left middle cerebral is the vessel most often affected. The point at which the embolus lodges depends upon its size. After the lodgment of an embolus the vessel usually goes into spasm and thrombosis may occur in it. When the embolus is infected, meningitis or cerebral abscess may subsequently develop or, when the infection is of low virulence, embolism may be followed by infective softening of the vessel wall and aneurysm formation – mycotic aneurysm. The changes in the brain after cerebral embolism are those of infarction (p. 289). Fat embolism may occur as the result of fat globules being set free into the circulation after the fracture of one of the long bones, passing through the pulmonary circulation, and so reaching the brain.

Symptoms

The onset of symptoms of cerebral embolism with blood clot is extremely sudden, the lodgment of the embolus producing symptoms more rapidly than either cerebral haemorrhage or thrombosis. Loss of consciousness is not very common unless the carotid artery is blocked, but the patient is usually somewhat confused. A convulsion may occur at the onset, and there is usually headache. The nature of the focal symptoms depends on the vessel in which the embolus becomes impacted. After the onset of embolism there may be a gradual increase in the severity of the symptoms due to spasm of the vessel, the development of oedema, or the extension of thrombosis.

Diagnosis

The CT scan may show evidence of cerebral infarction and sometimes an occluded vessel. No carotid atheroma was found on angiography in 40 per cent of one series of patients with cerebral embolic events.

See also pages 287 and 322.

Prognosis

Cerebral embolism as such is rarely fatal, unless the embolus lodges in the internal carotid artery. There is always, however, the risk that embolism of other organs may occur, and the prognosis of the condition causing the embolism must be taken into consideration. As shock passes off, and the oedema of the infarcted area of the brain diminishes, the extent and severity of the symptoms grow less, and the patient is finally left with such disabilities as result from destruction of the region of the brain exclusively supplied by the obstructed artery. Epilepsy also is a not uncommon sequel.

Treatment

The prophylactic value of anticoagulants in patients liable to cerebral embolism now seems established. Treatment of the cerebral lesion is the same as that of cerebral infarction from any other cause though in view of the risk of further embolization a good case can be made for the immediate use of heparin, followed by a coumarin derivative. Alternatively, anticoagulants may be delayed for three weeks as their prior use may run the risk of causing haemorrhage in the infarcted areas. Rest for several weeks is essential in order to diminish the risk of further emboli occurring.

INTRACRANIAL HAEMORRHAGE

Intracranial haemorrhage may be classified according to its anatomical site into four varieties, namely:
  1. Extradural.
  2. Subdural.
  3. Subarachnoid.
  4. Intracerebral.

Extradural haemorrhage is almost invariably traumatic and need not be considered further, and subdural haemorrhage is discussed elsewhere (p. 281). Subarachnoid haemorrhage and intracerebral haemorrhage, though anatomically distinct, overlap pathologically because the same haemorrhage may involve both the brain substance and the subarachnoid space.

SUBARACHNOID HAEMORRHAGE

Aetiology and pathology

Subarachnoid haemorrhage may occur as the result of any condition in which there is rupture of one or more blood vessels so placed that the extravasated blood can reach the subarachnoid space. Massive subarachnoid haemorrhage is usually due either to rupture of an intracranial aneurysm, or bleeding from a cerebral angioma, or the extension of an intracerebral haemorrhage in a hypertensive patient into the subarachnoid space either directly or, more often, through the

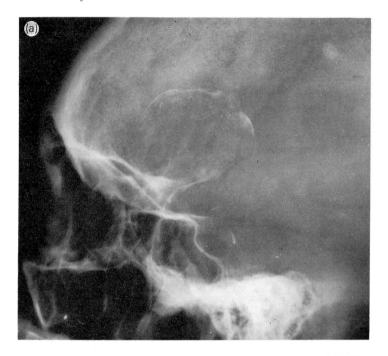

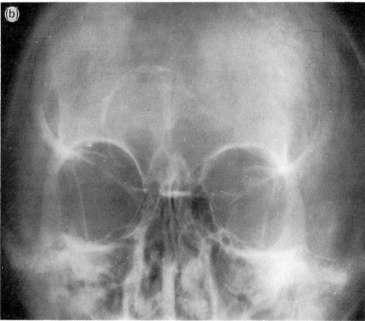

Fig. 14.10. Large calcified aneurysm of the anterior communicating artery. The lesion is usually large but the calcification is typically marginal. (a) Lateral view; (b) postero-anterior view.

ventricular system. Intracranial aneurysm is usually due to a congenital weakness in the media at the point of junction of two of the components of the circle of Willis, or at a bifurcation of one of the cerebral arteries (Figs. 14.10–14). Though the aneurysm may itself be congenital it is probable that it may develop at any period of life on the basis of the congenital structural deficiency. Whether hypertension plays a part in its causation is doubtful, but it may certainly contribute to its rupture. Congenital aneurysms may be single or multiple, and are most frequently encountered on the intracranial course of the internal carotid artery, on the middle cerebral artery, and at the junction of the anterior communicating with the anterior cerebral artery. The usual sites are either supraclinoid, at the origin of the posterior communicating artery, in which there is usually pain behind the eye and a third-nerve palsy or infraclinoid, causing pressure on the oculomotor nerves and a sympathetic paralysis because of involvement of the sympathetic plexus around the carotid artery. They range in size from smaller than a pin's head to 30 mm or more in diameter, but are usually about the size of a pea. They may be found at any age, and may even rupture in childhood, but more than half first cause symptoms between the ages of 40 and 55, and females suffer more often than males. A less common form of intracranial aneurysm which is nowadays becoming even rarer is a mycotic aneurysm caused by softening of the wall of an artery around an infected embolus which has reached it from the heart in subacute infective endocarditis. Such an aneurysm may also cause subarachnoid haemorrhage.

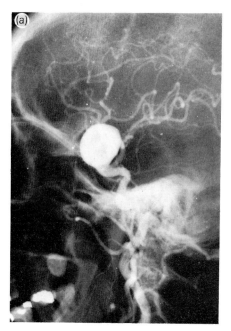 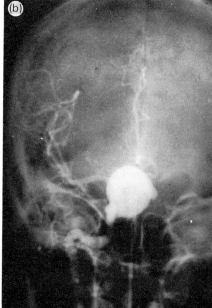

Fig. 14.11. Angiogram of large aneurysm which presented as a suprasellar mass. (a) Lateral view; (b) postero-anterior view.

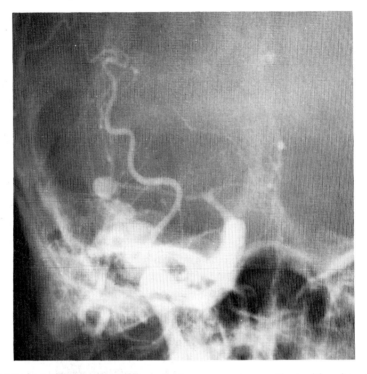

Fig. 14.12. Angiogram of middle cerebral aneurysm in a patient with subarachnoid haemorrhage showing local spasm of the terminal carotid and middle and anterior cerebral arteries.

Subarachnoid haemorrhage from a cerebral angioma is considerably less common than one from a ruptured aneurysm.

Subarachnoid haemorrhage from any cause spreads at first throughout the subarachnoid space from its point of origin and so extends into the subarachnoid space of the spinal cord. The haemorrhage may also invade the brain, which is especially common in the frontal lobe after rupture of an aneurysm at the junction of the anterior cerebral and anterior communicating arteries. There may also be areas of cerebral infarction. A cerebral angioma may also bleed simultaneously into the brain substance and into the subarachnoid space. Among the rarer causes of massive subarachnoid haemorrhage are the haemorrhagic diseases, and haemorrhage from an angioma of the spinal cord. In a small proportion of cases the source of the haemorrhage cannot be discovered.

Symptoms

The onset of subarachnoid haemorrhage from an intracranial aneurysm usually occurs without previous warning, but in a small proportion of cases there are focal symptoms produced by the aneurysm before rupture. There may be a

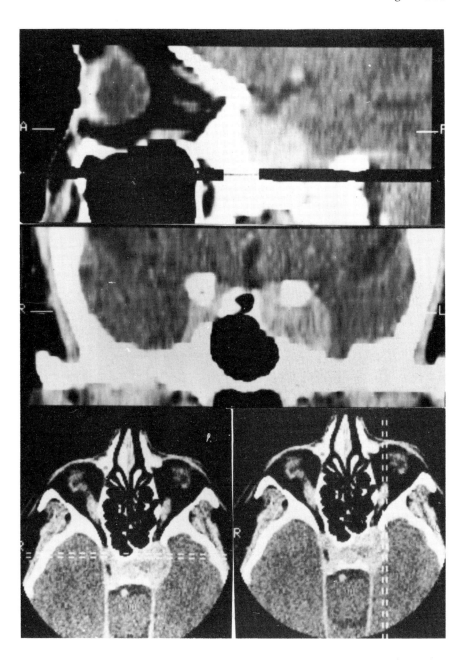

Fig. 14.13. CT scan of cavernous sinus aneurysm, with sagittal reconstruction (above) and coronal reconstruction (below); bottom, dotted lines show planes of reconstruction.

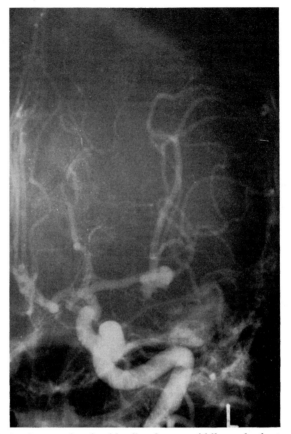

Fig. 14.14. Angiogram showing bleeding from a middle cerebral artery aneurysm.

history of migraine. Subarachnoid haemorrhage from a cerebral angioma may occur without previous warning, but is more often preceded by symptoms and signs of the cerebral lesion.

At one extreme subarachnoid haemorrhage may lead to immediate coma associated with profound shock, and cause death in a few hours, while at the other extreme it may cause only a headache which is not severe enough to interfere with the patient's occupation, and the cause of which is established only by examination of the cerebrospinal fluid. Loss of consciousness occurs rapidly when the leakage is considerable, and vomiting is not uncommon at the onset. In less severe cases the patient may not lose consciousness completely, but may pass into a semi-stuporose state, lying in an attitude of general flexion, resenting interference, and confused and irritable when roused. Headache is severe, and the presence of blood in the subarachnoid space produces signs of meningeal irritation, such as cervical rigidity and Kernig's sign. Moderate pyrexia is common at this stage.

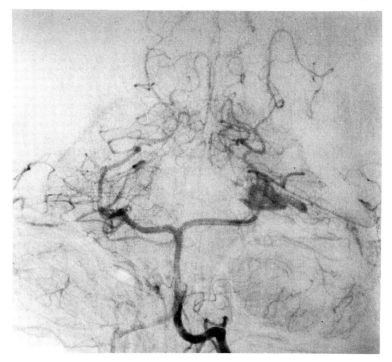

Fig. 14.15. Angiogram showing bleeding from cerebellar haemangioblastoma.

Changes are sometimes found in the fundus of the eye. Papilloedema is sometimes present, though slight in amount. Unilateral or bilateral retinal haemorrhages occur in some cases, and may be accompanied by subhyaloid or vitreous haemorrhages. Changes are most likely to be seen in the fundi when the subarachnoid haemorrhage is near the optic nerve (Plate 6(d)).

Other signs of subarachnoid haemorrhage include diminution or loss of the tendon reflexes, and of the abdominal reflexes, and extensor plantar responses in the absence of gross muscular weakness. Albuminuria and glycosuria occasionally occur.

Focal symptoms are due to compression of neighbouring cranial nerves by blood clot or to invasion of the cerebral hemisphere by the haemorrhage. The latter is likely to produce a crossed hemiplegia and increases the tendency to or the depth of coma.

Subarachnoid haemorrhage originating in the posterior fossa is likely to cause a degree of cervical rigidity disproportionate to the rest of the symptoms and may cause focal signs from disturbance of function of the cerebellum or one or more of the cranial nerves leaving the pons and medulla.

Diagnostic investigations

When the clinical diagnosis of subarachnoid haemorrhage has been made the next step, in order to confirm it, is to arrange for a CT brain scan (Figs. 14.16–18) which will confirm the presence of blood as certainly as examination of the spinal fluid, which was previously the critical diagnostic investigation. As in any form of intracerebral bleeding, a lumbar puncture is not without risk of causing possible fatal impaction of the brainstem in the foramen magnum ('coning'). A subarachnoid haemorrhage causes characteristic changes in the *cerebrospinal fluid*. The pressure is raised at first. In the first two or three days red cells are present, usually in sufficient amount to cause a deposit at the bottom of the test tube on standing. The supernatant fluid exhibits a yellow coloration which persists for from 2–3 weeks. The protein content of fluid is raised, though rarely above 0.1 g/l. Irritation of the meninges by the extravasated blood leads to a pleocytosis consisting usually of mononuclear cells. When polymorphonuclear cells are also present it usually means that the haemorrhage has invaded the substance of the brain.

A rupture of an intracerebral haemorrhage, due to hypertension, into the subarachnoid space or the ventricles may be very difficult to distinguish from a subarachnoid haemorrhage occurring in a hypertensive patient and invading one cerebral hemisphere. When the diagnosis of subarachnoid haemorrhage has been confirmed by CT scan or examination of the cerebrospinal fluid, therefore, it is necessary to exlude a ruptured aneurysm or a bleeding angioma as its cause. This may call for *angiography*, which raises the question of

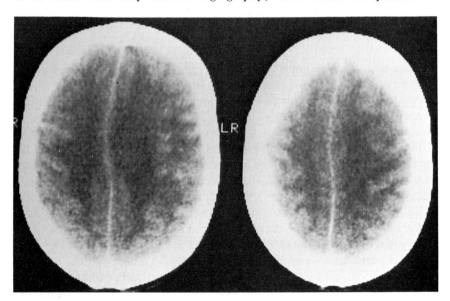

Fig. 14.16. CT scan showing blood over the surface of both hemispheres after a middle cerebral arterial haemorrhage.

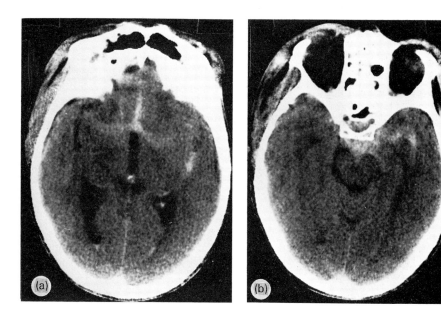

Fig. 14.17. Subarachnoid haemorrhage: (a) blood in right insular region and inter-hemisphere fissure; (b) blood in interpeduncular fissure and around right middle cerebral artery.

whether this should be done in every case, and if so when. There is a difference of opinion about this, some surgeons recommending that carotid angiography should be performed in every case of subarachnoid haemorrhage as soon as the diagnosis is made, while others are more selective. The rational answer seems to be that if there is a possibility that a life-saving surgical operation may be carried out as the result of information yielded by angiography, angiography should be performed. If, on the other hand, this is not the case because it is thought that the patient is too ill to stand operation or that either angiography or the operation is fraught with greater risks than expectant treatment, as may be the case particularly in patients over the age of 60 with evident atheroma, angiography should be postponed. There is no doubt, however, that surgery carried out sufficiently early may save lives which would otherwise be lost.

Carotid angiography may show not only the site, size, and shape of the aneurysm (see Fig. 14.12) but also whether, as sometimes happens, there is an associated spasm of important arteries which may be contributing to the clinical picture. A carotid angiogram which does not show an aneurysm on one

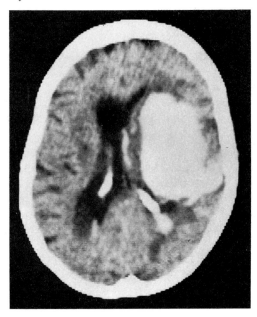

Fig. 14.18. CT scan showing intraventricular haemorrhage with blood in the ventricles and shift of midline to left.

occasion may nevertheless do so if repeated some days later. Carotid angiography will almost always show an aneurysm (see Figs. 14.10–14) if it is present. If neither an aneurysm nor an angioma is demonstrated by carotid angiography on either side, the possibility that the subarachnoid haemorrhage arises from an aneurysm or angioma in the posterior fossa should be considered (Fig. 14.15). It may be necessary to carry out vertebral angiography to demonstrate this. In some patients more than one aneurysm may be demonstrated. The clinical signs and angiographic appearances then usually indicate the aneurysm which is likely to have leaked. In some 10 per cent of patients with subarachnoid haemorrhage, investigated by carotid and vertebral angiography, no site of haemorrhage can be demonstrated. In some of these patients a subsequent haemorrhage, perhaps years later, may indicate that the first haemorrhage was likely to have occurred from an aneurysm which was not demonstrated at that time.

Diagnosis

See pages 287 and 322.

Prognosis

The prognosis of subarachnoid haemorrhage depends upon a number of factors – the size and site of the leakage, whether it can be found and treated surgically, the age of the patient, and the condition of the cardiovascular system, especially the presence or absence of hypertension and cerebral atheroma. The first rupture may prove fatal, or the patient may survive a series. About one-third of all patients with subarachnoid haemorrhage not surgically treated die in the first attack. About one-half of the survivors have a recurrence, in which two-thirds die. Most of these fatal recurrences occur within two to four weeks of the first attack: 90 per cent of those who survive for a month are alive at the end of a year, but the risk of a fatal haemorrhage remains. The prognosis as to recovery from an attack of subarachnoid haemorrhage must be based upon evidence as to whether the haemorrhage has been arrested. Increasing depth of unconsciousness, rising pulse and respiratory rate, and an increasing fever are bad signs, and the prognosis is worse when the cerebral hemisphere has been invaded. If after the haemorrhage appears to have stopped the patient fails to show signs of improvement within 48 hours, the outlook is bad. Even after recovery from the immediate effects of rupture, if the hemisphere has been invaded the prognosis is that of cerebral haemorrhage from any cause.

Treatment

The most urgent question is the suitability of the patient for surgery, which must be considered in the light of the angiographic findings if he has been considered suitable for angiography. The object of surgical treatment is to occlude the aneurysm by a clip or ligation if the aneurysm is accessible. Most surgeons favour carotid ligation for aneurysms of the terminal part of the carotid artery because of their inaccessibility, provided the patient is fairly alert and able to tolerate compression of the carotid artery in the neck on the same side for ten minutes. Middle cerebral artery aneurysms are usually tackled directly, preferably by clipping the neck of the aneurysm. So far aneurysms of the anterior cerebral artery have proved least easy to treat surgically. If the patient's level of consciousness deteriorates gradually watch must be kept for the development of communicating hydrocephalus which may need shunting (see p. 271). Hyponatraemia due to inappropriate antidiuretic hormone (ADH) secretion is a recognized complication of subarachnoid haemorrhage and can also lead to coma and fits. Recently the beneficial effects have been reported from the use of beta-adrenergic blockage in reducing cerebral arterial spasm. In the acute stage surgeons now use antifibrinolytic agents in the hope of reducing the incidence of bleeding but their benefit has not been proved in controlled trials. Aminocaproic acid with anexamic acid has been used. If comatose, the patient should be treated along the usual lines (p. 178). Headache will require analgesics, and if very troublesome may respond to a second lumbar puncture carried out a few days after the first. The patient should be kept completely at rest in bed for three weeks, and then if there has been no evidence of a recurrence, allowed to move about in bed and begin to get up at the end of another week. He must be advised to lead a quiet life as far as possible and avoid any activity likely to raise the blood pressure. The bowels should be regulated to prevent straining.

CEREBRAL HAEMORRHAGE

Aetiology and pathology

The commonest cause of cerebral haemorrhage is hypertension and the associated changes in the vessel walls. These have been much discussed and probably are not the same in every case. The most important are probably lipohyaline changes in muscle spasm, and atheroma with medial degeneration, both caused by microaneurysms. Cerebral haemorrhage is most likely to occur in the neighbourhood of the internal capsule, in the cerebellum, or in the pons. A capsular haemorrhage may burst into one lateral ventricle, or, much less frequently, into the subarachnoid space. After a large intracerebral haemorrhage the affected hemisphere is larger than the opposite one, and the convolutions are flattened. The site of haemorrhage is occupied by a red clot, and the surrounding tissues are compressed and may be oedematous. Later, if the patient survives, the clot is absorbed and may be replaced by a neuroglial scar, or by a cavity containing yellow serous fluid. Multiple haemorrhages sometimes occur.

Hypertensive cerebral haemorrhage usually occurs in late middle life. It is comparatively rare in younger hypertensives, and the vascular changes of old age more often lead to ischaemic cerebral infarction. Males suffer from cerebral haemorrhage more often than females, and a familial incidence is common.

Cerebral haemorrhage occurring in the first half of adult life is likely to be the result of a congenital vascular abnormality, either an angioma or an aneurysm. Other causes of cerebral haemorrhage include trauma and thrombocytopenic purpura. Petechial haemorrhages may occur in the brain in toxic and inflammatory states.

Symptoms

The onset of a cerebral haemorrhage is always sudden. The actual rupture of the vessel may be brought about by mental excitement or physical effort, or may occur during rest or sleep. Usually the patient complains of sudden severe headache and may vomit. He becomes dazed, and in all but the mildest cases loses consciousness in a few minutes. Convulsions may occur at the onset, but are exceptional. The physical signs produced by a cerebral haemorrhage depend upon its situation and its size.

Haemorrhage in the region of the internal capsule

The patient is usually unconscious, and there is often slight pyrexia. The pulse rate is generally slow – 50 to 60 – and the pulse full and bounding. The respirations are deep and stertorous, and the respiratory rate may be either slow or quickened, or there may be Cheyne–Stokes respiration. The head is usually rotated and the eyes are deviated towards the side of the lesion. This is due to paralysis of rotation of the head and of conjugate deviation of the eyes to the opposite side, as a consequence of unbalanced action of the undamaged cerebral hemisphere. The optic discs are usually normal, though slight papilloedema is not uncommon, and may or may not be accompanied by hypertensive retinopathy. The pupils may be unequal, but react to light unless that patient is very deeply comatose. A divergent squint is common. The corneal reflex is often lost on the side opposite to the lesion and will be lost on both sides when coma is profound.

A capsular haemorrhage causes paralysis of the opposite side of the body, but the comatose patient cannot be asked to carry out voluntary movements, so it is necessary to resort to indirect methods of demonstrating paralysis. Flattening of the nasolabial furrow may be evident on the paralysed side, and the cheek is usually distended more on the paralysed than on the normal side during expiration. If the patient is not too deeply comatose it may be observed that he moves the limbs spontaneously on the normal but not on the paralysed side. At first, after the haemorrhage, the limbs on the paralysed side are hypotonic and the arm and leg, if lifted up, fall to the bed inertly, whereas even in deep coma the normal arm and leg subside much more gradually. Pricking with a pin even in an unconscious patient usually causes contraction of the muscles of the face and movements of withdrawal of the limb which is pricked. These movements do not occur on the paralysed side. The absence of such movements, however, may also be due to hemianalgesia. This may often be demonstrated by the fact that reflex contraction of the facial muscles occurs when the patient is pricked on the normal side of the body but not when he is pricked on the analgesic side. The tendon reflexes are variable. They may be much diminished or abolished on the paralysed side, but sometimes they are exaggerated. The plantar reflex on that side is extensor. On the other side it may be flexor, or in deep coma extensor. Retention or incontinence of urine and faeces is the rule as long as the patient is unconscious.

Haemorrhage into the ventricles

If a haemorrhage in the region of the internal capsule bursts into the lateral ventricle, coma deepens and the signs of a pyramidal lesion are usually present on both sides of the body. There is often a tendency for the upper limbs to exhibit a posture of rigid extension, and cervical rigidity is likely to occur. The temperature frequently exhibits a marked terminal rise.

Pontine haemorrhage

If the patient is seen soon after the onset of a pontine haemorrhage the signs may be those of a unilateral lesion of the pons, namely facial paralysis on the side of the lesion with flaccid paralysis of the limbs on the opposite side. Owing to paralysis of conjugate ocular deviation and of rotation of head to the side of the lesion the patient lies with his head and eyes turned towards the side of the paralysed limbs. Even when the signs at the outset are those of a unilateral lesion of the pons, extension of the haemorrhage soon involves the opposite side, or the signs may be bilateral from the beginning. When both sides of the pons are thus affected there is paralysis of the face and limbs on both sides with bilateral extensor plantar reflexes. Marked contraction of the pupils – 'pinpoint pupils' – the result of bilateral destruction of the ocular sympathetic fibres, is characteristic of a pontine haemorrhage and there is often a terminal hyper-pyrexia.

Cerebellar haemorrhage

This is usually sudden with occipital headache and vomiting, and, sooner or later, loss of consciousness. Localizing signs are often absent.

The cerebrospinal fluid

Red blood cells are likely to be present in the fluid, and visible blood if the haemorrhage has ruptured into a ventricle or the subarachnoid space. As in a case of subarachnoid haemorrhage, lumbar puncture may be hazardous (see p. 147).

CT and NMR scanning in the diagnosis of cerebral haemorrhage

An acute intracerebral haematoma has increased density (see Figs. 14.4 and 14.16). Extradural haematomas have a convex appearance in contrast to a sub-dural haematoma which is more extensive and crescentic. Chronic subdural haematomas have an irregular striated appearance, the least dense areas cor-responding to a c.s.f. density. Intracerebral haematomas can always be identi-fied by increased density whereas chronic subdural haematomas have reduced density. In the main the CT brain scan has replaced cerebral angiography in the assessment of head injuries as virtually no false-positive or false-negative results for intra-cerebral haemorrhage have been observed after head injuries. CT scanning is also the best measure of subarachnoid bleeding and is in this situa-tion replacing the need for a lumbar puncture (see Fig. 14.17). Intracerebral haematomas are gradually absorbed between 10 and 30 days. Cerebral contu-sions have a 'pepper and salt' appearance. If a 'normal' pressure hydrocephalus is developing the scan will show enlarged cerebral ventricles.

Prognosis

A cerebral haemorrhage may prove rapidly fatal. A patient with a pontine haemorrhage or capsular haemorrhage which bursts into one lateral ventricle is unlikely to survive more than a day or two, a progressive haemorrhage in these sites proving fatal by causing brainstem compression. If the haemorrhage is continuing there is a progressive deepening of coma, indicated by inability to rouse a formerly responsive patient, and loss of the corneal and pupillary reflexes. The pulse tends to become rapid and irregular; the respiratory rate is often irregular and finally becomes rapid and shallow, and both the temperature and the blood pressure tend to rise. Bilateral paralysis of limbs is a bad prognostic sign, as is the presence of blood visible to the naked eye in the cerebrospinal fluid. In the past, a haemorrhage which ceased but left the patient unconscious for more than 48 hours was often fatal, but modern methods of treating and nursing the unconscious patient have made it possible in many cases to maintain the patient in a good state of nutrition for a long time and so make it possible for some patients who would previously have died to survive. However, if a patient shows no signs of recovery of consciousness within a week of the onset of the haemorrhage, the prospect of survival is poor. When the patient has recovered consciousness the degree of permanent disability will depend upon the situation of the haemorrhage and the extent of the resulting destruction of the brain tissue. With the disappearance of neural shock and oedema of surrounding areas of the brain some improvement may be expected in most cases. The mental efficiency of the patient is rarely as good after a cerebral haemorrhage as before. When a capsular haemorrhage has caused hemiplegia, some return of power always occurs in the lower limb, so that the patient is likely to be able to walk. If the upper limb exhibits some return of power at the end of a month, a considerable degree of recovery of movement at the larger joints will probably occur in it. If, however, there is no improvement at the end of three months, the paralysis is likely to be permanent. In any case movements of the hand recover last and least. When there is permanent loss of postural sensibility in the paralysed limb a useful degree of recovery is less likely, walking especially being much more difficult when sensation in the lower limb is impaired. Pain of thalamic origin on the opposite side of the body is a troublesome but fortunately relatively uncommon sequel of a capsular haemorrhage. The same is true of involuntary movements such as tremor and athetosis. Trophic changes are common in the paralysed limbs. The extremities are often cyanosed, and some oedema is common. The larger joints may be swollen and painful.

Treatment

The rational treatment of a cerebral haemorrhage would be the evacuation of the clot and control of the bleeding point, but the scope of surgery in treatment is still limited. The age of most patients, the extent of the damage caused by the haemorrhage, together with the oedema of neighbouring tissues, the condition of the rest of the cerebral circulation and of the cardiovascular system generally, all militate against successful surgery. Nevertheless, when these conditions are more favourable, especially when cerebral haemorrhage occurs before middle life, and may come from a congenital vascular abnormality or may be cerebellar in site, surgery should always be considered. Lumbar puncture aimed at lowering the intracranial pressure is probably not without risk. The intravenous injection of dexamethasone or a hypertonic solution, however, may do good by reducing cerebral oedema. If the patient is unconscious he should be treated as recommended on page 178. After recovery from the immediate effects of the haemorrhage, physiotherapy should be begun, special stress being laid upon passive movements at all joints. Orthopaedic supports for the affected limbs may be required as for a hemiparesis from any cause.

THE DIAGNOSIS OF LESIONS OF THE CEREBRAL ARTERIES

The diagnosis of lesions of the cerebral arteries covers a large part of the neurology of middle age and old age. The symptoms of such lesions may be those of:
1. Coma.
2. Meningeal irritation of sudden onset.
3. A focal cerebral lesion of sudden onset.
4. A focal cerebral lesion of insidious onset.
5. Recurrent cerebral lesions either in the same or in different areas.
6. Diffuse and progressive lesions.

Coma

For the diagnosis of coma see page 170.

Meningeal irritation of sudden onset

Subarachnoid haemorrhage is the only cerebral vascular lesion which leads to meningeal irritation of sudden onset, and which may therefore be confused with meningitis. Subarachnoid haemorrhage, however, is in most cases much more rapid in onset than meningitis, and the patient, though febrile, does not present the toxic appearance of a patient with an infection. The diagnosis can be rapidly settled by examination of the cerebrospinal fluid.

Focal cerebral lesions of sudden onset

Vascular causes of a focal cerebral lesion of sudden onset include hypertensive cerebral haemorrhage, haemorrhage from a ruptured aneurysm or angioma invading the substance of the hemisphere, thrombosis of a large artery, especially the internal carotid or middle cerebral artery, and embolism of one of these vessels. Coma is more likely to be present, and, if present, deeper in cerebral haemorrhage than in cerebral thrombosis or embolism, unless the internal carotid artery is occluded. Hypertension on the whole favours haemorrhage. When haemorrhage from an aneurysm invades the hemisphere it is almost always associated with subarachnoid haemorrhage. Cerebral embolism is rare without a demonstrable source for the embolus. The possibility the syphilitic endarteritis is the cause of hemiplegia, especially in the first half of adult life, should be borne in mind and can be excluded by serological tests. Endarteritis may also be the cause of hemiplegia in meningitis, especially tuberculous meningitis. Hemiplegia sometimes develops suddenly in general paresis, the usual physical signs of which will then be present. Transient hemiplegia of sudden onset may occur in migraine, when the diagnosis rests upon its association with the familiar symptoms of migraine, and the rapid recovery without residual symptoms or signs. Intracranial tumour rarely causes a sudden focal lesion; when this occurs it is probably usually due to a vascular disturbance, e.g. haemorrhage, associated with the neoplasm. Thus almost all focal cerebral lesions of sudden onset are in one way or another vascular in origin. An exception is multiple sclerosis, in which, however, it is rare for a lesion of sudden onset to cause a gross disturbance of function such as hemiplegia.

Focal cerebral lesions of insidious onset

Ischaemic brain disease, especially atheroma of one internal carotid artery, may cause a progressive focal lesion of gradual onset which it may be difficult to distinguish from a neoplasm. Conversely, a glioma in an elderly atheromatous subject sometimes progresses so slowly and with so little evidence of increased intracranial pressure as closely to simulate a cerebral vascular lesion. In cases like these the diagnosis can often be made only with the help of accessory methods of investigation such as computerized axial tomography, isotope encephalography, and angiography.

Recurrent cerebral lesions

Recurrent episodes of disturbance of cerebral function within the territory of a single artery occurring in an elderly person are characteristic of atheroma of that vessel, or the clinical picture may take the form of successive lesions involving different parts of the brain. These syndromes are unlikely to be confused with any other condition, but occasionally a glioma may simulate the former, while multiple metastatic neoplasms may produce symptoms resembling those of multiple vascular lesions. Again the accessory methods of investigation, combined with a careful search for a primary neoplasm, will usually enable the correct diagnosis to be made.

Diffuse and progressive lesions

The failure of the intellectual powers and impairment of memory characteristic of diffuse arteriosclerosis of the smaller cerebral vessels may simulate dementia due to any other cause (see p. 259). General paresis is distinguished by the characteristic physical signs, and positive Wassermann reactions in the blood and cerebrospinal fluid, in which there are also other characteristic changes.

Haemorrhage from arteriovenous malformations (see also p. 225)

Arteriorvenous malformations are a tangled group of blood vessels with both feeding arteries and draining veins. Several major arteries may supply the malformation. Smaller malformations which may present with epilepsy rather than haemorrhage may be associated with the congenital disorder ataxia telangectasia (p. 28), Sturge–Weber disease, and Von Hipple–Lindau disease. The bleeding from such malformations is under lower pressure than congenital arterial aneurysms and hence the mortality is lower. The malformation can usually be diagnosed from the CT scan, though angiography to identify the feeding arteries, often vertebral as well as carotid, is likely to be necessary. Surgery may be possible with the development of microsurgery and embolization techniques. Arteriovenous malformations are sometimes dural in site and may involve the blood supply from basal arteries and cause cranial nerve lesions, especially the third or sixth.

THE CEREBRAL VENOUS CIRCULATION

The venous sinuses

Within the brain the blood passes from the cerebral capillaries into the veins which drain into the venous sinuses. These, which are lined with endothelium, lie between layers of the dura matter. They communicate with the meningeal veins, and by emissary veins with the veins of the scalp. The *superior sagittal sinus* begins anteriorly at the crista galli and passes upwards, backwards, and finally downwards at the convex upper margin of the falx to end at the level of the internal occipital protuberance by turning, usually to the left transverse sinus. The superior sagittal sinus receives the superior group of superficial cerebral veins, and thus drains the upper part of the cerebral hemispheres. *The inferior sagittal sinus* lies in the free lower border of the falx for its posterior two-thirds, and terminates posteriorly by joining the great cerebral vein to form the *straight sinus,* which passes between layers of the dura along the line of junction of the falx with the tentorium and then turns to the left to become the left transverse sinus. The *transverse sinuses* arise posteriorly, the right from the superior sagittal sinus, the left from the straight sinus, and pass laterally and forwards in the attached border of the tentorium lying in a groove in the occipital bone. Each then turns downwards on the inner surface of the mastoid process, and leaves the skull by the jugular foramen to enter the internal jugular vein.

The *cavernous sinuses* lie on either side of the body of the sphenoid. They receive the ophthalmic veins and terminate posteriorly at the apex of the petrous portion of the temporal bone by dividing into superior and inferior petrosal sinuses. In the lateral wall of the cavernous sinus lie the internal carotid artery with its sympathetic plexus, the third and fourth nerves, the first and second divisions of the fifth nerve, and the sixth nerve (Plate 7). The *superior petrosal sinuses* run backwards and laterally from the cavernous sinus along the attached edge of the tentorium to end in the transverse sinuses. The *inferior petrosal sinuses* run from the cavernous sinuses backwards, outwards and downwards in the posterior fossa to join the internal jugular veins by passing through the jugular foramina. The superior and inferior petrosal sinuses receive the inferior cerebral veins which drain the lower halves of the hemispheres.

THROMBOSIS OF THE INTRACRANIAL VENOUS SINUSES AND VEINS

Aetiology and pathology

Primary sinus thrombosis is rare, and is chiefly seen at the extremes of life in wasted debilitated infants, and in cachectic conditions. Secondary sinus thrombosis may be the result of direct injury of a sinus through fracture of the skull or other trauma, or of spread of infection from some neighbouring site. The transverse sinus may thus become infected from mastoiditis, and the superior sagittal and cavernous sinuses may be involved in spread of infection from the skin of the face or scalp or nasal sinuses. Thrombosis may occur in the puerperium about the tenth day.

The affected sinus contains a reddish clot which may become purulent. Thrombosis may extend into tributary veins or other sinuses. The area of brain drained by the affected sinus exhibits congestive oedema, and in some cases softening. Meningitis, cerebral abscess, and septicaemia are occasional complications.

Symptoms

Cavernous sinus thrombosis leads to pain in the eye and forehead, exophthalmos, sometimes papilloedema, and paresis of the third, fourth, and sixth cranial nerves. It readily extends through the circular sinus to the opposite side. *Transverse sinus thrombosis* usually causes few focal cerebral symptoms. Papilloedema may be present, and slight signs of a corticospinal tract lesion on the opposite side of the body. *Thrombosis of the superior sagittal sinus* usually leads to a considerable rise of intracranial pressure, with headache, vomiting and papilloedema. There is often congestion of the veins of the scalp. Convulsions may occur, together with paraplegia due to infarction of the upper part of the cerebral hemispheres. In some cases the only symptoms are those of increased intracranial pressure. *Cortical thrombophlebitis*, which may be secondary to infection of the middle ear and mastoid, may cause focal convulsions and paresis.

The cerebrospinal fluid is likely to be under increased pressure, and when sinus thrombophlebitis leads to cerebral infarction the protein content of the fluid may be considerably raised, and the fluid may be yellow and even contain red blood cells. The presence of a slight excess of leucocytes, usually both polymorphonuclear and mononuclear, is not uncommon. When one transverse sinus is filled with clot, the pressure of the cerebrospinal fluid may fail to show the normal rise when the jugular vein on the affected side is compressed alone in Queckenstedt's test.

Diagnosis

The diagnosis of primary sinus thrombosis depends upon the characteristic distribution of the symptoms and signs and changes in the cerebrospinal fluid in the presence of a predisposing condition. Blood should be taken for culture.

Infective thrombophlebitis can be distinguished from meningitis as a rule by examination of the fluid. The diagnosis from cerebral abscess may be more difficult on clinical grounds, but is distinguished by CT scanning (see Fig. 12.1). Carotid angiography may demonstrate failure of one of the larger sinuses to fill, or alternatively may provide evidence of a space-occupying lesion.

Prognosis

Thrombosis of one of the major cerebral sinuses is a serious condition, but the prognosis has been considerably improved by modern methods of treatment. In primary sinus thrombosis the outlook is poor because the condition is usually a complication of a pre-existing state which is itself serious. In secondary thrombosis recovery may occur, provided the causal condition can be adequately treated and the thrombosis is not so extensive as to have caused severe cerebral damage. Even so, some residual disability, including epilepsy, may remain.

Treatment

In primary thrombosis anticoagulants may be called for, though their use may not be without risk of haemorrhage from an area of cerebral infarction. In secondary thrombosis the appropriate systemic chemotherapy should be used, combined if necessary with surgical treatment of the causal condition. Anticoagulants are unlikely to be required.

REFERENCES

Barnett, H.J.M., Jones, M.Q., Boughner, D.R., and Kostuck, W.J. (1976). Cerebral ischaemic events associated with prolapsing mitral valve. *Archs Neurol.* **33**, 777–82.

Caplan, L.R. and Schoene, W.C. (1978). Clinical features of subcortical arteriosclerotic encephalopathy (Binswanger's disease). *Neurology, Minneap.* **28**, 1206–15.

Christensen, P.C., Ovitt, T.W., Fisher, H.D., Frost, M.M., Nudelman, S., and Roehig, H. (1980). Intravenous angiography using digital video subtraction: intravenous cervico-cerebrovascular angiography. *Am. J. Neuroradiol.* **1**, 379–86.

Debono, D.P. and Warlow, C.P. (1981). Potential sources of emboli in patients with presumed transient cerebral or retinal ischaemia. *Lancet* **i**, 343–6.

Drake, C.G. (1981). Management of cerebral aneurysm. *Stroke* **12**, 273–83.

Garraway, W.M., Akhtar, A.J., Hockey, L., and Prescott, R.J. (1980). Management of acute stroke in the elderly: follow-up of a controlled trial. *Br. med. J.* **281**, 827–9.

Garraway, W.M., Whisnant, J.P., Kurland, L.T., and O'Fallon, W.M. (1979). Changing pattern of cerebral infarction 1945–74. *Stroke* **10**, 657–62.

Gillingham, F.J., Mawdsley, C., and Williams, A.E. (eds.) (1976). *Stroke.* Churchill Livingstone, Edinburgh.

Harrison, M.J.G. (1980). Vascular surgery. Surgery for ischaemic stroke. *Br. J. hosp. Med.* **24**, 108–12.

Harrison, M.J.G., Pollock, S., Kendall, B.E., and Marshall, J. (1981). Effect of haematocrit on carotid stenosis and cerebral infarction. *Lancet* **ii**, 114–15.

Harrison, M.J.G. and Marshall, J. (1975). Indications for angiography and surgery in carotid artery disease. *Br. med. J.* **i**, 616–18.

Hutchinson, E.C. and Acheson, E.J. (1975). *Strokes: natural history, pathology and surgical treatment.* Saunders, Philadelphia.

Licht, S. (1975). *Stroke and its rehabilitation.* Licht, New Haven, Conn.

Mendelow, A.D., Karmi, M.Z., Paul, K.S., Fuller, G.A.G., and Gillingham, F.J. (1979). Extradural haematoma: effect of delayed treatment. *Br. med. J.* **i**, 1240–2.

Meyer, J.S. and Shaw, T. (1982). *Diagnosis and management of stroke and TIAs.* Addison-Wesley, Menlo Park, California.

Millikan, C.H. and McDowell, F.H. (1981). Treatment of progressing stroke. *Stroke* **12**, 397–409.

Millikan, C.H. and McDowell, F.H. (1978). Treatment of transient ischaemic attacks. *Stroke* **9**, 299–308.

Ramirez-Lassepas, M. (1984). Antifibrinolytic therapy in subarachnoid haemorrhage caused by ruptured intracranial aneurysm. *Neurology, Minneap.* **31**, 316–22.

Ross Russell, W.R. (1983). *Vascular disease of the central nervous system,* 2nd edn. Churchill Livingstone, Edinburgh.

Samson, D.S., Hodosh, R.M., and Clark, W.K. (1979). Microsurgical treatment of transient cerebral ischaemia. *J. Am. med. Ass.* **241**, 376–8.

Shuping, J.R., Rollinson, R.D., and Toole, J.F. (1980). Transient global amnesia. *Ann. Neurol.* **7**, 281–5.

Stein, B. and Wolpert, A. (1980). Arteriovenous malformation of the brain: I Current concepts and treatment. *Archs Neurol.* **37**, 1–5.

Sundt, T.M. Jr and Whisnant, J.P. (1978). Subarachnoid hemorrhage from intracranial aneurysms. Surgical management and natural history of disease. *New Engl. J. Med.* **299**, 166–222.

Thomas, D.J. (1977). Effect of haematocrit on cerebral blood-flow in man. *Lancet* **ii**, 941–3.

Warlow, C.P. (1982). Transient ischaemic attacks. In *Recent advances in clinical neurology* (ed. W.B. Matthews and G.H. Glaser). Churchill Livingstone, Edinburgh.

Walter, P., Neil-Dwyer, G., and Cruickshank, J.M. (1982). Beneficial effects of adrenergic blockage in patients with subarachnoid haemorrhage. *Br. med. J.* **284**, 1661–4.

Weisberg, L.A. (1979). Computerized tomography in intracranial hemorrhage. *Archs Neurol.* **36**, 422–6.

Wilson, L.A. and Ross Russell, R.W. (1977). Amaurosis fugax and carotid artery disease: indications for angiography. *Br. med. J.* **ii**, 435–7.

Wintzen, A.R. (1980). The clinical course of subdural haematoma. *Brain* **103**, 855–67.

15 Diplegia and hemiplegia in childhood

CONGENITAL DIPLEGIA

Aetiology and pathology

The term congenital diplegia, or Little's disease, is now used to include a group of cases characterized by bilateral and more or less symmetrical disturbances of motility which are present from birth and which subsequently remain stationary or show a tendency towards improvement. Though commonly the lesion involves chiefly the corticospinal tracts, causing weakness and spasticity, which are most conspicuous in the lower limbs, mental defect, involuntary movements, and ataxia may be present either in association with spastic weakness or as the sole manifestations of the cerebral lesion.

There is no doubt that the causes of congenital diplegia are multiple. Earlier theories implicating brain injury or asphyxia at birth are now widely held, but it is believed that the damage, sometimes probably viral, occurs comparatively early in foetal life, and that an arrest of development or an actual degeneration of certain parts of the brain occurs *in utero*. Occasionally there is a gross maldevelopment. Two stages of normal brain development are shown in Fig. 15.1.

The commonest pathological finding has received the name of atrophic lobar sclerosis, and is characterized by a symmetrical atrophy of both cerebral hemispheres with destruction of nerve cells and glial proliferation. Microcephaly, when present, is the result of the cerebral hypoplasia and not its cause. Congenital diplegia is only exceptionally familial. Though usually not strictly congenital, erythroblastosis foetalis (see p. 333) may cause identical symptoms.

Symptoms

The symptoms depend upon the predominant situation of the lesions. In classic Little's disease, or spastic diplegia, there are bilateral weakness and spasticity, often remarkably symmetrical. Although the child is slow in reaching the usual landmarks of development, the spasticity does not usually become apparent until about the end of the first year of life. The lower limbs are always more severely affected than the upper, and become rigid in a position of plantar flexion of the ankle, extension of the knee, and adduction and internal rotation of the hip, the spasm being made worse by the child's attempts to stand and walk. Contractures develop in the spastic muscles, and the distribution of the hypertonia leads to a characteristic 'scissors gait' in which, owing to the adduction of the hips, the knees may rub together or be actually crossed. The

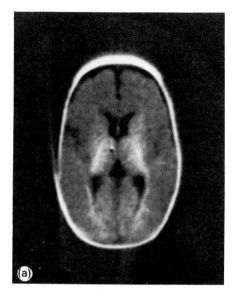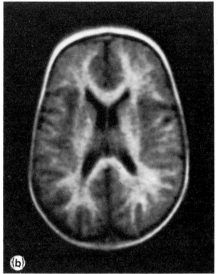

Fig. 15.1. Normal infant (a) six months old and (b) 20 months old: NMR(IR) scans show the normal process of myelination.

tendon reflexes in the lower limbs are much exaggerated and the plantar reflexes are extensor. The abdominal reflexes are frequently brisk in spite of the severity of the corticospinal tract lesion. Sensation is usually unimpaired.

In some cases involuntary movement, athetosis, chorea, or a blend of the two, are the predominant symptoms (these are described on page 93). Sometimes the clinical picture is that of cerebellar deficiency. Mental defect may accompany any form of congenital diplegia. Most diplegic children show some retardation of skeletal and sexual development. Epilepsy occurs in a small proportion of cases.

Diagnosis

Before spasticity develops, diagnosis may be difficult, and the condition has to be distinguished from simple mental defect and from congenital muscular disorders (p. 43). When spasticity has developed there is usually no difficulty in distinguishing congenital diplegia from the rare progressive degenerative disorders of infancy, since the diplegic child tends to remain stationary or to show slow improvement. In any child with apparent mental defect, screening for inherited biochemical defects is essential and may reveal diseases such as galactosaemia, phenylketonuria, fructosuria, Hartnup disease or maple syrup disease. Phenylketonuria can now be treated by a diet low in phenylalanine, galactosaemia by a lactose-free diet.

The CT or NMR scan may show evidence of unilateral cortical atrophy with ventricular dilation or possibly a calcified subdural, epidural, or intracerebral haemorrhage.

Prognosis

The prognosis depends upon the severity of the disorder and especially upon the degree of mental defect present. There is usually a very slow improvement in the motor symptoms, but this depends chiefly upon the mental state of the patient. In favourable cases it may be expected that a child will learn to walk even though it may not do so until it is five or six years old.

Treatment

Treatment consists essentially in the education of movement and the promotion of muscular relaxation combined with the removal as far as possible of the obstacles which result from contractures and deformities.

CONGENITAL AND INFANTILE HEMIPLEGIA

Aetiology and pathology

Congenital hemiplegia means hemiplegia which is present at birth. Infantile hemiplegia means hemiplegia acquired during the first few years of life, not necessarily during infancy. This is not a very logical distinction, however, since congenital hemiplegia may be due to a lesion acquired during birth. Indeed, an intracranial vascular lesion so produced is probably a common cause. Prematurity and postmaturity may be factors. Less frequently there is a congenital cerebral deformity, such as true porencephaly, or an intracranial angioma, or a lesion of unknown pathogenesis acquired during foetal life. Hemiplegia acquired after birth may occur as a complication of many acute infective disorders of childhood, especially whooping cough, and in such cases probably usually has a vascular origin. It may also be due to acute encephalitis, or complicate meningitis. When hemiplegia is associated with convulsions, the convulsions may be the cause of the brain damage. Intracranial tumour and tuberculoma are rare causes.

The pathology varies with the cause, and includes vascular lesions such as haemorrhage and arterial thrombosis, sinus thrombophlebitis, and the various forms of encephalitis. In brains examined long after the onset of hemiplegia, the changes commonly found are meningeal thickening, localized atrophic sclerosis, cysts, and pseudoporencephaly (see Figs. 15.2 and 15.3).

Symptoms

Congenital hemiplegia is usually detected at an early age, because it is observed that the infant does not move the affected arm and leg normally, or because these limbs feel rigid. *Infantile hemiplegia* usually develops suddenly and convulsions occur at the onset in a large proportion of cases. Convulsions may occur for the first time in the early teens. Consciousness is lost, and the convulsive movements frequently predominate upon and may be confined to the side which subsequently becomes paralysed. Usually a series of fits occurs during

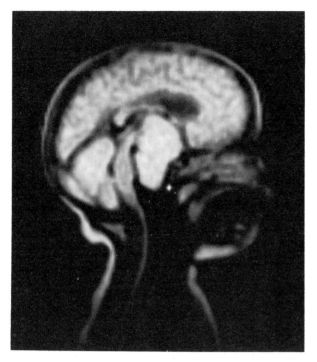

Fig. 15.2. Hamartoma of thalamus extending inferiorly anterior to the brainstem in a child of nine months. Sagittal NMR scan clearly shows the large tumour.

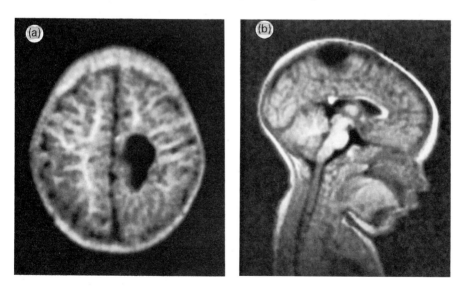

Fig. 15.3. Porencephalic cyst in a child of nine months: (a) NMR(IR) transverse and (b) sagittal scans. The cyst appears dark.

twenty-four hours, and the patient remains comatose for a variable period, sometimes for several days after the convulsions stop. Headache, vomiting, delirium, and fever frequently usher in the fits. During the stage of coma the limbs on the affected side are found to be flaccid and the plantar reflexes extensor. When the patient recovers consciousness he is hemiplegic, and when the right side of the body is paralysed, often dysphasic also, and sometimes mentally defective. The cerebrospinal fluid may be normal or may show an increase in the protein content, red cells, or a leucocytosis, depending upon the nature of the cerebral lesion. Epilepsy is much commoner as a sequel of infantile hemiplegia than in cerebral diplegia, and develops in over 50 per cent of cases.

Diagnosis

Congenital hemiplegia is readily recognized. The nature of the lesion may be apparent from the CT or NMR brain scan. Hemiplegia acquired in childhood must be distinguished from paralytic chorea, which is preceded by involuntary movements, and poliomyelitis, which is rarely limited to one upper and lower limb, and which is characterized by loss of tendon reflexes and muscular wasting. Hemiplegia of gradual onset is rare in childhood and is usually due to intracranial tumour or tuberculoma (see Fig. 15.4).

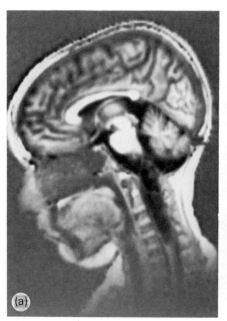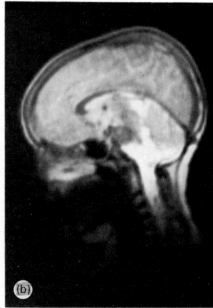

Fig. 15.4. Astrocytoma of the medulla and spinal cord in an eight-year-old boy. (a) NMR(IR) and (b) NMR(SE) scans, showing the extent of the tumour.

Prognosis

Little improvement is likely to occur in congenital hemiplegia. It is exceptional for the lesion responsible for an acquired infantile hemiplegia to prove fatal. The more severe the symptoms of the acute stage, the more likely are mental defect, dysphasia, and hemiplegia to be persistent. Nevertheless there are exceptions to this rule, and for several weeks after the acute stage there is no certain way of deciding how complete recovery will be. Hope of considerable improvement should not be abandoned until at least a year after the onset of the illness.

Treatment

During the acute stage of the illness which leads to infantile hemiplegia treatment is symptomatic. Cerebral oedema may be reduced by dexamethasone. Convulsions may be controlled by diazepam 5–10 mg intramuscularly according to the age of the patient. Naso-oesophageal feeding will be required as long as the patient is unconscious, and careful watch should be kept on the fluid intake and the blood electrolytes. Hyperpyrexia will call for hypothermia. An antibiotic should be given as a prophylactic against pneumonia. The usual after-treatment of the hemiplegia will be required, and the patient should be given regular small doses of phenobarbitone for a considerable time in the hope of preventing the development of epilepsy.

KERNICTERUS

Erythroblastosis foetalis, or haemolytic disease of the newborn, is secondary to Rh and ABO incompatibilities. There is a serum bilirubin exceeding 25 mg per 1000 ml which causes bile pigmentation in the nervous system, especially in the lenticular and caudate nuclei – *kernicterus*. The infant is usually normal at birth, but becomes jaundiced when two or three days old. Convulsions, rigidity, and coma mark the damage to the brain. Treatment by exchange transfusion with Rh negative blood gives good results if begun early enough. Residual brain damage may lead to mental deficiency, epilepsy and extrapyramidal syndromes, usually choreo-athetoid in type.

HEREDITARY METABOLIC DISEASES OF INFANCY

Cerebromacular degeneration will be described to illustrate the hereditary disorders of infancy which have a complex classification for which a textbook of paediatric neurology should be consulted. It is a disorder of the nervous system known also as amaurotic family idiocy and Tay–Sachs disease, in which there is a progressive deposition of lipids, mainly gangliosides, in the ganglion cells of the brain and retina. Several forms have been described, differing mainly in the age of onset. The infantile form develops during the first year of life, a late infantile form during the second and third year, a juvenile form between the ages of 3 and 10, and a late juvenile form between the ages of 15 and 25. The disease is frequently familial, and occurs in several siblings, being probably inherited as an autosomal recessive. The infantile form is confined to the Jewish race, but this is not true of the late infantile and juvenile forms.

The CT brain scan shows moderate general atrophy. At post mortem the ganglion cells of the cortex and thalamus, the cerebellum and spinal cord, show the characteristic degeneration with the formation of lipids and lipochrome. The white matter shows tract degeneration. Similar changes are found in the ganglion cells of the retina. One form of the disease is due to lack of the enzyme hexosaminidase A. Carriers can now be detected and so genetic counselling may be given. The enzyme deficiency can also be detected from cells in the amniotic fluid so that parents having the trait may be told if an unborn child will be affected and the mother may decide whether to bear the child.

The symptoms are essentially the same in all forms of the disorder. In the infantile form the child is normal at birth, and usually between the third and sixth months it becomes listless and apathetic. Myoclonus and epileptic seizures may occur. The retina and optic disc are atrophied and there is a cherry-red spot visible at the macula, which at this age is pathognomonic. In the late infantile and juvenile forms, the red spot at the macula is usually absent and may be replaced by fine pigmentation. Progressive flaccid paralysis of all four limbs develops and finally the child is completely blind and paralysed, and exhibits no mental activity.

The disease must be distinguished from diffuse sclerosis and from inclusion encphalitis. It is inevitably progressive, and the younger the patient at the onset the more rapid the downward course. In the infantile forms death occurs in from one to two years, but in the juvenile forms the patient may live for ten or fifteen years. If the cause of progressive cerebral degeneration in childhood is not clear from the clinical signs, a neurolipidosis or metachromatic leuco-dystrophy can sometimes be diagnosed from the degenerative changes in the myenteric plexus from rectal biopsy. Occasionally biopsy of the brain may be justifiable. In metachromatic leucodystrophy there may be an associated neuropathy and the diagnosis may be made in some cases by the finding of metachromatic lipid substances in the urine.

REFERENCES

Cohen, M.E. and Duffner, P.K. (1981). Prognostic indicators in hemiparetic cerebral palsy. *Ann. Neurol.* **9**, 353–7.
Hoskins, G. (1982). *An introduction to paediatric neurology.* Faber and Faber, London.
Kolata, G.B. (1980). Prenatal diagnosis of neural tube defects. *Science, NY* **209**, 1216–18.
Menkes, J.M. (1980). *Textbook of child neurology,* 2nd edn. Lea and Febiger, Philadelphia.

Swaiman, K.F. and Wright, F.S. (1982). *The practice of pediatric neurology,* 2nd edn. Mosby, St. Louis.

Vining, E.P.G., Accardo, P.J., Rubenstine, J.E., Farrell, S.E., and Royzen, N.J. (1976). Cerebral palsy: a pediatric developmentalist's overview. *Am. J. Dis. Child.* **130,** 643–59.

Williams, R.S., Hauser, S.L., Purpura, D.P., DeLong, G.R., and Swisher, C.N. (1980). Autism and mental retardation. *Archs Neurol.* **37,** 749–53.

16 Extrapyramidal syndromes

Anatomy and physiology

By extrapyramidal syndromes are meant those disorders which result from lesions involving those parts of the brain other than the corticospinal pathways which are concerned with movement. The principal such structures are those known as the basal ganglia, namely the corpus striatum and the nuclei which are anatomically and functionally associated with it. Diseases of the basal ganglia produce either reduction of movement (akinesis or rigidity) or excess of movement (hyperkinesis).

The corpus striatum consists of the caudate nucleus and the lenticular nucleus, which is divided into the putamen and the globus pallidus (Fig. 16.1).

The globus pallidus lies on the medial side of the putamen, and is separated from the optic thalamus and the caudate nucleus by the internal capsule. The caudate nucleus and putamen contain two types of ganglion cells, large and small; while the globus pallidus contains only one type. The caudate nucleus

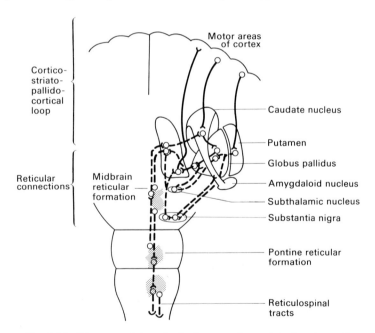

Fig. 16.1. Diagram of the principal connections of the basal ganglia.

and putamen are grouped together by some writers as 'the striatum', the globus pallidus being distinguished as 'the pallidum'.

On the medial side of the internal capsule and in the upper part of the midbrain lie three nuclear masses apparently intimately related to the corpus striatum. These are the red nucleus, the substantia nigra, and the subthalamic nucleus or corpus Luysi. Pathways connect the subthalamic nucleus and the substantia nigra with the globus pallidus and this in turn has what appears to be an efferent pathway running to the ventral part of the optic thalamus. There are also connections between the cerebral cortex and the corpus striatum and between that and the reticular formation of the brainstem.

Recent physiological studies in primates suggest that the major direct and indirect connections of the basal ganglia are with the cortex and not with the brainstem. Activity in pallidal neurones changes before the earliest electromyographic activity in moving limb muscles. The basal ganglia are more concerned with slow (ramp) movements than rapid (ballistic) movements, which are controlled by the cerebellum. The apparent increase in size of the pathways from the cortex to the subthalamic nuclei in primates suggests that these pathways have enabled the cortex itself to gain a direct control of the output from both the basal ganglia and spinal cord in order to control skilled limb movements. It is probably the function of the basal ganglia to recognize the likelihood that certain complex movements will take place and then to prepare the motor system for the successful accomplishment of these movements.

Neurotransmitters in the basal ganglia (Fig. 16.2)

One cell body in the substantia nigra has been estimated to have divergent projections on half a million striatal cells, the influence being inhibitory. The striatum has a high concentration of acetylcholine, mainly localized in intrinsic circuits which are mediated by muscarinic receptors which can be selectively blocked by atropine-like drugs. Other neurotransmitters also modulate basal ganglian function. Enkephalins utilize neurones whose effects are inhibitory and are blocked by naloxone. The major efferent pathway utilizes GABA, an inhibitory pathway blocked by bicuculline and excitatory projections contain substance P. Stimulation of the striatal dopamine receptors inhibits acetylcholine release and blockade of dopamine receptors with neuroleptics causes an increase in the turnover of striatal acetylcholine. The situation is further complicated by the existence of two types of dopamine receptor which can be differentially affected. The D1 involve stimulation of adenyl cyclase, leading to an increase in cyclic AMP levels whereas the D2 receptors can be activated independently of this enzyme. Specific D2 antagonists such as sulphride cause parkinsonian side-effects.

Although it is nearly fifty years since Kinnier Wilson first correlated symptoms with lesions of the basal ganglia, there are still large gaps in our knowledge of the functions of these structures. The established clinicopathological facts seem to be:

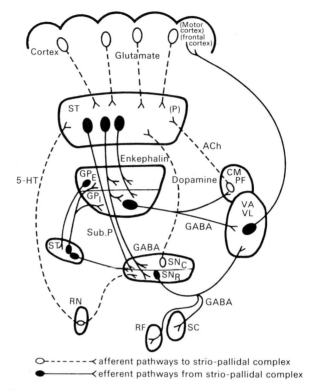

○----------◄ afferent pathways to strio-pallidal complex
●——————————◄ efferent pathways from strio-pallidal complex

Fig. 16.2. Diagram of the neurochemistry of the basal ganglia.

1. Degeneration of the substantia nigra is associated with the clinical picture of parkinsonism characterized by tremor and rigidity.

2. Destructive lesions of the subthalamic nucleus lead to hemiballismus characterized by violent choreiform involuntary movements on the opposite side of the body.

3. Chorea may also be associated with more diffuse degenerative processes, especially involving the caudate nucleus and putamen, as in Huntington's chorea.

4. There is evidence that surgical lesions of the globus pallidus, its efferent pathway, and the ventral nuclei of the thalamus, will relieve the tremor and rigidity of parkinsonism, the involuntary movements of hemiballismus, and also those of dystonia.

Of course the symptoms produced by disease of the nervous system must be mediated not by the structures destroyed but by the activity of the rest of the nervous system resulting from damage to those structures. It is a reasonable working hypothesis to suppose that the parkinsonian syndrome is the result of overactivity of the globus pallidus produced by loss of some control normally exercised over it by the substantia nigra, and that the syndromes characterized by chorea, dystonia and possibly athetosis are due to a disorganization of the normal activity of the globus pallidus. This would explain why in both instances improvement may follow destruction of the globus pallidus or its efferent pathway whereas deafferentation does not affect the tremor of a limb, but we are left with the mystery of why in such cases the patient is left with no disability which can be attributed to the loss of normal pallidal function.

THE PARKINSONIAN SYNDROME

The parkinsonian syndrome, named after James Parkinson, who first described paralysis agitans in 1817, is a disturbance of motor function characterized chiefly by slowing and enfeeblement of emotional and voluntary movements, muscular rigidity, and tremor. The importance of parkinsonism in neurology stems from the facts that it is a common disease and it is difficult to treat. On theoretical grounds, it represents a model of the type of neurological degenerative disease in which several types of receptor and transmitter defects can lead to a similar clinical appearance. In Parkinson's disease there is a loss of presynaptic function whereas after neuroleptic drugs or in certain primary striatonigral degenerations there is a postsynaptic defect.

Aetiology and pathology

There seems no doubt that the neuronal degeneration responsible for idiopathic parkinsonism (paralysis agitans) and encephalitic parkinsonism is situated in the basal ganglia. In the former, various types of cellular degeneration have been described, and in the latter the degeneration is secondary to inflammatory changes. Focal degeneration due to vascular occlusion is the basis of parkinsonism resulting from cerebral atherosclerosis.

Parkinsonism

The constant pathological lesion in idiopathic parkinsonism is loss of melanin pigment and degeneration of neurones in the substantia nigra. Biochemical and neurophysiological advances in the past few years have led to more precise knowledge of the basis of parkinsonism. Neurones from the substantia nigra pass to the striatum which has the highest dopamine content of the brain. This is reduced in parkinsonism, the loss paralleling the loss of cells in the substantia nigra. Topical application of dopamine to the caudate nucleus in animal experiments has been shown to inhibit the activity of neurones though acetylcholine increases it, suggesting a balance of excitatory and inhibitory influences on this part of the basal ganglia. In parkinsonism this balance is upset but can be redressed by increasing the dopaminergic activity or reducing the cholinergic activity in the brain.

In Parkinson's disease destruction of the nigrostriatal dopamine pathway also leads to denervation supersensitivity of the dopamine receptors in the postsynaptic receptors on the postsynaptic neurones in the striatum. This has been shown by an increased density of dopamine receptors assayed by ligand binding assays and increased sensitivity to the agonist. Other causes of parkinsonism are poisoning with carbon monoxide and manganese and heavy doses of drugs (and butyrphenones) such as haloperidol and tricyclic antidepressants, reserpine, alpha-methyldopa, and chlorpromazine, all of which deplete tissue catecholamines. Parkinsonian symptoms may arise during treatment with high doses of phenothiazines, and in the hope of preventing this complication anti-parkinsonian drugs are sometimes given prophylactically. Though parkinsonism has been observed to follow a head injury, this has not been established as a cause.

Paralysis agitans is a disease of late middle life and begins in most cases between the ages of 50 and 60, rarely before 40 or after 65. Males are affected slightly more often than females. Exceptionally the disorder is hereditary or familial.

During the epidemic of encephalitis lethargica (1916–26), parkinsonism sometimes developed acutely, or within a year or two of the acute illness. Since the greatest incidence of that disease was in early adult life, for many years after the epidemic most patients with encephalitic parkinsonism were under the age of 40. This, however, is now no longer true, but it is probable that most cases occurring before the age of 40 are examples of encephalitic parkinsonism.

Symptoms

Facies and attitude

In parkinsonism the facial muscles exhibit an unnatural immobility (Fig. 16.3). The eyes have a somewhat staring appearance, and spontaneous ocular movements are infrequent. The attitude of the limbs and trunk is one of moderate flexion. The limbs are moderately flexed and adducted, but the wrist is usually slightly extended. The fingers are flexed at the metacarpophalangeal, and extended or only slightly flexed at the interphalangeal joints, and adducted. The thumb is usually adducted, and extended at the metacarpo- and interphalangeal joints.

Tremor

Tremor is the characteristic involuntary movement of parkinsonism. It is usually the first symptom in paralysis agitans, but may be preceded by muscular rigidity in encephalitic parkinsonism. Tremor usually begins in one upper limb and later involves the lower limb on the same side; the other side being affected in the same order after a further interval. The head, lips and tongue often escape or are involved late. The characteristic features of parkinsonian tremor are described on page 95 and Fig. 3.1.

Muscular rigidity

In the early stages of parkinsonism the muscular rigidity may be limited to one upper limb, and may be only just detectable on passive movement. It is often

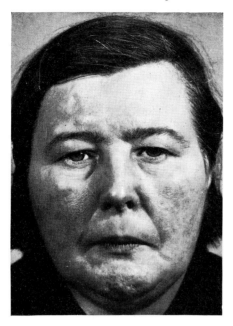

Fig. 16.3. Parkinsonism.

most evident on passive flexion and extension of the wrist and pronation and supination of the forearm. In advanced cases it is generalized and so severe that great resistance is offered to passive movement in all joints. Occasionally in such late cases muscular contractures occur, but this is exceptional.

Disorders of movement

Voluntary movement exhibits some impairment of power, but more striking is the slowness with which it is performed. In general the movements which are carried out by small muscles suffer most. Hence the patient shows weakness of the ocular movements which are characteristically jerky, of the facial movements, characteristically associated with tremor of the eyelids on closure of the eyes, and of movements concerned in mastication, deglutition, and articulation. The speech in severe cases is slurred and monotonous, owing to defective pronunciation of consonants and lack of variation in pitch. Movements of the small muscles of the hands are also markedly affected with resulting clumsiness and inability to perform fine movements. The patient has increasing difficulty in writing, and the handwriting tends to become smaller – *micrographia*. Certain associated and synergic movements suffer conspicuously. Swinging of the arms in walking is early diminished and later lost. Emotional movements of the face are reduced in amplitude, slow in developing, and unduly protracted. These motor symptoms constitute parkinsonian akinesia.

Gait

In the early stages the lack of swing of one arm may be the only noticeable feature. When parkinsonism is bilateral the gait is usually slow, shuffling and composed of small steps. The patient often exhibits a 'festiniant' gait, hurrying with small steps in a bent attitude, as if trying to catch up his centre of gravity. He may have difficulty in starting to walk, or stopping when pushed forwards or backwards – propulsion and retropulsion – or tend to move spontaneously in one of these directions. The patient who has great difficulty in walking, however, may be able to run quite fast.

The reflexes

Parkinsonism in itself does not affect the pupillary reflexes, but when it is due to encephalitis these may be impaired, especially the reaction on accommodation. Nor are the tendon reflexes directly affected, though muscular rigidity may render them difficult to elicit and reduced in amplitude. The plantar reflexes are flexor unless an independent lesion involves the corticospinal tracts. The glabella tap reflex is a facial reflex in which a brisk tap with the tip of the finger on the bridge of the nose of the patient causes a blink. This reflex habituates in normal individuals but not in patients with Parkinson's disease.

Other symptoms

There is no sensory loss in parkinsonism, but many patients in the later stages complain of pains in the limbs and spine, and extreme restlessness is a common symptom. Flushing of the skin and excessive sweating are occasionally seen, and excessive greasiness of the face, and salivation occur in encephalitic parkinsonism. This is also the cause of *oculogyral spasm*, now rarely observed. This symptom consists of spasmodic deviation of the eyes, usually upwards, which the patient is unable to overcome, which occurs paroxysmally and may last for minutes or even hours. Parkinsonism is not necessarily associated with any mental disturbance, though such may of course be an independent effect of the disorder causing the parkinsonism.

Diagnosis

Diagnosis of the cause of parkinsonism

It is often difficult to know whether parkinsonism is due to encephalitis or paralysis agitans, in the absence of a clear history of the former, which is rare. Encephalitis as a cause is suggested by the onset before the age of 40 and the occurrence of oculogyral spasms. A greasy skin, excessive salivation, and impaired pupillary reactions are suggestive of encephalitis. Arteriosclerotic parkinsonism is often fragmentary in the sense that it may remain limited indefinitely to one part of the body. There is usually hypertension and other evidence of vascular disease. A history of a sudden cerebral vascular lesion supports this diagnosis. The rarer causes of parkinsonism are usually obvious from the history.

Diagnosis of parkinsonism from other conditions

It is important to distinguish parkinsonian tremor from other forms of tremor having a more benign prognosis. This point is discussed on page 95. The features distinguishing parkinsonian from other forms of rigidity are described on page 90. The parkinsonian rigidity with an expressionless facies and loss of swing in one or both upper limbs, and frequently tremor, is so characteristic that difficulty does not usually arise. Rigidity due to joint disease, especially perhaps ankylosing spondylitis, may occasionally simulate parkinsonism. Rare causes of an extrapyramidal syndrome are multisystem atrophy associated with progressive autonomic failure (Shy–Drager Syndrome) (see p. 127) and progressive supranuclear ophthalmoplegia (Richardson–Steele–Olszewski syndrome, see p. 53). Progressive autonomic failure may also be associated with apparent Parkinson's disease.

Prognosis

Paralysis agitans is always progressive, though the rate of deterioration varies considerably. The symptoms may remain limited to one side of the body for months or years. Most patients with paralysis agitans, unless they die of some intercurrent disease, live for ten years, and many for much longer, even up to twenty years. The course of encephalitic parkinsonism is equally variable. In a few cases the disorder seems to become arrested, and this happens most often when the symptoms are predominantly unilateral. On the whole, the parkinsonism following encephalitis is a progressive condition often running a shorter course than that of paralysis agitans. The prognosis of arteriosclerotic parkinsonism is that of the underlying cerebrovascular disease.

Treatment

Dramatic improvements in treatment of idiopathic parkinsonism have followed recent advances in knowledge of neurotransmitters (Fig. 16.4). Since the dopamine content of the basal ganglia is reduced in parkinsonism to a level approaching 25 per cent of the normal value, it seems probable that the defect of dopaminergic transmission in striatal pathways has progressed gradually over several years before the onset of clinical symptoms. The traditional treatment of parkinsonism was to improve the symptoms by blocking cholinergic transmission, the excitatory effect of which in normal circumstances is balanced by dopaminergic inhibitory activity. Anticholinergic drugs which block muscarinic receptors, such as benzhexol (Artane) beginning with 2 mg and increasing to 8 mg or more a day, orphenadrine (Disipal) and benztropine (Cogentin), are undoubtedly effective in reducing parkinsonian symptoms, particularly tremor. The latter, which have antihistaminic as well as anticholinergic properties, may be particularly helpful if the patient is also anxious or depressed.

Treatment with dopaminergic drugs started from the observation that as dopamine given by mouth does not reach the central nervous system, there

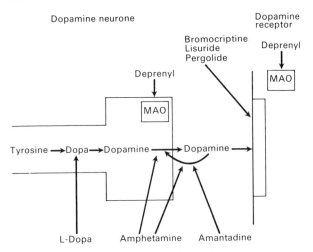

Fig. 16.4. Site of action of dopaminergic drugs.

should be attempts to give its precursor dihydroxy-phenylanine (dopa). It was then found that only the levo form of dopa crosses the blood–brain barrier to the central nervous system. In the past ten years levo-dopa has rapidly become the drug of choice in parkinsonian patients with a progressive disability in whom akinesis and rigidity are more prominent than tremor. It acts synergistically with their anticholinergic treatment. Levo-dopa caused a number of side-effects. The drug is a gastric irritant and should therefore be taken with food. Nausea may be reduced with cyclizine (50 mg by mouth). Other side-effects of the drug are postural hypotension and, rather more serious, the development of involuntary movements or dyskinesia which may affect the face, neck, or limbs. The development of such movements, or of mental agitation, sexual overactivity, which is extremely rare, or hallucinations, are clear indications for reducing the dose and these side-effects usually then subside, without loss of some benefit on the parkinsonian symptoms. Levo-dopa may also cause cardiac arrhythmia and is contra-indicated in patients with recent coronary disease. Care must be taken in combining levo-dopa with other drugs. Its effects may be dangerously potentiated by monoamine oxidase inhibitors and both sympatholytic and sympathomimetic drugs should be used with caution. The effect of levo-dopa is almost wholly blocked by pyridoxine. Despite these side-effects and precautions, levo-dopa represents a therapeutic advance and with this drug many parkinsonian patients with akinesis and rigidity can be helped so much that they are within weeks able to perform movements which were impossible for years previously.

Levo-dopa is now almost always combined with an extracerebral dopa decarboxylase inhibitor such as carbidopa, which does not cross the blood–brain barrier and prevents the destruction of levo-dopa outside the central nervous system. Hence it is possible to obtain comparable central nervous effects of levo-dopa by giving about one-fifth of the dose previously prescribed when it was given alone. A suitable starting dose of levo-dopa with decarboxylase inhibitor (either as Sinemet or Madopar) is 100 mg three times a day. Clinical benefits can be achieved in days rather than weeks as was necessary with levo-dopa alone. An average final dose is 200 mg three times a day. Nausea and vomiting occur less frequently than with levo-dopa alone. It has been suggested that the lack of an effective blood–brain barrier in the area postrema enables the decarboxylase inhibitor to gain access to the adjacent emetic centre so blocking catechol formation and associated nausea. Other adverse peripheral effects of levo-dopa alone, including postural hypotension and cardiac arrhythmias, also occur less commonly. Bromocriptine (Parlodil), a selective central dopamine agonist, may cause further improvement in some parkinsonian patients on maximum antiparkinsonian treatment, including levo-dopa. The side-effects of bromocriptine in addition to those of levo-dopa, are hallucinations and erythromelalgia, both of which are indications for stopping the drug. The dose of levo-dopa used must be reduced as the dose of bromocriptine is built up. Amantadine (Symmetrel), primarily an antiviral agent, appears to modulate the release of acetylcholine and dopamine and is valuable in patients who have difficulty in tolerating levo-dopa. Selegiline (Eldepryl) is a specific inhibitor of MAO-B, the enzyme which metabolizes dopamine in man, allowing the normal degradation of noradrenaline by MAO-A so avoiding catecholamine release, the so-called 'cheese' effect. In a dose of 5 mg twice daily it can smoothe the response in patients with end-dose akinesis, the commonest type of 'oscillation'.

These recent medical advances have reduced the place of surgical treatment. There are now seldom patients with idiopathic and postencephalitic parkinsonism having a marked unilateral tremor who need help by destructive stereotaxic surgery to the thalamus, which presumably reduces the afferent inflow to the disordered extrapyramidal system.

Despite these advances in treatment there remains no cure for parkinsonism; it is merely possible to replace, for a time, some of the transmitter deficiency, so making the symptoms more tolerable for a number of years. Cases of idiopathic parkinsonism vary in their severity; there are some benign cases with mild and often unilateral symptoms in whom progression may be slow over a period of some thirty years. At the other extreme there are rapidly progressive cases in which there is almost complete incapacity within some three years. Treatment with levo-dopa appears to slow down the rate of progression of the disease but after two or three years of levo-dopa treatment the benefits decline and the patient is more and more troubled by 'freezing' or akinesis on waking and also at times relatively suddenly during the day.

About 15 per cent of patients with Parkinson's disease do not respond to levo-dopa and this may possibly result from dopamine receptor degeneration which occurs progressively in all patients with parkinsonism. Half of those who respond initially to levo-dopa eventually develop severe 'on and off' effects. Some dyskinesias are thought to be due to dopamine receptor supersensitivity, possibly of a specific dopamine receptor subtype. It is important to recognize different types of dyskinesias as their management is different. The end of dose deterioration is due to inadequate stores of dopamine and requires either shorter intervals between doses or the addition of a longer-acting agonist. Peak-dose dyskinesias due to high plasma levels, need a reduction in individual doses. A failure to respond to the dose of levo-dopa may be due to delayed gastric emptying and may be helped by dissolving the levo-dopa before taking the tablets. Balancing the duration of action of the dopamine agonist drug and its relative effect on D1 and D2 receptors can be helpful. Dopamine is predominantly a short-acting D1 receptor agonist acting on striatal neurones whereas bromocriptine has the very important advantage that it is a long-acting drug. But dyskinesias are multifactorial and cannot all be controlled by maintaining a smooth plasma level of levo-dopa even by intravenous administration. In addition to the absorption problems there are also problems of brain uptake and subsequent synthesis and release of dopamine. The new drugs have undoubtedly helped many patients but much has yet to be learned about the management of these troublesome end-stage dyskinesias.

HEPATOLENTICULAR DEGENERATION

Aetiology and pathology

Hepatolenticular degeneration, or Wilson's disease, is a progressive disorder of early life which is frequently familial, and is characterized pathologically by degeneration of certain regions of the brain, especially the corpus striatum, and cirrhosis of the liver, and clinically by increasing muscular rigidity and tremor. The disease is caused by a disturbance of copper metabolism, though the metabolic disorder is complex and also includes aminoaciduria. It is believed that caeruloplasmin, which normally contains almost the whole of the copper in the blood, is deficient. This leads to a low serum copper level. The copper is carried loosely bound to the albumin. Hence it is deposited in the tissues and excreted in the urine. The disorder appears to be inherited as an autosomal recessive.

In the nervous system there is a degeneration of ganglion cells with neuroglial overgrowth, most marked in the putamen of the lenticular nucleus. Similar alterations are often present in other parts of the nervous system, including the cerebral cortex and the cerebellum. Macroscopically the lenticular nucleus appears shrunken, and may show cavitation. In the liver the changes are those of a multilobular cirrhosis, often associated with enlargement of the spleen.

Symptoms

The onset is usually between the ages of 10 and 25 years. In most cases tremor is the earliest symptom, but other types of involuntary movement have been observed. The early course is fluctuating. Rigidity soon develops, resembling that of parkinsonism in distribution and general character. Speech may become unintelligible, and there is almost always some degree of mental deterioration amounting to a mild dementia.

Corneal pigmentation – the Kayser–Fleischer ring – consists of a zone of golden-brown granular pigmentation about 2 mm in diameter on the posterior surface of the cornea towards the limbus. In advanced cases it is clearly visible to the naked eye; otherwise it may only be seen with the slit lamp and corneal microscope. It is due to the deposition of copper.

Symptoms of cirrhosis of the liver may be inconspicuous, but have sometimes proved fatal before the patient developed any nervous symptoms.

Biochemical tests of diagnostic value include a low serum copper (less than 13 μmol/l), a low caeruloplasmin in the blood (normal 1.3–2.9 μmol/l), and a high urinary copper (normal 24-hour excretion less than 4 μmol), especially if increased after BAL.

Diagnosis

There are few disorders with which hepatolenticular degeneration is likely to be confused, for no other disease is characterized by familial tremor and rigidity developing in the second decade of life, with corneal pigmentation and symptoms of cirrhosis of the liver. Difficulty may arise, however, in atypical cases when biochemical tests may be of value. These tests may also be abnormal in siblings who show no symptoms of the disease. Early diagnosis is important and in a child with obscure liver disease a liver biopsy is justifiable in order to make the diagnosis. Involvement of the lentricular nuclei is shown on CT and NMR scans (Fig. 16.5).

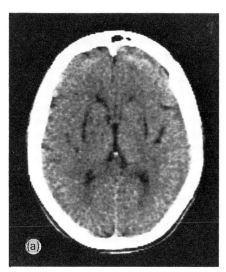 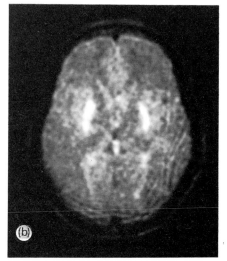

Fig. 16.5. Wilson's disease: (a) CT and (b) NMR (SE) scans: both scans show involvement of the lenticular nuclei.

Prognosis

The course of the disease may be acute, subacute, or chronic, and when it develops in early life it is probably invariably fatal. It is possible, however, that in some mild chronic cases it may remain stationary indefinitely.

Treatment

Apart from symptomatic treatment, an attempt may be made to reduce the absorption of copper from the alimentary canal by giving oral potassium sulphide. Penicillamine given by mouth with pyridoxine is an effective copper binding agent and it is now the drug of choice, though it is expensive and not free from the rare risk of side-effects such as myasthenia. Tri-ethylenetetramine is an alternative if patients cannot tolerate penicillamine. The possibility of identifying and treating prophylatically asymptomatic homozygous siblings of patients with this disease in under consideration.

CHOREA

Aetiology and pathology

Chorea is a type of involuntary movement the features of which have already been described (p. 93). It is thus a symptom which may be produced by a number of different pathological processes. In Sydenham's or rheumatic chorea, pathological changes, chiefly oedema and congestion, are diffuse, but most marked in the corpus striatum and related structures. The causation appears to be identical with that of acute rheumatism. Antibodies produced in response to the beta haemolytic streptococcus of acute rheumatism have been reported to cross-react *in vitro* with basal ganglia neurones. Huntington's chorea is a hereditary disorder characterized pathologically by degeneration of the ganglion cells of the forebrain and corpus striatum. Chronic chorea is occasionally the result of *kernicterus* produced by the haemolytic disease of the newborn. There is a rare association between polycythaemia and chorea and it may be a side-effect of drug treatment. Hemiballismus is usually the result of a vascular lesion involving the subthalamic nucleus on the opposite side to the involuntary movements. Less common causes of chorea include senile brain degenerations, thyrotoxicosis, and very rarely treatment with the oral contraceptive pill.

In chorea there is evidence of a reduction of dopamine and its metabolite homovanillic acid (HVA) in the caudate nucleus and a reduction of the cerebrospinal fluid HVA. Chorea probably results from an excessive stimulation of a damaged striatum by a relatively normal nigrostriatal dopaminergic pathway. There appears to be denervation hypersensitivity of excitatory dopaminergic receptors so that, in contrast to parkinsonism, drugs which depress dopaminergic function such as tetrabenazine (Nitoman) and haloperidol (Serenace) improve the movements and may reduce chorea from any cause. On the other hand, drugs which enhance cholinergic transmission aggravate the movements.

Special varieties of chorea

Sydenham's chorea

The onset of Sydenham's chorea occurs in the majority of cases between the ages of 5 and 15. Females suffer more than males, in the proportion of about 3 to 1. The onset is usually insidious, the first complaint being often that the child is clumsy and drops things. When the movements are noticed, the child is described as restless, fidgety, or unable to keep still. The characteristics of choreic movements have been described on p. 93. In mild cases of Sydenham's chorea voluntary power is little impaired, but muscular weakness may be very marked, as in so-called paralytic chorea, though complete paralysis never develops. Hypotonia is invariably present in chorea. The upper limbs are characteristically hyperpronated when outstretched and held above the head. When hypotonia is extreme the tendon reflexes may be difficult to elicit, but they are usually obtainable. Most choreic children exhibit some emotional instability.

Rheumatic involvement of the heart is not uncommon, but rheumatic arthritis is rarely associated with chorea.

Chorea must be distinguished from habit spasm or tic. This, however, consists of simple movements such as blinking or other grimaces, a quick jerk of the head, or shrugging of the shoulders, which are repeated again and again.

Death from Sydenham's chorea is very rare. Most patients recover in from two to three months, rarely in less than six weeks. Recurrences occur in about one-third of all cases, sometimes more than once. Chorea leaves no serious sequels, but slight involuntary movements are occasionally perpetuated as a habit.

Most patients respond well to rest in bed and sedatives. It is doubtful whether any of the newer methods of treatment is more effective. During convalescence suitable games and re-educational exercises and occupational therapy will help to re-educate the limb movements.

Huntington's chorea

This disease, being inherited as a Mendelian dominant, usually has a family history, though sporadic cases occur. It was originally described in 1872 by George Huntington who observed affected families in New England who were descendants of the seventeenth century immigrants from the Suffolk village of Bures. Both sexes are affected. The age of onset of symptoms is usually between 30 and 45, but may be either later or earlier. The first symptom is usually the involuntary movements, which develop insidiously, and are usually more rapid and jerky than those of Sydenham's chorea. As the disorder progresses they lead to dysarthria and ataxia of the upper limbs and of the gait. Mental changes gradually develop, usually a few years after the onset of the chorea, and consist of a progressive dementia. Either the involuntary movements or the dementia may exceptionally occur alone. Except in rare cases the disorder is progressive and terminates fatally, usually in from ten to fifteen years after the onset, though there is a wide variation in its duration.

Progressive degeneration of cell bodies in the striatum occurs affecting striatal cholinergic and striatonigral inhibitory GABA pathways which regulate the dopaminergic neurones of the substantia nigra. There is also a decrease in the striatal substance P pathways. The result is a relative hyperinnervation by the intact dopaminergic system leading to involuntary movements. These can be reduced by blocking dopamine receptors by neuroleptics or drugs which deplete dopamine such as reserpine or tetrabenazine.

Hemiballismus

The onset of hemiballismus is usually sudden. The unilateral movements differ from other forms of chorea in that they affect the proximal parts of the limbs to a greater extent and hence lead to wide excursions, and they are practically continuous except during sleep. Recently tetrabenazine (Nitoman) which blocks the re-uptake of monoaminergic transmitters, 25–200 mg daily, has been found to be helpful in some cases of hemiballismus and chorea. The operation of thalamotomy may also be successful in abolishing the movements.

Progressive supranuclear palsy (Richardson-Steele-Olszewski syndrome)

This disease of the elderly presents with gait disturbance, some memory and personality deterioration, supranuclear ophthalmoplegia, pseudobulbar palsy, and some truncal dystonia. Vertical eye movements are more restricted than horizontal eye movements. At first the extrapyramidal symptoms may be mistaken for Parkinson's disease but levo-dopa is of little benefit and the disease is steadily progressive. Pathological studies have shown neuronal loss and gliosis in the periaqueductal grey matter with more widespread neuronal loss and neurofibrillary degeneration in the basal ganglia. The cause of the disease is unknown.

ATHETOSIS

Bilateral athetosis is usually congenital, when it may or may not be associated with signs of corticospinal tract lesions, and is to be regarded as a form of congenital diplegia. Unilateral athetosis may also be congenital, being then usually associated with infantile hemiplegia. It may also occur, however, as the result of acquired focal lesions involving the corpus striatum at any age, but this is uncommon.

The characteristics of athetosis are described on page 93. Congenital athetosis is not usually noticed till the child is several months old, when abnormal postures or movements attracts the mother's attention. The resulting disability is often severe. The child is late in walking, and its gait is ataxic, and the normal control over upper limb movements is severely interfered with. The speech is dysarthric.

Medical treatment of athetosis is disappointing, but some improvement may follow re-educational exercises perseveringly carried out for a long period. A variety of operations have been devised with the object of reducing the involuntary movements, the most recent of which, pallidectomy and thalamotomy, are said to be beneficial, chiefly in cases of late onset, unilateral, and not associated with mental subnormality.

SPASMODIC TORTICOLLIS

Torticollis is the name for a rotated attitude of the head brought about by clonic or tonic contraction of the cervical muscles. Torticollis may occur as the result of organic disease of the nervous system, and in such cases it may be regarded as a limited form of dystonia musculorum deformans (p. 94). It has been seen, for example, as a sequel of encephalitis lethargica, or as part of other extrapyramidal syndromes. It may also, however, be a hysterical symptom, and organic and hysterical torticollis may be difficult to distinguish. Torticollis which arises in middle life in a patient of previously stable personality, and produces violent clonic movements of rotation of the head to one side, which persist when the patient does not know that he is being observed, and tend in time to produce hypertrophy of the contracting muscles, is much more likely to be organic than hysterical. It is always an intractable disorder. Medical treatment usually has little effect but benzhexol (Artane) used as for parkinsonism is worth a trial. Anterior cervical rhizotomy has been devised in order to put the contracting muscles out of action may relieve pain and the movements. Stereotaxic surgery seems to be less effective.

OCCUPATIONAL MOVEMENT DISORDERS

Neurologists now tend to think of writer's cramp as a form of partial torsion dystonia, though the response to the drugs used for dyskinetic movements (p. 353) is often disappointing. Occupational movement disorders are prone to afflict those whose occupation entails the persistent use of fine co-ordinated movements, especially of the hands, and characterized by a progressive occupational disability due to spasm of the muscles employed, which are often the site of pain and sometimes of tremor. Some prefer to explain occupational movement disorders in psychological terms, others postulate an underlying anatomical or physiological disability, but as in the case of obsessive-compulsive states this is perhaps an artificial distinction, and both causal factors may need to be taken into account. In this, occupational neurosis presents points of resemblance to stuttering, another functional disorder of finely co-ordinated movements.

Fatigue and the effort to carry out active work against time are important precipitating factors, and since in most cases the sufferer's livelihood depends upon his speed and accuracy, an impairment of his efficiency evokes anxiety, which probably plays a part in the genesis and maintenance of the disorder. Numerous occupational movement disorders have been described, writers', telegraphists', goldbeaters', violinists', and piano-players' cramps being the most familiar. Both sexes are affected, but males more often than females.

The symptoms of writers' cramp will alone be described, since the disorder is essentially the same in other occupations. The onset of symptoms is gradual, and the disorder shows itself at first only when the patient is fatigued, when difficulty in controlling the pen leads to inaccurate writing. When the condition is well-developed the attempt to write evokes a spasm of the muscles concerned in holding and moving the pen, and this may spread to the whole of the upper limb. The arm may thus become rigid so that the act is brought to an abrupt stop. More usually, the attempt to write leads to jerky and inco-ordinate movements of the fingers, so that the writing is completely illegible. Sensory symptoms are common and are the result of the muscular spasm, the patient complaining of fatigue or an aching pain in the muscles not only of the upper limb but sometimes also of the neck. Muscular wasting, sensory loss, and reflex changes are absent.

In most cases the disability is limited to the single act in which it originates, and this is of diagnostic importance, since there is no organic disorder of movement as such which severely interferes with writing but does not in any way impair such similar acts as shaving or cutting up food. Exceptionally, however, the disability extends to other acts which are carried out by the same hand, but it should be noted that it is always an act which is impaired, and not the power or co-ordination of the individual movements which compose it, tested in isolation.

In many cases the disability is progressive, though recovery may occur, and other patients may remain in a stationary condition but still able to continue their occupation.

Treatment consists of the trial of drugs used for dyskinesis (p. 353), biofeedback, rest from the occupation, psychological investigation and treatment, and relaxation and re-educational exercises.

TARDIVE OR DRUG-INDUCED DYSKINESIAS

Some of the earliest described were acute dystonic movements, often violent, with retrocollis or opisthotonos, after the first few doses of a phenothiazine drug. Some such movements cease spontaneously on withdrawal of the drug or after a short course of anticholinergic drugs, barbiturates or diazepam (Valium). Longer-term treatment with high doses of phenothiazines and other tranquillizers is often prescribed but is in general best avoided except in psychoses, and may cause tardive dyskinesias in which mainly the lips, mouth, and face but also the trunk and limbs are involved in continuous choro-athetoid movements. Such movements, which are commoner in the elderly, may not cease on withdrawal of the tranquillizer, sometimes indeed only starting on withdrawal of the drug, and may not be relieved by anticholinergic drugs. It is something of a paradox that these neuroleptics not only cause dyskinesias but they may also cause parkinsonian rigidity. The dyskinesias are similar to those occurring with levo-dopa therapy, which has led to the suggestion that they result from increased dopaminergic function. The mechanism is not clear but one possibility is that the drug induces irreversible denervation hypersensitivity of excitatory dopaminergic endings in the basal ganglia. Dopaminergic receptor blocking drugs such as haloperidol may reduce these dyskinesias, but only for a time. The normal transmitter balance, once disturbed, as in parkinsonism, is not easily re-established.

Other drug-induced dyskinesias include akathisia or restless, fidgety move-ments of the legs which occur with phenothiazines but are usually abolished on stopping the drug. Rather similar leg movements, known as dyslisis, occur in the restless legs syndrome (Ekbom's syndrome). A few cases are due to iron deficiency but in most the cause is obscure, possibly ischaemia causing hyper-excitability of spinal cord motor neurones.

Sometimes the dyskinetic movements may occur apparently without any preceding drug use as in Meige's syndrome (blepharospasm and orofacial dyskinesias).

In the treatment of dyskinesias a series of drugs should be tried in turn. After benzhexol (Artane) it is reasonable to use first haloperidol, then tetrabenazine then followed by pimozide (2–4 mg daily), clonazepam, and baclofen (see p. 92). To be realistic, with current drugs barely a half of the patients with dyskinesias can be helped.

REFERENCES

Boller, F., Mizutani, T., Roessmann, U., and Gambetti, P. (1980). Parkinson's disease, dementia and Alzheimer disease; clinicopathological correlations. *Ann. Neurol.* **7**, 329–35.

Cartwright, G.E. (1978). Diagnosis of treatable Wilson's disease. *New Engl. J. Med.* **298**, 1347–50.

Klawans, H.L., Goetz, C.G., and Perlik, S. (1980). Presymptomatic and early detection of Huntington's chorea. *Ann. Neurol.* **8**, 343–7.

Marsden, C.D. and Fahn, S. (1982). Problems in Parkinson's disease. In *Movement disorders* (ed. C.D. Marsden and S. Fahn). Butterworth, London.

Quinn, N., Marsden, C.D., and Parkes, J.D. (1982). Complicated response fluctuations in Parkinson's disease: response to intravenous infusion of levadopa. *Lancet* **ii**, 412–15.

Shapiro, E. and Shapiro, A.K. (1981). Tic disorders. *J. Am. med. Ass.* **245**, 1583–5.

Sheehy, M.P. and Marsden, C.D. (1982). Writer's cramp – a focal dystonia. *Brain* **105**, 461–80.

Shoulson, I. and Fahn, S. (1979). Huntington's disease: clinical care and evaluation. *Neurology, Minneap.* **29**, 1–3.

17 Disorders of the limbic system and hypothalamus

Anatomy and physiology

Limbic system (Fig. 17.1)

Limbus means the border of the cerebral hemisphere but it is a 'system' rather than a series of precisely defined brain structures. It includes the olfactory areas, hippocampus and amygdaloid complex, cingulate cortex and septal area, and regulates the hypothalamic area and is critical for emotional and affective display. In phylogenetic development it represents the older or palaeomammalian cortex as opposed to the neomammalian cortex. Its function is thought to be concerned with levels below cognitive behaviour and inductive and deductive reasoning, though it nevertheless is concerned with a feeling of individuality and identity. It seems to be the system which analyses the significance of the input of sensation to the organism in relation to the instinctive drives which promote the perpetuation of the individual by satisfying hunger and thirst. It is

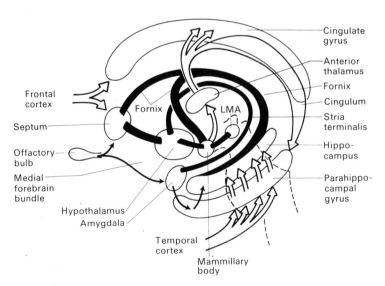

Fig. 17.1. Diagram of the afferent and efferent connections of the limbic system. LMA: limbic midbrain area.

concerned with maintaining homeostasis against a changing environment and also ensuring the perpetuation of the species by sexual and parental drive which can at times override more selfish self-perpetuating drives of the individual. The essence of its function is choice, based on sensory information, of patterns of behaviour, lying as it does between areas concerned with sensory perception and motor action. As it overlaps both with the sensory and motor systems it is essential for many aspects of memory, and learning.

Hypothalamus

The autonomic nervous system and many metabolic functions are under the control of nerve centres, many of which are situated in the hypothalamus, the region of the brain lying ventrally to the thalamus and constituting the floor of the third ventricle. The hypothalamus exerts its effect in two ways, by nervous pathways and by the release of hormones. The hypothalamus contains a large number of scattered ganglion cells, which have been differentiated into a number of nuclei. The projections of the hypothalamus are not yet completely known.

The hypothalamus is supplied by small branches from the circle of Willis. The neurones of the supraoptic and paraventricular nuclei of the posterior hypothalamus generate and conduct action potentials which depolarize the terminals in the posterior pituitary, causing release of oxytocin and vasopressin by calcium dependant excitation–secretion coupling. Neurosecretory granules are also transported down the fibres (Fig. 17.2).

The adenohypophysis or anterior pituitary is formed from the stomatodeum and is innervated only by postganglionic fibres that terminate on blood vessels which predominantly flow from the hypothalamus to the pituitary, transporting the hypothalamic releasing and inhibitory substances (TRH, LHRH, and GHRH (somatostatin)). The families of related peptides in the brain with neurotransmitter and neuromodulatory function now exceed 30 (see p. 9). Endorphins and substance P are discussed on page 10. Vasoactive intestinal peptide (VIP), first discovered in the gastro-intestinal tract, is present in nerves supplying the cerebral vessels. VIP has been shown to cause cerebral vasodilation of vessels in tonic contraction as a result of application of serotonin. Cholecystokinin, in addition to its presence in the gut from which it was first isolated, is widely distributed in the brain, especially in the cortex, and may have a role in appetite control. Vasopressin is present in higher concentration of the supraoptic and paraventricular nuclei in the hypothalamus but is also present in the spinal cord. ACTH is present in the hypothalamus and limbic systems. Experimental evidence points to a role of these hormones in the limbic system controlling memory functions quite distinct from their neuroendocrine role in salt and water metabolism and in anterior pituitary regulation. Thyrotrophin excretion by the pituitary is under feedback control by both T_3 (trithyronine) and T_4 (thyroxine), T_3 being is converted to T_4 in the pituitary. The TSH response to thyrotrophin releasing hormone (TRH) is valuable in the investiga-

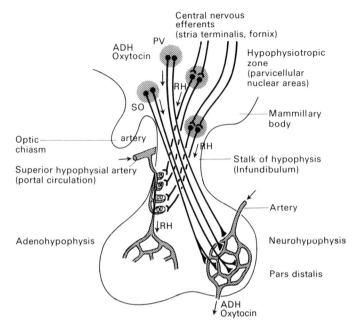

Fig. 17.2. Schematic drawing of the hypothalamic–hypophyseal system. ADH and oxytocin are produced in the large cells of the paraventricular (PV) and supraoptic (SO) nuclei; they travel through axons into the distal part of the neurohypophysis and there enter the bloodstream. The releasing hormones (RH) reach the sites of gland-otrophic-hormone production by way of the 'portal system'.

tion of hypothalamic and pituitary disorders. In hypothyroidism of hypothalamic origin responsiveness is present but is absent in pituitary failure.

Syndromes of the hypothalamus

The principal disturbances which may follow hypothalamic lesions are those of pituitary function, food and water balance, and temperature and blood pressure regulation. The lesion may be a tumour, such as craniopharyngioma, chronic basal meningitis, such as sarcoidosis, or a vascular lesion, particularly rupture of an aneurysm on the circle of Willis. Investigation follows the usual lines for an intracerebral lesion, with a range of endocrine tests added. The commonest cause of a hypothalamic lesion is a severe head injury, and diabetes insipidus, which may follow, is now described in more detail.

Diabetes insipidus

It has been shown experimentally that diabetes insipidus, in which there is excessive thirst and polyuria, follows bilateral destruction of the supra-optic nuclei, or removal of the posterior lobe of the hypophysis and its stalk. There is evidence that the antidiuretic hormone is produced by the nerve cells of the supra-optic nucleus, and reaches the hypophysis by their descending tracts. The hormone is necessary for the resorption of water by the renal tubules. The presence of the anterior lobe of the hypophysis and of the thyroid appears to be necessary for diabetes insipidus to occur.

Diabetes insipidus may be the result of any lesion in the neighbourhood of the hypothalamus, but it commonly arises either as the result of head injury or spontaneously. The sufferer may drink several gallons of water a day, and sleep is disturbed by thirst and the necessity for frequent micturition. Diabetes insipidus due to lack of the antidiuretic hormone must be distinguished from hereditary nephrogenic diabetes insipidus and psychogenic compulsive water-drinking.

When the cause is head injury, some patients improve or recover after a few months: in others, the disorder is permanent.

The synthetic analogue of pitressin, DDAVP, has high antidiuretic activity and low pressor activity and is effective treatment given by nasal insufflation.

REFERENCES

Appenzeller, O. (1982). *The autonomic nervous system,* 3rd edn. North-Holland, Amsterdam.

Bannister, R. (ed.) (1983). *Autonomic failure.* Oxford University Press.

Brodish, A. and Redgate, E.S. (eds.) (1973). *International Symposium on Brain–Pituitary–Adrenal Interrelationships.* Karger, Basel.

Johnson, R.H. and Spalding, J.M.K. (1974). *Disorders of the autonomic nervous system.* Blackwell, Oxford.

Reichlin, S., Baldessarini, R.J., and Martin, J.B. (eds.) (1980). *The hypothalamus.* Raven Press, New York.

18 Disorders of the spinal cord

Anatomy

The spinal cord lies within the vertebral canal, extending from the foramen magnum, where it is continuous with the medulla oblongata, to the level of the first or second lumbar vertebra. The concept of segmentation of the spinal cord is based upon the fact that the ventral and dorsal root filaments unite at intervals to form on either side a dorsal or posterior root, upon which is situated a ganglion, and a ventral or anterior root. One ventral and the corresponding dorsal root on one side join together just distally to the dorsal root ganglion to form a spinal nerve. Thus from each side there arises a series of spinal nerves, and the spinal cord is regarded as divided into segments, one corresponding to each pair of spinal nerves. The spinal roots, here forming the radicular nerve, emerge from the intervertebral foramina. Since the spinal cord terminates at about the lower level of the first lumbar vertebra, the lumbar and sacral nerve roots have to take an oblique course downwards to reach their respective intervertebral foramina, and the resulting leash of nerves constitutes the cauda equina, which occupies the spinal canal below the first lumbar vertebra.

The spinal cord, like the brain, is surrounded by three meninges. The pia mater forms the immediate covering of the cord; the arachnoid lies superficially to the pia mater, from which it is separated by the subarachnoid space, which contains the cerebrospinal fluid and extends as low as the second sacral vertebra. Outside the arachnoid lies the dura mater, which forms a lining to the vertebral canal, and extends a little lower than the arachnoid. The spinal cord is suspended within its dural sheath by a series of ligamenta denticulata, which extend laterally from the sides of the cord to terminate in a tooth-like attachment to the inner aspect of the dura.

The blood supply of the spinal cord

The arterial blood supply of the spinal cord is derived from several sources. There are two posterior spinal arteries, each coming from the corresponding vertebral or posterior inferior cerebellar artery. The single anterior spinal artery is formed by the union of a branch from each vertebral artery, and the spinal arteries are reinforced by segmental arteries which enter the spinal canal through the intervertebral foramina. Three of these, which are of particular importance, are situated in the lower cervical, the lower dorsal and the upper lumbar regions.

358

The spinal veins terminate in a plexus in the pia mater and pass upwards into the corresponding veins of the medulla oblongata. Segmental veins pass outwards along the nerve roots to join the internal vertebral plexus in which also blood flows upwards to the intracranial venous sinuses.

Paraplegia

Paraplegia means paralysis confined to the lower limbs. This may be caused by a disorder of function at different levels. It may be psychogenic, i.e. hysterical. It may occur as the result of a cerebral lesion, which is so placed as to damage the corticospinal tract fibres from the leg areas of the motor cortex only. In such cases the lower limbs are usually spastic in extension. Paraplegia due to a lesion of the spinal cord is very much commoner and may be associated with either extension or flexion of the lower limb, paraplegia-in-extension and paraplegia-in-flexion respectively. Paraplegia may also be caused by a lesion of the anterior horn cells of the lumbosacral region of the cord, e.g. in poliomyelitis or, rarely, motor neurone disease, or by a lesion of the cauda equina, or of the peripheral nerves to the lower limbs, as in polyneuritis, or may be the result of primary diseases of the muscles, myopathy. We are here concerned with paraplegia due to lesions of the spinal cord.

After a partial lesion of the spinal cord two mutually antagonistic reflex activities emerge, extensor hypertonia and the flexor withdrawal reflex. The former, being physiologically equivalent to decerebrate rigidity in the animal, is dependent upon the connections of the reticular nuclei with the spinal cord. The flexor withdrawal reflex, on the other hand, utilizes short spinal reflex arcs. After a lesion which involves the corticospinal tracts only, both sets of reflexes are potentially active, but extensor hypertonia predominates as a persistent tonic activity, giving way only occasionally to the flexor withdrawal reflex when a nocuous stimulus excites the latter. If, however, a spinal lesion involves a sufficient extent of the cord to destroy not only the corticospinal tract fibres but also the vestibulospinal and reticulospinal tracts upon which the extensor hypertonia depends, the flexor reflex, freed from its antagonist, manifests greatly heightened activity and dominates the picture. Violent flexor spasms occur in the lower limbs, which in severe cases finally become fixed in an attitude of flexion, with the heels approximated to the buttocks. Paraplegia-in-flexion may be the outcome of a slowly progressive lesion of the cord, in which case it follows paraplegia-in-extension after an intermediate phase in which the balance swings between the two reflex systems. After a traumatic lesion, however, which causes immediate and complete severance of the cord, paraplegia-in-extension never occurs, because the vestibulospinal and reticulospinal tracts are interrupted from the beginning. Hence, as soon as the stage of spinal shock has passed, paraplegia-in-flexion tends to develop, though careful management can prevent the development of flexor spasms.

The bladder and rectum in paraplegia

In paraplegia-in-extension impairment of voluntary control over the bladder is manifested in some difficulty in initiating micturition, or more frequently precipitancy with a tendency to incontinence. The rectum is usually less affected, but constipation is not uncommon.

During the stage of spinal shock which follows a rapidly developing severe lesion of the spinal cord, the normal reflex activity of the bladder and rectum is abolished, with the result that retention of urine and faeces occurs. When reflex activity of the divided spinal cord is well established, in traumatic cases about three weeks after transection, reflex evacuation of the bladder and rectum and reflex sweating occur. The volume of fluid required to evoke reflex contraction of the bladder varies in different cases, but is usually about 200 ml. Reflex emptying can be facilitated by deep breathing and aided by pressure over the hypogastrium. Reflex evacuation of the rectum occurs in response to a volume of about 200 ml.

THE SYMPTOMATOLOGY OF SPINAL CORD LESIONS IN THE LIGHT OF ANATOMY AND PHYSIOLOGY

Though there are many varieties of spinal cord lesion, the commonest and most important fall into certain well-defined groups.

1. Lesions which produce a focal interference with the functions of the cord at a particular level, for example spinal cord compression.

2. Massive lesions involving a number of adjacent cord segments, and sometimes a large extent of the cord, e.g. myelitis.

3. Multiple scattered lesions, e.g. disseminated sclerosis.

4. System degenerations involving particular spinal tracts, e.g. tabes dorsalis, vitamin B_{12} neuropathy (subacute combined degeneration).

Symptoms of a focal lesion at a particular level

What follows is an interpretation in anatomical and physiological terms of the symptoms which *may* follow a focal lesion of the spinal cord at a particular level. It must be borne in mind, however, that pathological processes rarely produce the clear-cut effects of a theoretical lesion.

Radicular symptoms

An irritative lesion of one posterior spinal root causes pain referred to the corresponding dermatome; that is, the area of skin innervated by that root (see Fig. 3.8, p. 116), and also to the muscles which receive from it their sensory supply. Such root pains are likely to be made worse by coughing and sneezing, which raise the pressure within the spinal canal, and by movements of the neighbouring part of the spine. The dermatome is likely to be hyperalgesic and hyperaesthetic until the lesion interferes with conduction in the root, when appreciation of light touch and pin-prick are impaired over the dermatome.

A lesion of an anterior spinal root causes the symptoms of a lower motor neurone lesion in the muscles innervated by the corresponding spinal segment.

Sensory impairment

A lesion of the posterior columns of the spinal cord leads to impairment of appreciation of posture, passive movement of the joints, and vibration below the level of the lesion on the same side. A lesion involving the spinothalamic tracts causes impairment of appreciation of pain, heat and cold on the opposite side of the body (see Fig. 3.6, p. 113). Since the pathways conducting these forms of sensation take several segments to cross the spinal cord, the upper level of the area of sensory loss will be a corresponding number of dermatomes below the segmental level of the lesion. This discrepancy will amount to two or three dermatomes in the thoracic and lumbar regions and one in the cervical region.

Corticospinal tract symptoms

Damage to the corticospinal tract will cause the symptoms of an upper motor neurone lesion, i.e. weakness, spasticity, increased tendon reflexes, diminished abdominal reflexes, and an extensor plantar response below the level of the lesion on the same side.

Co-ordination

It is not usually possible to detect the symptoms of a lesion involving the ascending spinocerebellar tracts, but co-ordination in a limb may be impaired as a result of loss of postural sensibility by a lesion of the posterior columns.

Anterior horn cells

Involvement of the anterior horn cells leads to the symptoms of a lower motor neurone lesion identical with those of a lesion of an anterior spinal root, except that a progressive lesion of the anterior horn cells is more likely to cause fasciculation in the muscles innervated than an anterior root lesion.

Reflexes

A lesion of the spinal cord will impair or abolish a reflex whose arc passes through the segment involved. Reflexes mediated by segments below the level of the lesion will show the changes characteristic of a corticospinal tract lesion.

Autonomic symptoms

Sweating will be abolished over the area of skin which receives its sympathetic innervation from the segment of the spinal cord affected. Excessive sweating may occur over the area which receives its sympathetic innervation from below the level of the lesion. Since the sympathetic outflow from the spinal cord is limited to the thoracic and first lumbar segments, a lesion of the cervical cord may cause excessive sweating over the whole of the body, while a lesion below the first lumbar segment will not lead to either excess or impairment of sweating.

When the symptoms just described are produced by a unilateral lesion involving one-half of the spinal cord, the resulting clinical picture is known as *Brown–Séquard's syndrome* (see p. 118).

COMPRESSION OF THE SPINAL CORD

Aetiology and pathology

The causes of spinal cord compression, excluding injury, are divided into extra-dural and intradural, the intradural being further divided into those which arise outside the spinal cord and are therefore called extramedullary, and those arising within the spinal cord, or intramedullary.

The principal extradural causes of compression are disease of the vertebral column, especially tuberculous osteitis (Pott's disease), secondary carcinoma, and cervical spondylosis with protrusion of intervertebral discs (Fig. 18.1). Less frequent causes include primary neoplasms arising from the vertebrae, and other forms of osteitis, especially the osteitis deformans of Paget. Other less common extradural causes of compression are extradural abscess, infiltration of the meninges with reticulosis and leukaemic deposits, and parasitic cysts.

The commonest extramedullary tumours are meningiomas and neurofibromas, which usually arise from spinal roots, the posterior more frequently than the anterior. Intramedullary tumours exhibit the same histo-logical features as the cerebral gliomas. Angiomatous malformations occasionally occur and may have a considerable longitudinal extent.

The sexes are equally likely to be affected by spinal compression. The age incidence depends upon the cause. Tuberculous spinal osteitis usually occurs in children and young adults, spinal tumour mostly between the ages of 20 and 60, and secondary carcinoma and Paget's osteitis usually in the second half of life.

The special pathological and clinical features of some of the commoner causes of spinal compression are separately considered below.

Effects of compression upon the cord

Spinal compression, however produced, affects the cord in several ways. Direct pressure interferes with conduction in the spinal roots and in the cord itself. Pressure upon the ascending longitudinal spinal veins leads to oedema of the cord below the site of compression. Compression of the longitudinal and radicular spinal arteries causes ischamia of the segments of the cord which they supply. As a result of these vascular disturbances, areas of softening may develop – so-called compression myelitis. Finally, obstruction of the subarachnoid space causes loculation of the cerebrospinal fluid below the point of compression and leads to characteristic changes in its composition (see p. 364).

Symptoms

The symptoms of compression of the spinal cord differ to some extent according to whether the source of compression is extradural, extramedullary or intramedullary; and according to its segmental level. However, is is by no means always possible to determine before operation the precise relationship of the source of compression to the cord.

Mode of onset

The onset is usually gradual, especially when the cause is a spinal tumour or cervical spondylosis, but is often rapid in secondary carcinoma of the spine. In tuberculous caries it is usually gradual, but paraplegia may develop acutely. About two-thirds of the sufferers from spinal tumour come to operation during the first and second years after the onset of symptoms.

The first symptoms are usually sensory, the commonest being pain radiating into the distribution of one or more spinal roots. Root pains are usually severe in vertebral collapse from all causes. In the case of spinal tumours they are most frequently encountered when the tumour is extramedullary, such as a neurofibroma. Root pains may be unilateral or bilateral, and have the characteristics described above (p. 118). Pain in the back may occur. Motor symptoms usually follow fairly rapidly, and may be the first to be noticed. Weakness, stiffness, and unsteadiness of one or both lower limbs may occur. When the source of compression is above the cervical enlargement, one upper limb may be affected before the lower. Sphincter disturbances are usually late in onset.

The clinical picture

The cardinal features of compression of the spinal cord are: (i) a slowly progressive impairment of function at (ii) a determinable and persistent segmental level, though, as we shall see, the second point needs qualification. It follows that the clinical picture will depend upon the level of the cord compressed, and the stage which the compression has reached. The symptoms of a severe degree of compression will be those enumerated above, bearing in mind the motor and sensory supply of the spinal segments (Fig. 3.8 (a) and (b), and pp. 116–17).

In the early stages of spinal cord compression the function of the corticospinal tracts tends to be impaired first. When the thoracic cord is compressed, it may be difficult to find evidence of a lower motor neurone lesion, and in the absence of sensory loss the clinical picture is that of a simple spastic paraplegia. The level of the lesion can then be established only by myelography. In some cases, especially when the cord is compressed in the cervical region, the upper level of the sensory loss may be some distance below that of the spinal segments compressed, for example in the mid-thoracic region. The level, however, tends to move slowly upwards.

The cerebrospinal fluid

Examination of the cerebrospinal fluid is of great diagnostic importance in spinal compression, but should only be undertaken when neurosurgical facilities are at hand. For a description of myelography see p. 153.

Manometry

The pressure of the fluid is frequently subnormal below an obstruction of the spinal subarachnoid space, and the normal variations corresponding to the pulse and respiration are often diminished or absent.

The presence of a tumour of the cauda equina may lead to a failure to obtain cerebrospinal fluid by lumbar puncture at the usual site if it completely fills the spinal canal at that point. When spinal subarachnoid block is due to a tumour, lumbar puncture may lead to a temporary exacerbation of symptoms and therefore should only be done when neurosurgical facilities are available for operation if necessary.

Chemical changes

The essential chemical abnormality is the rise in the protein content of the fluid, which usually lies between 1.0 and 2.0 g/l. The fluid may be yellow in colour – xanthochromia – and clot spontaneously. There is no excess of cells unless the source of compression is inflammatory. A rise in the protein content of the fluid is most marked in cases of extramedullary spinal compression, and may be slight in cases of intramedullary tumour. The protein tends to be lower when the cord is compressed in the cervical region, whatever the cause of compression, than when this is situated at a lower level. The protein content of the fluid may be raised *above* a tumour of the cauda equina.

The spine

The spine may exhibit angular deformity, local tenderness, and pain on movement when the vertebrae are diseased. In cervical spondylosis, however, both pain and limitation of movement are often slight.

Radiography

Radiography of the spine is necessary in all cases of suspected spinal compression. When this is due to disease of the vertebral column, only X-ray examination may enable the cause of the compression to be discovered. It renders visible the vertebral destruction due to tuberculous caries and other forms of osteitis, secondary carcinoma, primary vertebral neoplasm, and the changes associated with traumatic lesions. Chronic intervertebral disc protrusion is likely to be associated with narrowing of the corresponding disc space and bony spurs from the bodies of adjacent vertebrae. A tumour arising within the vertebral canal may by erosion lead to its diffuse enlargement, in which case the distance between the pedicles will be increased, or may pass outward through the intervertebral foramen with local destruction of bone – a dumb-bell or collar-stud tumour. CT scanning and myelography may be necessary.

SOME VARIETIES OF SPINAL CORD COMPRESSION

There are several causes of compression of the spinal cord which possess distinctive features and are sufficiently important to receive brief separate consideration.

Myelopathy due to cervical spondylosis

This is a very common disorder in the second half of life. Degeneration of one or more intervertebral discs in the neck leads to narrowing of the discs and production of bony and cartilaginous osteophytes which project backwards into the spinal canal, or laterally into the intervertebral foramina. Compression of the spinal cord leads to local softening with ascending and descending degeneration, and compression of the nerve roots to radiculitis.

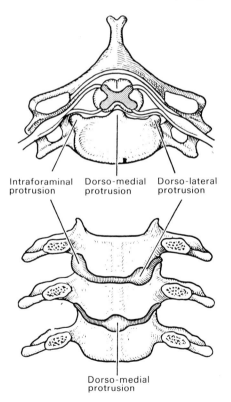

Intraforaminal protrusion   Dorso-medial protrusion   Dorso-lateral protrusion

Dorso-medial protrusion

Fig. 18.1. Sites of intervertebral disc protrusion.

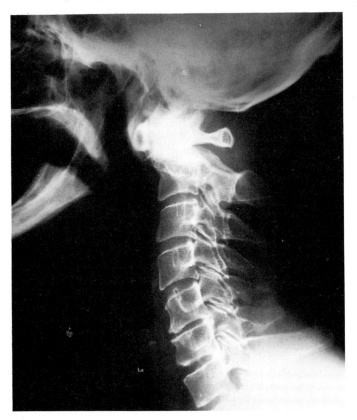

Fig. 18.2. Lateral X-ray of cervical spine showing atlanto-axial dislocation and degenerative osteoarthritic changes at the C5–6 level.

The onset of symptoms is usually insidious, and the clinical picture depends upon the level or levels at which the cord is compressed, and the extent of the damage. There is commonly a mixture of symptoms of upper and lower motor neurone lesions in the upper limbs with those of an upper motor neurone lesion in the lower. Sensory loss may be absent, but there is commonly impairment of appreciation of light touch and tactile discrimination and pin-prick over some of the digits, with or without loss of postural sensibility, which may also be present in the lower limbs. The tendon reflexes in the upper limbs may be diminished or exaggerated, and there is often an 'inverted' radial reflex, i.e. tapping the radius evokes only flexion of the digits. There is often little or no pain in the neck, but there is usually some limitation of active and passive movement, sometimes associated with crepitus. Plain X-rays and myelograms (Fig. 18.3) are characteristic. The dynamics and composition of the cerebrospinal fluid are usually normal.

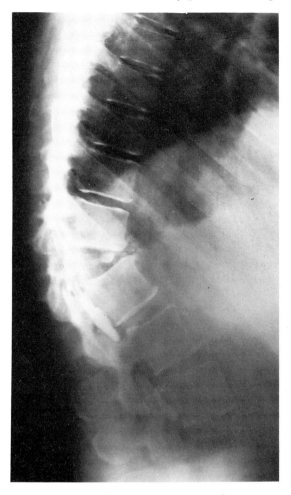

Fig. 18.3. Lateral X-ray of dorsal spine showing collapse of lower thoracic vertebra due to metastatic carcinoma.

Tuberculous spinal osteitis

The infective process usually begins in the body of the vertebra, and, spreading to adjacent bodies, leads to their collapse, and so produces an angular deformity of the spine. It is rare for the deformity as such to be an important factor in compression of the spinal cord, which is more frequently due either to an extradural tuberculous abscess or to tuberculous pachymeningitis. There is often interference with the vascular supply of subjacent segments, which is an important factor in the production of paraplegia, which occurs in about 10 per cent of patients with Pott's disease, usually within two or three years of the onset. The thoracic region of the cord is commonly affected.

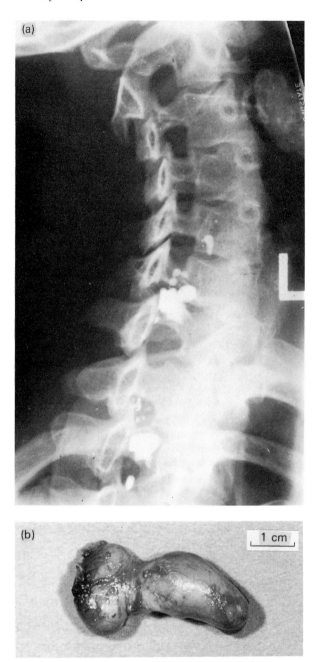

Fig. 18.4. (a) Lateral oblique X-ray of cervical spine showing widening of the exit foramen C7–T1. There is also calcification in cervical lymph glands. (b) 'Dumbell' neurofibroma removed at surgery.

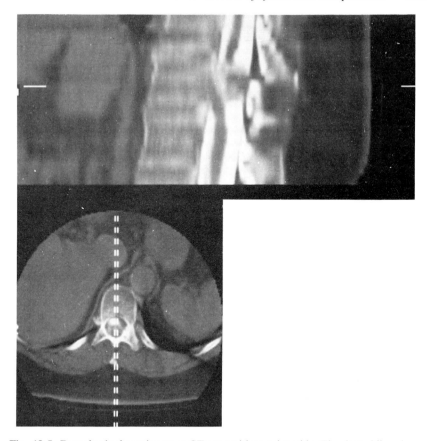

Fig. 18.5. Dorsal spinal meningoma: CT scan with metrizamide. The dotted line shows the plane of the sagittal reconstruction. The posteriorly placed meningioma is displacing the cord anteriorly.

The symptoms are usually those of gradual compression of the spinal cord, but sometimes symptoms develop acutely. They possess no distinctive features. The cerebrospinal fluid is likely to show the changes of spinal subarachnoid block. X-ray appearances are characteristic.

Secondary carcinoma of the spine

Neoplasms of the breast, prostate, thyroid, and kidney are particularly liable to metastasize into bone, and sometimes the collapse of a vertebra as the result of a metastatic deposit provides the first evidence of the existence of the cancer. Severe pain in the back and distribution of the compressed nerve roots is a prominent early symptom, and when the deposit is above the level of the first lumbar vertebra symptoms of paraplegia may develop in the course of two or three weeks. X-ray changes are usually characteristic, but it is not always easy

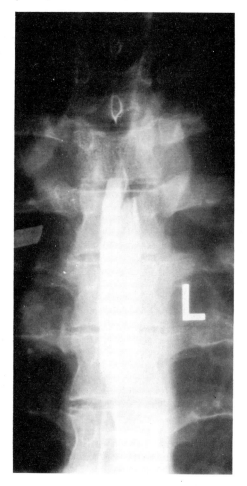

Fig. 18.6. Intradural extramedullary compression of the spinal cord causing complete spinal block on myelography. The lesion proved to be a meningioma.

to distinguish a secondary deposit from other causes of vertebral collapse. The cerebrospinal fluid is likely to show the changes of subarachnoid block.

The diagnosis of spinal compression

When the earliest symptom of spinal compression is root pain, it may be confused with visceral disorders, of which pain is a prominent symptom, for example pleurisy, angina pectoris, cholecystitis, gastric and duodenal ulcer, and renal calculus. This error can be avoided only by a thorough examination of the nervous system, which will usually yield some evidence of a lesion of the spinal cord, reinforced by the absence of any evidence of visceral disease. Spinal compression requires to be distinguished from other lesions of the spinal cord, particularly those giving rise to progressive paraplegia, e.g. spinal syphilis, disseminated sclerosis, syringomyelia, and motor neurone disease. On clinical grounds this distinction can usually be made with considerable certainty, but the diagnosis can only be clinched by examination of the cerebrospinal fluid and if necessary myelography and CT scanning.

In the localization of the segmental level of spinal compression, segmental symptoms, especially atrophic paralysis, root pains and hyperalgesia, are of the first importance. Next in value is the upper limit of the area of sensory loss, though this is not always easy to define and, as already mentioned, it may correspond to a lower segment than the uppermost compressed.

Since the spinal cord terminates at the level of the lower border of the first lumbar vertebra, spinal segments do not correspond numerically with the vertebral arches by which they are enclosed. Having localized the source of compression in terms of spinal segments, in order to ascertain which spinal segment is related to a given vertebra the following rule is roughly correct. For the cervical vertebrae, add one, for thoracic 1–6 add two, for thoracic 7–9 add three. The tenth thoracic arch overlies lumbar 1 and 2 segments, the eleventh thoracic arch lumbar 3 and 4, the twelfth thoracic arch lumbar 5, and the first lumbar arch the sacral and coccygeal segments.

The diagnosis of an extradural source of compression usually depends upon clinical and radiological evidence of changes in the vertebral column. The distinction between extramedullary and intramedullary compression is often difficult. Root pains favour an extramedullary source which also tends to cause a higher level of protein in the cerebrospinal fluid, and to produce spinal block earlier.

Prognosis

The prognosis of compression of the spinal cord depends principally upon three things:

1. The severity and duration of the disturbance of function when the patient comes under observation.

2. The nature of the source of the compression and the extent to which it can be relieved.

3. The level of the cord compressed. The more severe the interruption of conduction in the cord, the less likely is recovery to be complete. A patient with spastic paraplegia-in-extension, even when this has been present for some years, may show considerable improvement after removal of an extramedullary tumour. On the other hand, when the stage of paraplegia-in-flexion has been reached, little improvement can be expected, even though the cause may be removed. Little improvement usually follows an attempt to remove an intramedullary tumour, and when spinal cord compression of any kind has produced ischaemic softening of the cord, such changes are irreversible. On the whole, the prognosis is better when the cord is compressed in the thoracic region than in the cervical or lumbar regions. The natural tendency of the

myelopathy due to cervical spondylosis is to become arrested, but most patients are left with a varying degree of residual disability.

Treatment

The treatment of compression of the spinal cord involves: (i) the appropriate treatment of the source of the compression, and (ii) when paraplegia is present, adequate care of the paralysed limbs, skin, the urinary tract and the bowels along the lines laid down on page 385, for upon the careful treatment of the paraplegia may depend not only the patient's life but also the rate at which recovery of function occurs. The treatment of a spinal tumour is usually surgical, but X-ray irradiation may be of value in the treatment of an irremovable intramedullary growth. Laminectomy is rarely necessary in a case of tuberculous caries of the spine, because most patients do well on the appropriate chemotherapy and orthopaedic treatment. An exploratory operation, however, may be carried out when paraplegia has continued unimproved after several months of treatment, or when a sudden increase in its severity occurs. In most cases the myelopathy due to cervical spondylosis is best treated by immobilization of the neck in a suitable collar. Operation is usually contra-indicated in patients over the age of 60 or with severe changes in the spinal cord, or associated cardiovascular disease. It may be of value in younger patients, especially when there is a short history and protrusion of only a single intervertebral disc. Results have improved since the introduction of the anterior surgical approach to cervical discs.

COMPRESSION OF THE CAUDA EQUINA

Compression of the cauda equina may be due to a neoplasm, or one or more roots may be compressed by a displaced intervertebral disc. A small tumour may for a long time compress only one or two roots on one side. A large and massive growth may involve the whole of the cauda, but it is sometimes surprising how little function is disturbed by even a large tumour. In lumbar spondylosis apophysial arthritis and thickened ligamenta flava may cause compression as well as, or even without, disc protrusion.

In most cases pain is the earliest symptom, located in the lumbar or sacral regions of the spine, or referred to one or both lower limbs. Motor symptoms consist of atrophic paralysis, the distribution of which depends upon the roots affected, and which most frequently involves the muscles below the knee. The distribution of sensory loss also depends upon which posterior roots are involved. Disturbance of function of the bladder and bowels is usually a late development, and tends to lead to retention of urine and faeces, even though the external sphincters are paralysed. When the lowest sacral roots are com-pressed, the external genitalia become anaesthetic and the anal and bulbocavernosus reflexes are lost. Trophic symptoms may occur in the lower limbs, which are frequently cold and cyanosed, and tend to become oedematous if they are allowed to hang down.

INJURIES TO THE SPINAL CORD

The commonest spinal injuries in civil life today are the result of motor-car or industrial accidents. The commonest sites are the lower cervical region and the thoracolumbar junction. Most spinal injuries are the result of forcible flexion which may cause fracture dislocation at the site of greatest stress, or displacement of an intervertebral disc. The spinal cord may also be injured in the infant during birth as the result of violent traction.

The degrees of injury of the cord have been classified as concussion, contusion – which means bruising without rupture of the pia mater – and laceration. When cervical spondylosis is present, contusion of the cervical cord may follow an injury which would not have produced it had the neck been normal.

The symptoms of spinal injury depend upon the severity and situation of the lesion, and are those of a focal lesion of the cord (p. 308).

Complete interruption leads immediately to flaccid paralysis with loss of all sensation and most reflex activity below the site of the lesion, and paralysis of the bladder and rectum. Less severe lesions such as spinal contusion may lead to an equally severe immediate disturbance of function, or symptoms may increase in severity for several days. Slight spinal injuries cause motor symptoms of incomplete division, without complete sensory loss.

The diagnosis is usually obvious, the only question being the nature of the injury to the cord. Myelography may be necessary to determine the presence and degree of cord compression and its precise cause.

The prognosis of a severe injury of the spinal cord is always grave, but experience of the results of war injuries show that it is possible for a patient with a completely divided cord to retain good general health indefinitely under careful supervision. This is sometimes possible even when the lesion is as high as the fifth cervical segment. When the cord has been incompletely divided, the prognosis is obviously better.

The scope of surgery in the treatment of injuries of the spinal cord is limited by the fact that in most cases the maximal injury has been produced at the time of the accident, and the condition of the cord is both non-progressive and irreparable. When, however, there is radiographic evidence of gross bony deformity, disc protrusion, or the presence of a foreign body in the spinal canal, and clinical examination indicates that the cord has not been completely divided, or if recovery of function has begun but has become arrested, surgical intervention offers the hope of relieving compression or cicatricial contraction which may be retarding recovery. The general management of cases of injury of the spinal cord and cauda equina is described on page 384.

SYRINGOMYELIA

The term syringomyelia is derived from the Greek words, syrinx, a tube, and myelos, the marrow or spinal cord. It is characterized by elongated cavities lined by glia lying close to the central canal of the spinal cord and often extending upwards into the medulla, when it is known as syringobulbia. If the tube is lined with ependymal cells of the central canal it is described as hydromyelia.

Aetiology

Syringomyelia is due to a developmental abnormality in the formation of the central canal of the spinal cord. Though trauma to the neck can play a part in precipitating the emergence of symptoms, syringomyelia may also follow complete or incomplete transection in fracture dislocation of the spinal cord. Gardner has proposed a purely mechanical basis for the cystic excavation of the cord or hydromyelia based on two factors: first, obstruction to the outlets of the fourth ventricle, and, second, pulsation in the fourth ventricle due to the intracranial arterial pressure wave (Fig. 18.7). In many cases the obstruction to the fourth ventricle is due to protrusion of the tonsils of the cerebellum through the foramen magnum, the Arnold–Chiari malformation (p. 267). This may arise as a developmental defect that followed failure of perforation of the foramina of Luschka and Magendie in foetal life (the Dandy–Walker malformation), or may be associated with cerebellar ectopia, with or without the skeletal defects of Klippel–Feil (fusion of multiple cervical vertebrae), atlanto-occipital fusion or basilar impression. Other congenital skeletal abnormalities may be present, including kyphoscoliosis and spina bifida.

Pathology

The pathological changes are usually situated in the lower cervical and upper thoracic regions of the cord (Fig. 18.8). The cord is enlarged, mainly in the transverse plane, and transverse section reveals a cavity surrounded by a zone of translucent gelatinous material and containing clear or yellow fluid, and occupying the central grey matter near the central canal. In the medulla the region affected is usually the posterolateral part of the tegmentum. The expansion of the cavity and the surrounding gliosis lead to compression of the anterior horns of the grey matter causing atrophy of the anterior horn cells and degeneration of their axons. Compression of the long ascending and descending tracts of the cord occurs somewhat later and leads to secondary degeneration. Occasionally cavitation of the spinal cord is secondary to the presence of a tumour. Even though it may originate in a congenital abnormality, the symptoms of syringomyelia do not usually appear until adult life, usually between the ages of 25 and 40. The age of onset, however, may be as early as 10 or as late as 60.

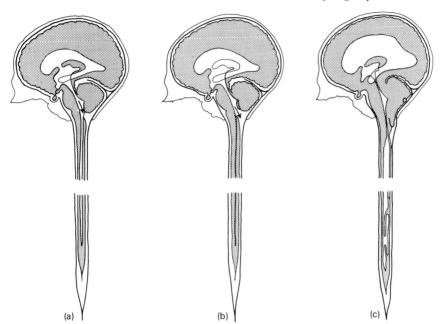

Fig. 18.7. Hydrodynamic mechanism of syringomyelia (Gardner).
(a) Outline of the embryonal neural tube superimposed upon the configuration of the mature nervous system. The outlet of the fourth ventricle is bridged by a permeable membrane that funnels the pulsations of the ventricular fluid into the central canal (arrow). Despite its vulnerable position, the persistence of this membrane may be demonstrated, not only in every Dandy–Walker malformation but also in many Arnold–Chiari malformations.
(b) Normal situation after the foramina open and the pulsations escape freely into the subarachnoid space (arrow) and to the outer surface of the spinal cord. As a result of this by-pass the central canal is compressed and becomes a vestigial structure.
(c) The neural tube in syringomyelia. The ventricles are sometimes large but the intracranial pressure is normal (compensated hydrocephalus). The foramina of the fourth ventricle are compressed by impaction in a congenital hindbrain hernia. The central canal at the level of the hernia is usually patent but cannot dilate because of impaction. Below the impaction the central canal is dilated. Dilatation is greatest in the cervical region where the transmitted ventricular fluid pulse pressure is widest. A false diverticulum of the neural tube as shown below the cut may develop at any level to form a 'true syrinx' that parallels the central canal and is entirely lacking in ependyma. It may originate from the floor of the fourth ventricle (syringobulbia) and by its downward extension collapse the central canal.

Symptoms

The patient usually first notices either the slow onset of wasting and weakness of one hand, or the loss of sensation of pain over one hand and forearm leading to injuries, especially burns, which are not noticed at the time. Examination at this stage is likely to show wasting, weakness, and hypotonia of

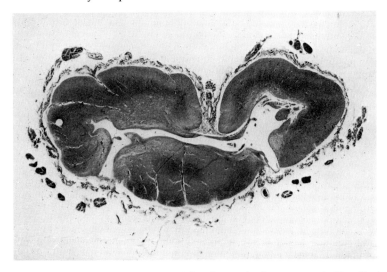

Fig. 18.8. Syringomyelia: spinal cord showing cavitation surrounded by gliosis.

one upper limb, chiefly distally. Fasciculation is inconstant and usually inconspicuous. The tendon reflexes in the affected limb are diminished or lost. Analgesia and thermo-anaesthesia to heat and cold are usually roughly coextensive. They tend to have a segmental distribution involving first the ulnar side of the hand and forearm, then spreading to the radial side and on to the neck and chest. Appreciation of light touch and postural sensibility are preserved. This selective disturbance of sensation, known as 'dissociated sensory loss', is due to the fact that the central position of the lesion in the spinal cord interrupts the decussating fibres concerned with appreciation of pain, heat and cold while sparing the fibres which run upwards in the posterior columns. Slight signs of a corticospinal tract lesion unaccompanied by much weakness are likely to be found in the lower limb on the same side.

Symptoms may remain unilateral for a long time before extending to the opposite upper limb, or they may be bilateral when the patient is first seen. The motor loss is reduplicated on the opposite side, though its extent and severity may not be symmetrical. Ocular sympathetic paralysis, leading to ptosis and small pupils, is often present.

The scars of burns or other injuries are usually to be found on the fingers and forearms (Fig. 18.9). Most syringomyelic patients have a dorsal kyphoscoliosis. Arthropathy of one or more of the joints of the upper limb is sometimes present and is seen in the cervical spine also in some cases. Sphincter function is usually unimpaired and the cerebrospinal fluid is normal.

Syringobulbia

A fine rotary nystagmus is often present in syringomyelia without other evidence of involvement of the medulla. The disease, beginning in the lower

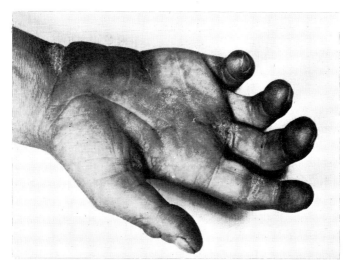

Fig. 18.9. Hand in syringomyelia, showing muscular wasting deformity and fleshy fingers with scars of burns.

cervical region, often spreads slowly upwards over a period of years to involve the medulla – syringobulbia. The spinal tract and nucleus of the trigeminal nerve are usually first affected on one or both sides. This causes the characteristic dissociated sensory loss to extend on to the trigeminal area, which it involves not in order of the sensory divisions but from behind forwards, converging on the nose and upper lip (Fig. 2.9, p. 60) – sensory loss of the so-called 'onion-skin' type. Vertigo is the next commonest symptom. Involvement of the motor functions of the cranial nerves innervated by the pons and medulla is not common. Exceptionally syringobulbia occurs without evidence of spinal cord involvement.

Diagnosis

The diagnosis in a patient with suggestive clinical signs is incomplete unless careful upper cervical and skull X-rays have excluded the skeletal abnormalities of cervical vertebral fusion (Klippel–Feil abnormality) or basilar impression (p. 374). Plain films should be followed by myelographic studies in the supine position, rather than the previously-used prone position, in order to demonstrate the presence of cerebellar tonsils partially obstructing the flow of metrizamide. Finally, a further useful technique is that of air myelography, which on changing the position of the patient from the head down position to the head up position may demonstrate the 'collapsing' of the spinal cord surrounding the syringomyelia or hydromyelia. CT scanning may be combined with myelography to show the extent of the Arnold–Chiari malformation or basilar invagination and a dilated cervical cord (Figs. 18.10–12).

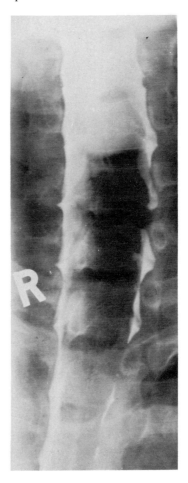

Fig. 18.10. Intramedullary lesion causing expansion of the spinal cord in the cervical region, due to syringomyelia.

Syringomyelia needs to be distinguished from conditions in which muscular wasting and cutaneous sensory loss are present in the upper limbs. When such symptoms are due to lesions of the spinal nerve roots or peripheral nerves, cutaneous sensory loss usually includes anaesthesia to light touch which is characteristically absent in syringomyelia. This fact, together with the characteristic distribution of the muscular wasting and sensory loss, distinguishes syringomyelia from compression of the median nerve in the carpal tunnel (p. 411), compression of the ulnar nerve at the elbow (p. 412) and cervical rib (p. 406). Cervical spondylosis may cause muscular wasting and sensory loss in the upper limb together with spastic paraplegia, and the X-ray changes in the cervical spine may be indistinguishable from those of syringomyelic arthro-

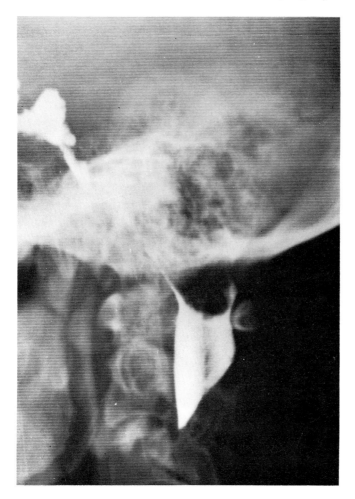

Fig. 18.11. Arnold–Chiari malformation: lateral film of myelogram showing abnormally low cerebellum.

pathy, but cervical spondylosis does not cause dissociated sensory loss over the upper limbs, and the impairment of sensation never extends to the trigeminal area. The history is usually shorter in relation to the severity of the symptoms, and the X-ray changes are constantly present, whereas cervical arthropathy occurs in less than half of all cases of syringomyelia. Tumour of the spinal cord may simulate syringomyelia, but, unlike the latter, usually causes symptoms with a well-defined upper level identical both for motor and sensory functions and accompanied by the changes in the cerebrospinal fluid characteristic of spinal block. Motor neurone disease is distinguished by the absence of sensory loss and the more rapid muscular wasting, accompanied by more obvious widespread fasciculation.

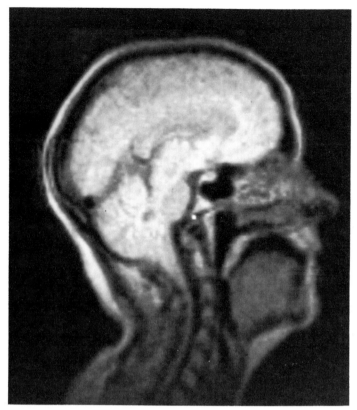

Fig. 18.12. Arnold–Chiari malformation: NMR(SE) scan showing abnormally low cerebellum (compare Fig. 0.2 (c)).

Course and prognosis

Syringomyelic symptoms tend slowly to extend and, without surgical treatment, to become worse in the course of years, and then may remain virtually stationary. The upper limbs become increasingly weak and wasted and cutaneous anaesthesia and loss of postural sensibility in the fingers may be added to the analgesia and thermo-anaesthesia. Trophic lesions of the fingers may call for amputation, and arthropathy of the shoulders may lead to spontaneous dislocation. Paraplegia tends to develop in the later stages, but the patient may not be completely disabled even twenty years after the onset.

Treatment

If the myelogram shows a complete block then an effort may be made by a neurosurgeon to aspirate fluid from the centre of the syrinx. The patient should be warned against the risks of unnoticed injury.

Many patients with a mechanical basis for the cystic excavation have been treated by upper cervical decompression, restoring the patency of the fourth ventricular outflow where this is occluded, blocking the entry to the central canal of the upper cervical cord, and aspiration of the central cavity where necessary. Some cases have improved following surgery and others have failed to progress postoperatively over a number of years. In a few patients without adequate proof of a congenital anomaly the defect appears to be due to arachnoiditis and such patients are probably better helped by ventriculo-atrial drainage.

MYELITIS

Aetiology and pathology

Myelitis is an inflammation of the spinal cord, usually involving both the grey and the white matter in a considerable part of its transverse extent. When the lesion is limited longitudinally to a few segments, it is described as transverse myelitis; when it spreads progressively upwards, as ascending myelitis.

Myelitis may be due to a large variety of causes, some of which have not yet been identified. It may be due to the spread of bacterial infection, pyogenic or tuberculous, to the cord, or a manifestation of meningovascular syphilis. It may be caused by some form of demyelinating disorder, acute disseminated encephalomyelitis occurring spontaneously or complicating an infection, neuromyelitis optica, or even an acute form of disseminated sclerosis. It may be due to a variety of viruses with known neurotropic propensities. But in many cases the cause is unknown, and its viral origin is hypothetical.

To the naked eye the spinal cord at the site of infection, which is usually the lower thoracic region, exhibits oedema and hyperaemia and in severe cases actual softening. Microscopically the leptomeninges are congested and infiltrated with inflammatory cells. The substance of the cord exhibits congestion or thrombosis of the vessels, with perivascular inflammatory infiltration and oedema. The precise details of the involvement of ganglion cells and white matter depend upon the pathogenesis.

Symptoms

The onset of symptoms is acute or subacute and there is usually some fever. Pain in the back at the level of the lesion is often prominent. Flaccid paralysis, partial or complete, develops more or less rapidly, being confined to the trunk and lower limbs when the thoracic region of the cord is the part involved. Sensory loss, which may be complete or incomplete, is present, and usually exhibits an upper level corresponding to the segmental site of the lesion. There may be a zone of hyperalgesia, and the spine may be tender in this region. There is an impairment of sphincter control, often amounting to complete paralysis of the bladder and rectum. The tendon reflexes are usually at first diminished or lost, and the abdominal reflexes are lost below the level of the lesion. The plantar reflexes may be absent at first, and later become extensor.

In the ascending form of myelitis there is a more or less rapid upward progression of the level of paralysis and sensory loss.

The cerebrospinal fluid usually contains a considerably increased protein content and an excess of cells which may be polymorphonuclear, lymphocytic, or mixed. Queckenstedt's test usually indicates an absence of obstruction in the subarachnoid space except in rare cases when meningeal adhesions develop, or the myelitis is secondary to an extradural abscess.

Diagnosis

The rapid onset of the symptoms of a transverse lesion of the spinal cord, often associated with the general symptoms of an infection, and without evidence of spinal block, renders the diagnosis easy. Myelitis is distinguished from acute infective polyneuritis by the presence of extensor plantar reflexes and of partial or complete sensory loss with a segmental upper level involving the trunk.

Syphilitic myelitis is distinguished by other signs of neurosyphilis when these are present, and by a positive Wassermann reaction in the blood and cerebrospinal fluid. When myelitis forms part of an attack of acute disseminated encephalomyelitis, symptoms of cerebral lesions may be present. In neuromyelitis optica the diagnosis may be in doubt until the optic neuritis develops. The bacterial origin of myelitis depends upon the discovery of the source of infection, usually in the neighbourhood of the spine. Though disseminated sclerosis may be suspected as the cause of the transverse lesion of the spinal cord, especially in a young adult, this diagnosis can only be established if there is a history of previous and characteristic symptoms, or if other signs of the disease are present.

Prognosis

The prognosis depends upon the nature of the infection and its severity, being most serious in the pyogenic variety and in the acute descending form. In myelitis forming part of one of the various forms of acute disseminated encephalomyelitis the prognosis is often good, and if the patient survives the acute attack a large degree of functional recovery may occur. In sporadic cases of myelitis a guarded prognosis should be given in view of the possiblity that the cord lesion may be the first symptom of disseminated sclerosis.

The general treatment of the patient must be carried out on the lines indicated for the treatment of paraplegia. Any specific cause must receive appropriate treatment, including chemotherapy. Even if the organism is unknown, a broad-spectrum antibiotic should be used. Whether or not to employ corticosteroids is often a difficult question. In the sporadic case of unknown aetiology, if the patient is deteriorating or his condition seems stationary, it is justifiable to use either a corticosteroid or corticotrophin.

THE DIAGNOSIS OF PARAPLEGIA

At this point it may be convenient to summarize the more important points in the diagnosis of paraplegia. The first basis of distinction is the time taken for the paraplegia to develop.

Paraplegia of acute onset

Apart from *trauma*, a really acute onset of paraplegia is rare, and should suggest a vascular cause. *Haematomyelia* means a haemorrhage into the spinal cord. When spontaneous, the source is probably often a small congenital vascular abnormality, but occasionaly a large angioma. A bruit may sometimes be heard on auscultation over the spine at the level of an angioma. The clinical picture is the sudden onset of severe and progressive destruction of the spinal cord, usually starting in the central part of the cervical region, and producing gross atrophic paralysis and impairment of all forms of sensibility over the upper limbs, together with paraplegia and sometimes sensory impairment over the lower limbs. Another uncommon cause of paraplegia of sudden onset is thrombosis of the anterior spinal artery.

Paraplegia of subacute onset

Paraplegia developing subacutely over the course of two or three days is usually inflammatory in origin, that is to say, it is due to one of the forms of acute myelitis described on page 381. It may be due to compression of the spinal cord, again often of infective origin, e.g. tuberculous spinal osteitis or a pyogenic extradural abscess, which is an acute neurosurgical emergency. Secondary carcinoma of the spine may also lead to subacute compression of the cord.

Paraplegia of insidious onset

When paraplegia develops slowly over a period of months, or even longer the first step is to exclude compression of the spinal cord as the cause. This depends upon clinical examination, plain X-rays of the spine, examination of the cerebrospinal fluid, and when necessary myelography (p. 153). Cervical spondylosis is one of the commonest causes of paraplegia of slow onset, which is not always associated with any abnormal physical signs in the upper limbs.

Motor neurone disease is usually diagnosed on account of the muscular wasting and fasciculation in the upper limbs. Difficulty may arise, however, when the symptoms of the lower motor neurone lesion appear first in the lower limbs, and in those rare cases in which spastic paraplegia of slow onset precedes the evidence of muscular wasting in any part of the body. In syringomyelia the characteristic muscular wasting and dissociated sensory loss in the upper limbs are almost invariably a much more prominent symptom than the spastic weakness of the lower limbs. Vitamin B_{12} neuropathy (subacute combined degeneration) is not difficult to diagnose when it presents with the characteristic sensory symptoms in the toes and fingers, sensory loss of the posterior column type, and diminution of the ankle-jerks. Exceptionally the presenting symptoms are those of corticospinal tract degeneration. In such cases the diagnosis must rest upon gastric achlorhydria and the appropriate haematological tests. Multiple sclerosis may present with the picture of a progressive spastic paraplegia, especially in middle-aged women. Points of help in the diagnosis are the past occurrence of transient symptoms, especially within the domain of the cranial nerves, the presence of abnormal physical signs above the level of the foramen magnum, and abnormal immunoglobulins in the cerebrospinal fluid. This mode of onset of multiple sclerosis appears specially likely to occur in patients who also have cervical spondylosis.

Among the less common causes of paraplegia of insidious onset is a hereditary degenerative form, hereditary spastic paraplegia, and an ischaemic degeneration of the spinal cord due to atherosclerosis in late middle life and old age.

Paraplegia of spinal origin may be simulated by cerebral disorders, especially a tumour involving the leg areas at the vertex, and symmetrical atheromatous ischaemic softening in that region.

THE CARE OF THE PARAPLEGIC PATIENT

The general management of a patient suffering from paraplegia requires much care, and is as important as the correct treatment of the cause of his disability, for his disorder renders him extremely susceptible to complications which may prove fatal, or even when less serious considerably retard recovery. In particular, pressure sores and urinary infection are not only potentially serious in themselves but they depress the patient's general health and also the functions of the injured spinal cord. Anaemia should be corrected, if necessary by transfusion.

Care of the skin

In paraplegia the skin is extremely liable to injuries which are slow in healing and readily become infected. The factors which lead to pressure sores are – shock in the early stages after injury, vasomotor paralysis, small traumas, and local ischaemia caused by pressure. Such sores are most likely to develop over the bony prominences, especially the heels, the tuber ischii, the sacrum, the greater trochanters, and the malleoli. The paraplegic patient should be nursed on an air or rubber bed, and the most important single measure in the prevention of pressure sores is that his posture should be changed every two hours, both by day and by night. Sir Ludwig Guttmann founder of the Stoke-Mandeville Spinal Unit once commented 'you can put anything you like on a pressure sore except the patient!' The lower limbs should be kept extended and the calves should rest upon small pillows with the heels projecting beyond them. When the patient is in the lateral position care should be taken that one leg does not press upon the other. The weight of the bedclothes is taken by means of a cradle. In acute cases the patient is propped up in bed after four weeks and should be able to sit out in a chair in from eight to twelve weeks.

The treatment of pressure sores

If an ulcer has already developed, all necrotic tissue should first be cut away to allow free drainage, and cultures should be made weekly. At first the sores may be cleaned with hydrogen peroxide and a dressing of a suitable antibiotic applied, for a few days. After that Eusol dressings should be used. Systemic chemotherapy may be required. When a discharge persists in spite of treatment, the possibility of infection of the deeper structures, including a bone, should be borne in mind. Skin grafting is sometimes helpful in the later stages.

Care of the bladder

The care of the bladder in paraplegia differs somewhat according to whether the patient is seen immediately after developing paraplegia as the result of a spinal injury, or comes under the observation with paraplegia of long standing.

Paraplegia of acute onset

Retention of urine will occur, and this must be treated in such a way as best to promote the development of an 'automatic bladder', that is a bladder which is uninfected and will empty itself automatically from time to time and so maintain a healthy urinary tract. In this way the use of an indwelling catheter can usually be avoided, and intermittent catheterization undertaken when necessary.

A careful watch is kept on the urine for evidence of infection which will require treatment with the appropriate antibiotics.

The bladder in established paraplegia

When a patient comes under observation with established paraplegia, it is necessary to investigate his bladder function. The first step is to determine the amount of residual urine, if any, whether the urine is infected, and the nature of the infecting organism. Cystometry provides useful information as to the state of reflex activity of the bladder wall, but the state of sphincter tone is equally important. In many cases cystoscopy, and in some cases cystography, are necessary. In paraplegia of long standing there may be vesical or renal calculi, pyelonephritis, or hydronephrosis. Excretion urography should therefore be carried out when necessary.

The treatment of the bladder will depend upon the situation disclosed by these investigations. When there is an active detrusor and spasm of the internal sphincter, fractional division of the sphincter may facilitate bladder emptying. When the bladder is much contracted and infected, the choice will lie between suprapubic cystostomy and an indwelling catheter. In all cases of impaired bladder function of neurological origin the patient must be instructed on the unreliability of bladder sensation, the need to empty the bladder at two- or three-hourly intervals, and the way in which this can be aided by posture, relaxation, suprapubic pressure, etc. During the phase of bladder re-education, carbachol by injection or orally may be useful. Bladder neck resection may reduce sphincter tone sufficiently to allow free drainage.

In spinal cord lesions the balance between precipitancy and hesitancy depends on the relative involvement of descending facilitatory and inhibitory pathways. Precipitancy with incontinence may be aided by anticholinergic muscle blocking drugs such as atropine (0.25 mg three times a day) or propantheline (30 mg three times a day) by mouth. The overdistended bladder with a lower motor neurone lesion is aided by cholinergic drugs such as carbachol (0.2 mg three times a day) or bethanechol (10 mg three times a day) by mouth.

Care of the rectum

The patient with paraplegia is likely to be constipated, but at the other extreme incontinence must be avoided. When constipation is troublesome, it is best treated by the administration of an aperient at night two or three times a week, followed by a suppository or an enema. Rectal examination should always be carried out, and it may be necessary to remove impacted faeces digitally.

Physiotherapy and compensatory training

After acute and especially traumatic lesions of the spinal cord, most paraplegic patients will be able to get about in a wheelchair, and many more can be taught to walk than was once thought possible. Physiotherapy therefore aims at the maximum development by means of exercises of all those muscles in which voluntary power remains, and the prevention of flexor contractures of the lower limbs by means of passive movements. These, together with massage, when begun sufficiently early, will do much to prevent the development of flexor spasms. With adequate physiotherapy and the avoidance of infection it is often possible to encourage extensor tone and reduce flexor spasms. If spasticity predominates diazepam (Valium) may be given in slowly decreasing dosages up to 30 mg a day with some benefit.

Surgical treatment

Surgical treatment may be called for, as already mentioned, to deal with the causative lesion. Orthopaedic surgery often has an important part to play in diminishing muscular spasms and reorganizing the muscular control of the lower limbs so as to make it possible for them to function again as supports for the body, with the aid of appropriate walking instruments and spinal supports. Finally, when hope of this has to be abandoned, it may be possible by means of the appropriate intrathecal injections, or by anterior ramisectomy, to abolish flexor spasms. Indeed, in some cases an intrathecal nerve block may make walking possible.

The treatment of spasticity (see p. 91)

Baclofen (Lioresal) is an analogue of GABA, the inhibitory transmitter. It is effective in reducing flexor spasms and pyramidal rigidity, probably by selectively reducing gamma fibre activity. The initial dose is 5 mg three times a day by mouth.

SPINA BIFIDA

Aetiology and pathology

Spina bifida means an incomplete closure of the vertebral canal, which is usually associated with a similar anomaly of the spinal cord. In the early embryo the nervous system is represented by the neural groove, the lateral folds of which unite dorsally to form the neural tube. An arrest in this process of development leads to defective closure of the neural tube, associated with a similar defect in the closure of the bony vertebral canal. A number of varieties of spina bifida are described, differing in respect of the nature and severity of the spinal defect. In severe cases a sac protrudes through the vertebral opening, which may contain meninges only or also the flattened opened spinal cord, meningomyelocele. In the least severe cases there is no protrusion, but a defect in the laminal arches may be palpable as a depression, which is sometimes covered by a dimple or a tuft of hair (spina bifida occulta). The commonest site of spina bifida is the lumbosacral region, but it is occasionally found in the neck. It may be associated with other congenital abnormalities, especially hydro-cephalus.

Spina bifida malformations occur with a frequency of approximately one in every two hundred pregnancies. In some 95 per cent of cases the amniotic alpha-fetoprotein levels is raised at the fifth month. The amniotic alpha-fetoprotein values give a false-negative reading in 0.5 per cent of cases and false-positive in 2 per cent of cases. Acetylcholinesterase concentration in the amniotic fluid is also increased. High-resolution diagnostic ultrasound is needed to confirm the abnormality before termination is recommended on the basis of biochemical tests. If further tests confirm the diagnosis, the mother can then be offered termination. This could reduce the need for more agonizing ethical decisions after birth.

Symptoms

There are two main clinical pictures associated with spina bifida. One is that presented by the newly-born infant with a protruding sac in the lumbosacral region. This is commonly associated with a severe degree of weakness and sensory loss in the lower limbs and sphincter paralysis. There may be other associated abnormalities, especially hydrocephalus and mental defect. In the other type of case there is spina bifida occulta, often with no abnormality of the overlying skin. The symptoms are due to an associated congenital abnormality of the lumbosacral spinal cord and cauda equina. Some symptoms are usually present from birth or an early age, but occasionally symptoms first appear, or become progressively worse at adolescence or in early adult life, the exacerbation being due to the effect of growth of the spine. Enuresis is a common symptom, and is often diurnal as well as nocturnal but retention of urine may occur. Motor symptoms range from slight to considerable weakness and wasting of the lower limbs, with diminution or loss of the tendon reflexes, especially the ankle-jerks. There is often cutaneous sensory loss over the sacral dermatomes. The feet are cold and cyanosed, and tend to develop trophic lesions.

In gross cases the X-rays show a large bony defect in the lumbosacral region. In spina bifida occulta the only radiographic abnormality may be defective fusion of one laminal arch.

Diagnosis

The diagnosis of spina bifida with a protruding sac is easy. Spina bifida occulta should be borne in mind as a possible cause of enuresis, especially diurnal enuresis in childhood, and its more severe manifestations need to be distinguished from those of other lesions of the cauda equina. X-ray examination of the lumbosacral spine may provide a valuable clue. Lumbar puncture may yield no cerebrospinal fluid in such cases, and if myelography is necessary it should be carried out by the cisternal route, bearing in mind, however, the possibility of an Arnold–Chiari malformation there.

Prognosis

Sufferers from the more severe degrees of spina bifida used not to survive long, but the outlook has been improved by modern surgery, including, when necessary, reconstruction of the urinary tract. In the case of spina bifida occulta, although no improvement can be expected in the condition of the spinal cord and vertebral column, considerable functional improvement may follow appropriate treatment, especially in childhood.

Treatment

Plastic repair of the spinal defect is justifiable if the extent of the deformity and the patient's ultimate mental and physical handicap is not too great. Orthopaedic treatment of the lower limbs will often be called for. The routine investigation of the urinary tract will show what surgical or other measures may be necessary to improve function and to combat infection. When symptoms develop late, laminectomy may reveal a cause for progressive deterioration which can be dealt with surgically.

REFERENCES

Barnett, J.J.M., Foster, J.B., and Hudgson, P. (1973). *Syringomyelia.* Saunders, Philadelphia.

Gardner, W.J. (1965). Hydrodynamic mechanisms of syringomyelia. *J. Neurol. Neurosurg. Psychiat.* **28,** 247.

Guttmann, L. (1976). *Spinal cord injuries,* 2nd edn. Blackwell, Oxford.

Hughes, J.T. (1978). *Pathology of the spinal cord,* 2nd edn. Lloyd-Luke, London.

Logue, V. and Edwards, M.R. (1981). Syringomyelia and its surgical treatment – an analysis of 75 patients. *J. Neurol. Neurosurg. Psychiat.* **44,** 273–84.

Sharr, M.M., Garfield, J.S., and Jenkins, J.D. (1976). Lumbar spondylosis and neuropathic bladder: Investigation of 73 patients with chronic urinary symptoms. *Br. med. J.* **i,** 695–7.

Silver, J.R. and Buxton, P.H. (1974). Spinal stroke. *Brain* **97,** 539–50.

Yates, D.A.H. (1970). Spinal stenosis. *J. R. Soc. Med.* **79,** 334–42.

19 Disorders of nerve roots and peripheral nerves

Anatomy and physiology

As elsewhere in the nervous system, accurate diagnosis rests upon anatomy and physiology, for the symptoms of a lesion depend upon the distribution of the motor and sensory fibres which happen to be grouped together in the nervous pathway at the site of which the lesion occurs. In the case of lesions of the nerve roots and peripheral nerves, however, the pathological nature of the lesion is particularly important, since it may influence both the character and the extent of the symptoms.

In the cervical region the ventral and dorsal spinal roots of each segment lie close together within the intervertebral foramen to form the radicular nerve. The dorsal root ganglion lies just peripherally in the gutter of the transverse process. Beyond that the two roots fuse to form the spinal nerve. In the lumbar region the ganglia lie in the foramina. Each radicular nerve has an investment of dura mater and the leptomeninges. An irritative lesion of a single dorsal root causes pain of a lancinating or burning character, which is often precipitated or intensified by coughing or sneezing, and sometimes by movements of the spine, and is associated with hyperaesthesia and hyperalgesia over the full segmental distribution of the root (Fig. 3.8, p. 116). Division of a single dorsal root, however, produces no detectable sensory loss owing to the overlapping of adjacent root areas. When more than one adjacent root is interrupted, the area of sensory loss is that area which is exclusively supplied by the combined roots involved, and the area of analgesia is larger than that of anaesthesia to light touch. A lesion of a ventral root causes atrophic paralysis of any muscle exclusively supplied by that root, and a partial lower motor neurone lesion of any muscle to whose innervation it contributes. A lesion of a radicular nerve produces the same symptoms as a lesion of the corresponding ventral and dorsal root combined.

Complete division of a mixed peripheral nerve causes motor, sensory, vaso-motor, sudomotor, and trophic symptoms corresponding in anatomical distri-bution to the region to which these functions are supplied by the divided nerve. Interruption of the motor fibres leads to a lower motor neurone paralysis of the muscles innervated. Division of a sensory nerve causes complete loss of cutaneous sensibility only over the area exclusively supplied by the nerve, the *autonomous zone*. This is surrounded by an *intermediate zone* which is the

390

area of the nerve's territory which is overlapped by the supply of adjacent nerves. The autonomous and intermediate zones together constitute the *maximal zone* which is the full extent of the nerve's distribution and to which pain and dysaesthesiae may be referred when the nerve is the site of an irritative lesion. When a sensory nerve is completely divided, the cutaneous area over which appreciation of light touch is lost is usually considerably greater than the area characterized by loss of appreciation of pin-prick. The term 'deep sensibility' is used to include the appreciation and localization of pressure and the pain induced by deep pressure and the recognition of posture and passive movements of the joints. Impairment of deep sensibility, when present as the result of nerve division, is confined to a peripheral area which is less extensive than the area anaesthetic to light touch.

After complete division of a nerve the analgesic area of skin becomes dry and inelastic and ceases to sweat. The affected area is blue and colder than normal, and the growth of the nails is retarded. Adhesions between tendons and their sheaths, and fibrous changes in the muscles and joints are to be regarded as complications rather than as direct results of the nerve injury, since they can be prevented by massage and movements of the joints.

Causalgia (see also p. 15)

Causalgia is a distressing symptom associated with incomplete lesions of a peripheral nerve, usually the median or the sciatic. It consists of intense and persistent burning pain excited by contact with the limb or even by the patient's emotional reactions. In median nerve causalgia the hand is pink and sweating, the skin tight, and glossy, and hyperaesthetic. The patient makes every effort to protect it from stimuli. The most effective treatment appears to be sympathetic block, with or without excision of the damaged area of the nerve and resuturing, though operative treatment whether at the nerve, cord, or thalamic level may not succeed in abolishing the pain.

Pressure neuropathy

In medical neurology complete lesions of the spinal nerve roots and individual peripheral nerves are rare, the common lesion being a pressure neuropathy. Repeated or prolonged pressure upon a nerve root or peripheral nerve leads to ischaemia, the response to which is oedema extending both above and below the source of pressure. If the pressure is not relieved, fibrosis tends to develop. This is the lesion underlying the neuropathy caused by pressure from a herniated intervertebral disc or within a narrowed intervertebral foramen, by cervical rib, compression of the median nerve in the carpal tunnel, of the ulnar nerve at the elbow, and of the lateral cutaneous nerve of the thigh in meralgia paraesthetica. All of these lesions are for a long time incomplete as far as their effect upon the function of the nerve is concerned, and all show individual differences in respect of the relative prominence of irritative and paralytic, motor and sensory disturbances.

The pathology of compression neuropathies

There are several types of acute compression injuries of nerves. With brief pressure on the lateral popliteal nerve, as in crossing the legs, the foot may 'go to sleep' but recover completely within a minute or so. This rapidly reversible physiological block of conduction is due to ischaemia of the nerve. With greater and more prolonged pressure recovery takes place within a few weeks, insufficient time for regeneration to occur following Wallerian degeneration. It is now thought that local demyelinating block takes place in these inter-mediate cases with fairly rapid recovery, and the histological lesion, by analogy from experimental work using a pneumatic cuff injury, is likely to be a mechanical displacement of the nodes of Ranvier with stretching of the paranodal myelin (Fig. 19.1). Thus local demyelinating block occurs at the edges of the pneumatic cuff. Though this type of lesion probably underlies the simple acute pressure palsy, where chronic recurrent pressure occurs, as with an ulnar nerve lesions at the elbow or median nerve lesions in the carpal tunnel, there is a more complicated picture of mixed segmental demyelination and remyelination, especially of large fibres, with regeneration 'clusters', which are outgrowths of axon sprouts through the Schwann tubes that enclose the original axon and sometimes small 'onion bulb' formations. Changes in the median nerve in the carpal tunnel similar to those seen in experimental entrapment neuropathies, may be found in patients apparently unaffected during life.

LESIONS OF THE SPINAL NERVE ROOTS

The principal causes of lesions of the spinal dorsal nerve roots are meningo-vascular syphilis causing spinal leptomeningitis, tabes dorsalis, extramedullary tumour, and herpes zoster, all of which operate within the spinal canal. Within the intervertebral foramen the roots may be compressed by an intervertebral disc protrusion or osteophytes projecting from the neurocentral joint, or by vertebral collapse due to primary or secondary neoplasm, tuberculous or other infection, Paget's osteitis, or traumatic fracture dislocation, or a neurofibroma.

SHOULDER-GIRDLE NEUROPATHY

In this condition, which is also known as *brachial neuralgia,* or *neuralgic amyotrophy*, neither the pathology nor the precise site of the lesion is known. Occasionally it may follow inoculations. Young males are most often attacked. Pain in the shoulder is usually the initial symptom, followed in a few days by muscular wasting and weakness on one or both sides involving serratus anterior, spinati, deltoid and trapezius in that order of frequency. In mild cases there is slow recovery, but some muscular wasting may be permanent.

SPINAL RADICULOPATHY DUE TO INTERVERTEBRAL DISC DISEASE

Disorders of the spinal column associated with lesions of the intervertebral discs are by far the commonest cause of radiculopathy. Such lesions are situated chiefly in the cervical and lumbar regions of the spine, though they occur occasionally in the thoracic region. Trauma tends to produce herniation of the nucleus pulposus through the annulus fibrosus. Degeneration, however, may produce an annular protrusion which becomes an osteophyte. Intervertebral disc protrusions may invade the spinal canal, either in the middle line or posterolaterally, or the intervertebral foramen.

CERVICAL DISC LESIONS AND BRACHIAL RADICULOPATHY

Acute protrusions

Acute disc protrusions in the neck may occur either spontaneously or as the result of trauma. A patient suffering from an acute protrusion of the spontaneous type usually gives a history of recurrent attacks of pain in the neck, often diagnosed as 'fibrositis'. Suddenly a pain more severe and lasting than the previous ones occurs. The neck may feel as though it is fixed, and both active and passive movements intensify the pain, which may be very severe. The pain is also referred within the distribution of the spinal nerve, which is compressed.

On examination the neck is usually held rigidly, sometimes slightly flexed towards the side of the lesion, and both active and passive movements intensify the pain. The muscles innervated by the spinal nerve compressed are usually somewhat wasted and hypotonic, and are sometimes the site of severe weakness. This seems especially common when the fifth cervical radicular nerve is involved. The tendon reflexes which the affected muscles mediate are diminished, and sometimes lost. There may be some hyperalgesia and hyperaesthesia within the dermatome supplied by the affected nerve, or some diminution of cutaneous sensibility.

Plain X-rays usually show little abnormality, though there may be slight narrowing of the affected intervertebral disc or the signs of pre-existing spondylosis. Myelography may show an obliteration of the corresponding root sheath and may be combined with CT scanning.

The treatment of spontaneous acute protrusion of an intervertebral disc involving one spinal nerve in the neck is a combination of traction on the head to relieve pressure upon the protruding disc with immobilization. After the acute phase has passed, immobilization may be continued by means of a collar. If these methods fail, surgical exploration may be required.

BRACHIAL RADICULOPATHY DUE TO CERVICAL SPONDYLOSIS

The production of brachial radiculitis or brachial neuritis, as it used to be called, by cervical spondylosis is complex. It has been pointed out that the

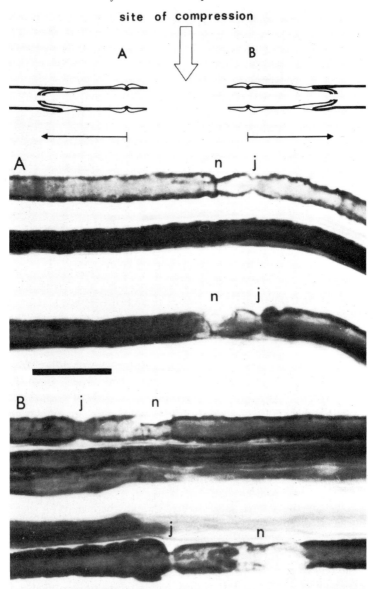

(a)

Fig. 19.1. (a) Single fibres from the human median nerve under the distal part of the flexor retinaculum to show displacement of the nodes of Ranvier (j, Schwann cell junction; n, new position of node. Bar – 30 μm).

(b) Human ulnar nerve from the elbow, showing small 'onion bulb' formations consisting of central thinly myelinated fibre surrounded by whorls of connective tissue and concentrically disposed nuclei (×1720).

(c) Ulnar nerve at elbow, small regeneration cluster containing six myelinated fibres (×6536).

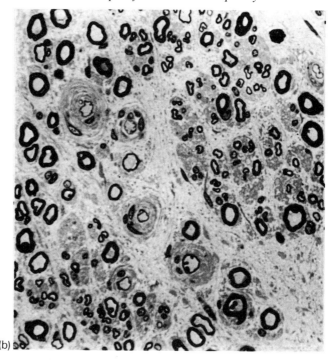

(b)

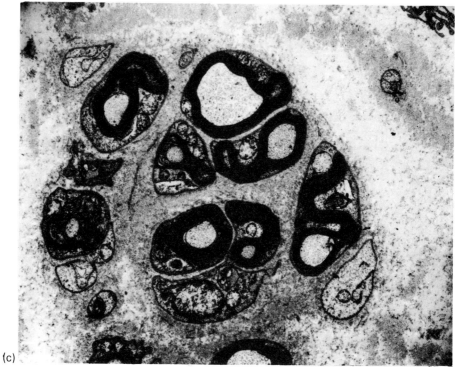

(c)

nerve roots occupy only a small part of the space of an intervertebral foramen, which would need therefore to be greatly narrowed before they became directly compressed. However, it has been shown that in cervical spondylosis adhesions form between the root sheath and the nerve roots themselves, leading to fibrosis, ischaemia, and degeneration of the root fibres. This appears to be the result of long-continued minor trauma resulting from movements of the limbs and the neck. It is also necessary to explain the frequent acute onset of symptoms in what is essentially a chronic condition. This may well be the result of trauma produced by traction upon the nerve roots already tethered in their foramina.

The duration and history of the symptoms of cervical spondylosis are extremely variable, and such symptoms may be acute, subacute, or insidious in their onset. Acute involvement of one spinal nerve leads to symptoms resembling those of a spontaneous acute protrusion of a single intervertebral disc described above. Pain, however, is not always limited to one dermatome, but may extend down the upper limb to involve to a greater or less extent all the digits, in which case a clinical picture resembling the classic one of 'brachial neuritis' is produced. An insidious onset is characterized by dysaesthesiae consisting of a burning and tingling sensation, sometimes accompanied by pain, radiating down the upper limb into one or more digits, and tending to be particularly troublesome at night. Motor symptoms are usually slight or absent, and only exceptionally is there a complaint of serious weakness, but occasionally wasting accompanied by fasciculation may be severe enough to simulate motor neurone disease.

On examination there is commonly some diminution of appreciation of light touch, tactile discrimination and pin-prick within the distribution of the dermatomes corresponding to the affected nerve roots. There may also be localized areas of tenderness in the corresponding muscles. Appreciation of posture and passive movement is usually unimpaired. There is likely to be slight muscular wasting, accompanied by hypotonia in the muscles innervated by the affected spinal nerves, but muscular weakness is usually slight. The tendon reflexes innervated from the affected segments are likely to be diminished or lost. Active and passive movements of the neck are somewhat limited in extent but relatively painless, though there may be some local tenderness upon pressure.

Plain X-rays usually show narrowing of intervertebral discs with posterior osteophytes, and, in the oblique views, of the intervertebral foramina owing to the projection of osteophytes from the neurocentral joints.

Treatment

In most cases there is a satisfactory response to immobilization in a collar, which is usually required for two or three months. Both traction and manipulation have their advocates, but the former is often disappointing and the latter probably not free from risk. Surgical treatment may be by a decompressive laminectomy or removing osteophytes by an anterior approach. Various forms of physiotherapy are useful adjuvants to treatment. In the acute stage, rest in bed is necessary with the arm supported on a pillow and, when the patient gets up, in a sling, but care should be taken that the arm itself is not immobilized, or a 'frozen shoulder' may result.

LUMBAR DISC LESIONS AND SCIATICA

The term sciatica has come to be applied to a benign syndrome characterized especially by pain beginning in the lumbar region and spreading down the back of one lower limb to the ankle, usually intensified by coughing or sneezing, and associated with little weakness or sensory loss, but with diminution or loss of the ankle jerk. During recent years is has been established that sciatica thus defined is usually due to herniation of one or more of the lumbar intervertebral discs. It seems best, therefore, to discuss sciatica under this heading, and to consider other causes of sciatic pain in relation to diagnosis.

Aetiology

Lumbar disc protrusion is usually in part at least the result of trauma, a history of which is obtainable in half of all cases. The commonest type of stress is that produced by lifting a heavy object in a bent-forward position, or by a fall in a similar posture. Since 75 per cent of patients are in or beyond the fourth decade, degenerative changes in the intervertebral discs which begin in the prime of life probably predispose towards herniation. Changes in the lumbar spine associated with pregnancy may also cause it. Most lumbar herniations occur between the fourth and fifth lumbar or fifth lumbar and first sacral bodies, with a relative frequency of 2 to 3. A disc protrusion compresses the spinal nerve, which is running to the foramen one segment below the fourth lumbar disc, the fifth lumbar nerve, and the fifth lumbar disc the first sacral nerve. Narrowing of a lumbar intervertebral foramen, however, will compress the nerve of the same denomination, as it passes through it. As elsewhere the initial result of compression of the nerve root is oedema, which may later go on to fibrosis.

Symptoms

In most cases the onset is subacute, and sciatica is frequently preceded by lumbar pain – 'lumbago' – which may have occurred intermittently for years. The sciatic pain may immediately follow an injury, such as a strain or fall, or there may be a latent interval of days or even weeks. After two or three days of pain in the lumbar spine the pain radiates down the back of one leg from the buttock to the ankle. It is often possible to distinguish three elements in the pain:

1. Pain in the back, aching in character, and intensified by spinal movements.

2. Pain deep in the buttock and thigh, also aching or gnawing in character, and influenced by the posture of the limb.

3. Pain radiating to the leg and foot, and momentarily increased by coughing and sneezing. When the first sacral root is compressed the pain radiates to the outer border of the foot. When the pressure is upon the fifth lumbar root it spreads from the outer aspect of the leg to the inner border of the foot. In general the pain is intensified by stooping, sitting, and walking, the patient being usually most comfortable lying in bed on the sound side with the affected leg slightly flexed at the hip and knee. There is often a feeling of numbness, heaviness, or deadness in the leg, especially along the outer border of the foot.

There are muscular hypotonia and slight wasting, not only of the muscles supplied by the sciatic nerve, but also of the glutei and sometimes of all the muscles of the lower limb. Compression of the first sacral root may cause weakness of the small muscles of the foot and the calf muscles, and the ankle-jerk is diminished or lost. Compression of the fifth root may cause weakness of the peronei, but the ankle-jerk is preserved. The knee-jerk may be slightly exaggerated, but if the fourth lumbar root is involved it may be diminished. The plantar reflex is flexor.

There is tenderness on pressure in the buttock and thigh, straight-leg-raising is limited by pain, and stretching the sciatic nerve by extending the knee with the hip flexed causes severe pain – Lasègue's sign. There is rarely much sensory loss, though often there is some blunting of light touch and pin-prick over the outer half of the foot and three outer toes and lower part of the outer aspect of the leg when the first sacral root is involved. The fourth and fifth lumbar cutaneous areas are shown in Fig. 3.8 (a) and (b) (pp. 116–17).

Scoliosis is often associated with sciatica, the lumbar spine being flexed towards the affected side, less frequently towards the opposite side. Some rigidity of the lumbar spine is usually present and there may be a tender spot at the level of the fifth lumbar transverse process.

An excess of protein up to 0.7 to 0.8 g/l is present in the cerebrospinal fluid in about 80 per cent of cases, but the cell count is normal.

X-ray examination should be carried out in all cases of sciatica, since many causes of sciatic pain are associated with bony changes visible in radiographs. Straight X-rays of the lumbar spine may show narrowing of the fourth or fifth lumbar disc with a posterior osteophyte. Disc protrusions may be outlined by selective CT scan pictures. In doubtful cases myelography may demonstrate a filling defect due to a disc protrusion (Fig. 19.2). CT scan is now the investigation of choice for detecting lumbar canal stenosis.

Diagnosis

Sciatica resulting from an intervertebral disc protrusion must be distinguished from other cause of lumbosacral nerve root compression, in particular a *tumour involving the cauda equina,* and *metastatic neoplasm* involving the lumbar spine or the pelvis or the internal iliac nodes. The principal points of distinction are that in herniated disc the onset of symptoms is fairly rapid, the buttock and posterior aspect of the thigh are tender on pressure, muscular wasting is slight, sensory loss is slight or absent, and the course of the disorder during the first months after the onset is stationary or tends to improvement. In sciatic compression, on the other hand, the onset is usually gradual, the nerve is not tender on pressure, muscular wasting is conspicuous, and sensory loss is always present, and both of these symptoms are progressive. The abdomen and pelvis must be thoroughly examined for sources of compression, and the lumbar spine and pelvis should be X-rayed. Attention should also be paid to the general condition of the patient, an inquiry made for symptoms suggestive of a pelvic neoplasm, and as to recent loss of weight. Rectal examination should be carried out, and in women vaginal examination also. If a tumour of the cauda equina is suspected, lumbar puncture should be carried out and evidence of spinal block sought in the dynamics and composition of the cerebrospinal fluid. Myelography is also likely to be required. Whether true sciatic 'neuritis' occurs is now doubtful. It is certainly very rare, and the diagnosis should be accepted with reserve even when investigations appear to exlude all other causes.

Vascular lesions within the distribution of the femoral artery, such as atheroma and thrombo-angiitis obliterans, are occasional causes of pain in the leg in middle age and later in life: intermittent claudication is not always present in these cases. The diagnosis is readily established by diminution in the volume of the femoral, dorsalis pedis and posterior tibial pulses.

Prognosis

In mild cases of sciatica the stage of severe pain lasts only for two or three weeks, and the patient recovers in a month or two, except that he may from time to time experience aching in the course of the leg, and stooping may still excite some pain. In more severe cases there may be slight improvement after several weeks, but the condition then becomes stationary and the patient continues to suffer from considerable pain for a number of months. Relapses are common. In some cases they occur at frequent intervals, in others the second attack may be delayed until ten or more years after the first.

Treatment

Most patients with lumbar intervertebral disc protrusion recover completely if treated conservatively. Operation should therefore be reserved for those whose symptoms do not respond after three weeks strict bed rest or after traction or manipulation and become chronic, those who relapse, and those with gross and persistent symptoms of root compression, sufficiently severe to cause disability. Probably not more than 10 per cent will require operation, but the percentage will be higher among manual workers, in whom inability to do the necessary physical work itself constitutes an indication for surgery.

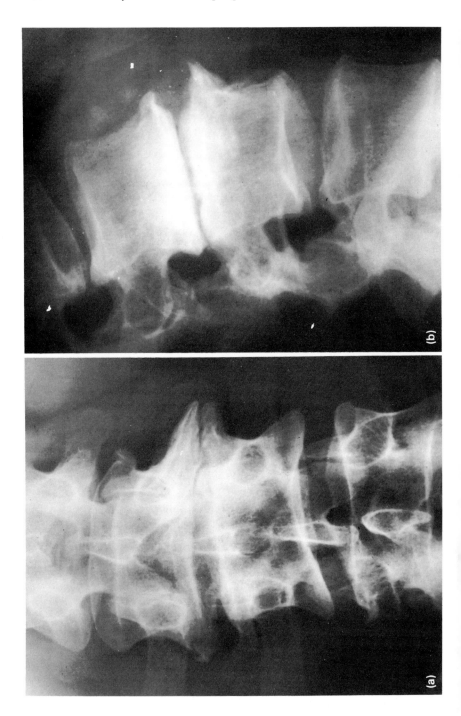

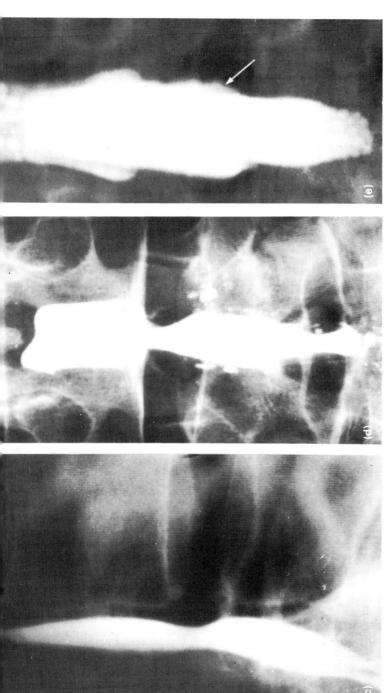

Fig. 19.2. (a) and (b) Spondolysosis. Narrowing of the disc space, sclerosis of adjoining vertebral surface and osteophytic growth. (c) Posterior disc protrusion in lateral view. The contrast column is indented at the level of the intervertebral space. (d) Posterolateral lumbar disc prolapse. Arrow: the root sheath is obliterated. Lateral film normal. (e) Disc prolapse in anteroposterior view in same patient. The contrast column is constricted at the level of the intervetebral space.

Conservative treatment consists of rest in bed, with a board under the mattress, and analgesics, to which may be added various measures designed to immobilize the lower part of the spine and the affected lower limb. These include a plaster jacket which fixes the lumbar spine in slight extension. In some cases benefit may be derived from stretching the nerve roots by epidural injection of procaine followed by saline at the sacral hiatus. Physical therapy in its various forms is merely palliative, but graduated exercises are of value when the pain has gone.

HERPES ZOSTER

Aetiology and pathology

Herpes zoster, or shingles, is an acute virus infection which attacks the first sensory neurone and the corresponding area of skin. Its results from the reactivation of the latent varicella-zoster virus in a patient who has had chicken pox at some time. Neutralizing antibody to varicella-zoster virus is absent or present in low titres but both complement fixing and neutralizing antibody appear more quickly than in chicken pox. There is no evidence zoster may be contracted as a reinfection with a virus from a patient with chicken pox or zoster. The pathological changes in the nervous system are those of an acute inflammation at some point in the course of the first sensory neurone. The dorsal root ganglia and the corresponding sensory ganglia of the cranial nerves are the commonest sites of the lesion, but the posterior horn of the grey matter of the spinal cord, the dorsal root, and less often the anterior root or the peripheral nerves may also be involved. One or more successive dorsal roots on the same side may be affected. The microscopical changes consist of haemorrhages and infiltration with mononuclear leucocytes and degenerative changes in the nerve cells. Fibrosis and secondary degeneration follow in severe cases. The cutaneous lesions consist of vesicle formation with inflammatory infiltration of the epidermis and dermis.

The virus responsible for zoster appears to be identical with that which causes chicken pox or varicella. Either disorder may give rise to the other in contacts. Zoster may occur without any evident predisposing cause, or as a complication of some other disease or toxic state, especially when this causes damage to the first sensory neurone. These two groups are distinguished as idiopathic and symptomatic zoster, but both are due to the same virus. Symptomatic zoster may be precipitated by disturbed autoimmune mechanisms including those due to immunosuppressant drugs, and may occur in tuberculosis, uraemia, the leukaemias and reticuloses. It may complicate any lesion of the posterior roots where the virus may have remained latent.

Zoster may occur at any age, but is rare in infancy and more frequent in the second half of life than the first. It is most often seen in patients over the age of fifty. The incubation period is usually about a fortnight.

Symptoms

The first symptom is usually pain in the distribution of the dorsal root or roots involved, often associated with hyperalgesia of the corresponding area of skin. Three or four days after the onset of pain the eruption appears as a series of localized papules which develop into vesicles grouped together upon an erythematous base, in patches within the distribution of the dermatome. After a few days the eruption fades, the vesicles drying into crusts which separate, leaving small permanent scars in the skin. The skin may become partially or completely analgesic, but often analgesic areas alternate with areas of hypersensitiveness. Pain may persist for weeks, or months, or indefinitely after the eruption, and this post-herpetic neuralgia is the more likely to occur the older the patient. The association of pain with sensory loss is sometimes described as anaesthesia dolorosa. Muscular wasting of segmental distribution is an occasional accompaniment of zoster. Encephalitis occurs very rarely.

General symptoms of zoster include fever, and there is occasionally a generalized vesicular rash.

The cerebrospinal fluid often contains an excess of mononuclear cells and a moderate rise of protein.

Ophthalmic zoster

When zoster attacks the first division of the trigeminal nerve the eruption appears on the forehead and the cornea may be involved. If the cornea becomes anaesthetic then the eye must be protected against risk of infection. Optic neuritis and ophthalmoplegia are rare complications.

Geniculate zoster

Geniculate zoster is the term applied to a syndrome in which one or more of the following symptoms occurs – pain in the ear and palatoglossal arch, vesicles with a similar distribution, loss of taste on the anterior two-thirds of the tongue, facial paralysis, giddiness and deafness (Ramsay Hunt's syndrome). Sometimes the eruption involves the trigeminal area or the occipital region and upper part of the neck.

Diagnosis

The diagnosis of herpes zoster offers little difficulty, at any rate as soon as the eruption has appeared. Herpes febrilis is less painful, is usually situated in the proximity of a mucous membrane, is often bilateral, and leaves neither residual pain nor scarring. Diagnosis of herpes zoster is impossible in the pre-eruptive stage, but its possibility should be suggested by root pains of sudden onset less than four days before examination.

Prognosis

Most sufferers from zoster recover without residual symptoms, and one attack usually confers permanent immunity, but second attacks sometimes occur. The most troublesome sequel is persistent intractable pain, which may endure for years in elderly patients.

Treatment

In most cases the treatment of zoster is simple; dusting powder and a dry dressing are all that is needed for the eruption. Chlortetracycline or chloramphenicol, applied locally, may help to combat the infection, or at least to prevent secondary infection. Treatment with a local application of 5 per cent idoxuridine in dimethyl sulphoxide as soon as possible aids healing and may reduce the likelihood of post-herpetic neuralgia. Acyclovir by intravenous infusion appears to be effective in limiting the spread of herpes zoster and may be used in immunosupressed patients. If the pain does not appear to be subsiding, a number of physical methods of treatment should be tried. These include the application of local vibration to the skin, local transcutaneous electrical stimulation, and local skin cooling with an ethylene chloride spray. Though attempts to destroy the pain pathways by means of local nerve block, deep X-ray radiation of the nerve root or operations to the spinal cord and thalamus are sometimes attempted, none of these is strikingly effective in the small percentage of patients in whom severe and persisting pain continues, because by then a widespread central disturbance of pain conduction has occurred (p. 11).

Though needless polypharmacy is to be avoided, the synergic effect of substances which act at different sites can often be exploited. A peripherally acting analgesic such as aspirin, which may act by affecting prostaglandin release, can be followed by a tranquillizer (pericyazine) or an antidepressant such as amitriptyline (Tryptizol) and a sedative such as promethazine (Phenergan). The progression can then continue to a centrally acting narcotic of a mild degree such as Codeine before resorting to drugs such as morphine which may cause dependence.

Corticosteroids and amantidine during the acute herpetic attack are reported to reduce the likelihood of post-herpetic neuralgia.

LESIONS OF THE BRACHIAL PLEXUS

The brachial plexus (Fig. 19.3) is normally formed from the anterior primary divisions of the fifth, sixth, seventh, and eighth cervical, and first thoracic spinal nerves. Variations in its position are not uncommon. In the so-called prefixed type there is a contribution from the fourth cervical nerve, the fifth cervical branch is large and there may be none from the second thoracic. In the postfixed type there may be no branch from the fourth cervical and that from the fifth is comparatively small, whereas the second thoracic branch is quite distinct. The spinal segmental representation of muscles may be slightly higher or slightly lower than normal according to whether the plexus is prefixed or postfixed.

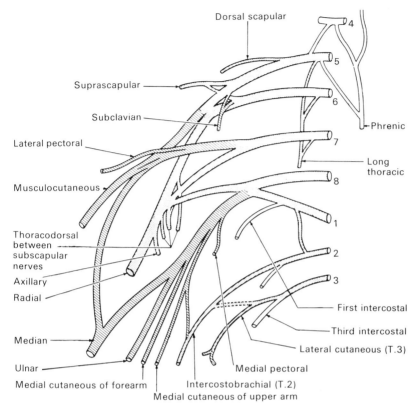

Fig. 19.3. Right brachial plexus.

TRAUMATIC LESIONS

The two principal traumatic lesions are upper and lower plexus paralysis. In *upper plexus paralysis* (the Erb–Duchenne type) the branch from the fifth and occasionally also the sixth cervical nerve to the plexus is involved, usually as a result of forcible separation of the head and shoulder. It occurs as a birth injury, and after falls. The muscles paralysed are those innervated by the fifth cervical segment (pp. 116–17) as a result of which the limb hangs at the side with the elbow extended and the forearm pronated. The arm should be put up in an abduction splint with a movable joint at the elbow. The prognosis is usually good.

In *lower plexus paralysis* (the Dejerine–Klumpke type) the contribution from the first thoracic nerve is torn as a result of traction on the arm in an abducted position. The resulting paralysis and wasting involves the small muscles of the hand, and a claw-hand results, with sensory loss in the distribution of the first thoracic dermatome.

COSTOCLAVICULAR SYNDROMES, INCLUDING CERVICAL RIB

The bony structure of the upper thoracic outlet is peculiarly liable to congenital abnormalities which may interfere with nerves and blood vessels. There may be a rudimentary rib derived from the seventh cervical vertebra – cervical rib – which may be associated with a prefixed brachial plexus. Or the relationship of the brachial plexus to the scalene muscles may be abnormal. The production of symptoms by these factors is complex. The eighth cervical and first thoracic contributions to the plexus, or the inner cord, may rest upon, and be compressed by, a cervical rib, or an enlarged seventh cervical transverse process, or a fibrous band uniting such a structure to the first rib, or an aberrant vessel. The subclavian artery may also be compressed. Sometimes even where there is no structural abnormality the functions of the brachial plexus are interfered with by a low level of the shoulder girdle. These syndromes are much commoner in women.

Symptoms

With structural abnormality

The onset is usually gradual and symptoms may be mainly sensory, motor, or vascular, or a combination of these. The commonest sensory symptom is pain, which is referred to the ulnar border of the hand and distal half of the forearm and may be associated with numbness, tingling, or other paraesthesiae. These symptoms may be temporarily relieved by raising the hand above the head. Careful sensory investigation usually reveals either hyperalgesia or relative analgesia in a narrow zone corresponding to the cutaneous distribution of the first dorsal dermatome along the ulnar border of the hand and of the distal part of the forearm. The ring finger may also be involved. Motor symptoms consist of weakness and wasting, the distribution of which depends in part upon the position of the plexus. It is usually confined to the small muscles of the hand and may begin either in those supplied by the median or by the ulnar nerve. Ocular-sympathetic paralysis may be present.

Vascular symptoms, due to compression of the subclavian artery, include blanching or cyanosis of the fingers, and sometimes even gangrene. The radial pulses are frequently unequal, that on the affected side being smaller in volume than its fellow.

A cervical rib may be visible or palpable as a bony swelling in the neck, pressure over which may cause pain or tingling referred to the ulnar border of the hand and forearm, or obliteration of the radial pulse. The presence of cervical ribs can be demonstrated radiographically, but it must be remembered that the symptoms may be due to a fibrous band which will not be seen in the X-rays, or to a normal first rib. The radiological signs may be bilateral but the symptoms unilateral, more commonly right sided.

Without structural abnormalities

Though the symptoms may be as severe as in the former group, they tend to be less so, and to be sensory rather than motor, and subjective rather than objective. Pain and paraesthesiae are referred along the ulnar border of the forearm and hand, or sometimes into the whole hand. Symptoms may be entirely nocturnal, developing only when the patient has been lying down for some time, or be noticeable chiefly in the daytime after carrying a heavy object. Most of the patients are women, and neurological abnormalities are slight or absent. A low shoulder girdle is usually present, and when the symptoms are unilateral the shoulder is lower on the affected than on the normal side. Owing to the position of the shoulders a lateral X-ray of the neck gives an unusually clear view of the upper thoracic vertebrae often as low as the intervertebral disc between the second and the third.

Diagnosis

A cervical rib is distinguished from motor neurone disease by the presence of pain and analgesia, and by the absence of muscular fasciculation. In syringomyelia wasting of the small muscles of the hands is associated with analgesia and thermo-anaesthesia, but the sensory loss is usually much more extensive than that associated with a cervical rib, and the tendon jerks are often lost in the upper limb. It must be remembered that a cervical rib is a congenital abnormality which may be present in cases of syringomyelia, and its presence is therefore not in itself proof that the rib is the cause of the symptoms. The inner cord of the brachial plexus is occasionally compressed by a tumour arising at the apex of the lung, which however should be demonstrable radiographically. Lesions of the median and ulnar nerves, especially when they arise from occupational pressure at the wrist or in the palms, may be confused with cervical rib, but the diagnosis is established by the characteristic distribution of the motor and sensory symptoms, and confirmed by electromyography (p. 411).

Treatment

When symptoms occur without any abnormality in middle life, rest in bed may give relief, and in suitable cases exercises designed to strengthen the muscles which lift the shoulder girdle are helpful. Only surgical treatment, however, affords permanent relief from a structural abnormality, and to obtain the best results it should be undertaken early. The precise operation required depends upon the nature of the abnormality present.

LESIONS OF PERIPHERAL NERVES

THE LONG THORACIC NERVE

The long thoracic nerve is derived by three roots from the fifth, sixth, and seventh cervical nerves. It supplies the serratus anterior. It may be injured alone as the result of pressure upon the shoulder, either from a sudden blow or from the prolonged carrying of weights. It is one of the nerves most frequently affected in shoulder-girdle neuropathy.

The serratus anterior muscle fixes the scapula to the chest wall when forward pressure is exerted with the upper limb. It brings the scapula forward when the upper limb is thrust forward, as in a fencing lunge, and it assists in elevating the limb above the head by rotating the scapula. Paralysis of the serratus anterior causes no deformity of the scapula when the limb is at rest. If, however, the patient is asked to push the limb forward against resistance, the inner border of the scapula becomes winged, especially in its lower two-thirds (Fig. 19.4). He is unable to raise the limb above the head in front of him. The usual treatment of the paralysed muscle is carried out, but if recovery does not occur, the sterno-costal portion of the pectoralis major muscle can be transplanted from the arm to the inferior angle of the scapula.

THE AXILLARY NERVE

The axillary nerve arises from the posterior cord of the brachial plexus. It innervates the teres minor and deltoid muscles, and supplies cutaneous sensibility to an oval area, the long axis of which extends from the acromion to half-way down the outer aspect of the arm (Fig. 3.8 (a) and (b), p. 116–17). The axillary nerve may be injured as the result of surgical lesions in the region of the neck of the humerus. It leads to wasting and paralysis of the deltoid muscle, with paralysis of abduction of the arm and anaesthesia and analgesia corresponding to its cutaneous supply. The arm requires splinting in a position of abduction at the shoulder.

THE RADIAL NERVE

The radial nerve constitutes the termination of the posterior cord of the brachial plexus, and is derived from the fifth, sixth, seventh, and eighth cervical spinal nerves. It innervates the following muscles in the order given: triceps, anconeus, brachioradialis, extensor carpi radialis longus, and, through the posterior interosseous nerve, extensor carpi radialis brevis, supinator, extensor digitorum, extensor digiti minimi, extensor carpi ulnaris, the three extensors of the thumb, and extensor indicis. It supplies sensibility to the lower half of the radial aspect of the arm and the middle of the posterior aspect of the forearm and to a variable area on the radial aspect of the dorsum of the hand (Fig. 3.8 (a) and (b), p. 116–17).

The position of the radial nerve as it winds round the humerus makes it specially liable to injury. Apart from penetrating wounds and fractures of the humerus, it may be compressed in the axilla through the use of a crutch, and when the arm of an anaesthetized patient is allowed to hang over the edge of the operating table. It may also be compressed during sleep, especially when the

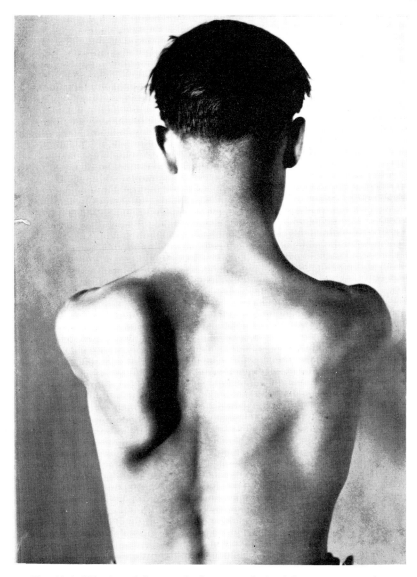

Fig. 19.4. Winging of the scapula due to paralysis of the serratus anterior.

patient is intoxicated. The nerve is occasionally the site of neuropathy, which may be confined to the posterior interosseous branch.

The symptoms of a lesion of the radial nerve depend upon the point at which it occurs. A lesion in or above the axilla leads to paralysis and wasting of all the muscles it supplies. When there is a pressure neuropathy of the nerve as it winds round the humerus, the triceps is often little affected and the paralysis is limited to the muscles below the elbow. Even so, the branch to the brachioradialis and less frequently that to the extensor carpi radialis longus may also escape, the distribution of the paralysis coinciding with that following a lesion of the posterior interosseous nerve. Typically there are wrist-drop and finger-drop due to paralysis of the extensors of the wrist and digits. In investigating extension of the thumb special attention must be paid to extension at the carpometacarpal and metacarpophalangeal joints, since extension at a terminal joint may be carried out by some of the intrinsic muscles of the hand. The long extensors of the fingers produce extension only at the metacarpophalangeal joints, extension at the other joints being brought about by the interossei and lumbricals. In pressure neuropathy sensory loss is variable and may be absent.

In radial nerve paralysis a splint must be used to maintain extension of the wrist, but although extension of the metacarpophalangeal joint must be ensured, these joints must not be rigidly fixed. A system of elastic extension should, therefore, be used for the fingers. The prognosis of lesions of the radial nerve is good. Even after suture, signs of returning muscular function are usually evident in from four to eight months, according to the level of the lesion. If the posterior interosseous nerve is thought to be the site of a neuropathy which does not respond to treatment, the nerve should be explored.

THE MUSCULOCUTANEOUS NERVE

The musculocutaneous nerve is a branch of the outer cord of the brachial plexus, its fibres being derived from the fifth and sixth cervical spinal nerves. It supplies the biceps and brachialis, the principal flexors of the elbow, and its sensory distribution is shown in Fig. 3.8 (a) and (b) (p. 116–17). Apart from trauma, lesions of this nerve are rare. They cause weakness of flexion of the elbow and sensory loss over its cutaneous distribution.

THE MEDIAN NERVE

The fibres of the median nerve are derived from the sixth, seventh, and eighth cervical and first thoracic spinal segments. It is formed by the union of two heads from the inner and outer cords of the brachial plexus. In the forearm it supplies the following muscles, to which branches are given in the order named: pronator teres, flexor carpi radialis, palmaris longus, flexor digitorium superficialis, flexor pollicis longus, flexor digitorum profundus, pronator quadratus. In the hand it usually supplies two radial lumbricals, opponens pollicis, abductor pollicis brevis, and the outer head of the flexor pollicis brevis. Sometimes it supplies the first dorsal interosseous.

Trauma may involve the median nerve at any point in its course, and a complete interruption above the elbow will cause paralysis of all the muscles just mentioned, together with the sensory loss shown in Fig. 3.8 (a) and (b). In medical neurology the only common lesion is compression of the median nerve in the carpal tunnel, which will now be described.

The carpal tunnel syndrome

The carpal tunnel lies beneath the flexor retinaculum and contains the median nerve and the flexor tendons. The pathogenesis of spontaneous compression of the median nerve in the carpal tunnel is not completely understood. It occurs principally in middle-aged women, and has been thought to be secondary to swelling of the synovial sheaths. It may also be secondary to narrowing of the tunnel as a result of fractures or arthritic changes in the neighbourhood of the wrist joint. It occasionally occurs during pregnancy, and in rheumatoid arthritis, myxoedema and acromegaly. Whatever the cause, the reaction of the median nerve to compression is to swell, which increases the pressure, and if the condition is not relieved the swelling is followed by fibrosis. The spontaneous variety is frequently bilateral, but often begins in one hand some months or longer before it starts in the other. Early symptoms are pain and tingling felt in the cutaneous distribution of the nerve in the digits, e.g. the thumb, index, middle and radial side of the ring finger (Fig. 3.8 (a) and (b), pp. 116–17). The tingling, which is often especially troublesome at night or on waking in the morning, constitutes one form of acroparaesthesiae. Cutaneous sensory loss over the affected digits renders the manipulation of small objects difficult, and is accompanied by weakness and wasting of abductor pollicis brevis and opponens pollicis, causing conspicuous hollowing of the outer half of the thenar eminence (Fig. 19.5). Weakness of opposition of the thumb adds to the clumsiness of the hand. Those areas of the digits innervated by the median nerve usually present the picture of incomplete division. Appreciation of light touch and tactile discrimination are impaired, and there is also impairment of appreciation of pain, heat, and cold, pin-prick, the threshold for which is raised, sometimes causing

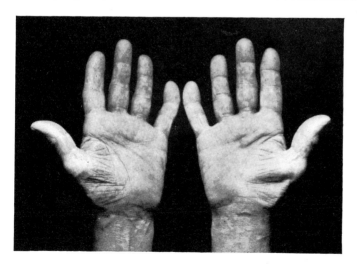

Fig. 19.5. Wasting of the outer thenar muscles due to compression of the median nerves in the carpal tunnels.

an unpleasant diffuse tingling sensation. Postural sensibility is unimpaired. The sensory changes are limited to the digits, the palmar skin escaping because the palmar branch of the nerve lies superficial to the retinaculum. The swelling of the nerve cannot usually be felt, but sometimes pressure over the ligament causes a tingling sensation to be referred to the affected digits.

When the carpal tunnel syndrome occurs in pregnancy, spontaneous recovery may be expected to follow delivery. In other cases, although improvement may result from rest or immobilization of the hand, or diuretics and the injection of 25 mg hydrocortisone acetate into the carpal tunnel, relapse is likely to follow the resumption of activity. Electrophysiological studies may help by demonstrating considerable delay in motor conduction at the wrist and point to the advisability of surgery rather than conservative treatment. Division of the flexor retinaculum gives rapid relief from the acroparaesthesiae, and, if the condition has not been left too long, full sensory recovery may be expected in the course of six to twelve months, and a high degree of recovery of muscular power.

THE ULNAR NERVE

The ulnar nerve is derived from the eighth cervical and first thoracic spinal nerves. It gives off no branches above the elbow, where it lies behind the internal condyle of the humerus. It supplies branches to the following muscles in the forearm in the order stated: flexor carpi ulnaris and the inner half of flexor digitorum profundus. In the hand it usually supplies the palmaris brevis, the muscles of the hypothenar eminence, the two inner lumbricals, the palmar and dorsal interossei, the oblique and transverse heads of the adductor pollicis, and the inner head of the flexor pollicis brevis. The first dorsal interosseous muscle is sometimes supplied by the median. The ulnar nerve supplies cutaneous sensibility to the little finger, the ulnar half of the ring finger and the corresponding area of the palmar and dorsal surfaces of the hand (Fig. 3.8 (a) and (b), pp. 116–17).

Traumatic lesions of the ulnar nerve may occur at any point in its course. In medical neurology the two common sites of ulnar nerve lesions are behind the elbow, and in the palm.

Lesions in the neighbourhood of the elbow

Pressure neuritis of the ulnar nerve at the elbow may be produced in several ways. A 'slipping ulnar' is particularly apt to occur in the presence of cubitus valgus. Flexion of the elbow causes the nerve to ride up on to the internal condyle and the repeated trauma produced in this way leads to a neuroma. A similar condition may result from bony thickening secondary to arthritis or old fracture. Less frequently the nerve is compressed by a ganglion.

Wasting of the flexor carpi ulnaris and the ulnar half of the flexor digitorum profundus is evident on the inner aspect of the flexor surface of the forearm. Weakness of the flexor carpi ulnaris causes the hand to deviate to the radial side on flexion of the wrist against resistance. Paralysis of the ulnar half of the flexor digitorum profundus abolishes flexion of the little finger at the inter-phalangeal joints, and weakens flexion of the ring finger at these joints. In the hand wasting is evident in the hypothenar eminence, the interosseous spaces, and the ulnar half of the thenar eminence. The fingers are semiflexed owing to paralysis of the interossei and the degree of flexion is greater in the ring and little finger than in the index and middle finger because, in the case of the latter, paralysis of the interossei is to some extent compensated for by the two radial lumbricals which are supplied by the median nerve. Paralysis of the muscles of the hypothenar eminence abolishes abduction of the little finger and impairs flexion of this finger at the metacarpophalangeal joint. Paralysis of the interossei abolishes abduction and adduction of the fingers. In examining this movement it is important that the hand should be kept up with the palm pressed against a flat surface, as the long extensors and flexors of the fingers act to some extent as abductors and adductors. Further, the fingers cannot be held with the metacarpophalangeal joints flexed and the interphalangeal joints extended. Paralysis of the adductors weakens adduction of the thumb, and this is most evident when the patient attempts to press the thumb firmly against the index finger.

After a lesion of the ulnar nerve at the elbow, loss of deep sensibility is usually limited to the little finger. The area of analgesia to pin-prick is variable, but usually covers the little finger and the ulnar border of the palm. The area of anaesthesia to light touch includes the little finger and the ulnar half of the ring finger, together with the ulnar border of the hand both on the dorsum and palmar aspects as far as the wrist, the area being bounded on the radial side by a line continuous with the axis of the ring finger (Fig. 3.8 (a) and (b), pp. 116–17).

Sensory symptoms are not usually prominent in cases of pressure neuritis of the ulnar nerve at the elbow. The patient may, however, notice some numbness and tingling of the two ulnar fingers and the ulnar border of the palm. Usually attention is drawn to the hand by the muscular wasting and the weakness.

Lesions of the deep branch of the ulnar nerve

Pressure neuropathy of the deep branch sometimes occurs in individuals whose occupation involves prolonged pressure upon the outer part of the palm. In such cases the muscles of the hypothenar eminence usually escape damage, and there is no sensory loss, the weakness and wasting being limited to the interossei and the adductors of the thumb. Electrophysiological studies are necessary to establish the precise level of the lesion of the ulnar nerve (see p. 162).

Treatment of lesions of the ulnar nerve

When the nerve is the site of chronic irritation and trauma at the elbow the nerve may be transplanted to be in front of the internal condyle of the humerus. In lesions of the deep palmar branch, without a history of trauma, exploration may reveal a ganglion compressing the nerve.

THE LATERAL CUTANEOUS NERVE OF THE THIGH

The lateral cutaneous nerve is derived from the posterior parts of the second and third lumbar nerves. Passing through the psoas major muscle it enters the thigh beneath the lateral end of the inguinal ligament, and, piercing the fascia lata of the thigh about four inches distal to the anterior superior iliac spine, it divides into an anterior and a posterior branch which supply sensibility to the lateral aspect of the skin of the thigh and the lateral part of its anterior aspect from the buttock almost as low as the knee (Fig. 3.8 (a) and (b), pp. 116–17). Either where the nerve emerges from the pelvis or where it passes through the fascia lata, it may become constricted by fibrous tissue with the production of pain, numbness, and paraesthesiae referred to the cutaneous distribution of the nerve. This condition, which is known as meralgia paraesthetica, usually occurs in middle life, and more often in men than in women, especially after putting on weight. The pain and numbness are often brought on by walking, which may suggest arterial disease. Part or the whole of the cutaneous area of supply of the lateral cutaneous nerve exhibits anaesthesia and analgesia. If the symptoms persist and are intolerable to the patient, it is usually possible to relieve them by decompressing the nerve where it emerges into the thigh.

THE FEMORAL NERVE

The femoral nerve arises from the posterior part of the second, third, and fourth lumbar nerves, which unite in the psoas muscle. It supplies the iliacus muscle and the pectineus, sartorius, and quadriceps. Its middle and internal cutaneous branches supply the medial and internal aspects of the thigh in its lower two-thirds, and by the saphenous nerve it supplies sensibility to the inner aspect of the leg and foot as far distally as midway between the internal malleolus and the base of the great toe (Fig. 3.8 (a) and (b), pp. 116–17).

The femoral nerve may be involved in psoas abscess or in new growths within the pelvis, or injured as a result of fractures of the pelvis or of the femur or by dislocation of the hip. The commonest lesion is compression of one or more of its roots by lumbar intervertebral disc protrusion.

A lesion of the nerve may produce slight weakness of flexion of the hip, but the principal motor disturbance is weakness of extension of the knee owing to paralysis of the quadriceps, which is wasted. As the result of this the leg gives way in walking and cannot be used to raise the body on stairs. The knee-jerk is lost, and sensibility is impaired over the cutaneous area innervated by the nerve.

THE SCIATIC NERVE

The sciatic nerve is derived from the sacral plexus. It is composed of two divisions which are destined to form the tibial and the common peroneal nerves. The tibial nerve comes from the anterior trunks of the fourth and fifth lumbar and first and second, and sometimes third, sacral nerves, and the common peroneal comes from the posterior trunks of the fourth and fifth lumbar and first and second sacral nerves. The sciatic nerve, in addition to its two principal components, contains nerves to the hamstring muscles and a nerve to the short head of the biceps. It leaves the pelvis by passing through the great sciatic notch and then descends in the back of the thigh, terminating at a variable point between the sciatic notch and the proximal part of the popliteal fossa by dividing into the common peroneal and tibial nerves.

The sciatic nerve may be damaged as the result of fractures of the pelvis and femur and gunshot wounds of the buttock and thigh. It may be compressed within the pelvis by neoplasm, or by the foetal head during delivery. The common peroneal division is much more susceptible to injury than the tibial. The commonest lesion of the sciatic nerve is compression of one or more of its roots by a lumbar intervertebral disc protrusion.

After complete interruption of the sciatic nerve there is paralysis of all muscles below the knee. Foot-drop occurs as the result of paralysis of the anterior tibial group of muscles and the peronei. The patient is able to stand and to walk, but drags the toes of the affected foot and is unable to stand on his toes on the paralysed side. When the lesion is in the buttock or higher, flexion of the knee is weak owing to paralysis of the hamstrings. Cutaneous sensory loss extends over the whole of the foot with the exception of the area supplied by the saphenous nerve on the inner aspect. On the leg, the area of sensory loss includes the outer aspect roughly from the middle line in front to the middle line behind as far up as two inches below the upper end of the fibula (Fig. 3.8 (a) and (b), pp. 116–17). Analgesia is less extensive than anaesthesia to light touch. Postural sensibility and appreciation of passive movement are lost in the toes. The knee-jerk is unaffected, but the ankle-jerk is lost and so also is the plantar reflex. Vasomotor and trophic changes are usually conspicuous. The leg is congested and swollen, especially when it is allowed to hang down. The skin is dry, and sweating is lost over the foot except along the inner border. Perforating ulcers may develop on the sole.

THE COMMON PERONEAL NERVE

The common peroneal nerve may be injured as the result of wounds in the neighbourhood of the knee joint and fractures involving the upper end of the fibula. It may suffer from compression by a tight bandage applied to the knee or pressure during sleep, and this type of pressure neuropathy is most likely to occur in elderly arteriosclerotics, especially diabetics.

After a lesion of the common peroneal nerve there is paralysis with wasting of the peronei and of the anterior tibial group of muscles. Dorsiflexion of the foot and toes and eversion of the foot are lost, and foot-drop results. Inversion of the foot is lost when it is dorsiflexed, but a weak movement of inversion is possible in association with plantar flexion. Cutaneous sensation is impaired over the dorsum of the foot, including the first phalanges of the toes, and over the antero-external aspect of the leg in its lower half or two-thirds (Fig. 3.8 (a) and (b), pp. 116–17). Deep sensibility is unimpaired.

THE TIBIAL NERVE

This nerve is rarely injured in isolation except by a traumatic lesion. The calf muscles and muscles of the sole are paralysed and wasted, and the foot assumes the position of talipes calcaneovalgus. The ankle-jerk is lost, and the plantar reflex may also be absent. There is anaesthesia to light touch over the skin of the sole, including the plantar aspect of the toes and the dorsal aspect of their terminal phalanges. The area of analgesia to pin-prick is less extensive and does not include the toes (Fig. 3.8. (a) and (b), pp. 116–17). There is usually no loss of deep sensibility.

Treatment of lesions of the sciatic and common peroneal nerves

After lesions of the sciatic nerve and of the common peroneal nerve it is important to prevent dropping of the foot and contracture of the calf muscles. The patient should therefore wear an aluminium night-shoe at night and during the day the foot-drop must be overcome by wearing a boot with toe-raising spring. After complete division of either nerve recovery is always slow and often incomplete. It may be necessary to carry out treatment for two or three years. After a pressure neuropathy of the common peroneal nerve, a satisfactory recovery usually occurs in from six to twelve months.

POLYNEUROPATHY

Polyneuropathy (or polyneuritis) is a clinical picture, the essential feature of which is an impairment of function of many peripheral nerves simultaneously, resulting in a symmetrical distribution of flaccid muscular weakness and wasting, and usually also of sensory disturbances, affecting as a rule the distal more than the proximal segments of the limbs, and sometimes also involving the cranial nerves. The term polyneuritis is now less commonly used since it suggests restriction to purely inflammatory disorders. Polyneuropathy thus defined may be caused by a very large number of agencies which may operate in several different ways and even at different points of the peripheral nerves. Among such agencies are numerous endogenous and exogenous toxins, acute infections which directly attack the nerves, and vitamin deficiency. It seems best, therefore, to begin by describing the pathology and symptomatology of polyneuropathy in general, and then to discuss its commoner causes and how they are to be recognized.

Pathology

Each nerve fibre consists of two types of cell, the *nerve cell* body with the axon arising from it and the satellite cell of *Schwann cell*. In myelinated fibres, myelin is formed by the invagination of the Schwann cell surface membrane round the axon. Each Schwann cell supports a length of myelin between two nodes of Ranvier which may be as much as 1 mm in length. Two kinds of pathological process occur in neuropathies. First the nerve cell body and axon may be primarily affected leading to *axonal degeneration*. The pathological appearances resemble those of 'Wallerian degeneration' which follows a crush injury to nerve. Secondly, the Schwann cell may be affected, causing demyelination without involvement of the axon. This process is termed '*segmental demyelination*' (Fig. 19.6). In many neuropathies either degeneration or demyelination predominates. In chronic neuropathies there is also evidence of partial regeneration of nerves. After axonal degeneration, regeneration is slow and incomplete;

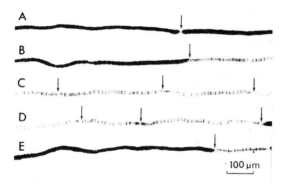

Fig. 19.6. Portion of isolated nerve fibre from a patient with diabetic neuropathy, after staining with osmium tetroxide.

The right-hand end of A is continuous with the left-hand end of B, and similarly from B to E. The nodes of Ranvier have been indicated by arrows. Other areas show evidence of segmental demyelination and remyelination.

after demyelination, recovery, if it occurs, is rapid and more complete. Examples of predominant nerve fibre degeneration include neuropathies resulting from crushing, ischaemia, nutritional neuropathies and poisons such as triorthocresyl-phosphate, lead, thallium, and acrylamide. Segmental demyelination occurs predominantly in diphtheritic polyneuropathy, diabetes (Fig. 19.6), metachromatic leucodystrophy and the Guillain–Barré syndrome.

A fresh light on the pathology of neuropathies has been thrown by electron-microscopic studies of experimental crush and toxic neuropathies in animals. Axonal degeneration occurs after a focal lesion in the nerve other than trauma, or after general insults. In some of these neuropathies distal terminals of the

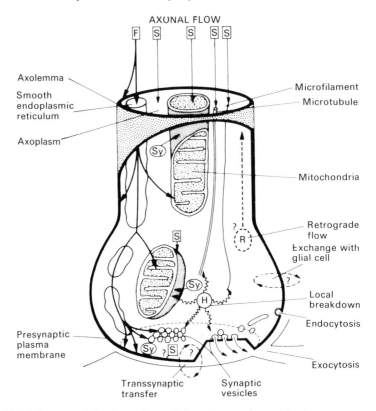

Fig. 19.7. Diagram of the dynamic condition of synaptic proteins in an axon terminal. F, fast phase of axonal flow; S, slow phase of axonal flow; Sy, sites of local protein synthesis; H, hydrolytic enzymes; R, retrograde flow.

longest fibres, perhaps because of the defect of axoplasmic flow, appear most affected – the so-called 'dying back' neuropathies, of which the toxic neuropathies are examples. An initial inhibition of protein synthesis has been shown before the appearance of distal degeneration in experimental toxic neuropathy (Fig. 19.7).

Experimental toxic neuropathy with acrylamide has suggested that neuronal damage is rapidly reversible when mild but when severer appears to progress for a time even after withdrawal of the toxin.

It is often difficult to distinguish between a process affecting the terminal part of longest fibres and a process affecting only the neurones with the longest fibres, as in porphyria. Sometimes both the neurone and axon are affected. Small scattered lesions such as occur in polyarteritis nodosa will result in proportionately more damage to the longer fibres. A feature of recurrent segmental demyelinating neuropathies is the development of hypertrophic neuropathy. Each episode of demyelination causes further division of the

Schwann cells, the new cells being unable to find a place on the axon, so leading to 'onion bulb' formation and sometimes clinically palpable thickening of the nerves. This occurs in the steroid-responsive recurrent polyneuropathy and also in hereditary sensory neuropathy.

Symptoms

The mode of onset varies according to the cause, ranging from acute or subacute in most infective and some metabolic disturbances to the slowly insidious. In a typical case sensory disturbances usually play a prominent part in the clinical picture. In the early stages the patient complains of numbness, tingling, and paraesthesia in the hands and feet, and often pain in the extremities, which may be severe, and involve both the superficial and deep structures. Cramp-like pains occur in the calves and are often troublesome at night. Following the early sensory disturbances the limbs become weak, the lower limbs usually being more noticeably affected than the upper.

Both motor and sensory symptoms affect predominantly the periphery of the limbs and in a symmetrical manner. In severe cases both wrist-drop and foot-drop are present, the latter causing a 'steppage' gait, and there is some wasting of the peripheral muscles of all four limbs. Weakness is most marked in the peripheral segments. If the patient can move his limbs, ataxia can usually be demonstrated, and in one form of disorder – the so-called 'pseudotabetic' variety – ataxia is conspicuous in the lower limbs and is due to loss of postural sensibility. There is a blunting of all forms of sensation in the periphery of the limbs, cutaneous anaesthesia and analgesia usually extending up to the elbows and knees. Postural sensibility and appreciation of passive movement are impaired in the fingers and toes. Vibration sense is also lost. Pressure upon the muscles, especially those of the calves, is usually intensely painful, and scratching the sole may also evoke severe pain, in each case after a slight delay.

The tendon reflexes are diminished or lost, the ankle-jerks disappearing before the knee-jerks. The plantar reflexes may also be lost, but if present are flexor. The skin of the extremities is often oedematous and sweating. Muscular contractures readily develop, and fibrous adhesions may occur in the tendon sheaths and around the joints. The sphincters are usually unaffected.

The muscles innervated by the cranial nerves may also be affected, most frequently the facial muscles, but sometimes ophthalmoplegia or bulbar paralysis occurs.

Electrophysiological studies (p. 162) show a mild reduction in motor conduction velocity in degenerative neuropathies but a marked reduction in velocity in demyelinating neuropathies.

THE CLASSIFICATION OF PERIPHERAL NEUROPATHIES

The classification of peripheral neuropathies cannot yet be based on precise and systematic knowledge of metabolic defects. In some cases the cause remains unknown even after full investigation. Howevei, a provisional grouping of some major causes follows and a few neuropathies will then be considered in more detail.

1. *Infective cause.* Only rarely is there direct involvement by bacteria, as in leprosy, or by a known virus as in herpes zoster or mumps. More commonly the relationship to the infection is indirect, resulting for example from the endotoxin as in diphtheria or from a more obscure interference by an infection as in 'infective polyneuropathy', also call the Landry–Guillain–Barré syndrome (p. 421) in which the myelin sheaths of peripheral nerves are attacked by immunologically activated cells after sensitization associated with a recent infection. In many cases there is a rising titre of cytomegalovirus antibody or sometimes there is a specific IgG antibody which is a good marker of acute infection. It is not known how a viral agent may cause an autoimmune response.

2. *Metabolic causes.* (a) Lack of essential vitamins such as B_1, the coenzyme in the metabolism of pyruvate (p. 493) and also other nutritional factors, as in alcoholic polyneuropathy and beriberi. Deficiency of vitamin B_{12} may also cause polyneuropathy (p. 493).

(b) Poisons, particularly the heavy metals arsenic, copper, thallium, mercury, and gold; organic compounds, triorthocresylphosphate, acrylamide, and disulphiram.

(c) Drugs may produce a polyneuropathy as a side-effect of their desired action, as, for example, isoniazid (by causing pyridoxine deficiency), thalidomide, sulphonamides, and nitrofurantoin.

(d) Porphyria. In acute intermittent porphyria peripheral neuropathy may follow episodes of confusion and abdominal pain during which urine is passed which becomes port wine coloured if allowed to stand. During latent periods between attacks there is usually an excess of porphobilinogen G and ō-amino-laevulinic acid in the urine. Attacks may be precipitated by drugs, particularly barbiturates. Autonomic involvement occurs.

(e) Uraemia. The increasing use of dialysis in the treatment of renal failure has led to recognition of a chronic polyneuropathy caused by the metabolic disturbance in renal failure.

(f) Endocrine disturbances. Diabetes is the commonest of these causes of polyneuropathy (p. 423).

3. *Vascular disorders.* These may be the result of atheroma, sometimes complicated by the presence of diabetes, Buerger's disease or a collagen disorder.

4. *Generalized disorders* in which there are abnormalities in the metabolism of serum proteins. These include collagen diseases, particularly polyarteritis nodosa, occasionally rheumatoid arthritis and disseminated lupus erythematosis, the reticuloses, amyloid disease, sarcoidosis, and carcinoma (p. 423).

5. *Genetically-determined disorders.* These, too, are metabolic disorders in which the precise defects are not as yet always known. They include peroneal muscular atrophy (p. 504), and the much rarer disorders hypertrophic interstitial polyneuropathy and Refsum's syndrome. In both the latter the peripheral

nerves are thickened due to an excess of collagen around each fibre. In Refsum's syndrome a chronic motor and sensory polyneuropathy occurs with other signs including deafness, cerebellar ataxia, and atypical retinitis pigmentosa. It is inherited by means of a rare recessive gene and recently a specific defect of lipid metabolism has been described in patients with this disorder. The defect may be circumvented by the use of a special diet which does not include phytanic acid and the plasma phytanic acid level lowered.

Other genetically determined neuropathies include hereditary sensory neuropathy, which may be of late onset and slowly progressive, and neuropathies associated with hereditary deficiency of high density lipoprotein (Tangier disease). All these disorders are inherited by recessive mechanisms. Undoubtedly further syndromes will be recognized, in view of the number of neuropathies in which, despite full investigations, no cause can at present be found.

ACUTE 'INFECTIVE' POLYNEUROPATHY – LANDRY–GUILLAIN–BARRÉ SYNDROME

Generalized polyneuropathy may develop acutely or subacutely, apparently spontaneously or following an inoculation procedure or a virus infection. This syndrome is thought to be due to an autoimmune response of the peripheral nervous system. In many cases no 'infective' causes can be identified. When the protein content of the cerebrospinal fluid is increased without any increase in cells – 'la dissociation albumino-cytologique' – the syndrome is named the *Guillain–Barré syndrome*. Other cases with similar onset but in which there is purely motor involvement with an ascending form of paralysis, were previously called the Landry syndrome. It is perhaps wisest to regard these eponymous syndromes as merely particular forms of acute 'infective' polyneuropathy and to use the term the *Landry–Guillain–Barré syndrome*. In some cases there may be evidence of involvement of the spinal cord or even brainstem in addition to the nerve roots and peripheral nerves. It may perhaps be thought of as the peripheral variety of acute 'allergic' reactions of the nervous system, though with some features in common with the more central variety – acute disseminated encephalomyelitis.

The model of the human disease – experimental allergic neuritis – is caused by injection of material including myelinated peripheral nerve with adjuvant, from which a myelin basic protein, named P_2, has been isolated. In both the natural and experimental disease the serum and mononuclear cells can cause demyelination *in vitro* and in both there is a marked elevation of c.s.f. protein. The effect of the serum is due to an antibody that attaches to Schwann cells.

The onset of symptoms is usually acute or subacute, and frequently febrile. In contrast with other forms of polyneuropathy, the proximal muscles of the limbs may suffer as severely as the distal ones, and the trunk muscles may also be involved. Sensory changes may be severe, slight, or even sometimes absent.

The cranial nerves often suffer, sometimes even the optic nerves with papill-oedema, and the eighth nerve causing deafness.

The protein in the cerebrospinal fluid is often greatly raised to 2.0 or 3.0 g/l or even higher, and may be yellow. There is no excess of cells. The pressure of the fluid may also be raised. There are patients, indistinguishable clinically, in whom there is an excess of cells, usually monocytic, with a mild rise of protein in proportion to the cell count. In some cases the pressure of the fluid may also be raised.

This is a serious disorder which may prove fatal, especially from respiratory paralysis. It is wisest to err on the side of tracheostomy early rather than late if there is progressive bulbar and respiratory weakness. Severe hypotension due to autonomic disturbances may require treatment with pressor drugs, particularly in elderly patients. Slight remissions are not infrequent, and are often followed by severe relapses. In most cases, however, the outlook is good, but improvement is slow, and the paralysis having reached its height tends to remain stationary for weeks or sometimes for months. Sometimes recovery is incomplete and recurrences occasionally occur. In the most favourable cases the patient is not likely to be convalescent in less than from three to six months.

The usual nursing care of polyneuropathy should be carried out. Bulbar and respiratory paralysis require special treatment (p. 466). Treatment aimed at interfering with presumed autoimmune disorder has not significantly improved the prognosis. Plasma exchange has been attempted and prednisolone which was frequently given has now been shown not to be beneficial.

ALCOHOLIC POLYNEUROPATHY

Though polyneuropathy may occur in chronic alcoholics, its relationship to the alcoholism is by no means clear. It has been thought to be a form of beri-beri, the deficiency of vitamin B_1, aneurine, being due chiefly to impaired absorption. While this may be true in some cases, other factors probably operate in others. Alcoholic polyneuropathy may result from the consumption of spirits or wine over long periods. Most patients are middle-aged, and males are affected more often than females.

The clinical picture is that of polyneuropathy (p. 419), and pain in and tenderness of the muscles are usually prominent symptoms. In alcoholic peripheral neuropathy there is also selective involvement of vagal fibres and the paravertebral sympathetic chain. Wernicke's encephalopathy, delirium tremens, Korsakoff's psychosis or alcoholic dementia (p. 257) may also be present. Gastritis is common and the liver is often enlarged.

Treatment is that of polyneuropathy in general, combined with that of alcohol addiction, the aim being the gradual withdrawal of the alcohol. Parenteral injection of a vitamin B preparation (such as Parentrovite) should be given promptly, with a fully balanced diet as soon as the patient can eat. It is helpful to give vitamin B_{12}, hydroxycobalamin, in addition.

DIABETIC POLYNEUROPATHY

Neuropathy in diabetes may take several forms.

1. The commonest form is a mild chronic symmetrical *motor and sensory neuropathy* affecting particularly the lower extremities. Severe burning pain in the legs is sometimes a striking complaint. The sensory disturbance may be associated with trophic lesions of the skin and joints which, unlike those of tabes, are usually distal. This form of neuropathy recovers partially with better control of the diabetes and is probably caused by the metabolic disturbance of diabetes.

2. The sudden onset of *cranial or peripheral palsies* in diabetics is likely to be the result of vascular lesions, either due to associated atheroma or diabetic microangiopathy.

3. The peripheral nerves and nerve roots in diabetes are abnormally susceptible to effects of *pressure* and *trauma*, which explains the liability of diabetics to the carpal tunnel syndrome and to radiculopathy secondary to cervical and lumbar spondylosis.

4. An *autonomic neuropathy* occurs in diabetics and may lead to impotence or disturbances of bowel control. Postural hypotension occasionally results from loss of autonomic reflexes which normally compensate for the tendency of blood to pool in the legs on standing (see p. 196).

5. Occasionally wasting may be strikingly restricted to the proximal leg muscles, so-called *diabetic amyotrophy,* with proximal leg pain and loss of tendon reflexes. Electrophysiological studies have shown slowed conduction in the nerves of the wasted muscles in such patients so that it is in fact a form of neuropathy.

CARCINOMATOUS NEUROPATHY

A neuropathy occasionally occurs in association with a carcinoma outside the nervous system, usually an oat-cell carcinoma of the lung, less often the stomach, or ovarian carcinoma or reticulosis. The neuropathy may be primary motor, sensory and motor, or purely sensory in its type. It may be only part of the neurological syndrome; there may be a cerebellar degeneration, polymyositis or a myopathy. There may also be a myasthenic syndrome (p. 444), motor neurone disease, encephalomyelitis, or metabolic disturbances, usually hypercalcaemia or hyponatraemia with inappropriate secretion of anti-diuretic hormone (p. 525). The relationship to the carcinoma is complicated. The neuropathy sometimes precedes the first symptoms of the carcinoma, occasionally by more than a year. Often the neuropathy progresses with the growth of the carcinoma and remits after the removal of the tumour. Occasionally the neuropathy remits before removal of the tumour and on rare occasions the neuropathy may progress despite removal of the tumour. The mechanism of the production of the remote neurological effects is unknown but a disturbance of 'auto-immunity' seems more probable than any direct toxic or metabolic effect of the tumour itself.

DIPHTHERIAL POLYNEUROPATHY

The exotoxin of *Corynebacterium diphtheriae* has an affinity for the peripheral nerves. Paralysis of the palate, usually the earliest nervous symptom, develops during the third or fourth week after infection. It causes the voice to assume a nasal character and leads to regurgitation of fluid through the nose in swallowing. Paralysis of accommodation develops usually during the fourth to sixth weeks, and leads to blurring of vision for near objects. Weakness of the lateral recti occasionally occurs. Generalized polyneuritis is less common and tends to make its appearance from the fifth to the eigth week after infection. The clinical picture in the limbs is typical of polyneuritis. Postural sensibility is often greatly impaired, leading to gross ataxia of the lower limbs – the so-called 'pseudotabetic' form. The sphincters usually escape. Paralysis of the pharynx and larynx and respiratory muscles constitutes a serious complication. In addition, a local form of paralysis of muscles supplied by the same spinal segment may occur when the organism infects a skin wound.

The nervous complications of diphtheria are very rare if adequate doses of antitoxin are given on the first day of the illness. If antitoxin has already been given it is doubtful if a further dose when polyneuropathy appears is of any value. Bulbar and respiratory paralysis will require treatment on the same lines as in poliomyelitis.

TETANUS

It has been estimated that tetanus is the cause of death in half a million people in the world annually. The toxin travels along peripheral nerves to the brain and probably causes spasms by blocking the release of glycine which has an inhibitory action at synapses.

After cleaning of the wound and starting treatment with penicillin, human tetanus immunoglobulin (30–300 international units per kg of body weight) is given intramuscularly to neutralize circulating toxin. It does not reverse toxins which has already started to have its effect and does not penetrate the CNS. Minor spasms can be controlled by intravenous diazepam (Valium). In severe cases incubation and tracheostomy will probably be needed and also partial curarization. Autonomic disturbances are common and those caused by sympathetic over-activity may be controlled by beta-adrenergic blocking agents.

LEAD NEUROPATHY

Lead neuropathy is usually encountered among lead workers, such as plumbers and painters, but its incidence has been much reduced by legislative restrictions.

It occasionally follows contamination of water, beer or cider, passed through lead pipes. Lead has a predilection for the motor fibres of the nerves supplying the muscles used in an occupation. It usually affects the extensor muscles of the wrist and fingers, bilaterally, causing wrist- and finger-drop, the brachioradialis escaping. An upper-arm type of paralysis involves the spinati, deltoid, biceps, brachialis and brachioradialis muscles. Involvement of the lower limbs is rare. There is no sensory loss. A progressive deterioration of the anterior horn cells of the spinal cord causing progressive muscular atrophy occasionally occurs, and there is sometimes degeneration of the corticospinal tracts as well.

The diagnosis rests on the presence of other signs of chronic lead poisoning, and an anaemia with basophilic stippling of red cells and a high blood lead level.

DRUGS CAUSING NEUROPATHIES

The type of neuropathy caused by drugs is usually a form of axonal degeneration prodominantly. A list of commoner drugs includes antineoplastic drugs such as vincristine, which also causes an autonomic neuropathy; antimicrobial drugs, such as nitrofurantoin and isoniazide if not 'covered' with pyridoxine; cardiovascular drugs, such as perhexilene maleate, hydralazine (in a high dose) and amioderone; antirheumatic drugs such as penicillin; psychotropic drugs, such as imipramine; anticonvulsants such as phenytoin and also antiparasitic drugs such as metronidazole.

THE DIAGNOSIS OF POLYNEUROPATHY

Usually the diagnosis of polyneuropathy is easy, owing to the characteristic symmetrical and peripheral distribution of the muscular weakness and wasting, pain, tenderness, and sensory impairment. The association of pain, ataxia, and loss of tendon reflexes in the lower limbs may simulate tabes. In polyneuropathy, however, the calves are tender on pressure, whereas in tabes they are insensitive, and the Argyll Robertson pupil is never found in polyneuropathy. The polyneuritic element may be prominent in the early stages of vitamin B_{12} neuropathy, but some signs of involvement of the spinal cord are usually to be found, and gastric achlorhydria, together with a megalocytosis in the blood, should enable the right diagnosis to be made. Occasionally the symptoms of a tumour of the cauda equina may simulate polyneuritis – a diagnosis which should always be accepted with reserve when the symptoms are confined to the lower limbs. Myelography will usually settle the matter.

The important points which are likely to lead to a diagnosis of the cause of the peripheral neuropathy include the manner of its development, whether acute, subacute, chronic or recurrent and whether the distribution is proximal, distal or diffuse and whether the neuropathy is associated with hypertrophy. On this basis it is often possible to make some prediction as to the likely fibre size involved and whether the process is axonal or demyelinating even before resorting to electrophysiological tests or nerve biopsy. The febrile onset and the changes in the cerebrospinal fluid will establish the diagnosis of the Guillain–Barré type. Alcoholism and diabetes are usually obvious as causes. The nature of the rarer forms of polyneuropathy can usually be established by means of the appropriate investigations, including electromyography, palpation of the peripheral nerves, which are usually palpably thickened in progressive hypertrophic polyneuritis, leprosy, amyloid disease, and possibly nerve biopsy.

TREATMENT OF POLYNEUROPATHY

It is obviously necessary to deal with the cause when that is treatable though in some half the cases of generalized neuropathy no specific aetiology can be discovered. Rest in bed is essential, not only on account of muscular weakness, but also because the heart may be involved. Local treatment consists of the prevention of muscular contractures, the maintenance of the nutrition of the muscles, and the promotion of recovery of voluntary power. Wrist-drop and foot-drop must be prevented by the use of appropriate splints. As long as the muscular tenderness is severe, splints cannot be borne, and the feet must then be supported by means of a sandbag placed beneath the soles, the weight of the bedclothes being taken by a cradle. Later, aluminium night-shoes may be used to support the feet at a right angle. Daily massage and passive movement should be instituted as soon as the patient is able to bear them, and the muscles may be stimulated electrically. Analgesic drugs may be required. It is doubtful whether any drug influences the rate of recovery. Vitamins appear to be of little value except in those cases when vitamin deficiency is known to be a cause of the polyneuropathy.

REFERENCES

Argov, Z. and Mastaglia, F.L. (1979). Drug-induced peripheral neuropathies. *Br. med. J.* **i**, 663–6.

Asbury, A.K. (1981). Diagnostic considerations in the Guillain–Barré syndrome. *Ann. Neurol.* Suppl., **9**, 1–5.

Arnason, B.G.W. (1971). Idiopathic polyneuritis (Landry–Guillain–Barré syndrome) and allergic neuritis: a comparison. *Res. Publs Ass. Res. nerv. ment. Dis.* **49**, 156–77.

Bannister, R. (ed.) (1983). *Autonomic failure.* Oxford University Press.

Dyck, P.T., Thomas, P.K., and Lambert, E.H. (1975). *Peripheral neuropathy.* Saunders, Philadelphia.

Medical Research Council Memorandum No. 45 (1976). *Aids to the examination of the peripheral nervous system.* HMSO, London.

Prineas, J.W. (1981). Pathology of the Guillain–Barré syndrome. *Ann. Neurol.* Suppl., **9**, 6–19.

Sunderland, S. (1978). *Nerves and nerve injuries,* 2nd edn. Churchill Livingstone, Edinburgh.

Winegrad, A.I. and Greene, D.A. (1976). Diabetic polyneuropathy. *New Engl. J. Med.* **295**, 1416–20.

20 Disorders of muscle

Anatomy and physiology

A voluntary muscle is composed of muscle fibres, each of which is a multi-nucleated cell, consisting of contractile substance with a sarcolemma and its nuclei, and a motor end-plate in which the nerve fibre terminates. The lower motor neurone ends in relation with a bundle of 150 or more muscle fibres. Skeletal muscle fibres are not homogeneous and contain two distinct types of fibre. The type I fibre is smaller and has a high concentration of enzymes which are concerned with aerobic metabolism. The type II fibre is large with coarse myofibrils and has a higher concentration of glycogen and of enzymes which are concerned with anaerobic metabolism. Postural muscles like the soleus which contract slowly are, particularly in animals, largely made up of type I fibres and are in macroscopic appearance 'red' muscle. Muscles concerned with rapid twitch activity have a higher proportion of type II fibres. In human muscles the proportion of each type of fibre is more equal (Plate 8). These histochemical characteristics of fibres have been shown to be dependent on their innervation.

At the myoneural junction the nerve impulse liberates acetylcholine which alters the end-plate potential and excites muscular contraction. The muscle fibre itself allows for the process of excitation-coupling and contraction using ATP to drive the actin–myosin crossbridge cycling and to support the membrane ionic pumps including the re-uptake of calcium ions during relaxation.

In tonic striated muscles (for example eye muscles) stimulation does not trigger a conducted action potential but causes local depolarization of the membrane. Such fibres do not obey the all-or-none law but the force they develop is regulated by varying the intracellular calcium ion concentration. Anticholinesterases act on the nerve endings and end-plates (Fig. 20.1). Potassium plays a complex part in muscle contraction, the important factor beging the ratio between the level of potassium in the blood and in the muscle cell. Muscular weakness may be a symptom of either a low or a high blood potassium.

Muscle diseases have different clinical features. Most are progressive with the occurrence of either weakness, fatigability, stiffness or cramps which may be more prominent at rest or on exercise. The age of onset and the distribution whether proximal or more occasionally distal finally determine the clinical

427

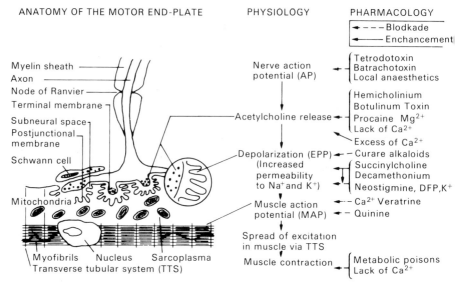

ANATOMY OF THE MOTOR END-PLATE   PHYSIOLOGY   PHARMACOLOGY

Fig. 20.1. Diagram of motor end-plate showing from the left, anatomy, sequence of events leading to contraction and modification of these processes by various agents.

diagnosis in conjunction with the rate of progression and the presence or absence of pseudohypertrophy.

Pathology of muscle disorders

In dystrophies the changes are a reduction in cell mass caused by repeated episodes of muscle fibre necrosis due to a muscle membrane fault associated with high intracellular calcium and replacement by fat and connective tissue. Muscle fibres may be acutely destroyed as in acute myoglobinuric myopathies or slowly as in the muscular dystrophies, possibly by an influx of calcium ions resulting from genetic faults in the muscle membrane. In polymyositis, necrosis is a result of humoral and cell-mediated auto-immune mechanisms. Other diseases affect the contractile mechanism, for example McArdle's disease and central core disease (Plate 8). Membrane excitability is lost in the periodic paralyses and in myotonia. Defects of excitation, contraction, and coupling with impaired calcium release also occur. In a variety of rare enzyme defects known as the mitochondrial myopathies there is a defect of release of energy from the muscle fibre.

POLYMYOSITIS

The onset of polymyositis often follows a viral infection which may initially sensitize lymphocytes and cause muscle cell damage and then further sensitization. Lymphocytes from patients with polymyositis show tissue specific cytotoxicity for muscle cells. A histologically similar inflammatory polymyositis can be produced in guinea pigs by immunization with muscle in Freund's adjuvant but no specific antigen has been isolated in the human disease. Polymyositis is not a single nosological entity. It is a clinicopathological diagnosis. Some authors distinguish acute dermatomyositis, in which an inflammation of the skin is associated with that of the muscles, from chronic polymyositis, but intermediate forms occur, ranging from an acute and progressive disorder to one which may not only be chronic but exhibit long remissions.

Polymyositis may also occur as a minor feature in association with other collagen diseases, particularly scleroderma, lupus erythematosus, and poly-arteritis. It may also be associated with a carcinoma. Other inflammatory disorders which very occasionally involve muscles may be classified with polymyositis and these include sarcoidosis, trichinosis and toxoplasmosis.

Pathology

Experimental work has suggested that polymyositis may be regarded as an auto-immune disease mediated by lymphocytes with organ specificity confined to muscles or affecting other tissues such as joints, skin or viscera. Carcinoma elsewhere may also affect the auto-immune process.

In the more acute cases the characteristic pathological changes consist of fragmentation of muscle fibres, and active phagocytosis of their contents. There is an intense cellular reaction in the connective tissue. When skin lesions are associated microscopical examination shows the dermis to be oedematous, with swollen and thickened collagen fibres. The small arteries have thickened walls and there is an infiltration of inflammatory cells beneath the epidermis and around the blood vessels and sweat glands. In more chronic examples of polymyositis the muscles are less abnormal but may show, at the periphery of each fasciculus, fibres which are vacuolated and reduced to thin sarcolemmal tubes containing large numbers of shrunken nuclei. In longitudinal section the contents of the muscle fibres are seen to be coagulated in a segmental manner, with pyknotic muscle nuclei. Small veins within the muscles are surrounded by aggregations of lymphocytes known as lymphorrhages, plasma, and other cells (Fig. 20.2).

Symptoms

In the more acute cases the muscles become tender, swollen, and weak, with an oedema of the overlying subcutaneous tissue, the proximal muscles tending to be more affected than the distal ones. The skin is swollen and there may be a diffuse erythema. Other muscles of the limbs are gradually involved, becoming weak or paralysed, and the tendon reflexes disappear. Eventually the oedema and induration of the muscles slowly subside, leaving them reduced in bulk, and shortened by fibrous tissue.

In the more chronic cases, wasting, weakness, and fatigability of the muscles, with diminution or loss of tendon reflexes, are slowly progressive. Either the proximal or the distal muscles may be mainly involved, sometimes mimicking a progressive dystrophy, and in some cases the bulbar muscles and even the ocular muscles. Myocarditis may occur, and there may be scleroderma. In

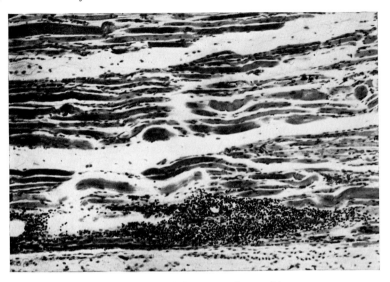

Fig. 20.2. Muscle in acute polymyositis.

the more acute cases, there is fever and a polymorphonuclear leucocytosis in the blood. There is a rise in the gamma globulin in the blood and in the erythrocyte sedimentation rate which parallels the activity of the disorder. Elevation of the levels of muscle enzymes such as creatine kinase is a more sensitive index of the extent of the muscle damage.

Diagnosis

Polymyositis has to be distinguished from motor neurone disease, in which fasciculation is much commoner, and in which the electromyogram is different (p. 164), and from two other muscular disorders, thyrotoxic myopathy, in which there is evidence of thyrotoxicosis, and myopathy complicating carcinoma. It must also be distinguished from polymyalgia rheumatica in which there is muscle pain, malaise and restriction of joint movement and the sedimentation rate is raised, but the serum muscle enzymes are normal. Muscle biopsy may be necessary to establish the diagnosis of polymyositis.

Prognosis and treatment

Polymyositis ranges from acute cases terminating fatally in a few months to chronic and remittent cases, the course of which extends over many years. Recovery, especially in patients under 30, has been commoner since treatment was introduced. Treatment is by immunosuppression using prednisolone (60 mg daily, enteric coated) and azothiaprine for six months before gradual reduction of the drugs. In older patients evidence of diffuse carcinomatosis often emerges.

THE MUSCULAR DYSTROPHIES

The muscular dystrophies are a group of disorders of which the essential feature is a progressive degeneration of certain groups of muscles. The disease is frequently familial or hereditary, and a number of forms have been distinguished by differences in the age of onset and variations in the distribution of the muscles affected. A given form usually breeds true. One variety is distinguished by the association of myotonia with the other symptoms of a muscular dystrophy.

Aetiology and pathology

Beyond inheritance nothing is known about the aetiology of the muscular dystrophies. The pseudohypertrophic form is usually inherited as a sex-linked recessive, while the juvenile and facioscapulohumeral forms tend to be dominant or recessive. Pathologically the essential changes in the muscles are the same in all, the most striking microscopical features being the great variation in the size of the individual fibres, and the large amount of connective tissue and fat cells. Both very large and very small fibres are seen scattered about the muscle at all stages of the disease. Swelling is the initial change, which is later followed by atrophy. The palpable enlargement of some of the muscles in the pseudohypertrophic form is due to an excess of fat (Fig. 20.3). As a result of the increased information obtained by muscle biopsy with electron microscopy, histochemical identification of fibre types, and more complex metabolic investigations, it has become clear that there are a large number of genetically determined muscular defects and many more probably remain to be discovered. The commonest causes of muscular dystrophy will be listed first followed by some rarer types and a few of the commoner varieties will be described in more detail to illustrate the presenting features, diagnosis and management.

Classification muscular dystrophies

1. X-linked pseudohypertrophic types.
   (a) Sex-linked recessive (severe) (Duchenne).
   (b) Sex-linked recessive (mild) (Becker).
2. Facio-scapulo-humeral (Landouzy and Dejerine).
3. Scapuloperoneal muscular atrophy, dominant or X-linked.
4. Limb girdle dystrophy, autosomal recessive or dominant.
5. Distal, autosomal dominant.
6. Ocular-pharyngeal.

Duchennne muscular dystrophy

This is the commonest variety, originally described by Duchenne. It is inherited as a sex-linked recessive and it is almost confined to males, though one-third of the cases arise by spontaneous mutation. Occasional cases occurring in girls are

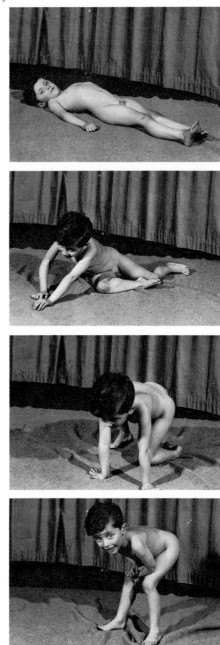

Fig. 20.3. Boy with muscular dystrophy rising from the ground by 'climbing up' his own legs (see p. 433).

the result of an autosomal recessive mechanism or a genetic defect such as Turner's syndrome or mosaicism. It usually appears in childhood about the middle of the first decade of life. The onset of symptoms is gradual. A child which has previously been normal begins to walk clumsily, tends to fall, and has difficulty in getting up unaided. Occasionally the history is that the child has never walked properly. Examination reveals enlargement, pseudohypertrophy, of some muscles and wasting of others. Those which most frequently exhibit pseudohypertrophy are the calves, the glutei, the quadriceps, the infraspinati, and the deltoids. The triceps and forearm muscles may also be enlarged. Pseudohypertrophied muscles are firmer than normal to the touch, and in spite of their appearance are usually weak, but there are exceptions to this. Wasting is almost always present in the sternal part of pectoralis major and in latissimus dorsi. The proximal muscles of the limbs are more liable to waste than the distal ones. The muscles of the face and hands escape.

The peculiar distribution of the muscular weakness causes the patient to assume an attitude of lordosis when standing, the trunk being thrown back to displace the centre of gravity behind the vertebral column. The gait is waddling. Weakness of the extensors of the spine and knees leads to the adoption of a characteristic method of rising from the ground, the patient turning over on to the hands and feet and assisting himself into the upright attitude by clasping his legs with his hands and 'climbing up' his own legs. Muscular fasciculation is absent, the tendon reflexes are diminished and ultimately lost. Sensation is unimpaired, and intelligence is usually normal.

MYOPATHIES WITH ABNORMAL MUSCLE FIBRE ACTIVITY

Dystrophia myotonica

This is a hereditary disorder characterized not only by muscular dystrophy but also by myotonia and other dystrophic disturbances, especially cataract and gonadal atrophy.

The histology of the muscle differs from other myopathies in that there are long chains of central nuclei within the muscle fibres and striated annulets or 'ring binden'.

A characteristic feature of this disease is the occurrence of cataract as the only abnormality in the family for several generations until there is a sudden outbreak in one generation of the dystrophic disturbances, subsequent generations being usually free from all symptoms of the disorder.

Symptoms of the fully developed form of the disorder first appear between the ages of 15 and 40, in most cases between 20 and 30, but may be found in childhood. Usually muscular weakness or myotonia is the first symptom noticed by the patient. Muscular wasting is most conspicuous in the facial muscles, the sternocleidomastoids, which may be completely atrophied, the muscles of the shoulder girdle, forearms and hands, the quadriceps, and the legs below the knees. The wasted muscles are weak. The weakness and wasting usually develop slowly over a number of years. Fasciculation is absent.

The face is expressionless and the forehead smooth. The eyelids often droop and the cheeks are sunken (Fig. 20.4). The tendon reflexes are lost in the wasted muscles.

The myotonia leads to a prolonged after-contraction of the affected muscles which persists after the voluntary effort to contract the muscle has ceased. Myotonia is increased by fatigue, emotion, and cold. It is usually most evident in the flexors of the fingers, so that the patient has difficulty in relaxing his grasp. It may also involve the facial and masticatory muscles, and occasionally the legs. It can usually be induced by percussion, and is then most easily seen in the muscles of the thenar eminence and the tongue. The electromyogram shows a characteristic declining discharge frequency on mechanical stimulation (p. 165). It has been shown that the muscle membrane potential in myotonia congenita has a greatly increased resting membrane resistance which is attributed to a decrease in membrane chloride permeability. Since an increase in the external potassium concentration further reduces permeability to chloride it will aggravate myotonia whereas increase in the internal potassium will prevent the repetitive spike discharges. The effect of procainamide and hydantoinate lies in their stabilization of the muscle membrane.

Other dystrophic symptoms include cataract and frontal baldness which is more conspicuous in males than in females. Atrophy of the testes and ovaries is

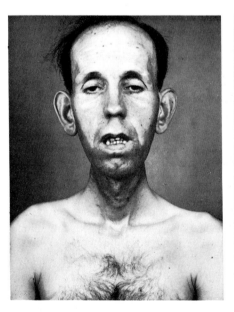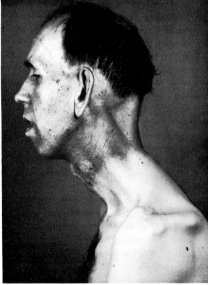

Fig. 20.4. Dystrophia myotonica. Note the frontal alopecia, myopathic facies and wasting of the sternocleidomastoids.

usually present, leading to impotence and sterility. Other endocrine disturbances which may occur include diabetes mellitus. The myocardium is
sometimes affected and heart block has been observed. Low intelligence and
mental subnormality are common in affected families.

Myotonia congenita

Myotonia congenita, or Thomsen's disease, is a rare hereditary disorder
characterized by prolonged tonic contraction and retarded relaxation of the
muscles which occur both at the beginning of, and after, voluntary movement.
The disorder is usually hereditary, and behaves as a Mendelian dominant. The
term *hereditary paramyotonia* describes a hereditary disorder characterized by
the occurrence of myotonia only when the sufferer is exposed to cold.

The myotonia in myotonia congenita is usually first observed in childhood
and constitutes a considerable handicap, particularly when the patient's
endeavour to change his attitude by making a movement is prevented by the
prolonged contraction of the muscles maintaining the existing posture.

Biochemical changes in myopathies

In all disorders in which muscular wasting occurs impairment of normal muscle
metabolism leads to creatinuria. The level of the serum enzyme creatine
phosphokinase is usually elevated in proportion to the rate of muscular
degeneration.

Diagnosis

The diagnosis of the muscular dystrophies rests upon the mode of inheritance
and the age of onset, usually at an early age, of symmetrical muscular wasting,
with a distribution which cannot be explained in terms of the innervation of the
muscles. In the pseudohypertophic form the presence and distinctive distribution of the enlarged, firm, but weak muscles is pathognomonic. Chronic
muscular dystrophies are sometimes difficult to distinguish clinically from the
spinal muscular atrophies (see p. 504). In dystrophia myotonica there is the
added symptom of delayed muscular relaxation, especially of the flexors of the
fingers, together with cataract and other dystrophic symptoms. In myotonia
congenita the myotonia is not associated with muscular wasting. Amyotonia
congenita is distinguished by the fact that it is present from birth. In spastic
diplegia, the symptoms of which become apparent during the first year of life,
the muscles are spastic instead of being hypotonic and there are signs of
bilateral corticospinal tract lesion. In peroneal muscular atrophy the muscular
wasting begins in the feet and hands and gradually ascends the limbs and
sensory changes are present, especially in the lower limbs. Poliomyelitis is
distinguished by the acute onset and the asymmetrical and non-progressive
character of the muscular wasting. Electromyography and muscle biopsy are
usually necessary to confirm the precise diagnosis. The biopsy should be taken

from a moderately weak muscle and processed for histochemistry and electron microscopy (see Plate 8).

Prognosis

The prognosis of the Duchenne pseudohypertrophic form of muscular dystrophy is bad. Increasing weakness and wasting of the limb and trunk muscles leads to the patient's becoming bed-ridden, with severe deformities, and the disorder ends fatally during the second decade of life as a rule. The prognosis in the juvenile forms of muscular dystrophy is considerably better. Deterioration is slower, and many patients remain in a virtually stationary condition during the third and fourth decades. The same is true of dystrophia myotonica, in which the rate of development of the muscular wasting is very variable. Sometimes the condition remains stationary for many years, but usually there is a slow deterioration. Most patients die during middle age of some intercurrent illness. Myotonia congenita does not shorten life, and the severity of the myotonia tends to decrease as the patient grows older.

Treatment

No treatment appears to influence the course of any of the muscular dystrophies. In the more rapidly progressive forms, neither orthopaedic appliances nor operations appear to have any value. Myotonia is to some extent alleviated by quinine, but much more by procainamide hydrochloride. A suitable initial dose for an adult is 0.25 g four times a day, which can be increased if necessary. The average maintenance dose is 4 g per day. Sodium hydantoinate 100 mg three times a day may also be effective.

Genetic counselling has an important place in the management of families with myopathy. For Duchenne dystrophy about one-third of new cases are the result of mutations. The diagnosis of the non-carrier state in the female at risk, such as the sister of an affected boy, is based on the clinical data, family history, prominence of calf size, presence of muscle weakness, combined with an estimate of the serum creatine phosphokinase, and muscle histology and electron microscopy. At present there is a hope that the application of recent advances in recombinant DNA technology will before long provide a reliable marker for the gene of Duchenne dystrophy, which would justify antenatal diagnosis from chorionic trophic biopsy or amniocentesis. Topical radioactive phosphorus nuclear magnetic resonance permits research into energy metabolism and has permitted diagnosis of, for example phosphofructokinase deficiency without muscle biopsy.

THE MYOPATHIES OF LATER ONSET

The occurrence of chronic muscular disease, beginning especially in and after middle age, has recently been increasingly recognized. The pathology of these conditions is still obscure, and some of them may well be forms of chronic polymyositis. Indeed, the pathological picture ranges from one indistinguishable from this to one in which little abnormality is detectable, and there is often no correlation between the apparent acuteness of the pathological changes and the clinical course of the disease. In these circumstances the only possible classification appears to be a clinical one, taking into account aetiological factors when these are known. The more important forms of acquired myopathy are the following.

Spontaneous: this variety is chiefly seen in middle-aged and elderly women who complain of progressive weakness and fatigability. Muscular wasting at first affects chiefly the shoulder- and hip-girdle muscles and the trunk muscles. The muscles innervated by the pons and medulla may be involved, and less frequently the ocular muscles. The course is usually very slowly progressive. Some are due to spinal atrophy not primary muscle disease.

Carcinomatous: the symptoms of carcinomatous myopathy may precede those of the causal carcinoma. The course is usually more rapid than that of the spontaneous variety. Weakness and fatigability of the limbs accompanied by an atrophic paresis, most marked in the limb girdles and proximal parts of the limbs, develops in the course of a few months. Sometimes ptosis, diplopia and even bulbar paralysis occur due to the myasthenic syndrome (Eaton–Lambert syndrome) (see p. 444). When muscular wasting is inconspicuous there may be fatigability which responds up to a point to neostigmine. Polymyositis and dermatomyositis may also complicate a neoplasm, particularly carcinoma of the lung.

Thyrotoxic: severe muscular weakness and wasting are common in acute thyrotoxicosis. Here again the proximal muscles of the limbs and the trunk muscles are those most frequently and severely affected. The tendon reflexes may be diminished. The condition appears to be the direct result of the thyrotoxicosis. Serum T_3 and T_4 tests are necessary. It should be recalled that the other muscular syndromes which sometimes occur in thyrotoxicosis include exophthalmic ophthalmoplegia (see p. 55), myasthenia, and hypokalaemic or normokalaemic periodic paralysis.

Myxoedema myopathy is a rare feature of hypothyroidism, though 'slow' reflexes which result from a change in the structure of the muscle are a constant finding. In primary thyroid deficiency the TSH level is raised. The T_4 is reduced if the myoxoedema is secondary to pituitary insufficiency.

Hypoparathyroidism: the muscle symptoms are due to hypocalcaemia. Tetany may occur.

Cushing's syndrome and steroid myopathy: in Cushing's syndrome there is often weakness which is greater than the degree of apparent wasting. Similar muscular weakness may occur following treatment with steroids with the fluorine atom in the nine alpha position (for example triamcinolone) in particular.

Acromegaly and gigantism may be accompanied by a myopathy.

Addison's disease: there is generalized muscular weakness and wasting in Addison's disease, and also in hypopituitarism. Electrolyte changes and hypotension aggravate the weakness.

Rarer types of myopathy

1. Myopathies with specific biochemical defects: in contrast to dystrophies these result from rare specific defects in the energy production pathways of muscle, leading to damage when energy supply fails to keep place with demand. They are rare and symptoms of weakness, fatigue, and aching are more obvious than wasting. They include lesions of the cell cytosol, for example McArdle's disease, and mitochondrial defects, the first of which was described by Luft, but both lists are growing fast. McArdle's disease presents with cramps on exertion and is inherited by an autosomal recessive mechanism. On biopsy there is a muscle phosphorylase deficiency with failure of lactate production on ischaemic exercise. There are also lipid myopathies which include muscle carnitine deficiency.

2. Myopathies with periodic 'metabolic' manifestations: hypo-, hyper-, and normokalaemic period paralysis, malignant hyperpyrexia and familial myoglobinuria.

3. Myopathies with abnormal mitochondria: as a result of muscle biopsy irregular or mishapen mitochondria sometimes too numerous or with inclusions have been described, often with congenital defects outside the muscular system. Examples are hypermetabolic myopathy, megaconial myopathy, and the Kearns–Sayr syndrome (which also includes associated retinal degeneration, deafness, cerebellar atrophy, and growth failure).

4. Myopathies with specific structural changes in muscle fibres: these include central core disease of several types and nemaline myopathy in which tiny rod bodies are found in the muscle fibres. Central core disease is a rare non-progressive congenital myopathy inherited by a dominant mechanism which has been distinguished from other chronic myopathies by muscle biopsy. The muscle, though looking normal on routine staining, consists almost entirely of type I fibres with a single central core (see Plate 8), devoid of mitochondria and oxidative enzymes.

5. Myopathies with changes in histochemical fibre types: the type I fibres are slow fibres used for oxidative postural activity and stain poorly for ATPases. Type II fibres are used for fast anaerobic activity and stain readily for ATPase.

6. Myopathies with abnormal muscle fibre activity: these include dystrophia myotonica and myotonia congenita (Thomsen's disease) already described, and congenital paramyotonia and myokymia with impaired relaxation.

Diagnosis

The chief problem in diagnosis is to recognize the muscular origin of the weakness and wasting and to distinguish it from those lesions of the nervous system which may produce similar symptoms, particularly motor neurone disease. Distinguishing features are the tendency of the myopathies to involve first the proximal muscles of the limbs and the trunk muscles, the fact that muscular fasciculation, while not unknown in the myopathies, is infrequent and usually scanty, the electromyographic changes (p. 162), and muscle biopsy, which is often helpful.

MYASTHENIA GRAVIS

Aetiology and pathology

Myasthenia gravis is a chronic disease with a tendency to remissions and relapses characterized by abnormal muscular fatigability, which may for a long time be confined to, or predominant in, an isolated group of muscles, and is later associated with permanent denervation and weakness of some muscles. The muscles may show a mixture of simple atrophy and inflammatory cellular exudate, collections of round cells among the muscle being known as lymphorrhages. Changes have been described in the motor nerve endings even of muscles not clinically affected. The thymus gland may be enlarged, and, in a small percentage of patients is the site of a tumour. There is evidence that autoimmune processes play a major part in pathogenesis.

An immunological test for myasthenia followed the demonstration of a factor in the globulin fraction from serum of patients with myasthenia which blocks the binding of the snake venom protein alpha-bungarotoxin (a-BuTx) to acetylcholine receptors (AChR) in extracts of human muscle. A radioimmunoassay precipitation test based on this shows anti-receptor (AChR) antibodies in up to 90 per cent of myasthenics with a zero response in normal people and neurological controls. Further proof that myasthenia is a true autoimmune disorder followed the production of experimental autoimmune myasthenia in animals immunized against purified AChR from the electric organ of the eel which cross-reacted against their own acetylcholine receptors. The development of the syndrome paralleled the rise in circulating AChR antibodies. Features of myasthenia can be induced in mice by passive transfer of an immunological fraction of the serum from patients with myasthenia gravis.

The HLA associations and the titres of anti-acetylcholine receptor antibodies are different in the different clinical types of generalized myasthenia. Young women with thymomas have the highest titres of anti-acetylcholine receptor antibody (90 per cent) but low association with HLA B8 or DRw3 or both. Older patients with thymitis have low titres of anti-acetylcholine receptor antibody but with high frequency of HLA A3, B7, and DRw3. Ocular myasthenia is mild, occurs in the elderly and does not respond to thymectomy and only a half of such patients have anti-acetylcholine receptor antibodies. The symptoms do not become generalized.

The presence of antinuclear factor in the serum of some myasthenics suggests common aetiological factors between myasthenia and systemic lupus erythematosus. The known facts have been linked in an immune hypothesis, in which it has been suggested that the thymic changes may be the primary disturbance, the muscle lesion resulting from a cross reaction against muscle cells by lymphocytes sensitized to the thymic epithelial or myoid cells. On this basis the delay of months in the observed remission following thymectomy could be explained by persistence of active T lymphocytes. But the presence of a humoral factor in addition is suggested by the rapid improvement which often occurs within hours of thymectomy.

The essential disorder of function therefore appears to be reduced responsiveness of the postsynaptic ACh receptor. This is temporarily relieved by physostigmine and its analogue neostigmine, and other drugs which are known to act by inhibiting the enzyme, cholinesterase, which breaks down the acetylcholine necessary for the conduction of the nervous impulse to the muscle. The spontaneous miniature end-plate potentials in myasthenia are smaller than normal and there are ultrastructural changes at the end-plate, including loss of ACh receptor sites, but normal vesicles in the motor nerve ending.

Symptoms

Myasthenia gravis is usually seen in adult life, most cases occurring between the ages of 20 and 50, but the age of onset ranges from 10, or rarely earlier, to 70. Females are affected more frequently than males.

The cardinal symptom of myasthenia gravis is abnormal muscular fatigability. This is most frequently first observed in the ocular muscles. Less often it begins in the muscles innervated by the pons and medulla, and sometimes it is generalized from the beginning. The onset is almost always gradual, and the disease tends to show its characteristic fluctuations from the start. Ptosis of one or both upper lids is often the first symptom, and is soon associated with diplopia due to paralysis of one or more of the external ocular muscles. These symptoms characteristically appear in the evening, when the patient is tired, and disappear after a night's rest. Difficulty in swallowing may be complained of, often only developing in the course of a meal which the patient begins to swallow without any trouble. Speech may become indistinct when the patient is tired.

On examination, unilateral or bilateral ptosis is often found, and is intensified by asking the patient to gaze upwards. Weakness of the external ocular muscles is asymmetrical and may progress to complete external ophthalmoplegia of one or both eyes. The pupillary reflexes are usually normal.

The facial muscles are almost always affected, causing weakness of closure of the eyes and of retraction of the angles of the mouth, with the production of a characteristic snarling appearance on smiling (Fig. 20.5). Weakness of the bulbar muscles leads to difficulty in chewing, swallowing, and articulation. The characteristic fatigability may be demonstrated by asking the patient to count up to 50, during which speech becomes progressively less distinct. Paresis of the soft palate often gives a nasal character to the speech. In severe cases, weakness

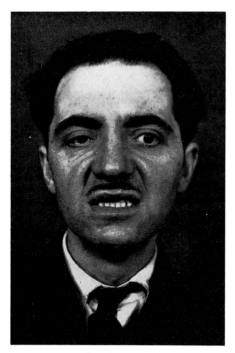 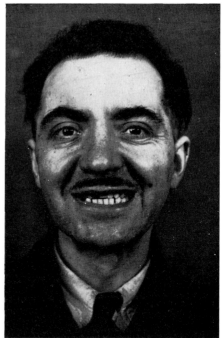

Fig. 20.5. Myasthenia gravis; facial movements before and after an injection of neo-stigmine. Note also the disappearance of ptosis and strabismus.

of the neck and limbs and trunk muscles occurs, and the patient may suffer from dyspnoea. Permanent paralysis sooner or later develops in some muscles which at first exhibit only abnormal fatigability. The tendon reflexes are usually normal, but sometimes exhibit fatigability.

A useful test is the rapid relief of symptoms by the intravenous injection of up to 10 mg of edrophonium (Tensilon) after an initial dose of 2 mg. Atropine may be used in a dose of 0.2 mg intravenously prior to the Tensilon injection in order to block the muscarinic effects. Some care is necessary in the use of the Tensilon test in patients with severe weakness who are already on large doses of anticholinergic drugs, as Tensilon may precipitate cholinergic block. In such patients resuscitation facilities should be on hand in case some deterioration is precipitated. A more delicate test is study of the electromyographic response to tetanic stimulation. In the carcinomatous variety electromyography often shows a paradoxical incremental response on tetanic stimulation.

A thymic tumour may be shown by appropriate radiological techniques.

Myasthenia requires to be distinguished from other conditions causing ptosis or diplopia, bulbar paralysis, or general fatigability. In cases of doubt the Tensilon test described above will usually settle the diagnosis. In *motor neurone* disease and the *myopathies,* the muscular weakness is associated with wasting,

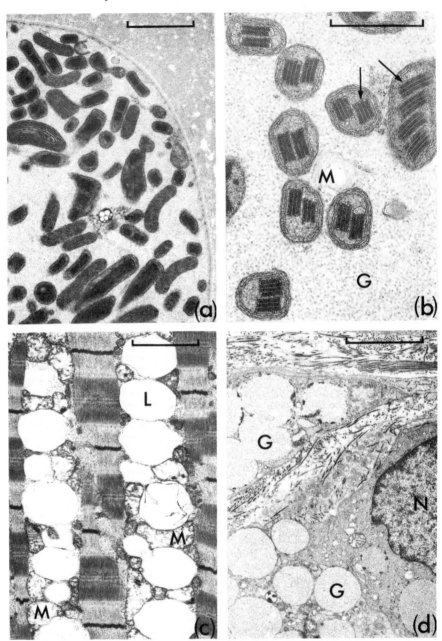

Fig. 20.6. Electron micrographs of mitochondrial myopathies. (a) Transverse section through the periphery of a 'ragged-red' fibre from a case of cytochrome b deficiency showing part of a large collection of abnormal mitochondria. Scale = 2 μm. (b) A higher magnification view of a similar aggregate of abnormal mitochondria (M) embedded in glycogen filled cytoplasm (G) from a case of chronic progressive external ophthalmoplegia.

and in the former with fasciculation. In *botulism* the toxin of *Clostridium botulinum* interferes with the production or release of acetylcholine causing profound muscle weakness resembling myasthenia. Bulbar weakness also occurs in *tetanus,* though it is then preceded by backache, back stiffness, and usually tetanic spasms. There are also certain *drugs* such as curare which block neuromuscular transmission by causing competitive block of the receptors on the end-plate. Naturally such drugs or any respiratory depressants should be avoided in myasthenics. *Neurosis* is sometimes a cause of fatigability, but is not accompanied by the objective signs of muscular weakness always evident in myasthenia.

Prognosis

The course of myasthenia is extremely variable. The onset is usually gradual, and ocular symptoms may recur at intervals or remain stationary over a period of many years without further symptoms developing. Even when the cranial and limb muscles are involved, striking remissions may occur and last for years. Crises of weakness may occur after unusual physical exertion, an infection, childbirth, or the unwise use of respiratory depressant drugs. If bulbar or respiratory weakness occurs in such crises urgent tracheostomy may be necessary. In the final stages the patient is bedridden and severely paralysed. Attacks of dyspnoea become increasingly frequent. Death usually results from bronchopneumonia or respiratory or cardiac failure. Pregnancy may improve or exacerbate the condition.

Rarer forms of myasthenia

Neonatal myasthenia is a transient illness due to the placental transfer of maternal anti-AChR antibodies and occurs in some 12 per cent of myasthenic mothers, responds to anti-cholinesterase, and remits within six weeks. This form of myasthenia must be distinguished from the rare case of congenital myasthenia, sometimes familial, which occurs within six months of birth and has none of the immunological abnormalities of myasthenia gravis, but is responsive to edrophonium. It may be progressive and end fatally. Myasthenia as a symptom occurs in some conditions other than myasthenia gravis, notably in some cases of carcinomatous myopathy, collagen disease, thyro-toxicosis and more rarely myxoedema, and occasionally after treatment with

---

The characteristic intramitrochondria crystals are indicated by arrows. Scale = 1 μm. (c) A longitudinal section through a muscle fibre from a case of carnitine deficiency, showing the arrays of neutral lipid droplets (L) and enlarged mitochondria (M) lying between the myofibrils which are typical of this condition. Scale = 2μm. (d) A transverse section through the periphery of a muscle fibre and part of the adjacent connective tissue from a case of acid maltase deficiency. Large membrane-bound collections of glycogen granules (G) are visible within both the muscle fibre (below), and an adjacent fibroblast (above). Scale = 3 μm.

drugs such as penicillamine. Penicillamine-induced myasthenia remits on stopping the penicillamine. The carcinomatous myasthenic syndrome, also known as the Eaton–Lambert syndrome, differs fundamentally from myasthenic gravis in that the defect is presynaptic. On electromyographic examination with rapid repetitive stimulation (greater than 20 Hz) there is a recruitment of muscle power from an initial low level. Electrophysiological studies have shown a reduction in the number of quanta of acetylcholine released by each impulse from the nerve terminal though paradoxically the number of quanta of acetylcholine released increases with repetitive stimulation. The postsynaptic acetylcholine receptors are normal in number and antibodies to acetylcholine receptors are absent. This form of myasthenia does not respond to pyridostigmine but guanidine is sometimes effective though it has serious side-effects including marrow depression and although no autoimmune basis for it is known immunosuppression with prednisolone and azothiaprine have been reported to be helpful.

Treatment

Neostigmine greatly improves the power of muscles still capable of responding to it but there is a poor response later in the disease when denervation has occurred. Oral administration of 1–3 or more 15 mg tablets of neostigmine bromide several times a day is often sufficient; 60 mg of pyridostigmine is equivalent to 15 mg of neostigmine, but lasts up to six hours and may be particularly useful given late at night to avert weakness on waking in the morning. In severe cases intramuscular neostigmine may be required three or four times a day and should be given an hour before meals. The full intramuscular dose is 2.5 mg of neostigmine methylsulphate. The unwanted side-effects of high doses of anticholinesterase drugs include abdominal colic, increased salivation, cardiac irregularities and, by crossing the blood-brain barrier, even mental confusion. Some of the side-effects due to muscarinic actions can be blocked with atropine 0.6 mg by mouth twice daily. The maximum effect is produced in an hour, and lasts for about six hours.

An important aspect of management is the avoidance of drugs which may exaggerate the defect of neuromuscular transmission. Antibiotics, such as neomycin, with the aminoglycoside group impair acetylcholine release. Penicillamine-induced myasthenia remits on stopping the penicillamine. Central nervous system depressants must obviously also be given with caution in myasthenia.

The management of a severe myasthenic calls for great care and the backing of artificial aids to respiration if a crisis supervenes. Sometimes it is difficult to judge whether an increase in weakness is due to a myasthenic crisis or to cholinergic drug blockade caused by drug overdose. A crisis may be precipitated by drugs with a muscular blocking action such as neomycin or by mere stress and fatigue. In the myasthenic crisis Tensilon will usually improve power but it has either no effect or an adverse effect on cholinergic block. Most myasthenic patients can only be improved up to a certain level. Problems arise when neuromuscular junctions in different parts of the body are differently affected so that myasthenic block may then occur in some parts of the body and cholinergic block in other parts, simultaneously. At all times bulbar and respiratory function must be observed. Sometimes resistance to anticholinesterase drugs occurs but recovers after a period of total drug withdrawal and artificial respiration, after curarization.

Ephedrine: when the maximum benefit from anticholinesterases has been obtained, further improvement may result from adding ephedrine up to 30 mg three times a day. This presumably aids neuromuscular transmission by acting on alpha and beta noradrenergic receptors adjacent to the neuromuscular junction.

Steroids: if a myasthenic patient deteriorates despite optimal doses of anticholinesterases, steroids should be started in a dose of 10 mg of prednisolone daily and increased slowly by 10 mg a week in order to avoid deterioration which may occur when high doses of prednisolone are started. The dose of prednisolone can be increased slowly up to 120 mg daily, with potassium supplements, and when control is achieved the steroids are given on alternate days and then gradually reduced.

Immunosuppression: Azothiaprine 2.5 mg per kg per day may have to be added if there is no remission on prednisolone alone but azothiaprine sometimes causes depression. It has been reported that plasma exchange can produce short-term clinical improvement in severe cases.

Thymectomy should be recommended, particularly in women with severe, progressive generalized myasthenia which is not controlled by drugs. Thymectomy is most effective when the patient is operated on less than five years from the onset of symptoms, and when there is no thymoma. Patients with thymomas require thymectomy because the tumour may become infiltrating but they do not respond as well from the point of view of their myasthenia as do patients without a tumour and they are likely also to require immunosuppression. The anti-AChR titre falls slowly after thymectomy which is an indication that the antibodies may not be directly produced from the thymus alone. Many patients will still need neostigmine after operation, but usually in smaller doses than before, and improvement may continue slowly for a long time. Carcinomatous myasthenia may respond to treatment with guanidine in a dosage of 30 mg per kg daily.

FAMILIAL PERIODIC PARALYSIS

This is a rare familial disorder, characterized by widespread paralysis which tends to occur in the early morning, either while the patient is asleep or shortly after he awakens. The most recent biochemical evidence suggests that it is due to an abnormal uptake of potassium by the muscles, which disturbs the normal ratio of intracellular to extracellular potassium. The blood potassium is low during the attack, which is cut short by giving a large dose of potassium by the mouth. Another familial disorder, *adynamia episodica hereditaria,* has been described in which attacks of periodic paralysis are associated with a raised blood potassium, and are treated by giving diuretics which promote excretion of potassium as well as sodium. A third type of hereditary periodic paralysis has been described in which the serum potassium is normal during attacks but the weakness responds to large doses of sodium chloride. Muscular weakness also occurs as a result of hypokalaemia in aldosteronism and 'potassium-losing' nephritis.

REFERENCES

Adams, R.D. (1975). *Diseases of muscle,* 3rd edn. Churchill Livingstone, Edinburgh.

Behan, A. and Peter, J.B. (1975). Polymyositis and dermatomyositis. *New Engl. J. Med.* **202,** 344–8, 403–8.

DeVere, R. and Bradley, W.G. (1975). Polymyositis: its presentation, morbidity and mortality. *Brain* **98,** 637–66.

Drachman, D.B. (1978). Myasthenia gravis. *New Engl. J. Med.* **298,** 136–42, 186–95.

Dubowitz, V. and Brooke, M.H. (1973). *Muscle biopsy: a modern approach.* Saunders, Philadelphia.

Dubowitz, V. (1982). The female carrier of Duchenne muscular dystrophy. *Br. med. J.* **284,** 1423–4.

Lang, B., Newsom-Davis, J., Wray, D., and Vincent, P. (1981). Autoimmune aetiology for myasthenic (Eaton–Lambert) syndrome. *Lancet* **ii,** 224–6.

Morgan-Hughes, J. *et al.* (1977). A mitochondrial myopathy characterized by a deficiency of reducible cytochrome B. *Brain* **100,** 617–40.

Newsom-Davis, J., Pinching, A.J., Vincent, A., and Wilson, S.G. (1978). The function of circulating antibody to acetylcholine receptor in myasthenia gravis: investigation by plasma exchange. *Neurology, Minneap.* **28,** 266–72.

Rowland, L.P. (1980). Controversies about the treatment of myasthenia gravis. *J. Neurol. Neurosurg. Psychiat.* **43,** 644–59.

Walton, J.N. (1981). *Disorders of voluntary muscle,* 4th edn. Churchill Livingstone, Edinburgh.

Part III
Infections

21 Encephalomyelitis

GENERAL CONSIDERATIONS

A very large number of living organisms may invade the nervous system or its membranes, thus causing many forms of encephalomyelitis, meningitis, and meningo-encephalomyelitis. The pyogenic organisms mostly cause pyogenic meningitis or cerebral abscess. The tubercle bacillus causes tuberculous meningitis or tuberculoma. *Treponema pallidum*, various yeasts and moulds also attack the nervous system. Though any of these by invading the brain may cause a disorder which can accurately be described as encephalitis, the process is not usually acute, and the term acute encephalomyelitis is in practice reserved for two groups of disorder, namely those due to the direct invasion of the nervous system by a virus, and those in which, although the primary cause is an infection of the body, usually with a virus, the changes which occur in the nervous system are not directly due to its invasion by the virus, but are the result of some incompletely understood hypersensitivity reaction to the systemic infection, which leads to acute disseminated or demyelinating encephalomyelitis, especially if the patient is immunosuppressed.

No hard-and-fast line can be drawn between encephalomyelitis and meningitis, but in general when the disorder is described as meningitis any damage to the brain or spinal cord which may occur is secondary to the inflammation of the meninges. Similarly in encephalomyelitis, if the meninges suffer at all they do so secondarily to the inflammation of the brain and spinal cord. There remain, however, a few disorders in which both the nervous system and the meninges seem to be attacked simultaneously, and this is appropriately called acute meningo-encephalomyelitis. Pathologically, in most virus infections and in the acute demyelinating disorders, both the brain and the spinal cord are involved. Occasionally the brunt of the damage falls on one or the other, more often on the spinal cord alone than on the brain alone. Acute myelitis and even infective polyneuropathy, therefore, may be nosologically a variant of acute encephalomyelitis.

ENCEPHALITIS DUE TO VIRUSES

Aetiology and pathology

Virus particles may reach the brain by the bloodstream or along nerves, having first caused varying degrees of systemic disturbance. The rate of spread may be

449

slowed by the development of the humoral type of immunity and by an intact blood–brain barrier. The site of the central nervous system primarily affected depends in part on the route of infection, whether by the blood and choroid plexus or by an olfactory route to the temporal lobes, as has been suggested in herpes simplex encephalitis. The brain response also depends on the predilection of the virus for certain brain cells, which itself may depend on the degree of cell-mediated immunity. At the acute end of this spectrum is primary invasion of the brain as in poliomyelitis and rabies, with early cell death, the virus being recoverable from the brain. In less acute infections such as measles encephalitis there is time for the development of antibodies, some of which may cause damage to nerve cells or glia. In post-infectious encephalomyelitis such as measles encephalitis, demyelination is the predominant pathological reaction and the virus is not recoverable.

The number of viruses known to be capable of attacking the nervous system is already large, and no doubt many more remain to be discovered. Few people infected with a particular virus develop neurological disease, presumably because of inherited or acquired immunity or factors concerned with the pathogenicity of the strain and the route of infection. Virus encephalitis occurs in all parts of the world, and is particularly common in the tropics. Viruses may be classified in three groups:

1. Neurotropic, that is those which primarily attack the nervous system.

2. Pantropic, those which attack both the nervous system and other tissues.

3. Viscerotropic, which do not usually attack the nervous system but may do so exceptionally. The distinction between the first two groups is perhaps not very clear-cut. Between them they account for the large majority of cases of encephalitis.

Varieties of encephalitis known to be due to *neurotropic* viruses in man include the Japanese type B, the St. Louis type, Russian Spring–Summer encephalitis, the Murray Valley encephalitis of Australia, and several forms of equine encephalitis. Rabies is also a form of viral encephalitis and the virus of herpes simplex, or febrilis, may attack the nervous system. Poliomyelitis is also caused by a virus, and since it may attack the brain might also be classed among the encephalitides. Three other diseases, encephalitis lethargica, inclusion encephalitis, and herpes zoster, are almost certainly due to neurotropic viruses.

Viruses of the *pantropic* type which chiefly attack the meninges but may also invade the brain or the spinal cord are those of mumps, lymphocytic chorio-meningitis, the Coxsackie group, and the Echo group. Infectious mono-nucleosis is due to infection with the Epstein–Barr virus and may cause encephalitic, meningitic, myelitic, or peripheral or cranial nerve involvement. The influenza virus is one of the *viscerotropic* viruses which occasionally attacks the nervous system.

Viruses are transmitted to man in a number of ways, some by human contacts and others by insect vectors such as mosquitoes and ticks from a wide variety of birds and animals, which sometimes, as in the case of rabies, may infect man directly.

All forms of viral encephalitis tend to show certain pathological features in common which, however, often have a distinctive distribution or some other special characteristics. The nerve cells show degenerative changes and occasionally eosinophil nuclear inclusion bodies. (Inclusion body encephalitis, though not the only form in which this feature is present, has derived its name from it.) Cellular infiltration is a characteristic, and may be present in grey matter, white matter, and meninges, involving the nervous tissue itself and collecting in the perivascular spaces, the cells being chiefly lymphocytes and plasma cells. Microglial cells play a part in the inflammatory reaction. In many forms of encephalitis the inflammation is limited to the grey matter, but in some there is also necrosis of the white matter, but this has not usually the characteristic perivascular distribution of the demyelinating types of encephalitis. Encephalitis may occur at any age, but is commonest in childhood, adolescence, and early adult life.

In the last few years an increasing number of chronic diseases of the nervous system have been thought to be due to chronic or 'slow' virus infections. The virus, or virus-like agent, appears to produce a gradually progressive neurological illness after an incubation period of several years. The list of such diseases already includes the subacute spongiform encephalopathies, Kuru and Creutzfeldt–Jakob disease, as well as subacute sclerosing leucoencephalopathy and progressive multifocal leucoencephalopathy. Clearly, other chronic and relapsing neurological disorders may ultimately prove to be due to similar transmissible agents though any final judgement at this stage would be premature.

Symptoms

Different forms of encephalitis differ somewhat in their clinical pictures, but that they have much in common is shown by the fact that it is much more often possible to make a diagnosis of encephalitis than it is to say what the cause is. The onset is usually that of a mild febrile illness, with viraemia, which is often missed, followed by a quiescent phase and then by the disturbance in the central nervous system, when isolation of the virus from the blood is rare. Headache and drowsiness are usually present, followed in severe cases by confusion developing into stupor and coma. Convulsions may occur, particularly in young children. Papilloedema is sometimes present, but is not likely to be severe. The pupils may be unequal and react poorly to light and accommodation. There may be a squint associated with some degree of ophthalmoplegia, and nystagmus is common. The motor functions of the cranial nerves and limbs may be little impaired, or there may be severe paralysis. If the cerebellum or its connections are damaged, there will be ataxia. Sensory changes are variable. Sometimes there is hyperaesthesia of part of the body, but severe degrees of loss of cutaneous or deep sensibility are uncommon. In the acute stage the tendon reflexes are likely to be diminished, and one or both plantars to be extensor. Cervical rigidity and Kernig's sign may or may not be present.

The blood commonly shows a polymorphonuclear leucocytosis. The cerebrospinal fluid may be under increased pressure, and a characteristic finding would be a moderate increase of cells, e.g. 10 to 40 per mm³, usually mononuclear. A large number of cells would suggest involvement of the meninges. Polymorphonuclear cells are uncommon. The protein will be correspondingly raised, but the sugar and chloride content will be normal.

The identification of the virus responsible for a case of encephalitis is often difficult. It may be impossible to grow any organism even from fresh post-mortem material. Occasionally a virus can be grown from the stools during the acute stage, but in general the most reliable method is the presence of an identifiable virus antibody in the blood serum, especially if a rising titre can be observed. Virus particles can now sometimes be detected by electron microscopy of fresh tissue and immunofluorescence may show the sites of virus and antibody concentration.

Special forms of encephalitis

Encephalitis lethargica

Encephalitis lethargica attracted much attention during the years after 1916–17, when it first appeared in epidemic form. Its characteristic features were the disturbance of sleep rhythm, the patients sleeping throughout the day and becoming wakeful, and often restless and excited at night, and the incidence upon the brainstem, leading to ptosis, pupillary abnormalities, and diplopia. During the epidemic parkinsonian symptoms were often noted during the acute stage, and progressive parkinsonism is a common sequel of the disease. One symptom, at one time peculiar to encephalitis lethargica, but now sometimes drug-induced, is oculogyral spasm – attacks of spasmodic deviation of the eyes, usually upwards lasting up to an hour or longer. Encephalitis lethargica is now rare, but patients exhibiting the clinical features of the acute attack are still seen from time to time.

Subacute sclerosing panencephalitis (inclusion body encephalitis)

This disease attacks principally children in the first decade of life who have usually had measles at an unusually early age. There is histological evidence of the presence of a polyoma-like virus in brain cells (Fig. 21.1(a)), the measles antibody titre is abnormally high in serum and cerebrospinal fluid and immunofluorescence has been demonstrated with anti-measles antibody but not anti-distemper antibody. The measles virus may have undergone some kind of transformation in the brain and this is now tentatively included in the list of slow viral infections (p. 455). The distinctive pathological lesion is widespread degeneration of ganglion cells, many of which show acidophil hyaline inclusion bodies in the nucleus and cytoplasm. The disease runs a slowly progressive course of from two to six months, in which three stages can be recognized, first mood changes with some intellectual deterioration, secondly akinetic mutism,

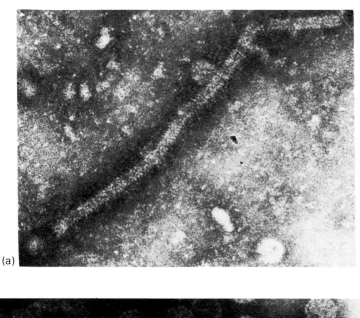

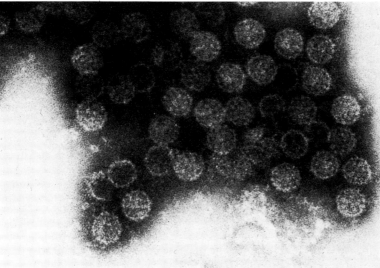

Fig. 21.1. (a) A preparation from the brain of a patient suffering from subacute sclerosing panencephalitis, the appearance of the measles-like viral helix being partly obscured by attached antibody molecules. (b) Empty and full particles of C–J virus from a patient suffering from progressive multifocal leucoencephalopathy.

with complex involuntary movements, especially myoclonic, and thirdly decortication. The cerebrospinal fluid contains an abnormally high level of gamma globulin and oligoclonal bands can be detected on electrophoresis. The electroencephalogram frequently shows synchronous periodic high-voltage complexes followed by electrical silence. The disease is usually but not always fatal. Steroids are frequently given but there is no proof that they affect the course of the illness.

Progressive multifocal leuco-encephalopathy

This disorder is an occasional complication of defective immune responses in chronic disease affecting the reticulo-endothelial system. The pathological features include multiple foci of demyelination and curious enlargement of astrocytic nuclei and abnormal mitotic patterns. There have been reports of particles resembling polyoma virus in the cells (Fig. 21.1(b)). The disease progresses rapidly to dementia and death.

Herpes simplex encephalitis

The herpes virus hominis (simplex) is a DNA virus almost universally distributed and the primary infection usually occurs in childhood, in 10 per cent with clinically apparent vesicles of the skin or mucocutaneous junctions. The type I affects the mouth and face and type II the genital region. After primary infection the virus is retained throughout life in sensory ganglia, causing occasional attacks of secondary herpes infection that are not usually serious. Rarely and in patients who are immunocompromised the herpes may spread beyond the dorsal root ganglia either centripetally, into the central nervous system or by causing a viraemia and then an encephalitis. The varicella zoster virus is another member of the herpes virus group.

Herpes simplex is a rare cause of aseptic meningitis in adults and in infants causes acute encephalitis with disseminated visceral necrosis. More important, herpes simplex also causes an acute necrotizing encephalitis without concurrent skin lesions. After a febrile illness lasting a few days the patient becomes confused with headache, convulsions and often progressive hemiparesis. A rapidly expanding cerebral lesion is usually suspected and a CT scan is likely to show bilateral extensive areas of loss of density (Fig. 21.2). A rising titre of herpes simplex antibody shows in the blood and cerebrospinal fluid by radioimmuno-absobent assay and this has now been developed as an early diagnostic test (within 10 days). However, the certain diagnosis of herpes simplex encephalitis usually rests on brain biopsy from patients with typical clinical features. It is not known whether the disease is caused by direct invasion with the virus or by an antigen–antibody reaction. The use of steroids in an attempt to lower intracranial pressure appears to have saved the lives of several patients though they have been left with a serious neurological disability. Recently idoxuridine, 200 mg per kg by intravenous infusion, has been used with apparent benefit.

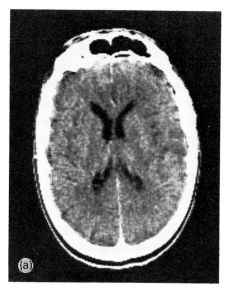 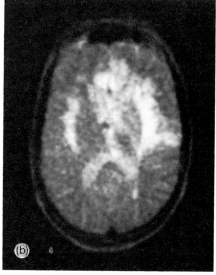

Fig. 21.2. Herpes encephalitis: (a) CT, contrast-enhanced, and (b) NMR(SE) scans. More extensive involvement is visible on the NMR scan.

Vidarabine (adenine arabinoside) has been reported to reduce the mortality without significant toxic side-effects.

Subacute spongiform viral encephalopathies

In the past few years an increasing number of chronic diseases of the nervous system have been thought to be due to chronic or 'slow' virus infections. The virus, or virus-like agent, appears to produce a gradually progressive neurological illness after an incubation period of several years. Kuru is a progressive extrapyramidal and cerebellar degeneration with dementia which is focally endemic in the highlands of New Guinea. It has been transmitted to chimpanzees by cerebral inoculation with material from the brains of kuru patients. It is thought that cannibalism of kuru victims was responsible for its spread, and since cannibalism has been suppressed the incidence has declined. Creutzfeldt–Jakob disease is a rare rapidly progressive dementia in the elderly with myoclonus and progressive paralysis, which leads to death within six months. The disease has been transmitted to chimpanzees by cerebral inoculation. The electroencephalogram shows an obliteration of normal rhythms, usually by high-voltage slow activity, and the CT scan shows both diffuse and focal changes. The cerebrospinal fluid is usually normal. The mode of spread of disease in man is unknown though in two cases transmission is thought to have occurred as a result of the use of depth electrodes in patients who later proved to have Creutzfeldt–Jakob disease. This underlines the extreme caution needed in dealing with material from such patients. No treatment has been reported to arrest the disease but it has been reported that life has been prolonged by use of the antiviral agent, inosiplex.

The pathological appearances of the brain in kuru and Creutzfeldt–Jakob disease consist of intracellular swelling of neurones and displacement of nuclei, which is indistinguishable from that which occurs in the animal disease scrapie. These two human diseases and scrapie (p. 508) are linked under the title subacute spongiform viral encephalopathies. It now seems that they are all the result of infection with small viruses with very low molecular weight which, because of their size and their cell membrane affinity, are exceptionally resistant to heat and radiation.

Rabies

The rabies virus is introduced accidentally through bite wounds or abrasions from rabid animals and probably spreads mainly up perineural spaces to the spinal cord and brain. An acute encephalomyelitis usually follows an ascending paralysis within a few days, after an incubation period which may be from two weeks to a year. The acute illness with thirst, hydrophobia, and excitement leads to coma, and without treatment, to death. Inactivated rabies vaccine prepared from virus grown on human diploid cells produces neutralizing antibody in most recipients in the second week of the course. There is much less risk of post-inoculation encephalomyelitis (p. 458) than after vaccine prepared from the brain of infected animals. Passive protection can also be obtained from a heterologous antiserum.

Diagnosis

The diagnosis of acute encephalitis rests upon the symptoms and signs of an infective illness involving the substance of the nervous system. Throat and rectal swabs together with serological tests are more important than the results of c.s.f. culture in herpes type 1 infection and poliomyelitis. Mumps and some echo and Coxackie viruses can be grown from cerebrospinal fluid and a positive culture may be available in a few days. Sometimes a positive viral culture may allow antibiotics to be stopped in a patient in whom treatment has been started on the supposition that it was a case of bacterial meningitis. Enteroviruses however have a high rate of culture in the c.s.f. and should be suspected in infants during summer, especially if associated with skin rashes. *Meningitis* is distinguished by the predominance of signs of meningeal irritation, to which any cerebral damage is secondary. The cell count in the cerebrospinal fluid is usually much higher in meningitis, and when that is due to a pyogenic organism predominantly polymorphonuclear. The sugar content of the fluid is very low in pyogenic meningitis, but normal in encephalitis. In *cerebral abscess* the signs are those of a focal cerebral lesion, and any general disturbance of cerebral function is secondary to the resulting rise in intracranial pressure. Both polymorphonuclear and lymphocytic cells may be present in the cerebrospinal fluid in cerebral abscess, but the protein content is usually raised to a greater extent than in encephalitis. CT scanning is necessary to demonstrate a focal lesion in a case of abscess and diffuse changes in encephalitis.

Prognosis

Prognosis depends upon many factors, especially the nature of the virus. In some epidemics the mortality rate has been from 20 to 50 per cent. In the sporadic case, a fulminating onset, deep coma, and hyperpyrexia, are bad signs. The risk of sequelae depends again upon the nature of the virus and the severity of the damage. In some epidemics the residual disability rate is as high as 30 per cent. In most sporadic cases of mild or average severity the patient makes a good recovery, though he may be left with some mild residual symptoms. Occasionally severe and permanent memory defects follow a viral encephalitis.

Treatment

The principle of treatment depends on recognition of the nature of the reaction to the virus within the brain (Fig. 21.3). If virus is replicating in the brain then anti-viral agents derived from cancer therapy may be given, but few have any proven success.

Antiviral agents

Interference with different parts of the infected cycle of the virus is the basis of current hopes for treatment. The virus attaches itself to specific receptors on the cell membranes and neutralizing antibodies can block the site. After penetrating the cells a nuclear capsid of the virus is uncoated by cellular enzymes

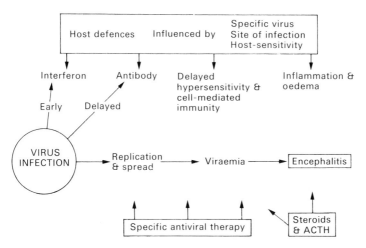

Fig. 21.3. Diagram showing the development of the clinical picture in a virus infection and the place of treatment.

and amantidine hydrochloride is thought to inhibit this. The next stage is the synthesis of messenger RNA by a specific virion which for the influenza virus is inhibited by interferon. The viral protein is then synthesized in the cell. Indoxuridine and cytosine arabinoside inhibit cellular and viral polymerase. The final stage is the assembly and maturation of the virus and its protein coat to form the nucleocapsid which buds at the cell membrane, a stage again inhibited for some viruses by interferon. Amantidine hydrochloride has been used in the treatment of the influenza A virus, idoxuridine has been used topically for herpes and the place of interferon with CNS infections is not yet established.

Acyclovir is the first antiviral agent that can be given systemically and safely. It inhibits the virus DNA synthesis, appearing to inhibit virus replication without damaging the host cell. Though less effective than idoxuridine for treating herpetic skin lesions it can be given intravenously with safety and appears to have an effect on herpes simplex and zoster.

In severe cases the treatment is that of the comatose patient (p. 178). Hyperpyrexia calls for hypothermia.

BENIGN MYALGIC ENCEPHALOMYELITIS

This name has been applied to a variety of encephalomyelitis which has recently appeared in epidemic form in many parts of the world. An epidemic in the Royal Free Hospital, London, some years ago led to its being also called the Royal Free disease. No causal organism has been isolated. It chiefly attacks young adults, and females more often than males.

The onset is usually that of a febrile illness, sometimes accompanied by sore throat, upper respiratory or gastrointestinal symptoms, and often a generalized lymphadenopathy. Depression and disturbances of sleep are common symptoms and tenderness, paraesthesiae, and hyperaesthesia or relative anaesthesia of irregular distribution. The fact that these symptoms and signs may be present with little change in the reflexes beyond slight depression or exaggeration of the tendon jerks has frequently led to the disorder having been diagnosed as hysterical. Cranial nerve palsies and extensor plantar reflexes, however, are sometimes encountered.

The cerebrospinal fluid has usually been normal. In the Royal Free Hospital epidemic toxic changes in the lymphocytes of the blood were observed.

The disease is not fatal and major persistent disability is rare. A striking feature has been the tendency for relapses to occur during the months, and even in some cases years, after the infection.

ACUTE DISSEMINATED ENCEPHALOMYELITIS

Aetiology and pathology

In the mid-1920s attention was directed to a rare complication of vaccination, in which the nervous system was attacked by a form of acute encephalomyelitis characterized by widespread areas of demyelination distributed particularly around blood vessels. It soon became clear that a similar disorder might follow other infections, particularly measles, German measles, and chickenpox, and it was known to occur in smallpox. It also occurs rarely following vaccination with pertussis. It was shown that unlike other forms of encephalitis, the lesions in the nervous system were not the direct result of the presence there of the virus causing the infection. Animal experiments showed that similar lesions (allergic encephalomyelitis) could be produced in animals by the subcutaneous injection of a purified extract of brain tissue, encephalitogenic fraction, and it was recalled that this had been observed in man as a rare complication of antirabic inoculation when brain tissue was used for that purpose. Pertussis vaccination in children with evidence of pre-existing brain damage or with febrile convulsions or a history of epilepsy has been thought to be associated with an increased risk of excephalitis following the vaccination.

While the pathogenesis of these acute demyelinating diseases of the nervous system is still incompletely understood, it is now believed that they are probably the result of some abnormal process of sensitization of the nervous system, initially excited by the causal infection. There is some reason to think that such reactions constitute a broad spectrum ranging from acute haemorrhagic leucoencephalitis to acute disseminated encephalomyelitis, and that while most of the known instances of the last-named have been due to vaccination or one of the exanthems, it is probable that sporadic cases are the result of other common infections; for example, of the upper respiratory tract.

Naked-eye changes consist merely of congestion and oedema of the nervous system. Microscopically there is marked perivascular infiltration of the brain and spinal cord, with lymphocytes and plasma cells both within the perivascular spaces and at a greater distance from the vessels. In the white matter the most striking feature is the presence of zones of demyelination, that is, loss of the myelin sheaths of the neurones around the vessels, especially the veins (Fig. 21.4). The most intense changes are usually found in the lumbar and upper sacral regions of the spinal cord and in the pons. Inflammatory changes of this kind may be present throughout the whole length of the nervous system. Meningeal infiltration is relatively slight.

Symptoms

In post-vaccinal encephalitis symptoms usually develop between the tenth and twelfth days after vaccination, though the incubation period may be shorter or longer. In measles encephalitis the onset is usually four to six days after the beginning of the illness, when the fever has fallen, and the rash is fading. In sporadic cases of acute disseminated encephalomyelitis, there may be no preceding general symptoms, or the neurological disorder may follow by a few days an infection of the upper respiratory tract or an influenza-like illness.

The onset is usually rapid and characterized by headache, vomiting, drowsiness, fever, and in some cases convulsions. When fully developed, the clinical

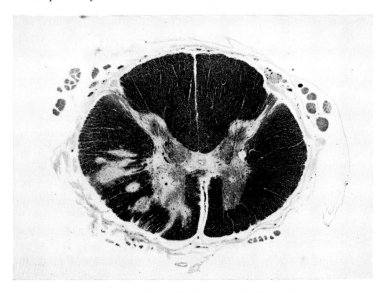

Fig. 21.4. Acute demyelinating encephalomyelitis.

picture is that of meningeal irritation associated with widespread disturbance of function of the brain and spinal cord. In severe cases drowsiness passes into stupor and coma. Cervical rigidity and Kernig's sign are often present. The ocular fundi are usually normal, but papilloedema due to optic neuritis is sometimes observed. Ocular palsies may be present, but the pupillary reactions are often normal. Trismus has frequently been described. There is often flaccid paralysis of some or all of the limbs, associated with loss of tendon reflexes and extensor plantar responses. Retention or incontinence of urine and faeces is the rule in severe cases. Sensory loss is inconstant, but may be marked when the spinal cord is severely affected. The cerebrospinal fluid may be normal in composition though under increased pressure, or an excess of mononuclear cells and of protein may be found.

Diagnosis

For the diagnosis of acute encephalitis see page 456. The diagnosis of acute disseminated encephalomyelitis is obvious when the illness follows vaccination or one of the exanthems, but is more difficult to establish in the absence of such a predisposing cause. However, it may be suspected when it is apparent that the brunt of the damage has fallen upon the white matter of the nervous system.

Prognosis

This is always a serious disorder. In post-vaccinal and measles encephalitis the mortality rate ranges from 10 to 30 per cent in different series. Perhaps 50 per cent of those surviving are left with some residual disability, for example mental defect or personality change, hemiplegia, paraplegia, or epilepsy. Complete recovery, however, may occur in spite of severe symptoms during the acute stage. In this group of cases the disease is self-limited. There is, however, some evidence that in the spontaneous form of the disease relapse may occur if the patient suffers from a further attack of the precipitating infection.

Treatment

Treatment is the same as that of virus encephalitis (p. 457). Corticotrophin (ACTH), 80 units daily in the acute phase, may possibly limit the spread of the inflammatory process.

REFERENCES

Beck, E., Bak, I.J., Christ, J.F., Gajdusek, D.C., Gibbs, C.J., and Hassler, R. (1975). Experimental kuru in the spider monkey. *Brain* **98**, 595–612.

Gajdusek, D.C. (1977). Unconventional viruses and the origin and disappearance of Kuru. *Science, NY* **197**, 943–60.

Gajdusek, D.C., Gibbs, C.J. Jr, Asher, D.M., Brown, P., Diwan, A., Hoffman, P., Nemo, G., Rohwer, R., and White, L. (1977). Precautions in medical care of, and in handling materials from, patients with transmissible virus dementia (Creutzfeldt–Jakob disease). *New Engl. J. Med.* **297**, 1253–8.

Illis, L.S. (ed.) (1974). *Viral diseases of the central nervous system.* Ballière Tindall, London.

Kennard, C. and Swash, M. (1981). Acute viral encephalitis; its diagnosis and outcome. *Brain* **104**, 129–48.

Roos, R., Gajdusek, D.C., and Gibbs, C.J. Jr (1973). The clinical characteristics of transmissible Creutzfeldt–Jakob disease. *Brain* **96**, 1–20.

Timbury, M.C. (1982). Acyclovir. *Br. med. J.* **285**, 1223–4.

22 Poliomyelitis

Aetiology and pathology

Poliomyelitis, or infantile paralysis, is an acute infective disease due to a virus with a predilection for the cells of the anterior horns of the grey matter of the spinal cord and the motor nuclei of the brain stem, destruction of which causes muscular paralysis and subsequent atrophy. Poliomyelitis had become rare but the fall in the number of immunized individuals has led to more increase in Western countries in recent years. Three strains of the virus have been isolated, known as Types 1, 2, and 3. These can be grown in tissue culture. The virus can be obtained from the nasopharyngeal mucous membranes of patients in the acute stage, of healthy contacts, and of convalescents, and also from the stools. It is believed that the usual route of infection in man is the alimentary tract. The neurotropism of the virus can be demonstrated by its inoculation into monkeys, usually into the spinal cord or brain. The virus is capable of ascending the peripheral nerves, but may also be disseminated through the bloodstream.

In the acute stage there is evidence of a general reaction to the infection particularly in the lymphoid tissue, and the spinal cord is congested, soft, and oedematous. Histologically the changes in the nervous system are usually most marked in the grey matter of the spinal cord and medulla, where there is degeneration of the anterior horn cells and an inflammatory reaction with small haemorrhages in the grey matter. This consists of perivascular cuffing, mainly with lymphocytes, but with a smaller number of polymorphonuclear cells, and a diffuse infiltration of the grey matter with similar cells and cells of neuroglial origin. In some cases the brunt of the infection falls upon the brainstem. During recovery from the acute stage, ganglion cells which have not been too severely damaged may be restored to normal. Others disappear completely, so that sections show a paucity of cells in the anterior horns, with secondary degeneration in the coresponding anterior roots and peripheral nerves. The muscles supplied by these segments show varying degrees of neural atrophy.

Epidemiology

In Great Britain poliomyelitis occurs for the most part sporadically, but till the introduction of inoculation there were considerable epidemics. It is no longer a major public health problem in Britain but cases are increasing in uninoculated individuals travelling abroad. The United States has been subjected from time to time to severe epidemics, and no part of the world is immune. The disease can be transmitted by healthy carriers and abortive cases, in which recovery occurs before the paralytic stage is reached, and there is evidence that most members of a household have been infected by the time a paralytic case appears, though multiple paralytic cases in a household occur in less than 10 per cent of infected families. Infants under the age of 1 year are rarely attacked, and after the age of 5 the susceptibility diminishes. In a country where the sanitation is poor, most individuals are exposed to the infection in early childhood, when they either develop the disease or acquire an immunity. In such communities, therefore, the disease is rare in adult life. The better the hygiene, the greater the chance of an individual escaping natural immunity and therefore developing the disease later in life, if he becomes exposed to it. In both Great Britain and the United States the age incidence has been rising, and cases in adults have become commoner. Protective inoculation may be expected to alter this. Males suffer somewhat more frequently than females. The incubation period appears to be usually from 7 to 14 days, but may be as long as five weeks. When the virus is prevalent in a community, there is evidence that the disease may be precipitated by operations on the nose, throat, and mouth, such as tonsillectomy and dental extractions, which presumably provide a portal of entry, and by inoculations for diseases other than polio-myelitis.

Symptoms

There are four possible ways in which a person may react to infection by the virus of poliomyelitis:

1. Through exposure to the virus he may become immune without any symptoms of illness.

2. The symptoms may be no more than those of a mild general infection.

3. In some epidemics as many as 75 per cent of the patients develop general symptoms, and at this stage may exhibit an excess of cells in the cerebrospinal fluid, perhaps with some symptoms of meningitis, yet never develop paralysis. The infection is overcome in the preparalytic stage, and these are called non-paralytic cases.

4. Only in a minority does the infection run its full course and cause paralysis.

The pre-paralytic stage

In this stage two phases can often be recognized. The first symptoms of infection are fever, malaise, headache, drowsiness or insomnia, sweating, flushing, faucial congestion, and often gastrointestinal disturbances. This phase, which lasts one or two days, is sometimes followed by temporary improvement with remission of fever for 48 hours, or it may merge into the second phase, in which headache is more severe and associated with pain in the back and limbs, together with hyperaesthesia, often of both the superficial and deep tissues. Delirium may occur. The child is often tremulous, and cervical rigidity and Kernig's sign may be present. The 'spinal sign' is of diagnostic value, especially in children. It is elicited by passive flexion of the spine when the patient is lying on his side, resistance being encountered because of pain in the back. A child may be asked to try to kiss its knee. A spontaneous sign is the reluctance of the child to extend the arms with the spine flexed and a tendency to use them to support the back behind.

In non-paralytic cases the patient recovers after exhibiting in mild or more severe form either or both of the phases of the pre-paralytic stage. This, however, may lead on to:

The paralytic stage

The onset of paralysis, which is often ushered in by muscular fasciculation, usually follows rapidly upon the pre-paralytic stage and is accompanied by considerable pain in the limbs and tenderness of the muscles on pressure. The paralysis may be widespread or localized. In milder cases its asymmetry and patchy character are conspicuous features. Usually the maximum of damage is done within the first 24 hours, but sometimes the paralysis is progressive, and in the ascending form it gradually spreads upwards from the legs and endangers life through respiratory paralysis. The lower limbs are more often affected than the upper. Careful watch should be kept for movements of the intercostal muscles and the diaphragm.

The brainstem may be involved as well as the spinal cord or in relative independence. The muscles of the face, pharynx, larynx, and tongue may be paralysed, and rarely the ocular muscles. Tremor and nystagmus may be present. It is of great practical importance to distinguish embarrassment of respiration caused by the accumulation of saliva and mucus in pharyngeal paralysis from true paralysis of the muscles of respiration. Difficulty of micturition may occur during the acute part of the paralytic stage.

Fortunately only a proportion of the muscles affected at the outset are likely to remain permanently paralysed. Improvement usually begins at the end of the first week after the onset of the paralysis. Wasting will not begin to be apparent for three weeks, and will be permanent in the paralysed muscles, and the reflexes which they mediate will be diminished or lost. When opposing muscle groups are unequally affected, contractures are liable to occur in the stronger muscles, causing limitation of movement at the joint. Fasciculation may continue for years in partially paralysed muscles. When the paralysis is permanent the affected limbs are blue and cold and may be the site of oedema or chilblains, and the growth of their bones is retarded.

The cerebrospinal fluid

From the pre-paralytic stage onwards the cerebrospinal fluid shows changes which are the outcome of meningeal irritation. The pressure is increased and there is an excess of cells, usually 50 to 250 per mm^3. During the first few days both polymorphonuclear cells and lymphocytes are present, but after the first week lymphocytes alone are found. The protein and globulin show a moderate increase, but the glucose and chloride content of the fluid is normal. During the second week protein may rise to between 100 and 200 g/l.

Diagnosis

In the pre-paralytic stage poliomyelitis has to be distinguished from other causes of meningeal irritation. In the *acute pyogenic* forms of meningitis the child is more ill, has greater neck rigidity. The glucose content of the fluid is reduced, the cells are exclusively polymorphonuclear, and organisms are likely to be present. *Tuberculous* meningitis may be difficult to distinguish but its onset is usually more gradual and the child is usually drowsy and apathetic and pale rather than flushed, as in poliomyelitis. In both conditions the cerebrospinal fluid may contain an excess of cells, both polymorphonuclear and lymphocytes, and also of protein. In poliomyelitis the sugar and chloride content of the fluid are normal, in tuberculous meningitis both are diminished, and tubercle bacilli may be found. Other forms of meningitis characterized by a lymphocytic pleocytosis in the cerebrospinal fluid may be impossible to distinguish, except by virological studies; when necessary the poliomyelitis virus may be sought in the stools.

The spinal form of the disease in the paralytic stage is usually easy of diagnosis, but when pain is severe other causes of painful lesions in a child's limb may need to be excluded. The bulbar form of the disease must be distinguished from other forms of encephalitis, but there is no other which produces only an acute lower motor neurone lesion in the pons and medulla associated with an inflammatory cell count in the cerebrospinal fluid.

Prognosis

The mortality varies in different epidemics and may be as high as 25 per cent. The risk is greatest in the first year of life, and in those who are attacked after the fifth year. The cause of death is usually bulbar paralysis or respiratory paralysis or a combination of the two. When the paralysis has ceased to progress it is safe to predict that considerable recovery will occur. Improvement once begun may be expected to continue for at least a year, and in some cases for longer. Second attacks, though very rare, are well authenticated.

Treatment

Immediate and complete rest should be insisted on in every suspected case of poliomyelitis, however mild, since there is evidence that physical activity in the pre-paralytic stage increases the risk of severe paralysis.

Four categories of paralytic case need to be distinguished, because in each form the treatment required is different. These are:

1. The patient with neither respiratory nor bulbar paralysis.
2. The patient with respiratory paralysis.
3. The patient with bulbar paralysis.
4. The patient with both respiratory and bulbar paralysis.

The patient without respiratory and bulbar paralysis

During the acute stage the patient's fluid balance should be maintained. Ordinary analgesics and sedatives may be required for the relief of pain and restlessness. Hypertonic saline baths diminish the hyperaesthesia. Gentle passive movements are the only form of physical treatment which is permissible at this stage. During the acute stage steps should be taken to prevent the stretching of paralysed muscles and contracture of their antagonists. The patient should be nursed on a firm bed and the limbs kept in the positions in which the paralysed muscles are relaxed by means of sandbags or improvised spints. The limbs, however, should not be kept immobilized. During the stage of convalescence prolonged rest in bed will be necessary in severe cases with appropriate physiotherapy and orthopaedic treatment.

Treatment of respiratory paralysis

A patient suffering from respiratory paralysis needs to be treated by some form of artificial respiration, which may be required for weeks, months, or even indefinitely. This may be carried out by means of negative pressure operating through some device which sucks the thoracic cage outwards, or by positive pressure which inflates the lungs by raising the pressure within the trachea. For uncomplicated respiratory paralysis a negative pressure method is on the whole the more suitable.

Treatment of bulbar paralysis

When bulbar paralysis occurs in the absence of respiratory paralysis, the danger to the patient arises from his inability to prevent fluids, or secretions in the pharynx, from being sucked into the lungs with inspiration. The dysphagia also leads to difficulty in feeding. Such patients should be nursed in the semi-prone position, being turned from one side to the other every few hours, while the foot of the cot or bed should be raised to make an angle of 15 degrees with the horizontal. A mechanical sucker is required to remove pharyngeal secretions, and feeding should be carried out by an oesophageal catheter preferably passed through the nose.

Combined respiratory and bulbar paralysis

This constitutes the most difficult and urgent problem of all, and is best treated by tracheostomy with positive pressure artificial respiration. The time to advise tracheostomy is before the patient's vital capacity is so limited that it has to become an emergency procedure. This has several advantages, one of which is that the use of a cuffed intratracheal tube effectively blocks the trachea to the downward passage of the pharyngeal secretions, and so protects the lungs.

Whatever method is used for the treatment of respiratory or bulbar paralysis, or the two combined, necessitates a team of experienced doctors and nurses. The efficiency of the lungs must be aided by postural drainage, physiotherapy to the chest wall, use of suction to remove the secretions accumulated in the pharynx, and when necessary also from the bronchi by bronchoscopy, prophylactic antibiotics against pneumonia, and X-rays of the chest when necessary.

Prophylaxis

The best prophylaxis is immunity, and it has now been established that a high degree of immunity is conferred by three injections of inactivated poliomyelitis virus vaccine. A live attenuated Sabin-type vaccine given orally has now virtually replaced it and appears to be as effective, without any higher incidence of neurological incidents complicating its use. Passive immunization with gamma globulin gives temporary protection during an epidemic. Since the nasopharyngeal secretions, the urine, and the faeces of the patient may contain the virus, appropriate nursing precausions should be taken. Virus may be present in the stools from five to six weeks after the onset, hence the patient should be isolated from other children for at least six weeks.

REFERENCES

Nicholas, D.D., Kratzer, J.H., Ofosu-Amaah, S., and Belcher, D.W. (1977). Is poliomyelitis a serious problem in developing countries? – The Danfa experience. *Br. med. J.* **i**, 1009–12.

Sabin, A.B. (1962). Oral polio virus vaccine: recent results and recommendations for optimum use. *R. Soc. Hlth J.* **82**, 51–9.

23 Meningitis

AETIOLOGY AND PATHOLOGY

By acute meningitis is meant acute leptomeningitis; that is, an infection of the pia mater and arachnoid, which inevitably involves the subarachnoid space and the cerebrospinal fluid. There are three principal ways in which the meninges may become infected:

1. After fracture of the skull. In the case of a penetrating injury of the cranial vault organisms may be carried in from the scalp. When the base of the skull is fractured, they may spread to the meninges from the nasopharynx, middle ear, or mastoid.

2. Extension to the meninges of a pre-existing pyogenic infection of one of the nasal sinuses, the middle ear, or mastoid.

3. Infection through the bloodstream. Sometimes meningitis is the only or the principal manifestation of a bacteraemia, as in meningococcal meningitis and some cases of pneumococcal meningitis, or the infection of the meninges may be secondary to focal infection elsewhere in the body, for example pneumonia, empyema, osteomyelitis, enteric fever, etc. Tuberculous meningitis may be part of a general miliary dissemination of the infection. Sometimes meningitis is secondary to a blood-borne infection which first settles in the brain, as in the case of metastatic cerebral abscess or tuberculoma. It is probable that the infection is blood-borne in most cases of meningitis caused by a virus.

Sometimes meningeal inflammation plays a subordinate part in the picture of encephalitis or myelitis, for example poliomyelitis. Such a condition may be described as a meningo-encephalomyelitis. Less frequently encephalitis is secondary to meningitis, as in some cases of meningococcal and tuberculous meningitis.

Spinal meningitis, that is meningitis arising in, and at first limited to, the spinal canal, is rare and is usually secondary to osteitis of the vertebral column. Rarely also meningitis may be caused by an organism introduced into the subarachnoid space at lumbar puncture.

The organisms commonly responsible for meningitis are *Neisseria meningitidis, Diplococcus pneumoniae, Haemophilus influenzae, Streptococcus, Staphylococcus, Escherichia coli,* all of which cause pyogenic meningitis; *Mycobacterium tuberculosis*; and various viruses which cause so-called 'acute aseptic' or 'lymphocytic' meningitis. Other organisms less frequently the cause of meningitis are *Salmonella typhosa, Bacillus anthracis, Brucella abortus,*

Pseudomonas aeruginosa, Leptospira, and yeasts such as *Cryptococcus neoformans (Torula histolytica).*

It is convenient to consider the commoner forms of acute meningitis under three headings:

1. Acute pyogenic meningitis.
2. Tuberculous meningitis.
3. Acute aseptic meningitis.

Pathology

Pyogenic meningitis

Whatever the causative organism, the pathological changes in acute pyogenic meningitis are similar in all cases. Whether the organism reaches the meninges by direct spread or through the bloodstream, inflammation and its products become rapidly diffused through the whole subarachnoid space of the brain and spinal cord. This becomes filled with greenish-yellow pus which may cover the whole cerebral cortex or may occasionally be confined to the sulci. When there is a local site of infection the pus may be most evident in its neighbourhood. The cortical veins are congested, and the cerebral convolutions are often flattened owing to internal hydrocephalus. Microscopically (Fig. 23.1) the leptomeninges show inflammatory infiltration, which in the early stages consists wholly of polymorphonuclear cells, though later lymphocytes and plasma cells are present. The cerebral hemispheres show little change except for perivascular inflammatory infiltration of the cortex. Internal hydrocephalus is most often due to inflammatory adhesions in the cerebellomedullary cistern obstructing the outflow of cerebrospinal fluid from the fourth ventricle.

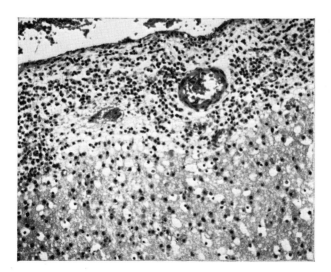

Fig. 23.1. Pyogenic meningitis.

In the 'adrenal type' of meningococcal infection haemorrhage, thrombosis, or toxic or inflammatory changes are found in the adrenals; and the internal ear is sometimes invaded by the infection.

Tuberculous meningitis

It is now believed that in most cases tuberculous meningitis is due to an infection of the meninges from a caseous focus in the brain, which in turn has been infected via the bloodstream from a focus which in children is often in the mediastinal or mesenteric lymph nodes, but may be situated in the bones, joints, lungs, or genito-urinary tract. It may occur at any age, but is most frequently encountered in children between the ages of 2 and 5. In about one-quarter of all cases the infection is with the bovine bacillus, in the remainder with the human bacillus.

In acute cases the brain is usually pale and the convolutions are somewhat flattened. A yellowish gelatinous exudate is found matting together the lepto-meninges at the base and extending along the lateral sulci. Miliary tubercles are visible on the leptomeninges, being most conspicuous along the vessels, especially the middle cerebral artery. Microscopically these consist of collections of round cells, chiefly mononuclear, often with central caseation. Giant cells are rare. The substance of the nervous system shows little inflammatory reaction, but marked toxic degeneration of nerve cells. After prolonged treatment with antibiotics the basal exudate becomes intensely hard and 'woody', the large arteries passing through it show an arteritis, and as the result infarction of the brain may occur. Adhesions may cause hydrocephalus, or obstruction of the spinal subarachnoid space.

Acute aseptic meningitis

Acute aseptic meningitis is a convenient term to apply to acute non-pyogenic meningitis due to a variety of causes, most if not all viruses. In so far as the cerebrospinal fluid usually contains an excess of cells which are predominantly, if not exclusively, lymphocytic, acute aseptic meningitis is identical with acute benign lymphocytic meningitis, but occasionally the cells are predominantly polymorphonuclear. This combined clinical and cerebrospinal fluid picture may also be due to the Coxsackie and echoviruses, mumps, infectious mononucleosis, herpes simplex virus, or the meningitic phase of poliomyelitis. The pathology is therefore mixed, consisting usually of round cell infiltration of the leptomeninges with the pathological changes in the central nervous system, if any, produced by the causative organism.

SYMPTOMS

All forms of acute meningitis, whatever their cause, possess a number of symptoms in common. The onset may be fulminating, acute, or, less commonly, insidious. Headache, increasing in severity, is usually the initial symptom. Fever is the rule, though the degree of pyrexia varies. The temperature is usually between 100 and 102°F, though hyperpyrexia may occur, especially in the terminal stages. The pulse rate may be slow in the early stages, but always rises as the disease progresses, and at the end is usually very rapid and often irregular. The respiratory rate is usually slightly increased, and various forms of irregularity occur in the later stages. Headache is usually very severe, possessing a 'bursting' character. It may be diffuse or mainly frontal, and usually radiates down the neck and into the back, being associated with pain in the spine which spreads to the limbs, especially the lower limbs. Vomiting may occur, especially in the early stages. Convulsions are common in children, but rare in adults. The patient tends to lie in an attitude of general flexion, curled up under the bedclothes and resenting interference. Photophobia is frequently present.

Signs of meningeal irritation

The following signs are of special value as indicating meningeal irritation.

Cervical rigidity

Cervical rigidity is present at an early stage in almost every case of meningitis. It is elicited by the observer's placing his hand beneath the patient's occiput and endeavouring to cause passive flexion of the head so as to bring the chin towards the chest. There is a resistance due to spasm of the extensor muscles of the neck, and an attempt to overcome this causes pain.

Head retraction (Fig. 23.2) is an extreme degree of cervical rigidity and is usually associated with some rigidity of the spine at lower levels.

Kernig's sign

Kernig's sign, though slightly less frequently encountered in meningitis than cervical rigidity, is of a somewhat similar nature. An attempt to produce passive extension of the knee with the hip fully flexed evokes spasm of the hamstrings and causes pain.

Other signs

The mental state of the patient varies according to the stage and progress of the disease. Delirium is common in the early stages, but tends later to give place to drowsiness and stupor which is followed by coma. The ocular fundi may be normal or show venous congestion or papilloedema. The pupils are often unequal and may react sluggishly. In the later stages they tend to be dilated and fixed. Squint and diplopia are often present. Difficulty in swallowing may occur in the later stages. Muscular power in the limbs is usually well preserved, but some incoordination and tremor are common, and there is considerable muscular hypotonia. A general flaccid paralysis is a terminal event. The tendon reflexes are usually sluggish and often are soon lost. The plantar reflexes are

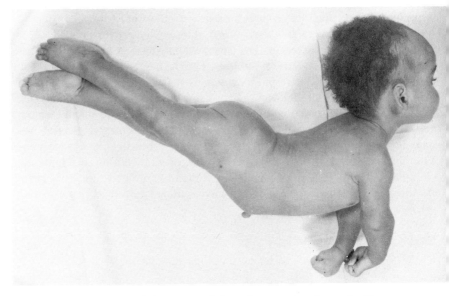

Fig. 23.2. Opisthotonus and decerebrate posture in meningitis.

usually flexor at first, though later one or both may become extensor. True paralysis of sphincter control occurs only late, but the mental state of the patient may lead to retention or incontinence of urine early in the illness, and constipation is the rule.

Special clinical features

Meningococcal meningitis

In meningococcal meningitis there is frequently a purpuric rash which is specially liable to occur on regions subjected to pressure. Somewhat less frequently the rash is maculopapular. Arthritis occurs in from 10 to 15 per cent of cases in most epidemics, and permanent deafness in under 5 per cent. In the adrenal type – the Waterhouse–Friderichsen syndrome – the characteristic features are grave hypotension and cyanosis, together with the biochemical changes of suprarenal cortical failure.

Tuberculous meningitis

The onset of symptoms is insidious, and there is almost always a prodromal phase of vague ill health. In children lassitude, anorexia, loss of weight, and change of disposition are present; in adults mental changes may be conspicuous. This prodromal phase usually lasts two or three weeks, and is followed by the development of symptoms of meningeal irritation. These are usually slighter than in pyogenic meningitis. Choroidal tubercles are present in about 50 per cent of patients, and are visible ophthalmoscopically as rather ill-defined rounded or oval yellowish bodies about half the size of the optic disc. Tuberculous lesions are usually discoverable outside the nervous system, especially in the lungs.

The cerebrospinal fluid

The cerebrospinal fluid is always under increased pressure. Table 23.1 shows its principal features in the three main types of meningitis.

Table 23.1. *The cerebrospinal fluid in meningitis*

Cerebrospinal fluid	Type of meningitis		
	Pyogenic	Tuberculous	Acute aseptic
Appearance	Turbid, yellow	Clear: sometimes cobwed clot	Clear: sometimes turbid
Cells	Polymorphs 1000–2000 per mm^3, or more	Mononuclears or mononuclears and polymorphs 10–350 per mm^3	Mononuclears, rarely polymorphs or mixed 50–1500 per mm^3
Protein	1.0–5.0 g/l	1.0 g/l	1.0–5.0 g/l, rarely more
Chloride	110–115 mmol/l	About 100 mmol/l	Normal, 120–130 mmol/l
Glucose	Much reduced or absent	Below 3.0 mmol/l	Normal, 4.0–6.0 mmol/l
Organisms	Present in smear or on culture	Present in smear: or on culture or guinea-pig inoculation	Absent in smear and ordinary culture media. May be demonstrable by special virological methods

DIAGNOSIS

Occasionally *acute general infections* may simulate meningitis, especially in childhood, if they cause severe headache and still more meningism, which is characterized by cervical rigidity and Kernig's sign, but the cerebrospinal fluid, though under increased pressure, is normal in composition. In all doubtful cases lumbar puncture should be performed and will settle the matter. The various forms of *acute encephalitis* are distinguished by the predominance of physical signs indicating severe damage to the nervous system, while signs of meningitis are often absent, or if present are relatively slight. *Cerebral abscess* may need to be distinguished from meningitis, but sometimes both are present. In abscess uncomplicated by generalized meningitis, the signs are those of a focal intracranial lesion. The cerebrospinal fluid usually contains an excess of cells, though not often more than 100 per mm^3, the majority being lymphocytes. The protein is often disproportionately increased. The chloride and sugar content of the fluid is normal, and organisms are absent.

Subarachnoid haemorrhage may simulate meningitis because it leads to meningeal irritation. Its onset, however, is usually much more rapid, and the true diagnosis is readily established by the demonstration of blood in the cerebrospinal fluid.

PROGNOSIS

The prognosis of meningitis depends upon a number of factors, of which the chief are the infecting organism and its sensitivity to antibiotics, the stage of the illness at which the patient comes under treatment, and the presence of fracture of the skull or cerebral abscess. In uncomplicated meningococcal meningitis treated early, the prognosis is excellent, the mortality rate being not more than 5–10 per cent, and the only serious sequel being the occasional occurrence of deafness. Meningitis due to other pyogenic organisms has a much higher mortality rate. It is difficult to compare different series of cases, because the basis of selection differs and there are so many variables. In meningitis complicating surgical conditions, the mortality rate is likely to lie between 25 and 50 per cent. In 'primary' pneumococcal meningitis and meningitis due to *H. influenzae*, the mortality rate in some series has been as low as 10 per cent. In tuberculous meningitis much depends upon the stage at which the patient is first treated. Of those comatose, only a small percentage survive, and they are left with neurological sequelae. Among patients treated early by modern methods, the mortality rate should be under 20 per cent, and of those who survive 70 per cent should be free from sequelae. In acute aseptic meningitis the prognosis is very good. The disorder is rarely fatal, and sequelae are uncommon.

TREATMENT

The management of a case of meningitis calls for a series of urgent interrelated diagnostic and therapeutic decisions, which can be made intelligently only if their pros and cons are known. These considerations will now be discussed as the rational basis of a plan of treatment.

We begin at the point at which a tentative diagnosis of meningitis has been made. No treatment should be given until lumbar puncture has been performed, since the administration of antibiotics before lumbar puncture may make it impossible to identify the causal organism. The first step, therefore, is to carry out lumbar puncture, measuring the initial pressure of the cerebrospinal fluid. At the time the cerebrospinal fluid is examined, blood should also be taken for blood culture and blood sugar estimation. Bacterial endocarditis sometimes presents as meningitis and some organisms, such as *Listeria monocytogenes*, are more easily cultured from blood than cerebrospinal fluid. Since the blood glucose level may be lowered in the course of meningitis, the finding of a lowered blood level removes some ambiguity in interpreting the cerebrospinal fluid level which is normally 30–40 per cent lower than the blood level. If the fluid is turbid it may be assumed that the meningitis is pyogenic. Remove 10 ml in two consecutive portions of 5 ml for examination and culture. Should an intrathecal injection of penicillin now be given? If there is clinical evidence that the meningitis is meningococcal, it is unnecessary. There is no doubt that some cases of 'primary' meningitis due to other pyogenic organisms can be treated successfully without intrathecal injections. However, the data upon which such a decision can be based are often not immediately available, and therefore it is wise in all cases of pyogenic meningitis other than meningococcal to give an intrathecal injection of benzyl-penicillin (penicillin G). The initial dose for an adult is 12 mg (20 000 units) in 10 ml of normal saline, that for a child being calculated in proportion to its weight. It need hardly be stressed that extreme caution in checking the dose of drugs for intrathecal injection is essential. Ampicillin, 150 mg per kg body weight per day, should then be given orally or intravenously until the bacteriological diagnosis is made.

If the cerebrospinal fluid is clear macroscopically, treatment may be left until the cytology and bateriology have been reported upon. Meningitis with a clear fluid is likely to be either tuberculous or acute aseptic. The differentiating points in the cerebrospinal fluid are shown in Table 23.1.

Treatment when the infecting organism is known

Penicillin in high dosage is the main line of treatment to be pursued in both meningococcal and pneumococcal meningitis. There is an increasing incidence of meningococci resistant to sulphonamides which were formerly the treatment of choice in meningococcal disease. For an adult at least 1 mega-unit of penicillin G should be given three-hourly intramuscularly or, in a severely ill patient, intravenously, up to a dose of 20 mega-units a day. On this higher dose, continuing intrathecal penicillin is not necessary. Streptococcal and staphylococcal infections should be treated in the same way, but substituting chloramphenicol 50 mg/kg and ampicillin 500 mg four hourly for penicillin should the organism be penicillin-resistant. Chloramphenicol is given in quantities of 100 mg per kg every 24 hours intramuscularly in four divided doses. The intrathecal dose for adults is 3–5 mg daily. *Haemophilus influenzae* infections should be treated by chloramphenicol intramuscularly. The treatment of meningitis due to other organisms will depend on their antibiotic sensitivity. How often should intrathecal injections be given in the treatment of pyogenic meningitis? This depends entirely on the condition of the patient. Their chief use is to deal with fulminating infections and to increase the power of the antibiotic when a patient is not responding satisfactorily. They should not be used unnecessarily when all is going well. Systemic antibiotic therapy should be continued for at least five days after the cerebrospinal fluid has become sterile.

In all cases of pyogenic meningitis careful search should be made for a possible source of infection, especially in the ear and nasal sinuses, and if such is found the possibility of the coexistence of a cerebral abscess should be borne in mind. Arrest of improvement may be due to the development of hydrocephalus.

Tuberculous meningitis

Since tuberculus meningitis is likely to be fatal if treatment is delayed while consciousness deteriorates, it is justifiable to start treatment on a strong clinical suspicion after setting up cultures. Each introduction of a new antibiotic effective against the tubercle bacillus has been followed by an improvement in recovery rate from tuberculous meningitis. The routine treatment, therefore, consists of the systemic administration of isoniazid and streptomycin in the following doses for an adult: isoniazid, 100 mg thrice daily by mouth, and streptomycin, 1 g twice daily by intramuscular injection. These doses are halved after three days and continued for up to six months. PAS can be added and rifampicin or ethambutol may have to be given if the organism is resistant to the commoner drugs. Rifampicin and ethambutol in too large doses for too long cause optic nerve damage. As in the case of pyogenic infections, tuberculous meningitis can usually be adequately treated without intrathecal injections. In some cases, there still appears to be a place for intrathecal injections, particularly in advanced cases and if a patient is not otherwise responding well. The intrathecal dose of streptomycin is from 20 to 50 mg daily or every other day for ten injections. Prednisone is a useful adjuvant to treatment and should be given to infants under 1 year and in advanced cases daily for a month to diminish the likelihood of adhesive arachnoiditis and communicating hydrocephalus. When a rise in cerebrospinal fluid protein and a fall in its pressure suggests that a spinal subarachnoid block is developing, an intrathecal dose of 10–25 mg of hydrocortisone, repeated daily if necessary for a week, is often valuable. Pyridoxine in doses of 40 mg daily is helpful to counteract the toxic effects of the antibiotics, and anticonvulsants should always be given. The development of hydrocephalus calls for surgical intervention.

Acute aseptic meningitis

This calls for no specific treatment. It is desirable to try to identify the virus and specimens of cerebrospinal fluid and blood should be sent to a virological laboratory. In a case of meningitis if the c.s.f. shows a normal glucose and less than 100 cells, all lymphocytes, then antibiotics can be withheld, though if after 24 hours the repeated lumbar puncture shows the presence of polymorphs, antibiotic treatment should be started.

Chronic meningitis

A subacute or chronic meningitis, which may relapse and remit, may sometimes prove difficult to diagnose and hence to treat. The cerebrospinal fluid shows a rise of protein, mild mononuclear or polymorph excess and a low sugar. Culture, using special techniques, or histological examination of the deposit may eventually lead to a diagnosis of sarcoidosis, cysticercosis, brucellosis, cryptococcal infection, or carcinomatosis of the meninges. Cryptococcal infections may be treated with flucytosine, 100–200 mg/kg body weight by mouth and amphotericin B given intravenously and continued for 10–20 weeks.

A number of other practical problems of treatment may occur. In children 'meningismus' may occur with an intercurrent infection but examination of the spinal fluid which is, in retrospect, unnecessary is preferable to delaying recognition of meningitis. In bacterial meningitis the cerebrospinal fluid is sometimes sterile as a result of partial prior treatment with antibiotics, but if other forms of meningitis can be excluded, effective appropriate antibiotic treatment should be continued. If, after starting antibiotic treatment for bacterial meningitis, consciousness deteriorates or focal neurological signs develop, it must be suspected that the meningitis is complicated by intracranial or subdural infection which needs locating by CT scan studies. Finally, if the patient's general condition is deteriorating and tuberculous meningitis is suspected but no bacilli can be found on smears, it is wise to start treatment with antituberculous drugs. Despite a normal chest X-ray, negative Mantoux, and mild polymorph in the cerebrospinal fluid, the infection may nevertheless be tuberculous.

General management

Good nursing is of the utmost importance, and in severe cases the long illness, often with relapses, and the need for repeated lumbar punctures, make heavy demands upon the skill and patience of the nurses. Patients should be nursed in a darkened room, and nasal feeding or the administration of fluids by intravenous drip will be required when swallowing is difficult. Sedatives will be needed to control restlessness. An unexplained rise of temperature should suggest the possibility of urinary infection, or of the development of a focus of infection somewhere outside the nervous system caused by the organism responsible for the meningitis. Constipation is often troublesome, and the abdomen should be examined daily for distension of the bladder. Acute adrenal insufficiency should be treated with intravenous saline and corticosteroids.

REFERENCES

Bell, W.E. (1981*a*). Treatment of bacterial infections of the central nervous system. *Ann. Neurol.* **9**, 313–27.

Bell, W.E. (1981*b*). Treatment of fungal infections of the central nervous system. *Ann. Neurol.* **9,** 417–22.

Delaney, P. (1977). Neurologic manifestations in sarcoidosis: review of the literature, with a report of 23 cases. *Ann. Intern. Med.* **87,** 336–45.

The Lancet (1976). Tuberculous meningitis. (Editorial.) *Lancet* **i,** 787.

24 Syphilis of the nervous system

AETIOLOGY AND PATHOLOGY

Neurosyphilis was becoming an uncommon disease but recently there has been an increase in incidence as a result of promiscuity in urban societies, in particular among male homosexuals. Only a small proportion – perhaps 10 per cent – of persons infected with the *Treponema pallidum* subsequently show evidence that the organism has invaded the nervous system. However, 30 per cent of patients with secondary syphilis have an abnormal cerebrospinal fluid. This may occur as early as during the secondary stage. On both clinical and pathological grounds, a distinction must be made between two groups of tertiary manifestations of neurosyphilis, one of which is known as meningovascular, or cerebrospinal syphilis, the other, which comprises tabes dorsalis and general paresis, being distinguished as parenchymatous syphilis. The essential lesion in meningovascular syphilis is a vascular and perivascular inflammation. The affected vessel exhibits endarteritis obliterans, and infiltration of the perivascular space. Impairment of blood supply to the nervous tissues through reduction of the lumen of the vessel, or actual thrombosis, together no doubt with the action of toxins produced by the organism, cause necrosis or caseation of neighbouring tissues. The result is a granuloma or gumma originating in an area of such necrosis and surrounded by a zone of fibrotic reaction. This characteristic reaction to *Treponema pallidum* is the pathological basis of all forms of meningovascular syphilis. Clinical manifestations depend entirely upon the site of the process. A cerebral gumma large enough to produce the symptoms of a space-occupying lesion is very rare.

Parenchymatous neurosyphilis, that is tabes and general paresis, differs from the meningovascular form in the comparative absence of gross vascular reactions and the tendency for the lesions to be selective in their distribution, though in other respects perhaps the differences between tabes and general paresis are as great as the resemblances.

In *tabes* there is macroscopical evidence of atrophy of the dorsal spinal roots and the posterior columns of the spinal cord are flat or even sunken – hence the name tabes dorsalis, or dorsal wasting. Microscopically the essential lesion is a degeneration of the exogenous fibres of the cord, that is, of the central processes of the dorsal root ganglion cells, which themselves are usually little affected. Since the only exogenous fibres which possess a long course within the cord are situated in the posterior columns, these exhibit a selective degeneration, and their demyelination is conspicuous, stained by stains for myelin (Fig. 24.1).

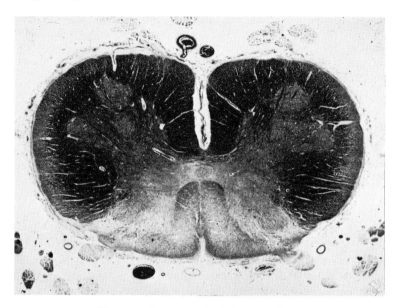

Fig. 24.1. Spinal cord in tabes dorsalis.

Although various theories have been proposed in explanation of the selective character of the degenerative lesions of tabes in the spinal cord, none is altogether unsatisfactory.

In *general paresis* the brain is macroscopically shrunken and there is a compensatory hydrocephalus. The atrophy is confined to the anterior two-thirds of the cerebral hemispheres. Microscopical changes are predominantly cortical and are found in the meninges, blood vessels, and neurones. The lepto-meninges show a diffuse infiltration with lymphocytes and plasma cells, which also occupy the perivascular spaces of the small vessels and capillaries of the cortex, the ganglion cells of which show a varying degree of degeneration going on to complete disappearance. These changes are most marked in the molecular layer and the layers of small and medium-sized pyramidal cells. There is a proliferation of the glia. These cortical changes are always diffuse, but the frontal and temporal regions usually suffer most severely. The organism is demonstrable in the cortex in some 50 per cent of cases, especially in the frontal region.

Primary optic atrophy may occur in any form of neurosyphilis but is commonest in tabes. Pathologically it is due to syphilitic inflammation of the sheath of the nerve.

Syphilitic aortitis is common in all forms of neurosyphilis.

Why one person infected with syphilis should develop the meningovascular form of the disease while another develops tabes or general paresis is unknown, but is has plausibly been suggested that the difference depends in some way upon the presence or absence of immune reactions. Males suffer from meningovascular syphilis somewhat more frequently than females, and the male to female sex ratio in tabes and general paresis is about four to one.

SYMPTOMS

Meningovascular syphilis

Meningovascular syphilis may cause symptoms within a few months of infection, or at any subsequent period in the patient's life, but usually about five years after the original infection. They are extremely varied, because the pathological changes may involve any part of the nervous system, and may be sharply focal or diffuse. *Diffuse cerebral leptomeningitis* mimics pyogenic meningitis and is likely to cause headache which is frequently severe – with nocturnal exacerbations – and papilloedema may occur. Mental changes are common and there may be convulsions, either generalized or focal. Paresis and incoordination of the limbs on one or both sides are common. *Basal meningitis* may cause optic atrophy and disturbances of the hypothalamus. Reflex iridoplegia is almost constant, and cranial nerve palsies may occur.

On the other hand, a *focal cerebral lesion* may be the result of syphilitic endarteritis, of which hemiplegia is a not uncommon manifestation. Or a single cranial nerve may be involved, especially the third, and syphilis should always be considered as a possible cause of a painless third nerve palsy. Cerebral gumma is rare.

The commonest spinal lesion due to meningovascular syphilis is *meningomyelitis,* which is not uncommonly an early tertiary manifestation. The dorsal region of the spinal cord is usually affected. Syphilitic amyotrophy, which may be a secondary or tertiary manifestation, is the term applied to muscular wasting developing as the result of localized spinal meningitis. It may be unilateral or bilateral and occur with or without pain. *Syphilitic radiculitis* may involve one or more posterior spinal roots, causing pain of the corresponding segmental distribution on one or both sides and associated with either hyperalgesia or analgesia. *Spinal paralysis* is the term applied to a form of progressive spastic paraplegia due to syphilis running a slowly progressive course and characterized by early involvement of bladder function, with comparatively slight sensory loss.

Tabes dorsalis

Patients with tabes frequently give no history of primary infection. The latent interval between infection and the development of symptoms is usually between eight and twelve years. Exceptionally it may be less, or much longer. The onset is usually gradual and insidious. Usually sensory symptoms, especially pain, precede ataxia by months or years. This has led to the distinction between pre-ataxic and ataxic stages. So-called *'lightning pains'* are the characteristic early symptom. They are stabbing in character, occur in brief paroxysms in the lower limbs and may be very severe. They are localized to one spot, each attack lasting only a few seconds, but attacks may occur repeatedly in the same place or may shift from place to place in the limb. Other forms of pain may be experienced, especially a constricting pain around the chest or abdomen – sometimes called *'girdle pains'*. *Paraesthesiae* are not uncommon, especially in the lower limbs, and impairment of sensation may lead to the complaint that the patient feels as though he is walking on wool, that he cannot feel the chair upon which he sits, that he is unaware when his bladder is full, or that he is unconscious of the act of defaecation.

Ataxia, the next symptom to develop, is due partly to loss of postural sensibility and partly to loss of unconscious afferent impulses concerned in the regulation of posture and movement.

The patient walks with a wide base, the feet are lifted too high and brought down to the ground too violently. Walking becomes impossible without a stick, and finally in severe cases the patient can walk only if he is supported on both sides.

Visual failure due to primary optic atrophy occurs in only a small proportion of cases, and is then usually a late development, but is sometimes the presenting symptom.

On examination, most patients with tabes are of spare build. There is no characteristic mental change. The facies is often distinguished by a wrinkled forehead due to contraction of the frontal belly of the occipitofrontalis muscle in association with a moderate degree of ptosis of both upper lids. The optic discs may be normal or may exhibit primary atrophy, with corresponding changes in the visual acuity and fields. The pupils are usually contracted and irregular and show the changes characteristic of the Argyll Robertson pupil; that is, the pupillary reaction to light is impaired or lost, while that to accommodation-convergence is retained. The iris shows areas of atrophic depigmentation. The ocular movements are usually full and there is no nystagmus, but diplopia may occur owing to defective balance of the ocular muscles. Sensation may be impaired over the face, and in particular there is often a characteristic area of analgesia on the nose on one or both sides. Anosmia, deafness, and laryngeal palsy occasionally occur.

In the limbs the symptoms are those which result from the *loss of afferent impulses.* There are always more pronounced in the lower than in the upper, and tend to affect the limbs symmetrically. Muscular tone is much diminished, but there is no muscular weakness or wasting save in rare cases. Co-ordination is impaired in the heel-knee test, and is worse when the eyes are closed. It leads to the disorder of gait already described. In Romberg's test, the patient, who can stand steadily with the feet together and the eyes open, sways when his eyes are closed, and he can no longer compensate with vision for his loss of afferent impulses from the lower limbs. Trunk ataxia may be present, and less often ataxia in the upper limbs. The tendon reflexes are diminished or lost, the ankle-jerks being usually affected before the knee-jerks, and it is not uncommon to find the reflexes unequal. The tendon-jerks of the upper limbs are usually diminished at an early stage, but are finally lost only after those of the lower limbs have disappeared. The plantar reflexes usually remain elicitable and are flexor, and the abdominal reflexes are also obtainable, and are frequently unusually brisk.

The forms of sensation which are first impaired are usually those which are mediated by the posterior columns. Appreciation of vibration suffers early and usually before recognition of posture and passive movement. As a rule the lower limbs suffer before the upper, though exceptionally the upper limbs are first affected – so-called 'cervical tabes'. Painful sensibility is also early impaired, the deep tissues becoming insensitive to pain before the skin. Forcible compression of the muscles and of the tendo calcaneus evokes no pain, and pain sensation is frequently lost in the testicles. Cutaneous painful sensibility is not uniformly impaired, but is usually first lost in certain situations, namely the side of the nose, the ulnar border of the arm and forearm, the region of the trunk between the nipples and the costal margin, the outer border of the leg and dorsum and sole of the foot, and the region surrounding the anus. In these regions even when pin-prick is appreciated as painful there is often a long delay, which may reach several seconds, between the application of the stimulus and its perception. Cutaneous sensibility to light touch, heat, and cold is usually unimpaired until a late stage, and the patient may even be hypersensitive to cold.

Disturbances in bladder control may occur early when the sacral roots are early involved. The patient may complain either of difficulty of micturition or of incontinence, but frequently he is for a long time unaware that anything is wrong. The bladder's sensation being lost, and with it normal reflex activity, it becomes large and atonic, and catheterization in such cases usually reveals several hundred millilitres of residual urine. Cystitis may bring the situation to light. Constipation is the rule, but faecal incontinence may occur, especially when the patient is unconscious of the act of defaecation. Impotence is frequently an early symptom.

Trophic lesions are an important part of the symptomatology. Arthropathies – Charcot's joints – are not uncommon. They appear to be the result of a loss of pain impulses from the joint, associated with wear and tear and sometimes trauma. The affected joint is swollen and almost always painless, and fluid may be present. X-ray changes show a combination of atrophic and hypertrophic changes. The joints of the lower limbs are most frequently affected, especially the knee, and after that the hip. Involvement of the lower dorsal and lumbar spine is common.

The commonest trophic change in the skin is the painless perforating ulcer, which is usually seen beneath the pad of the great toe or at other pressure points on the sole (Fig. 24.2).

Tabetic crises are paroxysmal painful disorders of function of various viscera which may occur in tabes, but are uncommon. The gastric crisis is the com-

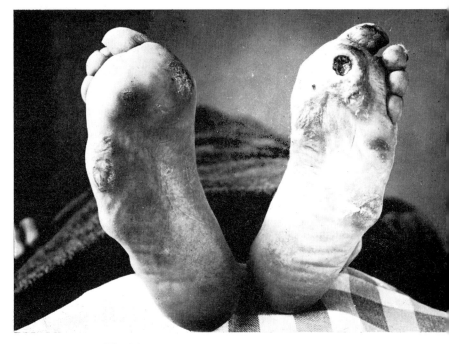

Fig. 24.2. Perforating ulcers in tabes dorsalis.

monest of these: it is characterized by attacks of epigastric pain associated with severe vomiting, lasting from a few hours to several days. Laryngeal, rectal, and vesical crises have also been described.

General paresis

The earliest symptoms are usually *mental*, and are frequently so slight at first as to be apparent only to those who know the patient well. It is important therefore, always to obtain a history from a relative or friend. The earliest mental change is usually an impairment of intellectual efficiency, with loss of the power to concentrate, and impairment of memory. The patient, however, lacks insight, and his inefficiency, though apparent to others, is not evident to himself. Exceptionally, however, anxiety may be prominent. As the condition progresses the patient's behaviour becomes more abnormal, and he is likely to become careless about his dress and personal appearance and about money, as the result of which he may throw large sums away in extravagant or ill-judged speculations. Alcoholic excess and sexual aberrations may occur. The commonest early mental changes are thus symptoms of dementia. Other clinical pictures, however, occur. The grandiose form, though frequently regarded as typical, is less common. Other emotional states may dominate the picture, leading to so-called depressed, agitated, and maniacal, types. As the patient becomes worse the symptoms of dementia become more prominent, and in the terminal stage there is little evidence of any mental activity. Speech exhibits a degradation parallel with that of other mental functions. Generalized or focal epileptiform attacks occur in approximately 50 per cent of cases and such attacks may suggest the diagnosis and may bring the patient under observation.

The facial expression is often vacant or fatuously smiling, sometimes somewhat mask-like. Optic atrophy is much less common than in tabes. The pupils are typically Argyll Robertson. Voluntary power becomes progressively impaired, and weakness is usually associated with tremor, which is most conspicuous on voluntary movement and is best seen in the facial muscles, especially the lips and the tongue, and in the outstretched fingers. The slow slurred speech is highly characteristic. In addition, incoordination usually develops during the later stages, rendering the gait unsteady and the movements of the upper limbs ataxic. Owing to bilateral degeneration of the corticospinal tracts, the tendon reflexes are usually exaggerated, the abdominal reflexes diminished or lost, and the plantar reflexes extensor. Loss of control over the sphincters is common at a comparatively early stage, but is then the outcome of the mental deterioration and not of a disorder of innervation at lower levels. There is usually a progressive loss of body weight.

Taboparesis is the term applied to a combination of the symptoms of tabes and general paresis in the same patient. In cases so described clinically the lesions are usually those of meningovascular syphilis associated with tabes.

Modified neurosyphilis

The classical forms of neurosyphilis are now less often encountered but possibly because of the use of antibiotics other unrelated diseases, patients present with atypical or modified symptoms including epilepsy and psychiatric disorders.

Congenital neurosyphilis

Active neurosyphilis occurs in from 8 to 10 per cent of congenitally syphilitic children. It does not differ either pathologically or clinically in any essential respect from the acquired form. Both meningovascular and parenchymatous neurosyphilis occur. The meningovascular form is much commoner than the parenchymatous. Both mental deficiency and convulsions are common. Mild hydrocephalus is common. Optic atrophy may be due to direct involvement of the optic nerves, or secondary to choroidoretinitis. Reflex iridoplegia is common, and the deafness of congenital syphilis may be present. Destruction of the corticospinal tract fibres may lead to diplegia or hemiplegia. Moderate degrees of infantilism are not uncommon.

Parenchymatous neurosyphilis is rare and it has been estimated that general paresis occurs in 1 per cent of congenital syphilitics. The symptoms are similar to those of the acquired form, and usually develop during the first half of the second decade. Congenital tabes usually develops somewhat later, and may not make its appearance until early adult life.

CHANGES IN THE CEREBROSPINAL FLUID AND BLOOD (see p. 000)

The c.s.f. specific serology and a high titre of c.s.f. VDRL indicate active disease and are negative in yaws which is endemic in the West Indies. The blood and c.s.f serology may remain negative in a few treated patients and in burnt out tabes but after specific treatment tests are usually positive. The cellular response in neurosyphilis is mononuclear with up to 200 cells, mainly lymphocytes. The c.s.f protein is almost always abnormal with an increase in total protein and a rise in the c.s.f IgG which was reflected by the previously used colloidal curve of Lange. This shows a first-zone elevation in paresis, a mid-zone rise in tabes and an end-zone rise in the meningitic form. These abnormalities may persist despite treatment.

An excess of globulin is usually found in the fluid when the protein content is raised, particularly in general paresis. An exceptionally acute meningeal reaction will lead to a greater excess of cells than usually found, and this is especially likely to occur in syphilitic meningomyelitis, when also the protein may be as high as 2.0 or 3.0 g/l, and exceptionally blockage of the spinal subarachnoid space may be present.

In congenital neurosyphilis the blood serology is usually positive when the condition is progressive, but may otherwise be negative. The cerebrospinal fluid usually shows the changes associated with the same form of the acquired disorder.

DIAGNOSIS

The clinical manifestations of neurosyphilis are so varied that its diagnosis covers a wide field. The diagnosis is of course considerably simplified by the serological reactions, and it is a wise plan to have the blood VDRL examined in the case of every patient suffering from a neurological disorder, the cause of which is not obviously non-syphilitic. It must be remembered, however, that syphilis leading to a positive blood VDRL may co-exist with a non-syphilitic condition such as a brain tumour, and, further, that a positive blood VDRL is not invariably even an indication of syphilitic infection (biological false-positive reaction). The treponemal microhaemagglutination test (MHA-TP) and the fluorescent treponemal antibody absorption test (FTA-ABS) are more specific and sensitive methods of detecting treponemal infection and remain positive after treatment, usually for the rest of the patient's life. Positive serological reactions in the blood or cerebrospinal fluid or both are particularly valuable in the case of patients with neurosyphilis in the following groups:

1. Those with mild mental disturbances as the presenting symptom, and few or no abnormal physical signs.

2. Those presenting with epilepsy.

3. Those presenting with the symptoms of a focal vascular lesion such as hemiplegia.

4. Cases of isolated cranial nerve palsy or optic neuritis.

5. To distinguish syphilitic amyotrophy from other conditions associated with muscular wasting.

Since meningovascular syphilis frequently causes multiple lesions of the cerebrospinal axis it may perhaps be confused with *multiple sclerosis*, in which, however, the pupillary reflexes are normal. Nystagmus and incoordination of the limbs in the absence of sensory loss are rare in syphilis and common in multiple sclerosis, in which also the tendon jerks are exaggerated, whereas in neurosyphilis thay are more often diminished or lost.

General paresis needs to be distinguished from other causes of dementia.

The lightning pains of tabes should not be mistaken for arthritis or sciatica if the nervous system is properly examined. In polyneuropathy the tendon reflexes are diminished or lost, the lower limbs are frequently ataxic and are the site of pain and impaired postural sensibility. In polyneuropathy, however, weakness of the peripheral muscles is conspicuous, and the deep tissues, especially the muscles, are tender on pressure and not, as in tabes, analgesic.

When ataxia is absent the prominence of some other symptom in tabes may lead to a mistake in diagnosis; for example, root pains in the trunk may be attributed to lesions of underlying viscera, gastric crises to ulceration of the stomach or duodenum, disturbances of the vesical sphincter to enlarged prostate, arthropathy to arthritis, and optic atrophy to toxic amblyopia. These mistakes can be avoided only by systematic examinations of the nervous system, and in doubtful cases examination of the blood and cerebrospinal fluid. On clinical grounds it should usually be possible to distinguish the tonic pupil (Holmes–Adie syndrome) from tabes.

PROGNOSIS

The introduction of penicillin has greatly reduced both the incidence and the mortality of neurosyphilis. The prognosis of meningovascular syphilis is on the whole good, and excellent results are often obtained from energetic treatment.

Tabes is extremely variable in its rate of progress and the extent to which it responds to treatment. A rapidly progressive course is rare, and usually the duration of the pre-ataxic stage lies between two and five years. Untreated general paralysis is fatal within five years.

Adequate treatment of general paresis with penicillin may be expected almost invariably to bring the infection to an end and to stabilize the patient in a condition somewhat better than that at which treatment was begun. Obviously, therefore, the earlier the diagnosis is made the better the outlook. The response to the treatment of congenital neurosyphilis is usually disappointing when it is symptoms of the nervous disorder which bring the patient for treatment.

TREATMENT

General management

Penicillin destroys the treponema, but only if treatment is adequate. This is therefore the foundation of treatment. After a preliminary examination of the blood and cerebrospinal fluid, an adult should be given 1–2 mega-units of procaine penicillin intramuscularly daily for at leat 12 days. Is there any risk of a Herxheimer reaction, that is a severe exacerbation of symptoms resulting from the widespread destruction of the organism? It occurs in 5 per cent of cases and can be avoided by treatment with tetracycline 2 g daily for 20 days or erythromycin, though the long-term effectiveness of these drugs is uncertain. If there is any special reason to fear it, the patient may be given a preliminary course of prednisolone, 30 mg/day by mouth for 10 days. After treatment the patient is kept under clinical observation, and it is wise to examine the blood and cerebrospinal fluid every six months for two years. A cerebrospinal fluid initially abnormal is not likely to have become normal at the end of six months, so an abnormality persisting then is not in itself a reason for further treatment. Sometimes patients in whom the clinical course of the disease appears to be arrested continue to manifest a positive serology reaction in the blood or the cerebrospinal fluid or both. Such patients may benefit from a further course of penicillin, but if their clinical condition remains satisfactory a positive serology reaction by itself is no indication for the indefinite continuance of treatment. Erythromycin, 500 mg four times daily for 20 days, is the drug of choice in patients unable to tolerate penicillin.

Treatment of special symptoms in tabes

Pain

When severe, tabetic pains are sometimes alleviated by penicillin. Carbamezepine may also be effective. If these drugs fail, it may be necessary to have recourse to spinal cordotomy.

Ataxia

Co-ordination of the limbs may be improved by suitable re-educational exercises.

The bladder

The residual urine should be estimated, and, if the bladder is uninfected, the patients should be instructed to empty the bladder every three hours during the day, if necessary with the aid of manual pressure on the hypogastrium. The atonic bladder should not be treated surgically unless there is impairment of renal function or infection of the urinary tract which has failed to respond to chemotherapy. The choice will then lie between transurethral division of the internal sphincter which sometimes succeeds, and suprapubic cystostomy (p. 385).

Crises

Patients subject to gastric crises should take a bland, non-irritating diet together with alkalis. A crisis can frequently be cut short by the slow intravenous injection of phenobarbitone, repeated if necessary. When pain is very severe, cordotomy may be necessary.

Perforating ulcer

Tabetic patients should wear well-fitting shoes and should be warned against cutting their corns on account of the risk that a perforating ulcer may follow a slight injury. When an ulcer has developed the foot must be rested and the thickened epidermis should be softened by repeated hot fomentations and carefully pared away with a sharp razor.

Arthropathy

The object of treatment is to relieve the strain on the damaged joint. The knee and ankle may be supported by a leather corset strengthened with steel. When the hip or knee is affected, a walking caliper will be required. Spinal arthropathy necessitates a leather corset or spinal brace.

REFERENCES

Luxon, L., Lees, A.J., and Greenwood, R.J. (1979). Neurosyphilis today. *Lancet* **i**, 90–3.

Oates, J.K. (1979). Serological tests for syphilis and their clinical use. *Br. J. hosp. Med.* **21**, 612–17.

Oriel, J.D. (1982). Serological tests for syphilis. *Br. med. J.* **285**, 759–61.

Sparling, P.F. (1971). Diagnosis and treatment of syphilis. *New Engl. J. Med.* **284**, 642–53.

Tramont, E.C. (1976). Persistence of *Treponema pallidum* following penicillin G therapy. *J. Am. med. Ass.* **236**, 2206–7.

Part IV
Diffuse and system disorders

25 Deficiency disorders

In starvation and malabsorption neurological symptoms and signs may be caused by a wide variety of deficiencies. In addition to lack of vitamins, there may be a lack of glucose and minerals, particularly calcium, potassium, magnesium, sodium, or iron. The relationship of dietary deficiency to toxic factors is sometimes complex. For example, excessive cyanide intake from foods or from smoking may play a part in the production of the neurological symptoms of 'tobacco' amblyopia and Leber's optic atrophy, because vitamin B_{12} is concerned in the detoxication of cyanide. Cyanide may also play a role in the production of neurological symptoms in vitamin B_{12} neuropathy. In some neurological syndromes found in the tropics it is difficult to separate dietary factors and the effects of certain chronic inflammatory disease, such as syphilis. Sometimes a deficiency may be induced or aggravated by drugs. For example isoniazid may cause a deficiency of pyridoxine (B_6) and anticonvulsants may lead to a deficiency of folate and B_{12}.

THE B GROUP OF VITAMINS

Experimental work has led to the isolation of a number of factors in the vitamin B complex, some of which are important in relation to nervous diseases. The B group of vitamins are present in greatest amount in brewers' yeast, in the germ (aleurone) layer of ripe wheat, and also in egg yolk and mammalian liver, and in smaller amounts in milk, green vegetables, potatoes, and meat.

Vitamin B_1 (aneurine or thiamine) plays an important part in the metabolism of carbohydrates. A deficiency of this vitamin leads to an accumulation of pyruvate in the blood, and is the cause of polyneuropathy (beriberi) and Wernicke's encephalopathy. Nicotinic acid acts as a co-enzyme in intracellular oxidation processes. Deficiency of nicotinic acid is probably the most important factor in the causation of pellagra, and it has also been held responsible for confusional states in elderly patients with arteriosclerosis.

Pyridoxine: B_6 (pyridoxine) is needed for a co-enzyme involved in decarboxylation and transamination and deficiency can result from a dietary insufficiency, malabsorption, or from drugs which antagonize its action such as isoniazid or penicillamine. The clinical syndrome which results is a sensory neuropathy, so-called 'burning feet', and optic neuropathy.

Deficiency of cyanocobalamin (vitamin B_{12}) is the cause of subacute combined degeneration, better described as vitamin B_{12} neuropathy. In conditions of gross malnutrition there is often a lack of more than one vitamin, and the clinical picture is correspondingly mixed.

BERIBERI

Beriberi is due to deficiency of thiamine. In the tropics it is usually caused by lack of this vitamin in the diet. In temperate climates it is rare, and when it occurs is usually the result of conditioned deficiency due to defective absorption caused by some form of gastrointestinal disease or alcoholism. What part vitamin B_1 deficiency plays in the causation of alcoholic polyneuropathy is uncertain.

The pathological changes in the nervous system in beriberi are those of axonal degeneration (p. 392). There may also be myocardial degeneration and the changes in the viscera associated with myocardial failure.

The clinical picture is that of polyneuropathy (p. 419), which may develop acutely or more insidiously. The 'wet form' is also characterized by congestive cardiac failure.

The blood pyruvic acid is raised from a normal content of 40–80 mmol/l to an average of 120 mmol/l in subacute cases and 200 mmol/l in fulminating cases. A rise in the blood level after giving glucose is the basis of the pyruvate tolerance test.

The diagnosis of polyneuropathy is discussed on page 419.

In untreated fulminating cases, death may occur within a few days from heart failure, but most patients who receive early and thorough treatment during the acute stage make a complete recovery.

Treatment consists of rest in bed. The diet should consist of frequent small feeds with a minimum of carbohydrate and fluid. Aneurine should be injected intravenously. As much as 50 mg may be given in this way if necessary on the first day, and smaller doses on subsequent days as required. 10 mg should be given daily by mouth, together with yeast and Marmite. In gross malnutrition when the vitamin deficiency is multiple, vitamin B complex should be given by intramuscular injection (for example Parentovite). The usual treatment of polyneuropathy should be carried out, and the underlying cause of the vitamin deficiency should be dealt with.

TROPICAL ATAXIC NEUROPATHY

A generalized neuropathy associated with optic atrophy (p.42) has been described in the indigenous peoples of southern Nigeria. This 'tropical ataxic neuropathy' is of great interest because the principal element in these patients' diet is cassava which contains the cyanogenetic glycosides, linamarin, and their plasma cyanide level is abnormally high. The neuropathy may therefore result from interference with B_{12} metabolism.

Other tropical nutritional disorders cause neurological syndromes. For example, in central India, eating the seeds of the sweet pea (*Lathyrus sativus*) causes a spastic paraparesis. The toxic factor is oxalyl aminoalanine.

ALCOHOL AND THE NERVOUS SYSTEM

Wernicke's encephalopathy

This syndrome appears to be due mainly to thiamine deficiency. Its causes are the same as those of beriberi and include persistent vomiting of pregnancy and malnutrition associated with carcinoma of the stomach. In the alcoholic it is usually associated with the Korsakoff's syndrome (p. 422). The lesions are present in the paraventricular part of the medial thalamic and hypothalamic nuclei, the mammillary bodies, the periaqueductal grey region around the fourth ventricle, and the anterior superior vermis of the cerebellum. The posterior and posterior lateral hypothalamic lesions are probably the cause of the hypothermia which sometimes occurs. Patients also have a high cardiac output, low peripheral resistance, and low blood pressure which are due to the sympathetic efferent lesion and associated denervation supersensitivity to sympathetic drugs (see p. 124).

Optic atrophy and peripheral neuropathy

These are due to thiamine deficiency resembling beriberi with a prominent autonomic component. An associated nicotinic acid deficiency probably contributes both to the neuropathy and mental changes which are similar to those occurring with a pure nicotinic acid deficiency in pellagra.

Other central degenerative changes whose precise cause is unknown and which occur in alcoholism, include diffuse cerebral cortical atrophy, cerebellar degeneration, myelopathy, myopathy, and a 'flapping' tremor.

Rare central disturbances include mental deterioration associated with degeneration of central white matter, particularly of the corpus collosum (Machiafava–Bignami disease), possibly caused by some toxic factor in certain Italian red wines.

Central pontine myelinolysis is a rapidly progressive deterioration to coma and death with demyelination of the central pons, which also occurs in terminal carcinoma and other debilitating diseases.

Other neurological disturbances in the alcoholic include acute intoxication, head injury, subdural haematomas, hepatic encephalopathy, and B_{12} deficiency.

Withdrawal states in the alcoholic include hallucinations, delirium tremens, tremors, and epileptic seizures. Many of the withdrawal symptoms are essentially sympathetic overactivity with dilated pupils, tremor, tachycardia, sweating, anxiety, and circulatory collapse. Similar tremors can be induced by adrenaline or isoprenaline. The withdrawal syndrome may in part result from overactivity of beta-adrenergic receptors in the intrafusal fibres of the muscles spindles, though the beneficial affect of the beta blockers is probably the result of a central not a peripheral action. It is also possible that alcohol causes a progressive blockade of central adrenergic receptors and on withdrawal of alcohol the receptors become hypersensitive to catecholamines.

VITAMIN B$_{12}$ NEUROPATHY (SUBACUTE COMBINED DEGENERATION OF THE SPINAL CORD)

Aetiology and pathology

Vitamin B$_{12}$ or cyanocobalamin appears to be essential for normal haemopoiesis and for the nutrition of the nervous system. Its absorption from the intestine depends primarily upon the presence of a glycoprotein secreted by the parietal cells of the normal gastric mucosa known as the intrinsic factor. Intrinsic factor is also a normal constituent of the diet and with B$_{12}$ is necessary for the normal synthesis of DNA which is in turn necessary for the normal division of bone marrow cells. Vitamin B$_{12}$ deficiency therefore may be due to an absence of the intrinsic factor or to a failure of absorption from some other cause. The commonest cause of absence of the intrinsic factor is Addisonian pernicious anaemia, in which there is a hereditary tendency to atrophy of the gastric mucosal glands leading to gastric achlorhydria and later to disappearance of the intrinsic factor. The same result may follow other disorders causing atrophy of the gastric mucosa, and total gastrectomy, less frequently partial gastrectomy, and occasionally carcinoma of the stomach. Defective absorption of vitamin B$_{12}$ may be the result of disease of the small intestine, especially tropical sprue and idiopathic steatorrhoea, regional ileitis, and resections, diverticulosis and fistulae of the small intestine, or in countries such as Finland, infestation with a fish tapeworm *Diphyllobothrium latum*. Very occasionally B$_{12}$ intake may be inadequate in strict vegetarians. Neurological disturbances similar to those in vitamin B$_{12}$ neuropathy have occasionally been described in patients with a megaloblastic anaemia due to anticonvulsants or malabsorption syndromes, in whom there is a folate deficiency but not a vitamin B$_{12}$ deficiency.

The neurological symptoms associated with B$_{12}$ deficiency are not likely to be due to a folate inter-related process because the anaemia and subacute combined degeneration frequently present independently of each other. Also, unlike the anaemia, subacute combined degeneration is not associated with folate deficiency and whereas B$_{12}$ deficiency responds to folic acid therapy, subacute combined degeneration either fails to respond or become worse. The precise nature of the B$_{12}$ dependant process that underlines the subacute combined degeneration remains unknown. Folate deficiency occurs in pregnancy, after a poor diet and as a result of drugs, including the oral contraceptive drugs and anticonvulsants.

The term subacute combined degeneration, invented to describe the combination of changes in the posterior and lateral columns of the spinal cord, is a

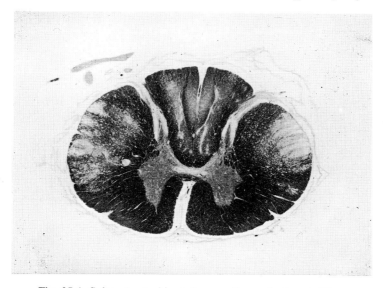

Fig. 25.1. Subacute combined degeneration; spinal cord, C3.

bad one for various reasons, but chiefly because the nervous system is much more widely affected than that would imply. Degeneration occurs in the peripheral nerves. In the spinal cord (Fig. 25.1) there are necrotic foci and degeneration of the long tracts, which is most marked in the posterior columns and the cortico-spinal and ascending cerebellar tracts; in the upper part of the cord in the ascending tracts, and in the lower part in the descending tracts. Both types of lesion are characterized by demyelination and the disappearance of both myelin sheaths and the axis cylinders leaves vacuolated spaces separated by a fine glial meshwork. Similar focal and more diffuse degenerative changes have been described in the cerebral association fibres.

Vitamin B_{12} neuropathy is a disorder chiefly of middle life, the average age of onset being about 50, but with a spread of twenty or more years on either side. The sexes are equally affected, in contrast to the female preponderance in pernicious anaemia.

Symptoms

The clinical picture in most cases is a mixture of signs of the peripheral nerve and spinal cord degeneration, with, on occasion, cerebral signs. The onset is insidious, the patient first noticing tingling and numbness of the extremities, the toes usually being affected before the fingers. The parasethesiae tend to spread slowly up the lower limbs towards and up the trunk, and similarly up the upper limbs. Pains of a stabbing character sometimes occur. Motor symptoms consisting of weakness and ataxia develop at a variable period after the paraes-thesiae and begin in the lower limbs. Cutaneous sensibility to light touch, pin-prick, heat and cold is impaired at first over the periphery of the extremities, leading to the characteristic 'glove-and-stocking' distribution of superficial sensory loss. Postural sensibility and appreciation of passive movement and of vibration are impaired first in the lower and later in the upper limbs. In some cases weakness and spasticity predominate in the lower limbs, in others ataxia, leading to an ataxic gait and the presence of Romberg's sign. Moderate muscular wasting is usually present, especially in the peripheral muscles of the limbs.

The reflexes vary considerably. In more than half the cases the ankle-jerks are absent when the patient comes under observation; the knee-jerks are lost rather less frequently. Occasionally both are exaggerated. The plantar reflexes are flexor at first in about 50 per cent of cases, but later become extensor in all but a small proportion. Impotence occurs early, and the sphincter disturbances are characteristic of a spinal cord lesion. Mental deterioration and primary optic atrophy are among the less common symptoms. Mental symptoms may occasionally be a presenting feature of B_{12} deficiency. The symptoms range from irritability and mild confusion to frank psychosis, often with paranoid features. Vitamin B_{12} deficiency is one of the possible organic causes of 'psychiatric' symptoms which may be overlooked.

When vitamin B_{12} neuropathy is a symptom of Addisonian anaemia, gastric achlorhydria is constantly present, and the blood and bone marrow show the changes characteristic of the anaemia, though the actual degree of anaemia may be slight. Glossitis appears to be more closely related to the anaemia than to the neuropathy.

Diagnosis

In a classical case the insidious onset and slow spread of the sensory symptoms should suggest the diagnosis and call for a gastric test meal and blood examination. Vitamin B_{12} neuropathy may occur without anaemia or even obvious changes in the blood film or bone marrow. However, even in the non-anaemic patient, it may be diagnosed by estimating the serum vitamin B_{12} level. The normal level of vitamin B_{12} in the serum is from 100 to 960 pg per ml. In vitamin B_{12} neuropathy it is usually below 80 pg per ml. The cause of the deficiency can usually be established by the radioactive B_{12} absorption test. In pernicious anaemia the absorption of oral vitamin B_{12} is improved when the dose is given with intrinsic factor, but there is no improvement if the defect is due to an intestinal lesion. The association of megaloblastic anaemia and neurological symptoms and signs does not always mean that the signs are due to vitamin B_{12} deficiency. In patients with a poor diet or who have been receiving prolonged treatment with barbiturates or other anticonvulsant drugs the serum folate level should also be estimated. Moreover, there is a recognized association between Addisonian pernicious anaemia and diabetes, myxoedema and rheumatoid arthritis, all of which may also cause neuropathy.

If the spinal cord symptoms are minimal or even absent the condition may be confused with other forms of polyneuropathy. If the polyneuropathic element is slight or absent, it may simulate disseminated sclerosis or compression of the spinal cord. Difficulty may arise from the coexistence of cervical spondylosis with vitamin B_{12} neuropathy, the spondlyosis being regarded as the sole cause of the symptoms. The ataxic gait and loss of ankle-jerks may be attributed to tabes dorsalis, especially if pain is a symptom, but the normal pupils and serological reactions enable that to be excluded.

Prognosis

The average duration of the illness of Addisonian anaemia before the introduction of treatment with vitamin B_{12} was about two years. Now it is possible to maintain the patient in good health indefinitely, and there is no reason why such patients should develop vitamin B_{12} neuropathy. When this has already developed it can always be arrested, but the degree of recovery depends upon the stage at which the degeneration of the nervous system has reached. The peripheral nerves can regenerate, but not the spinal cord, though even there already damaged fibres may be restored to normal. A striking improvement may therefore be expected in the polyneuritic symptoms, but extensor plantar reflexes, spastic weakness and gross loss of postural sensibility usually persist unchanged.

Treatment

Treatment consists of giving the patient vitamin B_{12} parenterally, which must be continued for life. When the patient first comes under treatment, 1000 μg of hydroxocobalamin can be given by injection two or three times a week for the first two weeks, and thereafter a dose of 500 μg every three months. Folic acid should never be given alone in megaloblastic anaemia with neurological signs because the sudden uptake of the little available vitamin B_{12} by the marrow for erythopoiesis will further deplete the nervous system of vitamin B_{12} and may provoke a neurological crisis. Re-educational exercises are helpful, and in advanced cases the usual care of the skin, bladder, rectum and paralysed muscles necessitated by paraplegia will be required.

REFERENCES

Huddin, V. (1980). Impairments of the nervous system in alcoholics. In *Addiction and brain damage* (ed. D. Richter) pp. 168–200. Croom Helm, London.

Harper, C. (1979). Wernicke's encephalopathy: a more common disease than realised. *J. Neurol. Neurosurg. Psychiat.* **42,** 226–31.

Le Quesne, P.M. (1981). Toxic substances and the nervous system: the role of clinical observation. *J. Neurol. Neurosurg. Psychiat.* **44,** 1–8.

Lishman, W.A. (1981). Cerebral disorder in alcoholism: syndromes of impairment. *Brain* **104,** 1–20.

McEntee, W.J. and Mair, R.G. (1978). Memory impairment in Korsakoff's psychosis: a correlation with brain noradrenergic activity. *Science, NY* **202,** 905–7.

Pallis, C.A. and Lewis, P.D. (1974). *The neurology of gastrointestinal disease.* Saunders, Philadelphia.

Scott, J.M., Dinn, J.J., Wilson, P., and Weir, D.G. (1981). Pathogenesis of subacute combined degeneration: a result of methyl group deficiency. *Lancet* **ii**, 334–7.

Shorvon, S.D., Carney, M.W.P., Chanarin, I., and Reynolds, E.H. (1980). The neuropsychiatry of megaloblastic anaemia. *Br. med. J.* **281**, 1036–8.

Victor, M., Adams, R.D., and Collins, G.H. (1971). *The Wernicke-Korsakoff's syndrome.* Blackwell, Oxford.

26 Genetically determined degenerations of the nervous system

Certain regions of the nervous system are, for reasons which we do not yet clearly understand, particularly vulnerable to genetically determined degenerative disorders. These structures include the optic nerves, the cerebral cortex, the cerebellum, the olives, the long tracts of the spinal cord and the peripheral nerves. The different systems of the nervous system which appear to be vulnerable will be grouped under separate headings but though in any particular syndrome the most prominent damage affects one part of the nervous system, there is frequently less obvious involvement of other vulnerable parts of the nervous system. Degenerative processes which affect the optic nerve (p. 42) and cerebral cortex (p. 256) are considered elsewhere in the book.

The age of onset ranges from childhood to middle life, and the course of the disease is slowly progressive. The commonest and best known is Friedreich's ataxia. Hereditary ataxia and paraplegia may be inherited either as a dominant or as a recessive. As in the case of other inherited disorders, sporadic cases are not much less common than familial ones. The sexes are affected about equally.

SPINOCEREBELLAR DEGENERATIONS

In these genetically determined degenerations there is predominant involvement of the cerebellum but the sensory and motor systems from the peripheral nerve up to the spinal cord and brainstem are also at risk. These systems are clearly vulnerable to a number of different biochemical defects of which only a few are known. The main different types will be listed and a few of the commonest will be described to illustrate the whole group. No satisfactory classification exists.

PREDOMINANTLY CEREBELLAR ATAXIAS

1. Friedreich's ataxia.
2. Roussy–Levy syndrome, similar to Friedreich's ataxia but onset in childhood without as much evidence of spinal cord involvement.
3. Olivo-ponto-cerebellar atrophy.
4. Refsum's syndrome (see p. 28).
5. Late-onset hereditary cerebellar degeneration.

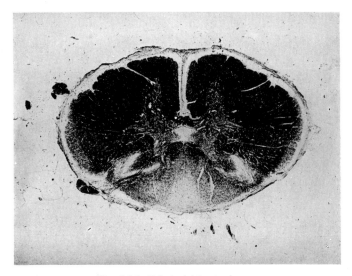

Fig. 26.1. Friedreich's ataxia.

6. Hereditary dentatorubral degeneration, sometimes with myoclonus.
7. Some cases of hereditary spastic paraplegia.

Friedreich's ataxia

Pathology

The spinal cord is unusually small. Histologically the degeneration is most marked in the posterior columns and next in the lateral columns, especially the corticospinal tracts and the posterior spinocerebellar tracts. The dorsal root fibres also exhibit degeneration (Fig. 26.1). The heart may show a diffuse change, enlargement being caused by thickening of the muscle and a diffuse fibrosis.

Symptoms

The age of onset, interpreted as the age at which symptoms first bring the patient under observation, is usually between 5 and 15 years. It is the ataxic gait which usually first attracts attention. In the later stages movements of the upper limbs also become ataxic, and intention tremor is present. Speech also is dysarthric in the later stages. Nystagmus is present in most cases, and weakness due to the corticospinal tract degeneration complicates the ataxia, the plantar reflexes being extensor. The tendon reflexes tend to be lost, the ankle-jerks before the knee-jerks. Sensory changes are inconstant, but postural sense and appreciation of movement are not infrequently impaired, especially in the lower limbs. The sphincters are usually unaffected. Pes cavus and scoliosis are present in almost all cases, the former being usually associated with a slight contracture of the muscles of the calf. Optic atrophy occasionally occurs and retinal pigmentation has been described. Wasting of the hands, occasionally being present, has been held to indicate a relationship to peroneal muscular atrophy. The cardiac changes may lead to heart failure, heart block, and electrocardiographic abnormalities.

Prognosis

Friedreich's ataxia is in most cases slowly but steadily progressive. Occasionally, however, it appears to become arrested, and abortive cases are encountered, for example in apparently healthy members of affected families. Few patients, however, live for more than twenty years after the onset of symptoms.

Progressive cerebellar degeneration

Not all forms of progressive cerebellar degeneration are familial or hereditary, but they exhibit a considerable clinical and pathological similarity. In primary parenchymatous degeneration of the cerebellum, which appears to be identical with delayed cortical cerebellar atrophy, there is a degeneration of the ganglion cells of all three cortical layers of the cerebellum, with atrophy and gliosis of the olives. In olivopontocerebellar atrophy there is atrophy of the ganglion cells of the olives with degeneration of the middle cerebellar peduncles, and the cerebellum itself suffers mainly secondarily.

It is difficult to distinguish these conditions clinically. They are essentially degenerative disorders, beginning in early life or late middle life, and characterized by symptoms of cerebellar deficiency, mainly dysarthria, ataxia and tremor of the limbs, and an ataxic gait. Mental deterioration may occur in the later stages.

Hereditary spastic paraplegia

This is a disorder, allied to the hereditary ataxias, in which the maximal degeneration is found in the corticospinal tracts of the spinal cord, with slighter changes in the posterior columns. The age of onset varies from childhood to middle age. The initial symptoms are those of a progressive spastic paraplegia, which later extends to involve the upper limbs and the bulbar muscles. The disorder usually affects several siblings, with or without a history of cases in previous generations.

Diagnosis of the hereditary ataxias

The diagnosis of the hereditary ataxias rests upon the onset early in life of progressive symptoms, of which ataxia is the most conspicuous, and which occur in several members of the same family. The presence of scoliosis, pes cavus, and loss of the knee- and ankle-jerks, distinguishes Friedreich's ataxia from disseminated sclerosis, while the presence of these deformities, the absence of pain, the normal pupils, nystagmus and extensor plantar responses, distinguish it from tabes dorsalis. The progressive cerebellar degenerations of later life must be distinguished from tumours in the posterior fossa.

Treatment

No treatment influences the course of these degenerations, but re-educational exercises may help to keep the ataxia under control.

PREDOMINANTLY SPINAL MUSCULAR ATROPHIES

1. Acute infantile spinal muscular atrophy (Werdnig–Hoffmann), autosomal recessive.
2. Pseudo-myopathic familial spinal muscular atrophy (Kugelberg–Welander) autosomal recessive, other types being dominant.
3. Scapulo-peroneal form of spinal muscular atrophy, may be recessive or dominant.
4. Distal spinal muscular atrophy.
5. Amyotrophy in the heredofamilial ataxias (Friedreich's ataxia, hereditary spastic paraplegia, and hereditary cerebellar degeneration).

PREDOMINANTLY MOTOR NERVE ROOT GENETICALLY DETERMINED DEGENERATIONS

1. Peroneal muscular atrophy (Charcot–Marie–Tooth disease) an autosomal dominant, recessive or X-linked disturbance, either of the demyelinating type, with hypertrophy of nerves, enlargement of myelin sheaths with Schwann cell proliferations or axonal or intermediate type; the intermediate type with axonal degeneration is also known as the Roussy–Levy syndrome.
2. Hereditary hypertrophic interstitial neuritis (Dejerine and Sottas).
3. Heredopathic atactica polyneuritiformis (Refsum's syndrome).

In addition there are familial recurrent neuropathies sometimes with recurrent pressure palsies. The numbers of conditions in this group are growing as more metabolic defects are revealed. They include alpha-lipoproteinaemic neuropathy (Tangier disease), glycosphingolipoidosis (Fabry's disease), familial dysautonomia, primary hyperoxaluria, and primary amyloid.

PERONEAL MUSCULAR ATROPHY

Peroneal muscular atrophy, or Charcot–Marie–Tooth disease, is a hereditary form of progressive muscular atrophy. The pathological change is widespread segmental demyelination and hypertrophic changes with Schwann cell proliferation and interstitial neuritis, chiefly affecting the branches of the common peroneal nerve, together with degeneration of the ganglion cells of the anterior horns, the corticospinal tracts, and the posterior columns of the spinal cord.

Wasting and weakness, symmetrically on both sides, begin usually in the second decade in the peronei, extensor digitorum longus and small muscles of the feet. 'Claw feet' and a steppage gait result. Some years later wasting of the hand muscles begins. Characteristically the wasting spreads proximally, not involving the muscles longitudinally but transversely, and usually stopping at the elbows and mid-thighs. Fasciculation may be present and the tendon jerks and plantar reflexes are lost. There is usually distal impairment of cutaneous, less often of postural, sensibility.

Several members of the family are usually affected, but abortive forms of the disease, limited perhaps to claw feet, are sometimes encountered in siblings. The disease runs a very slow course and may become arrested at any stage. It is uninfluenced by treatment, but does not usually shorten life.

NEUROFIBROMATOSIS

Neurofibromatosis, or von Recklinghausen's disease, is inherited as a Mendelian dominant, though its severity varies greatly in different members of the same family. It is characterized by cutaneous pigmentation, and tumours in various situations, especially the peripheral nerves (neurofibroma) and the skin (cutaneous fibroma and molluscum fibrosum). The neurofibromas are tumours usually situated upon peripheral nerves, and probably derived from perineural fibroblasts thus differing from the acoustic schwannoma derived from cells of the neurilemma. Neurofibromas may also occur on spinal nerve roots, and meningiomas and gliomas are occasionally found in neurofibromatosis.

Neurofibromas upon the peripheral nerves are seen and felt as movable, firm, bead-like nodules along the course of the cutaneous nerves. They may be tender and are rarely painful. Cutaneous pigmentation is the most constant symptom and consists of brownish spots, *café au lait* in colour, ranging in size from a pin's head to large plaques, occasionally with a spinal segmental distribution. Cutaneous fibromas are soft pinkish sessile or pedunculated swellings varying in size from a pin's head to an orange. Kyphoscoliosis is often present. Neurofibromatosis is unimportant except when symptoms arise from a tumour within the cranial cavity or spinal canal, or when a neurofibroma becomes sarcomatous. The peripheral lesions rarely need treatment.

REFERENCES

Baraitser, M. (1982). *The genetics of neurological disorders.* Oxford University Press.
Greenfield, J.G. (1954). *The spino-cerebellar degenerations.* Blackwell, Oxford.
Harding, A.E. (1981). Friedreich's ataxia: a clinical and genetic study of 90 families with an analyses of early diagnostic criteria and intrafamilial clustering of clinical features. *Brain* **104**, 589–620.
Harding, A.E. (1983). Classification of the hereditary ataxias and paraplegias. *Lancet* **i**, 1151–5.

27 Multiple sclerosis

Multiple sclerosis is one of the commonest nervous diseases. It is characterized by the widespread occurrence of patches of demyelination followed by gliosis in the white matter of the nervous system (Fig. 27.1). A striking feature is the tendency to remissions and relapses, so that the course of the disease may be prolonged for many years. The early symptoms are those of focal lesions of the nervous system, while the later clinical picture is one of progressive dissemination. The cause of the disorder is not known.

Aetiology and pathology

The pathological 'unit' in multiple sclerosis is a patch in the white matter of the brain or spinal cord (Fig. 27.1). Some plaques are perivenular and the acute changes include a perivenular lymphocytic response. In the acute stage the myelin sheaths degenerate and the perivascular spaces contain fat-granule cells and lymphocytes. The axis cylinders are less affected. In the late patches the damaged myelin has been removed, and a glial overgrowth leads to a sclerotic plaque which to the naked eye looks slightly sunken, greyish, and more translucent than normal nervous tissue. There is pathological similarity to the

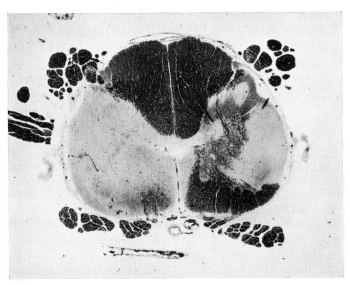

Fig. 27.1. Multiple sclerosis.

demyelination occurring acutely in acute disseminated encephalomyelitis (p. 458) though the tempo of the process clearly differs.

The physiology of conduction block in multiple sclerosis

The safety factor for conduction of a nerve impulse depends on the ratio of the action current generated by the impulse to the action current needed to maintain conduction. This is normally between 5 and 10, enough to excite the second adjacent node of Ravier or a distance of approximately 4 mm. As demyelination occurs and the safety factor approaches zero a marked lability occurs. Warming shortens the action potential duration. Signs of multiple sclerosis can be modified both favourably (by cooling) and unfavourably, by excessive warming by a hot bath. This is the basis of Uithoff's sign: a deterioration in symptoms by warming the patient. Exercise has a similar adverse affect.

The fundamental nature of the disturbance which leads to multiple sclerosis is unknown, and hence has been the subject of much speculation. It is characteristic of this elusive disease that we know some facts about its causation in some cases, but these do not at present add up to a complete picture. The main facts may be grouped under several headings.

1. *Geographic distribution.* Multiple sclerosis is common in temperate climates, particularly in the northern hemisphere and is rare in the tropics. Immigrants who have spent their childhood in countries with a low or high incidence seem to carry their susceptibility from their country of origin. Conversely, negroes, who migrated to colder northern areas centuries ago, though relatively immune in Africa and Jamaica, now seem to share the higher risk with white men. The Japanese with a low risk of multiple sclerosis carry the same risk wherever they live.

2. *Genetic factors.* Some 10 per cent of cases are familial, usually in siblings. The concordance rates are double in monozygotic as opposed to dizygotic twins. Early antecedent exposure of a family seems to be more important than any genetic influence. Conjugal cases are extremely rare. The relative risk of developing MS in people who have HLA-DR2 is approximately five times that in people without DR2. There is as yet no significant association between multiple sclerosis and organ specific autoimmune disease.

3. *Precipitating factors.* A large variety of events may immediately precede the onset of the illness and may reasonably be regarded as precipitating factors, though their mode of operation is unknown. These include influenza and infections of the upper respiratory tract, the specific fevers, pregnancy, the puerperium and lactation, surgical operations, the extraction of teeth, and electric shock. Trauma may occasionally act as a precipitant, but the large number of war-wounded men who do not develop the disease shows that the causal importance of trauma is slight.

4. *Biochemical factors.* Myelin is 75 per cent lipids and 25 per cent proteins, the basic protein being a single folded chain of about 170 amino acids. This basic protein is one of the first components to be broken down in demyelination and

enzymes that do so have been found at the edge of plaques. Fatty acid metabolism is abnormal in patients with multiple sclerosis, with a reduction in serum and brain polyunsaturated fats even in apparently structurally normal areas of the brain. Dietary intake of polyunsaturated fats is low in geographical areas where multiple sclerosis is commoner. Other unexplained biochemical defects in multiple sclerosis patients include an increased platelet adhesiveness.

5. *Immunological factors.* Abnormal humoral and cell mediated responses to encephalitogenic factor, one of the basic constituents of myelin, can be detected in many cases of multiple sclerosis. The abnormality seems to be an immunological hyperactivity towards brain antigens, including basic myelin protein, towards leucocytes, and towards viruses (especially measles). Measles and possibly other viruses may have antigens which share the same determinants as central nervous system antigens, like encephalitogenic protein. In addition, there is evidence of a demyelinating antibody present at the edge of a plaque where demyelination is proceeding, which is toxic to glial cells in culture, so causing demyelination but not axonal destruction. Further antibodies have been described with a synapse blocking effect. There is also evidence of abnormal immunoglobulin synthesis and many patients' sera have antibodies of the IgM class but of low titre. The level of T suppressor lymphocytes in the peripheral blood has been reported to fall in a relapse.

6. *Viral factors.* Evidence linking viruses with the aetiology of multiple sclerosis consists of the increased incidence of high antibody titres to viruses including measles, herpes simplex virus, mumps, and vaccinia in both the blood and c.s.f. The presence of paramyxovirus particles resembling measles virus has been reported in cultures of pathological specimens in multiple sclerosis but these reports are unconfirmed. Brains and lymph nodes from multiple sclerosis patients have been reported to have a granulopenic effect in rodents which can be transmitted, therefore suggesting the possibility of a virus particle. Interest in viruses as possible aetiological agents first arose from a study of scrapie, a disease of sheep. The scrapie agent is a 'slow' virus and scrapie was produced in sheep after injection of material containing nervous tissue from patients with multiple sclerosis. Such experiments probably represent no more than activation of a latent infection by non-specific stimuli.

7. *'Models' of multiple sclerosis.* Experimental allergic encephalomyelitis, produced in animals by intradermal injection of heterologous brain homogenate with adjuvant, consists of demyelination, but the course is progressive and either fatal or self-limiting; it is therefore unlike the human disease of multiple sclerosis, but resembles post-infective or allergic encephalomyelitis. The antigen responsible for experimental allergic encephalomyelitis has been shown to be a basic protein of myelin, now purified and identified.

A possible link between the virus and allergic and genetic factors could be provided by the capacity of the presumed virus to modify the cell membranes so that the neurones or glia would be regarded as 'non-self'. If the virus is attached to oligodendrocytes which produce myelin, these cells may be

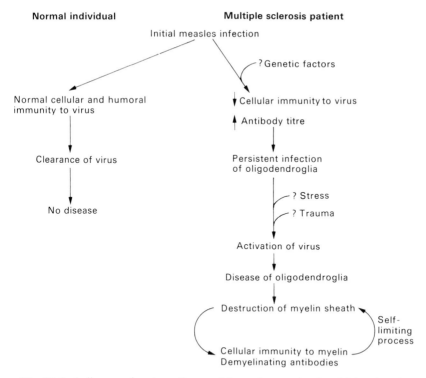

Fig. 27.2. A diagram showing a theory of the pathogenesis of multiple sclerosis.

sufficiently damaged by an immunological response for the myelin to break down. This could lead to the release of protein fractions thus stimulating a further anti-myelin reaction (Fig. 27.2). Genetic factors can be built into this hypothesis in that the nature of the immunological reactions – acute, subacute, and chronic – is probably in part at least genetically determined. The HLA A3, B7, and DR2 histocompatibility determinants which are linked to the immune response genes are some three times less common in patients with multiple sclerosis.

Its prevalence in England and Wales is about 1 in 2000 of the population. The disease principally attacks young adults. In two-thirds of all cases it begins between the ages of 20 and 40, and rather more often in the third than the fourth decade. It is occasionally seen in children between the ages of 12 and 15, and in an ageing population an onset between the ages of 50 and 60 will sometimes be encountered.

Symptoms

There are two chief modes of onset. In most cases the disease begins with the symptoms of a single focal lesion, or sometimes of several such lesions occurring within a short time. Unilateral acute *optic neuritis* (pp. 38 and 40) is often the first symptom. Other such symptoms include *numbness* of some part of the body, usually part of a limb or one side of the face or both lower limbs, or *double vision,* or *weakness* of a limb, particularly a lower limb with dragging of the foot, or *precipitancy* of micturition. The other mode of onset is an insidious and slowly progressive weakness of one or both lower limbs.

When the onset is acute or subacute, the tendency is for the initial symptoms to diminish over a period of weeks or months, and either to disappear completely or to leave behind some residual disability. The findings on examination, therefore, will vary greatly according to the mode of onset and the stage of the disease at which the patient is examined. During an early remission the abnormal physical signs may be slight, or even absent. Later the cumulative effect of multiple lesions produces permanent changes in the nervous system and this is also the case when the onset is insidious and progressive.

In the early stages, therefore, the diagnosis may depend upon the *history,* supported by slight abnormal physical signs, particularly pallor of the temporal half of one or both optic discs, slight sustained nystagmus on lateral fixation to one or both sides, slight intention tremor in one or both upper limbs, a diminution or absence of the abdominal reflexes, exaggeration of the tendon reflexes, and an extensor plantar response on one or both sides.

In the insidiously progressive type of case, the abnormal physical signs are usually predominantly spinal, consisting of *spastic paraplegia* with some degree of superficial sensory loss over the lower limbs and trunk, or of impairment of postural sensibility and vibration sense or sometimes of both combined, the patient exhibiting a spastic and ataxic gait. In such cases it may be difficult to be sure that the symptoms are due to multiple sclerosis unless there is a history or there are physical signs of lesions within the territory of the cranial nerves, or characteristic changes in the cerebrospinal fluid.

In a *typical advanced case,* the patients will be bedridden with scanning or staccato speech and slurring of individual syllables, pallor of both optic discs, nystagmus, and a dissociation of conjugate lateral movement of the eyes, the abducting eye moving outwards further than the adducting eye moves inwards. The upper limbs will be weak and grossly ataxic. There will be severe paraplegia, either in extension interrupted by flexor spasms, or in flexion. Cutaneous or deep sensory loss, or both, may be present in upper and lower limbs, and there is likely to be incontinence of urine and faeces.

The characteristic sense of mental and physical well-being – euphoria – is well known, but is often absent. Sometimes, on the other hand, depression and irritability are conspicuous. Some loss of control over emotional movements is common, especially in the later stages of the illness.

Characteristic clinical pictures are associated with a predominance of lesions in the brain stem, or cerebellum, and with a plaque in the fasciculus cuneatus in the cervical region, causing loss of postural sensibility and astereognosis in the hand on the same side and leading to the 'useless hand' of Oppenheim. Trigeminal neuralgia is a rare symptom. Exceptionally epileptiform convulsions may occur.

The cerebrospinal fluid (see p. 151)

Some abnormality is found in the cerebrospinal fluid in at least 50 per cent of cases. An excess of lymphocytes is found in about 10 per cent. The protein content may be normal or moderately raised, there may be an abnormally high gamma globulin and oligoclonal bands on electrophoresis. The relative proportion of IgG fraction in the cerebrospinal fluid is increased, particularly in cases with recent acute episodes and is almost certainly produced within the central nervous system. IgG production in the cerebrospinal fluid could result from an auto-immune process or could represent a reaction to an extrinsic antigenic stimulus. The Wassermann or VDRL reaction is of course negative.

Serial lumbar punctures are neither practical nor acceptable in multiple sclerosis and have not shown changes that correlate well with the clinical state of the patient. Current research in multiple sclerosis has centred on the use of non-invasive techniques to demonstrate the site of lesions. The CT and NMR scans will show low-density areas, particularly around the ventricles and on occasions high-density enhancing areas during an acute relapse (Figs. 27.3 and 27.4).

Other investigations in multiple sclerosis

The search continues for tests which increase the diagnostic certainty beyond the clinical symptoms and signs which are often inconclusive. An oligoclonal IgG in the cerebrospinal fluid is helpful when positive. Most useful are the *visual evoked potentials* (see p. 160). Medium-frequency flicker shows a clear-cut delay in patients with optic neuritis up to twelve years previously in whom the visual acuity is apparently normal. This shows the usefulness of visual evoked responses in detecting earlier and possibly subclinical attacks of optic neuritis. The high chance of a multiple sclerosis patient with, for example, a progressive paraplegia having had a subclinical attack of retrobulbar neuritis gives a high index of positivity for multiple sclerosis in such patients.

In one study more than two-thirds of a group of patients with clinically probable multiple sclerosis but without any history of visual symptoms had abnormal visual evoked potentials. Auditory evoked responses may also be helpful in confirming the presence of a brainstem lesion in multiple sclerosis. Sensory evoked potentials recorded from surface electrodes over the cervical cord and somatosensory cortex may also show objective evidence of the presence and site of lesions in multiple sclerosis.

Diagnosis

No diagnostic difficulty arises in a typical case with multiple lesions running a remittent course. The progressive spinal type of the disease must be distin-

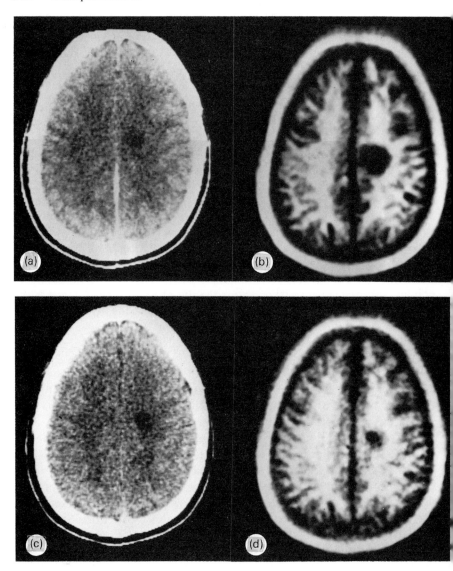

Fig. 27.3. Acute multiple sclerosis: (a) initial contrast-enhanced CT scan. Low attenuation area on CT scan corresponds in position to lesion seen on (b) NMR(IR) scan. (c) Follow-up CT; (d) NMR(IR) scans: lesion has diminished.

guished from other causes of progressive paraplegia, especially *compression of the spinal cord*. In doubtful cases myelography may be necessary. *Cervical spondylosis* may be distinguished by the characteristic X-ray changes, but may co-exist with multiple sclerosis. The *hereditary ataxias* are often familial and symptoms tend to begin at an earlier age and to run a slow progressive course.

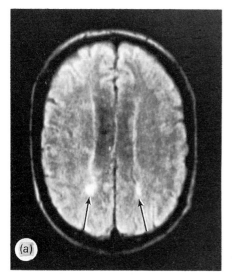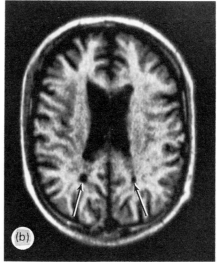

Fig. 27.4. Multiple sclerosis: (a) NMR(IR) and (b) NMR(SE) scans. Two lesions are demonstrated.

Diminution or loss of the ankle-jerks and later of the knee-jerks, scoliosis, and pes cavus are features found in Friedreich's ataxia but not in multiple sclerosis. The ataxic gait of *tabes dorsalis* may possibly lead to confusion, but in tabes the knee- and ankle-jerks are absent and not, as in multiple sclerosis, exaggerated, and there are Argyll Robertson pupils. *Vitamin B_{12} neuropathy* may lead to confusion as a cause of ataxic paraplegia. It begins, however, later in life than most cases of multiple sclerosis; paraesthesiae appear early and persist, the tendon reflexes of the lower limbs are often lost, and gastric achylia and megalocytic anaemia are distinctive features. *Hysteria* can be confused with multiple sclerosis only through neglect to make a thorough examination of the nervous system. Such early symptoms as giddiness, paraesthesiae, and paresis may superficially suggest hysteria, but these are rarely present in multiple sclerosis without some of the characteristic signs of organic disease. It is not rare, however, for a patient to develop hysterical symptoms in addition to those of multiple sclerosis.

Prognosis

There is no other disease which runs such a variable course. In cases verified at autopsy death has occurred three months, and six months, after the first symptoms. On the other hand, one patient was still doing her housework 39 years after the onset of the disease. When retrobulbar neuritis is the first symptom, the next may not follow for many years. A remission may last 20 or even 25 years in exceptional cases. The average number of fresh 'attacks' is about 0.4 per year for patients of both sexes. Frequently the length of remissions gives a clue to the outlook, but there are exceptions to this. The average duration of life in fatal cases is about 20 years.

In current multiple sclerosis research several questions in relation to prognosis are being pursued. Is it possible to make a diagnosis of multiple sclerosis with an apparent single lesion, for example, unilateral optic neuritis, in which the overall incidence of development of multiple sclerosis is approximately 50 per cent (see p. 40). If the patient has HLA DR2 antigens but has c.s.f. oligoclonal bands and abnormal evoked potentials outside the affected eye, then the chances of developing multiple sclerosis obviously increases. A second attack of optic neuritis has been shown to increase the risk fourfold.

Treatment

There is no specific treatment. The general management of the patient requires tact and judgement. The problem of when to tell a patient can be particularly difficult but, in general, secrecy is unwise when the diagnosis is certain, if only because the patient will soon come to know and may then feel lack of trust in doctors. Contact can be made with various bodies supporting multiple sclerosis patients. This may bring many benefits though there is the danger of the emotional shock of the discovery of the incapacity of seriously afflicted patients and also of a patient being overwhelmed by information about various forms of suggested treatment. As with any serious disease of unknown cause, it is sometimes the physician's duty to protect his patient from treatment suggested on a theoretical basis but of unproven benefit. It is, of course, much easier to suggest such treatments than to prove their efficacy in a controlled trial.

Several modern immunological treatments for multiple sclerosis depend on the adoption of different causal hypotheses. If the persistence of an altered virus in the brain, which is normally kept in check by immune mechanisms, is assumed, then it would be reasonable to try to enhance a defective immune response with transfer factor. Long-term steroids on the other hand would be undesirable because of the risk of favouring spread of the virus. In an acute exacerbation of multiple sclerosis, external stress or intercurrent infection might act by temporarily inhibiting the immunosuppression of the virus, so facilitating further damage. The vicious circle of destruction of myelin and development of demyelinating antibodies might be reduced by steroids or immunosuppressant treatment. Several treatments may be listed in the unproven but, possibly, helpful category.

1. *Steroids.* Prednisone is often given in an acute relapse in a dosage starting with 60 mg daily and reducing over the course of two to three weeks to a maintenance level. The use of steroids has already been discussed (see p. 17).

There is no evidence that the synthetic oral glucocorticoids, prednisone or prednisolone, which are interconvertible in the body, and cross the blood–brain barrier, are less effective than ACTH which must be given parenterally.

When a course longer than two months is planned, then there are good reasons for giving alternate-day treatment so that the suppression of pituitary-adrenal function is reduced.

2. *Immunosuppressant drugs* (such as azathioprine or cyclophosphamide). The complications of treatment and the relapse rate on ceasing treatment hardly justify the use of this treatment in benign cases in whom the prognosis is even better than the mean survival rate in multiple sclerosis of twenty years. Further control trials are needed.

3. *Vitamin B$_{12}$* has been given as hydroxocobalamin (Neo-Cytamen) 1000 μg by intramuscular injection but without any proof of benefit.

4. *The avoidance of animal fat* and the addition of polyunsaturated fatty acids such as linoleic acid, which are preserved in vegetable oils like sunflower seed oil. The observation which led to this treatment was that in the serum and tissue from patients with multiple sclerosis there was a reduction in the content of polyunsaturated fatty acids. Trials suggestive of a benefit have not been conclusive.

5. *The elimination of gluten from the diet.* The toxic factor in gluten is thought to be alpha gliaden, which might either act as an allergen or cause an epithelial peptide deficiency. No evidence of benefit has been shown in controlled trials.

6. Spinal cord stimulation by electrodes inplanted in the epidural space is still under review. Reduction in spasticity and improvement in bladder function after stimulation have been reported.

Fatigue is to be avoided, but short of this every effort should be made to keep him at his usual occupation as long as possible. In the later stages encouragement and suggestion may long postpone the bed-ridden state.

Impaired bladder function is a particularly distressing symptom. Propantheline bromide, 30 mg three times daily, helps to increase control over micturition, if precipitancy is a problem. At a later stage, if outflow resistance is increased, surgical resection of the bladder neck helps to reduce the residual urine and hence the risk of infection. Patients with severe and painful flexor spasms may sometimes be helped by dantrolene sodium (Dantrium) 25 mg three times daily initially or diazepam (Valium) in increasing dosage up to 10 mg three times daily until side-effects of drowsiness or hypotension occur (see p. 91). Occasionally such patients may need treatment with an intrathecal injection of phenol. It is possible to manipulate the small dose of phenol so that it damages selectively mainly the small diameter gamma fibres in the nerve roots carrying impulses maintaining the spasticity. A successful injection may not only abolish the flexor spasms but may, by relieving spasticity, cause an apparent increase in the power of the limb. This may be achieved with only mild loss of cutaneous sensation, or, if the sacral roots are involved, some deterioration in bladder function. Massage and passive movements may help to relieve spasticity, and re-educational exercises control incoordination. For other methods of dealing with the paraplegia (see page 384).

NEUROMYELITIS OPTICA (DEVIC'S DISEASE)

Neuromyelitis optica, also known as disseminated myelitis with optic neuritis, is a rare disorder characterized by massive demyelination of the optic nerves and spinal cord. Its aetiology is unknown, but in some cases the nervous symptoms follow a febrile illness or what appears to be a mild infection of the upper respiratory tract. For these reasons it should perhaps be grouped with acute disseminated encephalomyelitis (p. 458) rather than disseminated sclerosis. Either the ocular or the spinal lesion may develop first, and these events may be separated by days or weeks, or both may occur simultaneously. Both eyes are affected with either optic or retrobulbar neuritis, the characteristic field defect being a bilateral central scotoma and in severe cases blindness may be complete or almost so. The spinal cord lesion, the onset of which may be associated with severe pain in the back and limbs, leads to the usual symptoms of transverse myelitis with paraplegia, loss of some or all forms of sensibility below the level of the lesion, and loss of sphincter control.

The cerebrospinal fluid may show no abnormality or there may be an increase of protein and globulin and an excess of cells which are usually mononuclear, though occasionally polymorphonuclear cells have been described.

The association of optic or retrobulbar neuritis with a lesion of the spinal cord may suggest multiple sclerosis. In that disease, however, optic neuritis is very rarely simultaneously bilateral and the coincidence of bilateral optic neuritis with myelitis is unknown. This clinical picture sometimes occurs in cases of acute disseminated encephalomyelitis following one of the exanthemata, but to differentiate Devic's disease from this may be artificial.

Devic's disease has a high mortality rate, but, if the patient survives, recovery may be remarkably complete. The disease is usually self-limiting, but a relapsing form has been described.

In the absence of knowledge of the cause, treatment can only be empirical. In some cases the response to corticotrophin or steroids has been good.

DIFFUSE SCLEROSIS

Diffuse sclerosis is a group of disorders probably of mixed pathogenesis and called by a variety of names of which various leucodystrophies and Schilder's disease are perhaps the best known. They are characterized pathologically by widespread and usually symmetrical demyelination of the white matter of the cerebral hemispheres (Fig. 27.5), tending to begin in the occipital lobes and spread forwards, and clinically in typical cases by visual failure, mental deterioration and spastic paralysis. Both sporadic and familial cases are encountered, and the cause of these disorders is unknown. The disease is invariably progressive and almost always terminates fatally. It may run an acute course leading to death within one or two months, and few patients survive more than three years after the onset of symptoms. No effective treatment is known.

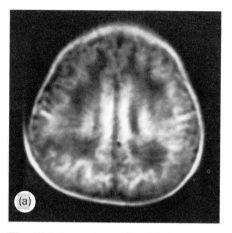 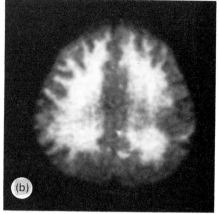

Fig. 27.5. Leucodystrophy: (a) NMR(IR) and (b) NMR(SE) scans. Extensive abnormal areas are seen in the cerebral white matter.

REFERENCES

Arnason, B.G.W. and Waksman, B.H. (1980). Immunoregulation in multiple sclerosis. *Ann. Neurol.* **8**, 237–40.

Cohen, S. and Bannister, R. (1967). Immunoglobulin synthesis within the central nervous system in disseminated sclerosis. *Lancet* **i**, 366–7.

Cook, S.D. and Dowling, P.C. (1980). Multiple sclerosis and viruses: an overview. *Neurology, Minneap.* **30**, Suppl., 80–91.

Davison, A.N., Humphrey, J.H., Liversedge, A.L., McDonald, W.I., and Porterfield, J.S. (1975). Multiple sclerosis research. HMSO, London.

Dean, G., McLoughlin, H., Brady, R., Adelstein, A.M., and Tallett-Williams, J. (1976). Multiple sclerosis among immigrants in Great Britain. *Br. med. J.* **i**, 861–4.

Graham, J. (1981). *Multiple sclerosis. A self-help guide to its management.* Thorsons, Wellingborough.

Halliday, A.M., McDonald, W.I., and Mushin, J. (1973). Visual evoked responses in diagnosis of multiple sclerosis. *Br. med. J.* **iv**, 661–4.

Kurtzke, J.F. (1980). Epidemiological contributions to multiple sclerosis: an overview. *Neurology, Minneap.* **30**, 61–79.

McAlpine, D., Lumsden, C.E., and Acheson, E.D. (1972). *Multiple sclerosis—a reappraisal,* 2nd edn. Churchill Livingstone, Edinburgh.

Matthews, W.B. (1978). *Multiple sclerosis: the facts.* Oxford University Press.

Nathan, P.W. (1959). Intrathecal phenol to relieve spasticity in paraplegia. *Lancet* **ii**, 1099–102.

Reinherz, E., Weiner, H.L., Hauser, S.L., Cohen, J.A., Distaso, J.A., and Scholossman, S.F. (1980). Loss of suppressor T cells in active multiple sclerosis. *New Engl. J. Med.* **303**, 125–9.

Reisner, T. and Maida, E. (1980). Computerized tomography in multiple sclerosis. *Archs Neurol.* **37**, 475–7.

Robinson, K. and Rudge, P. (1975). Auditory evoked responses in multiple sclerosis. *Lancet* **i**, 1164–6.

28 Motor neurone disease

Motor neurone disease, or amyotrophic lateral sclerosis, is so called because it is characterized by a selective degeneration of the motor neurones involving both the corticospinal pathways and those which originate in the motor nuclei of the brainstem and the anterior horn cells of the spinal cord.

Aetiology and pathology

It is one of the commonest purely neurological disorders, after multiple sclerosis. Except that in a very small proportion of cases it may be hereditary, the cause of motor neurone disease is entirely unknown. There are, however, certain facts which any theory must explain. Syndromes resembling motor neurone disease may occasionally occur in a number of other situations.

1. Chronic poisoning with mercury, lead, triorthocresylphosphate or manganese.

2. A variety of metabolic disturbances which include the post-gastrectomy state, hypoglycaemia, uraemia, and macroglobulinaemia.

3. In a few cases the first wasting has been observed after trauma to a limb and typical generalized motor neurone disease has then developed.

4. In association with certain other progressive degenerative diseases of the nervous system of unknown cause, including Pick's disease, parkinsonism, and Creutzfeldt–Jakob disease.

5. There is a familial incidence of several rare varieties of motor neurone disease. For instance there is a variety which is endemic among the Chamorro tribe on the island of Guam, where it may sometimes occur with parkinsonism and dementia. A rare hereditary spinal muscular atrophy in childhood which is only slowly progressive and of proximal distribution, and therefore super-ficially resembling a myopathy, was described in Sweden (the Kugelberg–Welander syndrome). Similar cases have been described elsewhere, though this may be no more than a late onset and more chronic variant of progressive muscular atrophy of infants (Werdnig–Hoffman disease).

The most that can be said concerning causation at present is that a variety of influences, hereditary, traumatic, toxic, or viral, appear to bring to light this progressive system degeneration in susceptible subjects.

Males are affected more often than females in the proportion of two to one, and symptoms usually begin between the ages of 50 and 70, occasionally as early as the third decade or as late as the eighth.

Naked-eye changes in the spinal cord are slight, but on section the grey matter of the anterior horns appears smaller than normal and the anterior roots are wasted. Microscopically there is severe degeneration of the motor neurones of the anterior horns, usually most marked in the cervical enlargement, but always widespread. Chromatolysis is present in the ganglion cells, the total number of which is much reduced. The Weigert–Pal stain reveals degeneration of the white matter which is most marked in, and often confined to, the anterior and lateral columns (Fig. 28.1). The corticospinal tract fibres suffer

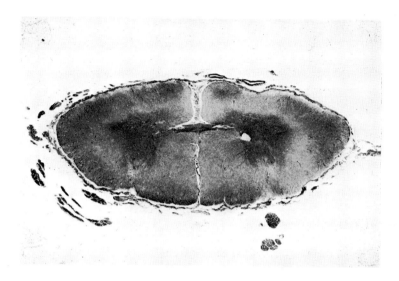

Fig. 28.1. Spinal cord in motor neurone disease.

most, both the direct and the crossed corticospinal tracts being affected, but corticospinal tract degeneration is never equally severe at all levels. The other long tracts of the spinal cord suffer to a varying extent, sometimes even the posterior columns. The ganglion cells of the motor nuclei of the medulla show degenerative changes which are in all respects similar to those of the anterior horn cells of the spinal cord and are most marked in the hypoglossal nucleus, the nucleus ambiguus, and the trigeminal motor nucleus. The third and fourth nerve nuclei in the midbrain almost invariably escape. There is marked degeneration in the pyramids of the medulla.

Symptoms

The mode of onset is usually insidious, rarely subacute. The clinical picture depends upon the relative prominence of symptoms of the lower and upper motor neurone lesions and the distribution of both. There are four main clinical varieties, though most cases show the features of more than one variety.

1. Progressive muscular atrophy

Usually the initial symptoms are those of the *lower motor neurone lesions* – progressive muscular atrophy. Commonly the first abnormality is observed in the hands, where the patient may be conscious of weakness, stiffness, or clumsiness of movements of the fingers, or his attention may be drawn to the wasting, or the twitching of fasciculation. Cramp-like pains in the limbs are often an early symptom. When degeneration begins in the bulbar motor nuclei, the first symptom to be noticed may be dysarthria or difficulty in chewing or swallowing.

Usually muscular wasting begins in the hands (Fig. 28.2), the muscles of the thenar eminences being first affected. Not uncommonly one hand may begin to waste some months or even a year before the other, or the onset may be symmetrical. Usually after the hands the forearm muscles are next involved, the flexors suffering before the extensors. Less often the muscles of the shoulder girdle and upper arm are those first affected. Early involvement of the muscles of the lower limbs is rare. The anterior tibial group and the peronei are usually first affected, and bilateral foot-drop results. Weakness of the trunk muscles and finally the muscles of respiration characterize the terminal stage.

Fasciculation is a prominent symptom. It may be limited to a few groups of muscles, or much more widespread, and its extent is an indication of the diffuseness of the degenerative process. When it is not immediately evident it can often be evoked by sharply tapping the muscle or by the observer's moving the limb so that the muscle becomes passively relaxed.

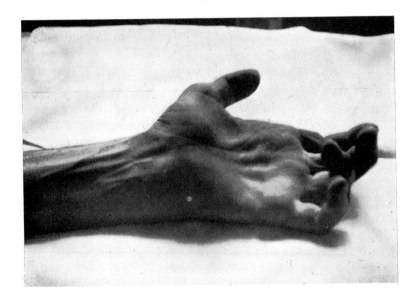

Fig. 28.2. Wasted hand in motor neurone disease.

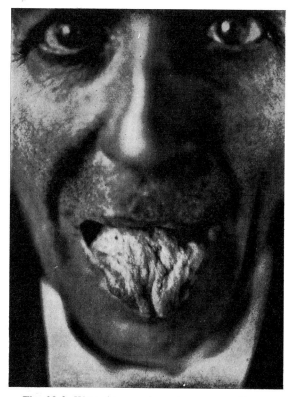

Fig. 28.3. Wasted tongue in motor neurone disease.

2. Progressive bulbar palsy

As the degeneration spreads, the bulbar muscles become affected. The tongue wastes and becomes shrunken and wrinkled and shows conspicuous fasciculation (Fig. 28.3). The orbicularis oris also suffers, usually at the same time as the tongue, but the orbicularis oculi and other facial muscles are affected later and less severely. The palate is usually involved shortly after the tongue, together with the extrinsic muscles of the pharynx and larynx. Protrusion of the tongue is first weak and later lost. Speech suffers from paresis of the lips, tongue, and palate. Swallowing becomes increasingly difficult, and food tends to regurgitate through the nose.

3. Amyotrophic lateral sclerosis

Degeneration of the *upper motor neurones* adds to the muscular weakness and contributes certain features of its own. Since lower motor neurone lesions are rarely present at an early stage in the lower limbs, these usually for a long time present an uncomplicated picture of corticospinal tract degeneration, with weakness and spasticity which is not as a rule severe. In the upper limbs the effect of the addition of an upper to a lower motor neurone lesion is to cause a degree of weakness which is disproportionately great in comparison with the severity and extent of the wasting. The condition of the reflexes depends upon the relative preponderance of upper and lower motor neurone degeneration. Degeneration of the lower motor neurones causes impairment, and finally loss, of the tendon reflexes. Corticospinal tract degeneration, on the other hand, leads to their exaggeration. Hence it is not uncommon to find exaggerated tendon jerks in the upper limbs in spite of considerable muscular atrophy, an association which led to the term 'tonic muscular atrophy' being applied to such cases.

4. Bulbar-pseudobulbar palsy

But it is in the muscles innervated from the medulla that the effects of cortico-spinal tract degeneration are of the greatest importance. Here we may encounter *lower motor neurone degeneration* only – *progressive bulbar palsy; upper motor neurone degeneration* only – *'pseudobulbar palsy'*; or a combination of the two, which is the most frequent occurrence. A lesion of both corticospinal tracts above the medulla, so-called 'pseudobulbar palsy', causes weakness of the bulbar muscles and hence leads to dysarthria and dysphagia. The weak muscles are not wasted and hypotonic, as in progressive bulbar palsy, but spastic. The tongue may appear somewhat smaller than normal, but is not wrinkled and exhibits no fasciculation. The jaw-jerk, palatal and pharyngeal reflexes are exaggerated, and sneezing and coughing may be excited reflexly with abnormal readiness. The dysarthria resembles that which results from a lower motor neurone lesion. Pseudobulbar palsy, when severe, also leads to an impairment of voluntary control over emotional reactions, as the result of which paroxysmal attacks of involuntary laughing and crying occur, unrelated to the patient's emotional state.

In the early stages the sphincters are not as a rule severely affected, though slight precipitancy or difficulty of micturition is not uncommon. Ocular sympathetic palsy may occur. There is no sensory loss. The subcutaneous fat tends to disappear as the muscles waste and marked emaciation characterizes the later stages. For electromyographic changes see page 162.

Diagnosis

Motor neurone disease requires to be distinguished chiefly from other conditions leading to muscular wasting, especially in the upper limbs. In *syringomyelia* fasciculation is rarely observed in the wasted muscles, and the characteristic dissociated sensory loss develops at an early stage. In *syphilitic amyotrophy* the onset of the weakness and wasting is often accompanied by pain of considerable severity and of radicular distribution. Pupillary abnormalities may be present and the characteristic serological changes are likely to be found. *Intramedullary tumour* of the spinal cord is likely to cause sensory loss and the changes characteristic of spinal block in the cerebrospinal fluid. *Cervical spondylosis* may give rise to real difficulty. In most cases sensory changes will be present, but occasionally cervical spondylosis causes muscular wasting in the upper limbs accompanied by spastic weakness of the lower limbs which closely resembles motor neurone disease. The rate of progress of myelopathy due to cervical spondylosis is usually much slower than that of motor neurone disease. The characteristic X-ray changes are present and protrusions of the cervical discs will be demonstrable on myelography. There are, however, rare cases in which both cervical spondylosis and motor neurone disease co-exist.

Cervical rib is an occasional cause of wasting of the hand. In such cases fasciculation is absent and pain along the ulnar border of the hand and forearm is usually a prominent symptom, often associated with sensory loss in this area. A cervical rib can be demonstrated radiographically. Lesions of *peripheral nerves* causing muscular wasting usually give rise to little difficulty since the distribution of the wasting is recognizable as corresponding to the supply of the nerve, and does not spread beyond that. In the case of the median and ulnar nerves it is usually associated with sensory abnormalities possessing an equally distinctive distribution.

Various muscular disorders by leading to wasting of the muscles may cause difficulty in diagnosis. The various *hereditary myopathies* usually appear at a much earlier age than motor neurone disease, and possess their own distinctive features, particularly of distribution. The same is true of peroneal muscular atrophy, which is also associated with sensory loss. It has recently been recognized that some of these apparent myopathies are in fact spinal muscular atrophies. *Myopathy* associated with *carcinoma* and some of the more chronic forms of *polymyositis* occurring in middle-aged persons may simulate motor neurone disease. If the possibility is borne in mind, the cause can usually be ascertained by the appropriate investigations, including electromyography and muscle biopsy. *Myasthenia* may cause bulbar palsy but does not usually lead to muscular wasting, and the symptoms rapidly respond to anticholinesterase drugs.

Prognosis

Motor neurone disease is invariably progressive, but its rate of progress varies from case to case. In one case, verified by autopsy, the patient died six months after the onset. Most patients survive for two or three years, exceptionally for longer, but it is probable that instances of survival for five to ten years recorded in the past have been in cases of cervical spondylosis or chronic polymyositis mistaken for motor neurone disease.

Treatment

The cause of the disease being unknown, treatment is limited to dealing with the symptoms. The patient should avoid fatigue and exposure to cold, but should be encouraged to continue at a light occupation as long as possible. When dysphagia occurs, food of the consistency of porridge is usually swallowed better than either solids or liquids. Physiotherapy may be of psychological value, but electrical stimulation of the muscles probably does harm. Vitamin E has been tried and found useless.

REFERENCES

Adams, R.D. (1975). *Diseases of muscle: a study in pathology* 3rd edn. Harper and Row, New York.
Kurtzke, J.F. (1982). Motor neurone disease. *Br. med. J.* **284,** 141–2.
Rosen, A.D. (1978). Amyotrophic lateral sclerosis; clinical features and prognosis. *Archs Neurol.* **35,** 638–42.
Walton, J.N. (1981). *Disorders of voluntary muscle,* 4th edn. Churchill Livingstone, Edinburgh.

29 Neurological syndromes associated with malignant diseases

An increasing variety of neurological syndromes have been recognized in association with malignant disease. These syndromes are not due to direct invasion, and the causes are in the main unknown. Nutritional and metabolic effects, viral infections, and immunological disorders have all been proposed and are not mutually exclusive. Although some of these syndromes are described elsewhere under the region of the nervous system affected, it may be useful to review here their different manifestations because search for underling malignant disease is part of the investigation of a patient with many different neurological disabilities. The list of syndromes occurring singly or in combination includes dementia, encephalomyelitis, progressive multifocal leuco-encephalopathy (PML), meningitis, cerebellar degeneration, spinal cord degeneration, motor or sensory peripheral neuropathy, myasthenia, Eaton–Lambert syndrome (see p. 444), myopathy, and myositis. All are considered elsewhere in this book. The prevalence of these syndromes is difficult to assess but, in some half the patients with cerebellar degeneration or myopathy occurring in middle life, there is an underlying malignancy. The combination of myasthenia with myopathy is particularly suggestive of malignancy; half the cases of carcinomatous neuromyopathy occur in lung cancer, and neuromyopathy occurs in some 15 per cent of men with lung cancer.

The carcinomas most frequently associated with neurological syndromes are, in order, bronchus, stomach, and ovary. The course of the syndrome is usually progressive, occasionally remits spontaneously or after removal of the underlying carcinoma, but it is not often obviously influenced by steroids or other forms of treatment. Lymphomas, though rarer than carcinomas, are even more commonly associated with both direct and indirect neurological syndromes. PML is due to a virus and is the most bizarre of the disturbances associated with neoplasia.

It is possible that carcinomas produce these effects either by synthesizing polypeptides which inhibit immunological mechanisms or by releasing genetic material which has been repressed in mature and specialized body cells. These polypeptides may also have metabolic effects of relevance in neurology, as when they mimic the action of hormones. The most important is ectopic production of antidiuretic hormone, usually secreted by oat-celled bronchial carcinoma, in which plasma sodium is low (below 110 mEq/l) with low plasma osmolality in the presence of high urinary osmolality. The clinical picture is one of lethargy, confusion, and even epileptic fits and coma. If the tumour cannot be removed, treatment is attempted either by water restriction or by causing a water diuresis with fludrocortisone.

REFERENCE

Henson, R.A. and Urich, H. (1982). *Cancer and the nervous system. The neurological manifestations of systemic malignant disease.* Blackwell, Oxford.

Part V
Psychological factors in neurology

30 Psychological factors in neurology

Introduction

The brain and the mind constitute a unity, and we may leave to the philosophers, who have separated them in thought, the task of putting them together again. In practice, there are two ways of explaining disorders of the mind. They may be the result of damage to the brain; for example, by transmitter defects, trauma, inflammation, tumour, impaired blood supply, etc. In such cases the cause itself is not mental, though its result is a disorder of mental function. In the other group of cases, the cause is mental, because the patient's present mental symptoms can be traced back to, and explained in terms of, one of his previous mental experiences, or a whole series of such experiences, which constituted his reactions to what happened to him in the past. In the first group of cases the cause of the mental disorder is said to be *organic*, while in the second it is described as *psychogenic* or sometimes, using the misleading but convenient euphemism, as *'functional'*. It is not to be supposed that there are not physiological processes occurring in the nervous system and corresponding to the pschological events underlying a psychogenic disorder, but this disorder still has to be explained in terms of psychological causation and not as a result of some physical interference with the physiological functions of the nervous system.

This fundamental distinction having been made, it is now necessary to qualify it by pointing out that there is often a place for both kinds of causation in the interpretation of a particular mental illness. For example, it is probable that recurrent attacks of 'endogenous' depression are the outcome of recurrent disorders of transmitter function within the nervous system, yet *psychological stress* may precipitate such an attack. Similarly, *inherited predisposition*, which presumably operates through genetic influence upon the structure and function of the nervous system, may explain why a similar degree of psychological stress provokes psychological symptoms in one individual but not in another. Many doctors who have had much experience of hysterical patients will take the view that hysteria is often at least the expression of a psychological constitution which may in time be interpreted in terms of disordered neurophysiological function. This, however, does not in the least invalidate the interpretation of particular hysterical symptoms or reactions in psychological terms.

Hence every patient who complains of psychological symptoms requires consideration from the physical as well as the psychological standpoint, and in this connection other bodily systems besides the neurological are often important, particularly the endocrine. And since the patient's physical constitution includes his genes, his family history is highly relevant. It also follows that even if the psychogenesis of the symptoms is clear, physical methods of treatment may be of great value. This has always been obvious so far as sedatives have been concerned, and the rapidly increasing range of drugs acting upon the nervous system is greatly adding to the possibility of what is now called psychopharmacology. In a sense, most psychiatric illness may be regarded as due to an imbalance in the amount of transmitter available for action at postsynaptic receptor sites. There is a prospect of more successful manipulation of most psychiatric disorders in this way. But equally electroshock therapy may be a necessary adjunct to the psychotherapy of depression, or the recognition and treatment of mild myxoedema may facilitate a psychological adjustment previously impossible.

The recognition of the psychogenesis of psychological symptoms is of course extremely old: what is modern is the development of this idea, particularly by Freud, into a most elaborate conceptual system which is often given scientific status. However Freud's ideas may need to be modified in detail, as many of them have been already, there can be little doubt that he has made a permanent contribution to our knowledge of the human mind by stressing the profound and lasting effects of the experiences of early childhood. But this has led to some psychotherapeutic conclusions which seem to be fallacious. However causally important infantile experiences may have been, it does not follow that they are reversible by trying to live through them again in adult life. Life cannot thus be reversed, and the adult cannot be put back into infancy to develop again differently. This is not a criticism of the value of psychotherapy in general, but it means that however much account it may take of their past, it must always deal with people as they are now, and its methods must therefore often resemble those of the orthopaedic surgeon, who aims to make life easier for his patients by correcting deformities and giving support, though he can rarely hope to restore them to the state in which they would have been if they had not suffered from congenital deformity or an acquired illness.

HYSTERIA

Aetiology

The distinguishing feature of hysteria is the peculiar tendency of the hysterical personality to mental dissociation. As the result of this, certain psychophysiological elements become separated from the conscious life. In the most severe cases this dissociation is so extensive that the patient may be regarded as suffering from dissociated personality. A similar profound dissociation is responsible for the state known as hysterical fugue, in which the patient may disappear from home and wander about, having lost his sense of identity. More superficial or less extensive forms of dissociation lead to hysterical paralyses and sensory loss and convulsions. Pain may also be a hysterical symptom. As already stated, it is probable that the tendency to mental dissociation is in many cases inborn. Hysterical symptoms may be precipitated by some particular emotional conflict, or they may be a more general mode of reaction to life in general with its difficulties and responsibilities or to anxiety or depression. The hysterical symptom may sometimes be regarded as serving a purpose in that it provides an escape from some emotional difficulty, while the patient's propensity for mental dissociation allows him or her to disclaim any responsibility for the symptom. Certain organic nervous disorders, especially disseminated sclerosis, seem to predispose to the development of hysterical symptoms which in general sometimes mask the onset of some organic disease. Indeed, cerebral lesions, especially in the temporal lobe, may cause symptoms indistinguishable from hysteria. Perhaps because of the tendency to mental dissociation, hysterical patients are very susceptible to suggestion, which may therefore play a part in the production of their symptoms.

Symptoms

Amnesia and dissociated personality

Hysterical loss of memory and multiple personality in outspoken forms are rare. The commonest example is the hysterical fugue, in which the patient wanders about having lost his sense of identity, and when he comes to himself remembers nothing of what has happened.

Hysterical convulsions

These are described on page 197, and *hysterical trance* on page 174.

Paralysis

Hysterical paralysis may affect any part of the body over which there is normally voluntary control. Most commonly it involves one limb or part of a limb, the movements at one joint often alone being affected. Less frequently more than one limb is involved, as in hysterical hemiplegia, paraplegia, and diplegia. Hysterical paralysis of the face and tongue is rare, and is usually associated with spasm of the corresponding muscles on the opposite side.

The diagnosis of hysterical paralysis rests upon the following points.

Anomalies of distribution. Since the paralysis corresponds to the patient's idea, there are inevitably discrepancies between hysterical paralysis and that produced by organic lesions of the nervous system. The distribution of the weakness is often anomalous, and paralysis limited to the movement of one joint is unknown in organic disease.

Contraction of antagonistic muscles. It is very common in hysterical paralysis to find that when the patient attempts to move the limb, he contracts the antagonistic muscles as well as the prime movers. For example, if he is asked to flex the lower limb, the quadriceps is felt to contract. Antagonistic contraction is absent only when the paresis is so great that the prime movers hardly contract at all.

Wasting and contractures. Muscular wasting and contractures are absent except in cases of long standing in which these phenomena may supervene upon the prolonged muscular inactivity. Electromyograms reveal no abnormality.

The reflexes

Extreme muscular rigidity may make the tendon reflexes difficult to elicit, but if adequate muscular relaxation can be obtained they are never asymmetrical and never diminished. The same is true of the abdominal reflexes, and the plantar reflexes are flexor.

Gait

Hysterical disorders of gait may be associated with hysterical paralysis of one or both lower limbs. A hysterical gait is usually easily recognized on account of its bizarre character and its dissimilarity from any disorder of gait produced by organic disease. There is often a tendency to fall, especially when other patients are present, but the fall does not lead to injury. In severe cases there is complete inability to stand, and a patient with hysterical unsteadiness is always more difficult to support than a patient of normal mentality whose difficulty in walking is due to organic disease.

Rigidity

Hysterical rigidity may be localized to a paralysed limb, or generalized, as in hysterical trance. It is distinguishable from all forms of rigidity due to organic disease by the fact that it increases in proportion to the effort made by the observer to move the rigid part.

Involuntary movements

Tremor is a common hysterical involuntary movement, and coarse tremor is often associated with hysterical paralysis. It is increased when attention is directed to it, and may be absent in movements carried out when the attention is distracted.

Sensory symptoms

Hysterical sensory loss is common, and is most often confined to a limb which is the site of hysterical weakness. It may involve only cutaneous sensibility, or all forms may be lost. When cutaneous sensibility is lost over the peripheral part of the limb, the anaesthetic area is demarcated from the area of normal sensibility by a sharp upper border which encircles the limb and often coincides with a joint. Sensation may be lost over one half of the body, and in such a case there may be loss of smell and taste on the same side. Hysterical sensory loss is distinguished from that due to organic nervous disease by failure to correspond with the distribution of the loss resulting from lesions of the sensory tracts, spinal segments or peripheral nerves. Moreover, hysterical patients often exhibit striking discrepancies in their sensory symptoms which are incompatible with an organic origin. For example, co-ordination may be perfect in spite of complete loss of postural sensibility and appreciation of passive movement in a limb. Hysterical sensory loss can readily be produced and modified by suggestion. Hysterical deafness may disappear during sleep, so that the patient can be aroused by sounds and the blinking reflex on auditory stimulation may be retained by the hysterically deaf. Hysterical blindness may be unilateral or bilateral, and may be complete or consist merely of a reduction of visual acuity. In hysterical blindness the optic discs and the pupillary reactions are normal, and it may be possible to evoke blinking by a sudden feint with the hand towards the eyes. Moreover the blind hysteric may avoid obstacles in his path. Various ophthalmological tests have been devised to detect hysterical blindness.

Speech disturbances

Hysterical mutism and aphonia are described elsewhere (p. 113).

Visceral disturbances

Hysterical dysphagia is rare. Globus hystericus, described as a sense of constriction or lump in the throat, is a common complaint. Hysterical vomiting, when severe, may cause loss of weight and may be a serious disorder, as may hysterical anorexia or anorexia nervosa, a disorder affecting young women and associated with amenorrhoea. Hysterical hyperpnoea may occur and lead to tetany. Retention of urine occasionally occurs, usually in young girls.

The skin

Dermatitis artefacta is the term applied to cutaneous lesions produced by an hysterical patient, either by scratching or rubbing, or by the use of external agents including corrosives. These lesions are usually easily recognized by their appearance and by the fact that they quickly heal when covered by an occlusive dressing.

Pyrexia

Probably in most cases of apparent pyrexia occurring in hysteria the thermometer is manipulated by the patient. Very rarely an actual rise of body temperature may occur in hysteria.

Hysterical pain

Hysterical pain may occur in any part of the body, but probably the head is the commonest site. Such pain is most intractable, usually failing to respond to all physical measures, and since the patient lacks insight he is resistant to psychotherapy also.

Diagnosis

Diagnosis of individual hysterical symptoms has already been considered. In general it may be said that the diagnosis of hysteria depends upon the presence of positive signs of hysteria already described, and the absence of those of organic disease. As already pointed out, however, the one does not invariably exclude the other. Eliot Slater warned about the diagnosis of hysteria in the context of neurological symptoms presenting in a neurological department, commenting that 'the diagnosis of hysteria is not only a snare but is a delusion'. However, this does not discount the presence of conversion hysteria occurring rarely under conditions of extreme stress such as occur in war.

Prognosis

While recovery from an individual symptom often takes place, the constitution which is the basis of the hysterical reaction to difficulties remains in most cases. Sometimes an hysterical symptom lasts indefinitely because the situation to which it is a reaction also persists, e.g. in a patient who has developed hysterical symptoms after an injury which entitles him to compensation.

Treatment

Since a hysterical symptom is a neurotic solution of a psychological difficulty, symptomatic treatment alone is inadequate. It is essential that the cause of the difficulty should be discovered if possible, and that the patient should be induced to deal with it in a less abnormal manner. Many hysterical patients fail to develop insight into the nature of their symptoms, and exhibit a strong resistance to doing so. Narco-analysis is sometimes helpful. In some cases recovery is best brought about by a gradual process of persuasion and re-education extending over a considerable time. Some prefer to attempt to remove a symptom at one sitting, but this method is not without risks, since the failure of a protracted attempt to cure will only reinforce the patient's belief in the intractable nature of his disorder. Anorexia nervosa requires admission to hospital and skilled nursing. Chlorpromazine in large doses is useful in overcoming resistance to eating.

ANXIETY STATES

Anxiety may occur in an individual who is otherwise mentally normal, and be directed towards some object or situation which does not normally excite it, or be experienced as an undirected emotional state, the cause of which the patient is unable to explain. Anxiety directed against a specific external object or situation is known as a phobia. Some patients are subject to paroxysmal exacerbations of anxiety, known as anxiety attacks, in which an overwhelming sense of fear dominates consciousness, and is associated with its bodily manifestations in an intense form. Other mental symptoms which are often associated with anxiety include irritability, depression, lack of concentration, and insomnia, and anxiety may find expression during sleep in terrifying dreams and nightmares.

It has been estimated that 8 per cent of adults of the United Kingdom currently take drugs for treatment of anxiety for at least a month in the year. The high number of people who are maintained on such drugs for years shows the dangers of development of pharmacological dependence and it is now appreciated that on attempted withdrawal, symptoms resembling the initial anxiety symptoms may occur with increased prominence.

Neurotransmitters and anxiety

GABA is an important inhibitory transmitter and is facilitated by the benzo-diazepines which selectively reduce arousal and alleviate anxiety, without causing central depression. There are binding sites which appear to be receptors for benzodiazepines similar to opiate receptors and there may be naturally occurring endogenous ligands involved in the control of anxiety, just as opiate peptides are related to opiate receptors. A current hypothesis is that anxiety is related to stimulation of GABA-ergic fibres and receptors in the limbic system. This system may compare actual stimuli with expected ones and if there is a 'mismatch', anxiety is engendered until successful matching occurs.

Physical symptoms

Anxiety is often attended by over-activity of the sympathetic nervous system, and many of its physical manifestations are directly or indirectly the result of this. The patient often complains of palpitations, weakness and fatigability, dyspnoea, giddiness, a sensation of falling, or of pressure at the vertex, loss of appetite, epigastric discomfort, flatulence, constipation, diarrhoea, frequency of micturition, and seminal emissions. The pupils are often dilated, the pulse rapid, and the extremities cold, sweating, and tremulous. The tendon reflexes are exaggerated.

Diagnosis

The anxiety attack must be distinguished from other paroxysmal disorders, especially from epilepsy, syncope, and aural vertigo. There is usually little difficulty in this in view of the prominence of anxiety, the absence of loss of consciousness and true vertigo, and the presence of symptoms of sympathetic over-activity. Anxiety states must be distinguished also from minor impairment of mental function resulting from organic disease of the brain, especially cerebral syphilis and atherosclerosis. Thyrotoxicosis is a common cause of anxiety, but should be recognized by its characteristic physical signs. Anxiety states must also be distinguished from more serious mental disorders. Endogenous depression, though sometimes itself giving rise to anxiety, is characterized by the cardinal symptoms of true depression, which is usually worst in the early morning, early awakening, and difficulty in concentration. Anxiety may occur in schizophrenia. Here the correct diagnosis may be suggested by the previous seclusive character of the patient, the lack of emotional contact with the outside world, and the disturbed character of the thinking.

Prognosis

The prognosis of anxiety states is on the whole good. When the neurosis is of recent origin and a reaction to a well-defined source of fear, a cure can often rapidly be effected. Those patients in whom anxiety is an habitual reaction of long standing may require prolonged treatment, but, provided they are co-operative and intelligent, they will be much benefited and in some cases cured.

Treatment

The treatment of anxiety states must always be primarily psychological, directed to discovering the cause of the anxiety and bringing the patient to a realization of its relationship to his symptoms, and inducing him to alter his emotional attitude to the source of his fears. Physical measures, however, have their place, especially in the treatment of more severe cases, and it is sometimes necessary to isolate a patient from his usual environment in a nursing home or hospital. Rest, sedatives and physiotherapy may all play a useful part in treatment. Sedative and tranquillizing drugs have a place in the treatment of anxiety in that their use for a short time may suppress symptoms or reduce tension sufficiently to break the vicious circle of anxiety. If successful, the patient may be given the confidence necessary for him to resolve the conflicts which underlie the symptoms. However, the use of these drugs in anxiety states associated with chronic personality disorders carries the risk of producing a state of dependence on the drugs. Barbiturates reduce anxiety but have the disadvantage of producing sleepiness and an overdose, either accidental or deliberate, is likely to be serious. Amylobarbitone sodium (Amytal), 30 to 60 mg three times a day, relieves tension more than phenobarbitone which also has the disadvantage of being a mild depressant. On the other hand, tranquillizers with predominantly antihistaminic, anti-adrenergic and anticholinergic properties, though they do not cause much drowsiness, may have other side-effects and the effect of alcohol or other drugs may be potentiated. The phenothiazine derivatives may cause hypotension, peripheral vasodilatation and, in large doses, lowered body temperature. Promethazine (Phenergan), chlorpromazine (Largactil), and trifluoperazine (Stelazine) are commonly used, though the latter in large doses may cause extrapyramidal signs. The diazepine derivatives have a muscle relaxant effect, but in high doses may cause ataxia. Chlordiazepine (Librium) and diazepam (Valium) are commonly used, particularly in anxiety states associated with phobic, obsessional, or depressive symptoms.

DEPRESSION

The depressed patient may complain of a number of symptoms which must be distinguished from similar symptoms due to organic brain disease. Headache (p. 212) and facial pain (p. 62) are common but the pain often has a steady quality without the periodic features of pain caused by raised intracranial pressure, migraine or trigeminal neuralgia. Sometimes the sensory symptoms are not truly painful but consist of paraesthesiae, usually over a site which does not correspond to any particular anatomical distribution. The depressed patient often complains of lack of concentration, which must be distinguished from the earliest signs of a progressive organic dementia.

Neurotransmitters and treatment of depression

There are several clues that noradrenaline and serotonin metabolism are deranged in endogenous depression. For example, the serotonin precursors tryptophan and 5HT have antidepressant effects. Exogenous tyrosine leads to increased dopamine and noradrenaline synthesis in man and tyrosine enhances the antidepressive action of 5HT. The cholinergic and peptidergic systems have yet barely been studied in depression. Hypersecretion of cortisol and an incomplete failure to suppress after Dexamethasone have been observed in 50 per cent of patients with endogenous depression and if present this suggests noradrenergic hypoactivity and makes it more likely that the patient will respond to an adrenaline augmenting tricyclic antidepressant. The persistance of an abnormal tests indicates the likely need for lengthy treatment.

Prolonged use of tricyclic antidepressants in one group of patients with depression may lead to blunting of a noradrenergic regulatory feedback, which is mediated by postsynaptic alpha-receptors, because of a 'desensitization' of alpha-2-presynaptic receptors. These patients may represent a special subgroup of depressive patients. There has also been interest in the part played by beta-adrenoreceptors in depression. Propranolol a classical beta-receptor blocker, occasionally causes the side-effect of depression.

There has been a considerable limitation of the use of monoaminoxidase inhibitors because of the tyramine reaction. However, it is now possible selectively to inhibit only monoaminoxidase B which deaminates dopamine so avoiding the tyramine reaction. Deprenyl the selective MAO-B inhibitor introduced for the treatment of Parkinson's disease, may also be useful in the treatment of depression.

The management of the severely depressed patient, with a suicidal risk, is clearly a psychiatric problem. However, since mild depression often complicates or is mistaken for organic neurological disease, some knowledge of its diagnosis and treatment is a help to the neurologist. The predominantly *endogenous* and *reactive* types may be distinguished. In *endogenous* depression, there is no clear precipitating cause. Certain symptoms such as early wakening are often present and there may be a past history of similar episodes or perhaps a family history of similar disorder. The tricyclic group of antidepressant drugs is most likely to be successful. Imipramine (Tofranil) or amitriptyline (Tryptizol) are commonly used, the dosage of imipramine being increased slowly from 25 mg three times daily up to 50 mg three times daily if necessary over the course of a month. These drugs appear to act by increasing the concentration of noradrenaline at receptor sites and their side-effects are mainly anticholinergic reactions, such as dry mouth, dizziness, orthostatic hypotension, constipation, hesitancy of micturition, and occasionally impotence. *Reactive* depression on the other hand may follow some external triggering event. The prognosis is least good when there is a severe personality disorder in addition. The tricyclic antidepressant drugs are less likely to be effective and under psychiatric advice the patient may require treatment with a monoaminoxidase inhibitor such as phenelzine (Nardil), isocarboxazid (Marplan), or tranylcypromine (Parnate). The latter drugs appear to act by increasing the available noradrenaline and hydroxytryptamine within the nervous system. Apart from their anticholinergic side-effects, these drugs require great care in combination with other drugs, many of which they potentiate. Because of the risk of accumulation of noradrenaline, amphetamine-like substances should never be given intravenously. The strictures concerning diet have already been mentioned (p. 213). Lithium, which is effective in manic depressive illness, probably acts by substituting potassium ions in the sodium pump mechanisms, so reducing the efficiency of catecholamine transmission.

OBSESSIVE–COMPULSIVE STATES

An obsessive–compulsive state is characterized by the persistent obtrusion into consciousness of ideas or emotional states – obsessions – or impulses to action – compulsions – often linked together, which occur independently of the patient's will, without a cause which is evident to his consciousness, and in spite of his recognition of their irrational character and efforts to resist them. Thus defined, obsessions and compulsions occur in a wide range of mental disorders and vary in severity from the trivial to the grossly incapacitating. It has often been pointed out that mild obsessions and compulsions are common enough in normal people, especially in children; for example, a wish to avoid stepping on the cracks between paving-stones. Tic or habit spasm is a common form of compulsion, again chiefly in childhood. Obsessions and compulsions also occur in severe mental disorders; for example, in association with endogenous depression, and sometimes in schizophrenia. Leaving those on one side, obsessive-compulsive states are seen in their purest form in tics and habit spasms and in what is sometimes called obsessive-compulsive neurosis. The fact that obsessions and compulsions are sometimes produced in previously healthy people by organic disease of the brain, as was seen after the epidemic of encephalitis lethargica, suggests that we may in time be able to interpret them in physiological as well as in psychological terms. Indeed, the fact that we can speak of an obsessional temperament points to the importance of constitutional predisposition. The obsessional temperament is commonly characterized by a certain rigidity of outlook, laying stress upon precision and accuracy of performance, and demanding compliance with a high standard. Different schools of medical psychology have their own interpretations of the psychological nature of obsessions and compulsions.

Habit spasm

Habit spasm, or tic commonly seen in childhood, is a repetitive involuntary movement which may originate as an automatic or voluntary reaction to a local stimulus or external situation, and is perpetuated as a compulsive symptom. Thus conjuctivitis may initiate a blinking tic, which persists after the inflammation has subsided. Tics frequently involve the facial muscles, as in blinking or movements of the eyes or mouth. Rotation of the head is a common tic, and spasmodic torticollis is sometimes a symptom of a compulsive neurosis (p. 351). Respiratory tics include sneezing, coughing, and hiccup, and in some complicated tics the limbs and the whole body may be involved. Dr Johnson's elaborate gesticulations were of this kind. The sufferer from a tic experiences a conscious compulsion to carry out the movement, and increasing discomfort until he yields to it.

The obsessive-compulsive neurosis

Some adult patients continuously, and others periodically, suffer from a more complex type of compulsive symptom, namely a compulsion to carry out an elaborate set of movements animated by a strongly felt but unexplained emotional state. Compulsive washing is a good example of this. A constant fear of contamination leads to frequent washing, or such a patient may have a compulsion to add up the numbers of all the cars which he sees in the street. Obsessive doubts may lead the bank clerk to go back repeatedly to assure himself that he has locked the strong room, or the housewife that she has turned off the gas. At the ideational level obsessions may consist of fears, of which syphilophobia is a not uncommon example. The obsessive-compulsive state is sometimes linked with anxiety and sometimes with depression, and in its recurrent form recalls recurrent attacks of endogenous depression.

Most children who suffer from tics recover, though a few continue to twitch throughout their lives. The more serious obsessional symptoms, especially compulsive ideas and elaborate compulsions, are difficult to treat. Tics in children are often reactions to difficulties in the home or at school, and have often been injudiciously treated by the parents. The tic will usually disappear if no allusion is ever made to it. In adults suffering from long-standing and disabling obsessions and compulsions, leucotomy may relieve the tension associated with these symptoms, but relief following this is sometimes only temporary.

An interesting rare disorder is the syndrome of Gilles de la Tourette. Symptoms usually first occur in childhood and there is a compulsion to utter curious sounds including profanities. It has been suggested Dr Johnson had this syndrome though in his case there were facial and other movements with expiratory laryngeal noises but no utterance of profanities. A view that in such syndromes there is a prominant organic component has gained ground and a response to haloperidol in dosages lower than those used for schizophrenia has been reported. This suggests that they should perhaps be more properly classified under dyskinesias (see p. 352).

REFERENCES

Eccleston, O. (1982). Biochemistry of affective disorders. *Br. J. Hosp. Med.* **27**, 627–30.

Lishman, W.A. (1978). *Organic psychiatry: the psychological consequences of cerebral disorder.* Blackwell, Oxford.

Merskey, H. (1979). *The analysis of hysteria.* Baillière Tindall, London.

Nee, L.E., Caine, E.D., Polinsky, R.J., Eldridge, R., and Ebert, M.H. (1980). Gilles de la Tourette syndrome: clinical and family study of 50 cases. *Ann. Neurol.* **7**, 41–9.

Trimble, M.R. (1981). *Neuropsychiatry.* Wiley, Chichester.

Segmental innervation of the muscles

SEGMENTAL INNERVATION OF MUSCLES OF UPPER EXTREMITY

		CERVICAL SEGMENTS			THORACIC SEGMENTS
	5	**6**	**7**	**8**	**I**
SHOULDER					
Supraspinatus	▦				
Teres minor	▦				
Deltoid	▦	▦			
Infraspinatus	▦				
Subscapularis	▦				
Teres major	▦	▦			
ARM					
Biceps brachii	▦	▦			
Brachialis	▦	▦			
Coracobrachialis		▦	▦		
Triceps brachii			▦	▦	
Anconeus			▦	▦	
FOREARM					
Brachioradialis	▦	▦			
Supinator		▦	▦		
Extensores carpi radialis		▦	▦		
Pronator teres		▦	▦		
Flexor carpi radialis		▦	▦		
Flexor pollicis longus		▦	▦		
Abductor pollicis longus			▦	▦	
Extensor pollicis brevis			▦	▦	
Extensor pollicis longus			▦	▦	
Extensor digitorum communis			▦	▦	
Extensor indicis			▦	▦	
Extensor carpi ulnaris			▦	▦	
Extensor digiti minimi			▦	▦	
Flexor digitorum superficialis			▦	▦	▦
Flexor digitorum profundus			▦	▦	▦
Pronator quadratus			▦	▦	▦
Flexor carpi ulnaris				▦	▦
Palmaris longus			▦	▦	▦
HAND					
Abductor pollicis brevis				▦	▦
Flexor pollicis brevis		▦	▦		
Opponens pollicis		▦	▦		
Flexor digiti minimi brevis			▦	▦	▦
Opponens digiti minimi			▦	▦	▦
Adductor pollicis				▦	▦
Palmaris brevis				▦	▦
Abductor digiti minimi				▦	▦
Lumbricales				▦	▦
Interossei				▦	▦

542

SEGMENTAL INNERVATION OF TRUNK MUSCLES

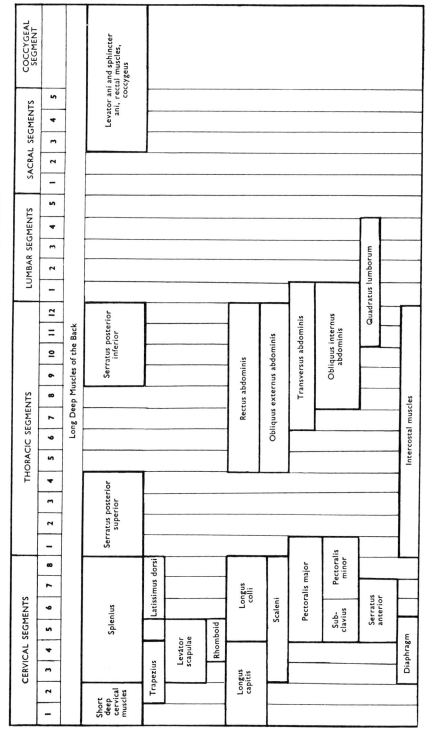

SEGMENTAL INNERVATION OF MUSCLES OF LOWER EXTREMITY

	T₁₂	L₁	L₂	L₃	L₄	L₅	S₁	S₂

HIP

- Iliopsoas
- Tensor fasciae latae
- Gluteus medius
- Gluteus minimus
- Quadratus femoris
- Gemellus inferior
- Gemellus superior
- Gluteus maximus
- Obturator internus
- Piriformis

THIGH

- Sartorius
- Pectineus
- Adductor longus
- Quadriceps femoris
- Gracilis
- Adductor brevis
- Obturator externus
- Adductor magnus
- Adductor minimus
- Articularis genu
- Semitendinosus
- Semimembranosus
- Biceps femoris

LEG

- Tibialis anterior
- Extensor hallucis longus
- Popliteus
- Plantaris
- Extensor digitorum longus
- Soleus
- Gastrocnemius
- Peroneus longus
- Peroneus brevis
- Tibialis posterior
- Flexor digitorum longus
- Flexor hallucis longus

FOOT

- Extensor hallucis brevis
- Extensor digitorum brevis
- Flexor digitorum brevis
- Abductor hallucis
- Flexor hallucis brevis
- Lumbricales
- Abductor hallucis
- Abductor digiti minimi
- Flexor digiti minimi brevis
- Opponens digiti minimi
- Quadratus plantae
- Interossei

Selected references of historic interest

Creed, R.S., Denny-Brown, D., Eccles, J.C., Liddell, E.G.T., and Sherrington, C.S. (1932). *Reflex activity of the spinal cord.* Oxford University Press, London.

Gowers, W.R. (1901). *Epilepsy and other chronic convulsive diseases.* Churchill, London.

Haymaker, W. (ed.) (1970). *Founders of neurology,* 2nd edn. Thomas, Springfield, Ill.

Head, H. (1920). *Studies in neurology,* Vols. 1 and 2. Oxford University Press, London.

Holmes, G. (1954). *The National Hospital, Queen Square, 1860–1948.* Livingstone, Edinburgh.

Penfield, W. and Jasper, H. (1954). *Epilepsy and the functional anatomy of the human brain.* Churchill and Livingstone, London.

Sherrington, C.S. (1947). *The integrative action of the nervous system.* Cambridge University Press.

Symonds, C.P. (1970). *Studies in neurology.* Oxford University Press, London.

Taylor, J. (ed.) (1931). *Selected writings from John Hughlings Jackson.* Staples Press, London.

Walshe, F.M.R. (1947). On the role of the pyramidal system in willed movements. *Brain* **70**, 329.

Index